HANDBOOK OF DEVELOPMENTAL DISABILITIES

Handbook of
DEVELOPMENTAL
DISABILITIES

Edited by
SAMUEL L. ODOM
ROBERT H. HORNER
MARTHA E. SNELL
JAN BLACHER

THE GUILFORD PRESS
New York   London

© 2007 The Guilford Press
A Division of Guilford Publications, Inc.
72 Spring Street, New York, NY 10012
www.guilford.com

Paperback edition 2009

Printed in the United States of America

This book is printed on acid-free paper.

Last digit is print number: 9 8 7 6 5 4 3 2

The authors have checked with sources believed to be reliable in their efforts to provide information that is complete and generally in accord with the standards of practice that are accepted at the time of publication. However, in view of the possibility of human error or changes in medical sciences, neither the authors, nor the editor and publisher, nor any other party who has been involved in the preparation or publication of this work warrants that the information contained herein is in every respect accurate or complete, and they are not responsible for any errors or omissions or the results obtained from the use of such information. Readers are encouraged to confirm the information contained in this book with other sources.

Library of Congress Cataloging-in-Publication Data

Handbook of developmental disabilities / edited by Samuel L. Odom ... [et al.].
    p. ; cm.
  Includes bibliographical references and indexes.
  ISBN 978-1-59385-485-0 (hardcover: alk. paper)
  ISBN 978-1-60623-248-4 (paperback: alk. paper)
  1. Developmental disabilities—Handbooks, manuals, etc. I. Odom, Samuel L.
  [DNLM: 1. Developmental Disabilities—therapy. 2. Developmental Disabilities—
etiology. 3. Disabled Children—education. 4. Disabled Persons—rehabilitation. 5. Early
Intervention (Education)—methods. 6. Social Support. WS 350.6 H23648 2007]
  RJ506.D47H356 2007
  616.85′88—dc22
                                                          2007018356

To Ed, Mary Lou, and Angela Otting,
whose lives have been affected by developmental disabilities
and have responded by enriching the lives of others

About the Editors

Samuel L. Odom, PhD, is Director of the Frank Porter Graham Child Development Institute at the University of North Carolina at Chapel Hill. He is the author or coauthor of numerous refereed journal articles and editor or coeditor of five published and two forthcoming books on early childhood intervention and developmental disabilities. Dr. Odom's recent articles, cowritten with his doctoral students, have addressed the efficacy of a variety of focused intervention approaches (e.g., peer-mediated interventions, sibling-mediated interventions, parent–child intervention to promote joint attention, independent work systems approach to promote learning) for children with autism spectrum disorder. His current work focuses on the efficacy of preschool readiness programs for at-risk children, treatment efficacy of early intervention for young children with autism, and professional development related to autism spectrum disorder. In 2007, Dr. Odom received the Outstanding Research Award from the Council for Exceptional Children.

Robert H. Horner, PhD, is Alumni–Knight Professor of Special Education and interim Associate Dean for Research in the College of Education at the University of Oregon. He is coeditor of the *Journal of Positive Behavior Interventions*, past editor of the *Journal of the Association for the Severely Handicapped*, and past associate editor for the *Journal of Applied Behavior Analysis* and the *American Journal on Mental Retardation*. Dr. Horner has written or edited seven texts and over 150 peer-reviewed journal articles. His research interests focus on positive behavior support, applied behavior analysis, stimulus control, instructional technology, severe disabilities, and sustainable systems change.

Martha E. Snell, PhD, is Professor in the Curry School of Education at the University of Virginia, where she is also coordinator of the Special Education Program. Dr. Snell teaches teacher preparation courses in severe disabilities, intellectual disabilities, and early childhood special education. She is a member of the current and the past two committees on terminology and classification for the American Association on Intellectual and Developmental Disabilities (AAIDD), a recent AAIDD board member, and past president of TASH. She has participated as an expert witness in court cases addressing the appropriateness of special education programs and the diagnosis of mental retardation. Dr. Snell's research has focused on instruction, data-based decision making, and teachers' roles in inclusion. Her current research addresses positive behavior support and beginning communication. She is the author of textbooks on severe disabilities and strategies for including students with disabilities in general education, as well as a recipient of the Education Award from AAIDD.

Jan Blacher, PhD, is Professor of Education and Faculty Chair of the Graduate School of Education at the University of California, Riverside. She is known nationally for her research on intellectual disability/mental retardation and other developmental disabilities, as well as for her expertise in special education programming. Dr. Blacher is frequently asked to appear as an expert witness in contested cases involving right-to-education suits for children with autism, mental retardation, or other learning disorders. She has served as consulting editor for the *American Journal on Mental Retardation* and *Mental Retardation* and as a reviewer for numerous other journals focused on child development and developmental disabilities. Dr. Blacher was recently appointed to the National Research Council of the National Academy of Sciences and the Johnson & Johnson/Rosalynn Carter Institute Caregivers Program, and is a newly elected Fellow of the American Association for the Advancement of Science. Since February 2002, she has been writing a monthly column for *Exceptional Parent* magazine.

Contributors

Linda M. Bambara, EdD, Department of Education and Human Services, College of Education, Lehigh University, Bethlehem, Pennsylvania

Cecily L. Betz, RN, PhD, Center of Excellence in Developmental Disabilities, University of Southern California, and Children's Hospital Los Angeles, Los Angeles, California

Jan Blacher, PhD, Graduate School of Education, University of California, Riverside, Riverside, California

Wanda J. Blanchett, PhD, School of Education and Human Development, University of Colorado at Denver, Denver, Colorado

Nick Bouras, MD, PhD, Institute of Psychiatry, King's College London, and Estia Centre, London, United Kingdom

Diane M. Browder, PhD, Department of Counseling, Special Education, and Child Development, University of North Carolina at Charlotte, Charlotte, North Carolina

Edward G. Carr, PhD, Department of Psychology, Stony Brook University, Stony Brook, New York

Judith J. Carta, PhD, Juniper Garden's Children Project, University of Kansas, Kansas City, Kansas

Erik W. Carter, PhD, Department of Rehabilitation Psychology and Special Education, University of Wisconsin, Madison, Madison, Wisconsin

Janis Chadsey, PhD, Department of Special Education, University of Illinois, Champaign, Illinois

Glen Dunlap, PhD, Department of Child and Family Studies, Florida Mental Health Institute, University of South Florida, Tampa, Florida

Carl J. Dunst, PhD, Orelena Hawks Puckett Institute, Asheville, North Carolina

Eric Emerson, PhD, Institute for Health Research, Lancaster University, Lancaster, United Kingdom

David Felce, PhD, Welsh Centre for Learning Disabilities, Cardiff University, Cardiff, United Kingdom

Brenda Fossett, MA, Department of Educational and Counseling Psychology and Special Education, University of British Columbia, Vancouver, British Columbia, Canada

Georgia C. Frey, PhD, Department of Kinesiology, Indiana University, Bloomington, Indiana

Glenn T. Fujiura, PhD, Department of Disability and Human Development, College of Applied Health Sciences, University of Illinois at Chicago, Chicago, Illinois

Susan L. Gibbs, PhD, Department of Counseling, Special Education, and Child Development, University of North Carolina at Charlotte, Charlotte, North Carolina

Randi J. Hagerman, MD, Developmental–Behavioral Pediatrics, UC Davis Health System, M.I.N.D. Institute, University of California, Davis, Sacramento, California

Robin L. Hansen, MD, Developmental–Behavioral Pediatrics, UC Davis Health System, M.I.N.D. Institute, University of California, Davis, Sacramento, California

Amber A. Harris, MS, Department of Counseling, Special Education, and Child Development, University of North Carolina at Charlotte, Charlotte, North Carolina

Beth Harry, PhD, Department of Teaching and Learning, University of Miami, Coral Gables, Florida

Chris Hatton, PhD, Institute for Health Research, Lancaster University, Lancaster, United Kingdom

Robert H. Horner, PhD, College of Education, University of Oregon, Eugene, Oregon

Carolyn Hughes, PhD, Departments of Special Education and Human and Organizational Development, Peabody College, Vanderbilt University, Nashville, Tennessee

Kara Hume, PhD, School of Education, Indiana University, Bloomington, Indiana

Pam Hunt, PhD, Department of Special Education, San Francisco State University, San Francisco, California

Ann P. Kaiser, PhD, Peabody College, Vanderbilt University, Nashville, Tennessee

Aaron S. Kemp, BA, Department of Psychiatry and Human Behavior, University of California, Irvine, Irvine, California

Janette K. Klingner, PhD, School of Education, University of Colorado at Boulder, Boulder, Colorado

Na Young Kong, MEd, Department of Special Education, University of Kansas, Lawrence, Kansas

K. Charlie Lakin, PhD, Research and Training Center on Community Living, University of Minnesota, Minneapolis, Minnesota

Julie J. Lounds, PhD, Waisman Center, University of Wisconsin, Madison, Madison, Wisconsin

David Mank, PhD, Indiana Institute on Disability and Community, Indiana University, Bloomington, Indiana

John McDonnell, PhD, Department of Special Education, University of Utah, Salt Lake City, Utah

Christopher J. McDougle, MD, Department of Psychiatry, Indiana University School of Medicine, Indianapolis, Indiana

Gail McGee, PhD, Department of Psychiatry, Emory University Medical Center, Atlanta, Georgia

Molly McKenzie, MEd, Department of Education and Human Services, College of Education, Lehigh University, Bethlehem, Pennsylvania

Pat Mirenda, PhD, Department of Educational and Counseling Psychology and Special Education, University of British Columbia, Vancouver, British Columbia, Canada

Tim Moore, MS, Department of Educational Psychology, University of Minnesota, Minneapolis, Minnesota

Wendy M. Nehring, RN, PhD, College of Nursing, Rutgers, The State University of New Jersey, Newark, New Jersey

Samuel L. Odom, PhD, Frank Porter Graham Child Development Institute, University of North Carolina at Chapel Hill, Chapel Hill, North Carolina

Dimitrios Paschos, MRCPsych, South London and Maudsley NHS Foundation Trust, and Estia Centre, Guy's Hospital, London, United Kingdom

Jonathan Perry, PhD, Welsh Centre for Learning Disabilities, Cardiff University, Cardiff, United Kingdom

Denise Poston, PhD, Beach Center on Disability, University of Kansas, Lawrence, Kansas

Sally Rogers, PhD, M.I.N.D. Institute, University of California, Davis, School of Medicine, Sacramento, California

Curt A. Sandman, PhD, Department of Psychiatry and Human Behavior, University of California, Irvine, Irvine, California

Mary Suzanne Schrandt, JD, Arthritis Foundation, Prairie Village, Kansas

Marsha Mailick Seltzer, PhD, Waisman Center, University of Wisconsin, Madison, Madison, Wisconsin

Martha E. Snell, PhD, Department of Curriculum, Instruction and Special Education, Curry School of Education, University of Virginia, Charlottesville, Virginia

Roger J. Stancliffe, PhD, Research and Training Center on Community Living, University of Minnesota, Minneapolis, Minnesota

Zolinda Stoneman, PhD, Institute on Human Development and Disability, College of Family and Consumer Sciences, University of Georgia, Athens, Georgia

Matthew J. Stowe, JD, Beach Center on Disability, University of Kansas, Lawrence, Kansas

Jean Ann Summers, PhD, Beach Center on Disability, University of Kansas, Lawrence, Kansas

Frank Symons, PhD, Department of Educational Psychology, University of Minnesota, Minneapolis, Minnesota

Nicole R. Tartaglia, MD, Developmental–Behavioral Pediatrics, UC Davis Health System, M.I.N.D. Institute, University of California, Davis, Sacramento, California

Travis Thompson, PhD, Department of Pediatrics, University of Minnesota School of Medicine, Minneapolis, Minnesota

Katherine Trela, MS, Department of Counseling, Special Education, and Child Development, University of North Carolina at Charlotte, Charlotte, North Carolina

J. Alacia Trent, PhD, Peabody College, Vanderbilt University, Nashville, Tennessee

Ann P. Turnbull, EdD, Beach Center on Disability, University of Kansas, Lawrence, Kansas,

H. Rutherford Turnbull, III, LiB/JD, LiM, Beach Center on Disability, University of Kansas, Lawrence, Kansas

Shawnee Wakeman, PhD, Department of Counseling, Special Education, and Child Development, University of North Carolina at Charlotte, Charlotte, North Carolina

Steven F. Warren, PhD, Institute of Life Span Studies, University of Kansas, Lawrence, Kansas

Barbara A. Wilson, PhD, Department of Exceptionality Programs, Bloomsburg University, Bloomsburg, Pennsylvania

Nina Zuna, MEd, Beach Center on Disability, University of Kansas, Lawrence, Kansas

Preface

Books spring from different sources. This book arose from a critical mass of research literature on developmental disabilities and an invitation from The Guilford Press to edit a handbook that would summarize the most current information on developmental disabilities. We crafted the handbook through coffee shop conversations, conference calls, and hundreds of e-mail communications. As coeditors of this book, our lives and focused effort overlapped in this common purpose, and yet through the wonders of technology, several of us still have not met in person.

Our vision for the book has been to gather and summarize the most current research on multiple dimensions of developmental disabilities, which was no small task. The charge we gave to contributing authors (with the exception of the initial "Foundations" section) was to focus their writing on the extant research base in their focal area; to summarize key past research studies that would provide a historical context for their current review; and to determine the implications of the current research for practice, social policy, and future research. In the initial section, authors addressed general issues in developmental disabilities, such as definition and classification, social policy, research methods, and cultural influences. Although the book chapters focus most often on psychological, educational, and human services practices, the biomedical research on neuroscience, genetics, and health has expanded rapidly in recent years. Thus several chapters in the second section of the book summarize the biomedical science of developmental disabilities in an authoritative and accessible manner. The succeeding sections of the book are practice- and age-related, as authors focus their chapters on early intervention, school-age intervention, and adult issues. For some individuals with developmental disabilities, there are concerns about problem behavior and/or mental health. To address these concerns, one section of the handbook covers the topics of positive behavior support, dual diagnosis, and pharmacological/behavioral treatment approaches. This is followed by a section addressing the long and active research literature on multiple aspects concerning the families of individuals with developmental disabilities. The book concludes with a section on international perspectives and practices in developmental disabilities and future directions for research and policy development.

As we were compiling the book, a historical event took place regarding terminology pertaining to mental retardation. When we began the book, there was ongoing discussion in the United States about this terminology. This discussion culminated with the American Association on Mental Retardation (AAMR) officially changing its name to the American Association on Intellectual and Developmental Disabilities (AAIDD), thus shifting terms and broadening their constituent interest to developmental disabilities. Later the Association's Terminology and Classification Committee clarified that the term "intellectual disability" would replace the term "mental retardation."

These changes presented a conundrum for us in that we wondered what terminology we should use in the handbook. In Chapter 1, we include a description of developmental disabilities as an umbrella term that may encompass a range of more discretely defined conditions such as intellectual disability, autism and associated spectrum disorders, cerebral palsy, and traumatic brain injury. We chose to continue with the original "developmental disabilities" term rather than introduce the term "intellectual disabilities" in order not to narrow the broader population of people included under developmental disabilities. Terminology matters, however, and to avoid confusion we go to some length here explaining our rationale.

There are two notable limitations in this handbook: First, the concept of "developmental disabilities" transcends national boundaries and is viewed differently in different cultures. In this book we have attempted to draw from the international literature and invited authors from other countries. We were generally limited, however, to the English language literature, so the international chapters and literature on developmental disabilities comes from English-speaking countries, with the United Kingdom being the most prominent. Second there are two topics (prevention and self-determination) that are deserving of chapter-length coverage but, due to space constraints, we were not able to include as chapters. The general area of prevention of developmental disabilities is a critically important topic that stretches across the public health, biomedical, and educational/intervention literature. Although Emerson, Fujiura, and Hatton discuss prevention in Chapter 29, a focused chapter on this topic would have been relevant. Self-determination is another important area of research in developmental disabilities. There is greater recognition and appreciation that individuals with developmental disabilities should have the power and right to make decisions about their own lives, and a literature has grown around self-determination issues. However, discussion of these issues is limited to chapters in the section on adult issues.

Any book of this magnitude requires the work of others beside the coeditors and authors, and to these other individuals we offer our gratitude. In particular, we acknowledge Monica Boyd, who spent long hours keeping us organized as a group and sending information across the country, and Rochelle Serwator, our editor at The Guilford Press, who has patiently supported the compilation of this book. Last, we thank our families for putting up with us when our professional work, particularly editing this book, at times intruded on our personal lives.

Contents

I

FOUNDATIONS

Laying the groundwork for a thorough review of research, practice, and policy in developmental disabilities is a central goal of this foundation section, and not an easy one to attain. There is much change afoot in the conceptualization of developmental disabilities, and the shifting definitions, terminology, and labels represent a challenge in establishing a firm foundation. In the first chapter, Odom, Horner, Snell, and Blacher examine the range of conceptualizations of developmental disabilities and the more discretely defined disabilities that are grouped within this "umbrella" construct. They propose that definitions are created for specific purposes and review terminology and classification systems that address those varying purposes. The authors extend this reflection into the future by suggesting challenges that lie ahead and implications for public policy.

Taking the theme of public policy forward, H. R. Turnbull, Stowe, A. P. Turnbull, and Strandt provide a novel view of core concepts that underlie policy, legislation, and services for individuals with developmental disabilities in the United States. After a description of the core-concept approach to policy analysis, the authors identify 18 core concepts associated with public policy and services that have emerged over the past 35 years. The core concepts represent the essential policy elements that underlie service provision in the field today. To name a few, empowerment, liberty, protection from harm, and autonomy are rights normally accorded to all members of society; and for individuals with developmental disabilities, these rights are ensured by specific legislation and policies.

A central focus of this *Handbook* is research in developmental disabilities and its implications for policy and practice. In her eloquent and provocative chapter on research in developmental disabilities, Stoneman reflects on the key components of the research process and the challenges faced by researchers interested in addressing meaningful questions. She returns to themes of definition, discussed in the initial chapter, as they relate to selection of participants in research studies. The historical model of research, based on a biomedical model and laboratory science, is examined, and Stoneman speculates on its relevance for social science research that addresses questions about developmental disabilities. Importantly, she describes the direction in the field toward evidence-based practice and the need for research that addresses causal questions, and she also notes the challenges for conducting such studies in naturalistic settings with participants who have low-prevalence disabilities. This chapter sets the stage for discussions of research that occur in nearly every chapter in the subsequent sections.

Cultural and linguistic diversity in society interact directly with conceptualizations of developmental disabilities and public policy. Klingner, Blanchett, and Harry examine the cultural definitions of disability, the defining nature of schooling for individuals of color, and faulty assumptions made about assessment and classification. Such faulty assumptions and their resultant practices are identified as primary culprits in the overidentification and overrepresentation of individuals of color as having developmental disabilities. The interplay of access to services for individuals of color who need them and overidentification of some children of color as having mental retardation is a subtle and paradoxical issue that the authors explore. Summarizing their review, the authors offer recommendations for working with individuals of color who have developmental disabilities and their families.

1

The Construct
of Developmental Disabilities

Samuel L. Odom
Robert H. Horner
Martha E. Snell
Jan Blacher

Developmental disabilities have a history as old as humankind. They have been viewed as possessions by the evil spirits, retributions for past sins, scientifically identified syndromes, culturally situated social phenomena, and portals for accesses to supports and services (Harris, 2006). The construct is dynamic in that (1) it changes over time as scientific knowledge of and cultural perspectives on disabilities evolve and (2) it may serve multiple purposes, with the purposes influencing the specific definition established. Perhaps more importantly, the term "developmental disabilities" is more than an academic concept—it affects the lives of real individuals with a wide array of characteristics and abilities. The purpose of this chapter is to propose a working definition for developmental disabilities, as well as a framework for understanding the construct of developmental disabilities based upon function and purpose, and to examine the future implication for this construct on social policy, practice, and research.

A NOTE ON TERMINOLOGY

A reflection of the dynamic and evolving nature of developmental disabilities is the change that is occurring in terminology, as of this writing. In the United States, developmental disabilities has been broadly construed as an umbrella term that includes other more discretely defined disability classifications sharing some common characteristics. For example, the Administration on Developmental Disabilities (ADD) at one time grouped within the developmental disabilities classification, mental retardation, autism, cerebral palsy, traumatic brain injury, and epilepsy, with the rationale that people with these disabilities had significant life limitations across several developmental areas. Yet, in the United States, terminology is changing to represent a broader conceptualization. Recently, the American Association on Mental Retardation (AAMR) changed the terminology of its constituent interest to intellectual and developmental disabilities. This change brings the U.S. definition into closer conformity with terminology used in the United Kingdom and other parts of the world, and more in line with the international research organization pertaining to developmental disabilities, the International Association for the Scientific Study of Intellectual Disability (IASSID; see *www.iassid.org/*).

For this chapter, we define developmental disabilities as a set of abilities and characteristics that vary from the norm in the limitations they impose on independent participation and acceptance in society. The condition of developmental disabilities is developmental in the sense that delays, disorders, or impairments exist within traditionally conceived developmental domains such as cognitive, communication, social, or motor abilities and appear in the "developmental period," which is usually characterized as before 22 years of age. While low IQ scores are typically associated with and can even be markers for developmental disabilities, other conditions (e.g., cerebral palsy, Asperger syndrome) may impose limitations on individuals with developmental disabilities whose intelligence is at or above average. Typically, in establishing the parameters of developmental disabilities, limitations associated with sensory impairments (i.e., deafness, blindness) are not folded into the definitions unless these impairments occur in combination with impairment in intellectual functioning (e.g., multiple disabilities). Similarly, the focus on developmental and adaptive abilities may distinguish developmental disabilities from most psychiatric conditions, although it is widely acknowledged that individuals may have a dual diagnosis (see Paschos & Bouras, Chapter 24, this volume for a thorough review).

SOCIAL CONSTRUCTION OF DEVELOPMENTAL DISABILITIES

Having offered a working definition of developmental disabilities, we also have to acknowledge that developmental disability is a social construction. As a species, humans are social beings. The evolution of language as a mode of communication created a capacity to share information and construct a shared sense of what is real in the world. In any discussion, the social construction of reality can be reduced to its most solipsistic form, but to live, work, and exist in the world, most humans come to explicit or tacit agreements about what exists. In fact, this agreement is functional in that it allows society to operate as a social system. Science, one of humankind's most important social constructions, emerged from an Aristotelian tradition based on logic and during the "Age of Reason" evolved into an empirical tradition that gathers information from the world to verify one's understanding of a phenomena. Yet even the understandings we construct from medical science, which is considered a most highly empirical science, change over time. One needs go no further than the cradle of a newborn baby to see an example. Twenty years ago, parents and caregivers would routinely place their babies on their stomachs to sleep, based on medical, scientific advice. Subsequent research found that babies sleeping on their stomachs were more likely to experience sudden infant death syndrome (SIDS), and in 1992 the American Academy of Pediatrics recommended placing babies on their backs to sleep. Since then there has been a 40% drop in SIDS (Schmidt, 2006). The point here is that as we learn from science, the understandings we construct and that guide our actions sometimes change.

Perhaps a more relevant example may be seen in our understanding of autism. As originally conceived, autism was a psychiatric disorder (Asperger, 1944; Kanner, 1943) with an etiology based in the psychodynamic relationship between the child with autism and his/her mother (Bettelheim, 1967). It was originally proposed as a low incidence disorder (1 to 2 per 10,000 children) and treatment recommendations were psychotherapeutic and focused on "fixing the mother." Scientific evidence related to treatments, as well as reactions of individuals involved in the therapeutic process, have led to a different conceptualization of autism as a broad spectrum of disorders sharing common characteristics, a different perspective on etiology, and an awareness that the incidence is much greater than ever imagined. In the 21st century, the social context of autism is much changed from Kanner's and Asperger's day, yet many children seen in autism diagnostic clinics today bear similar characteristics to those reported by Kanner and Asperger in the 1940s.

The social construction of developmental disabilities allows individuals to communicate in ways that are useful for accomplishing certain purposes. We propose that because of these different purposes, developmental disability is a multidimensional construct. Drawing on an earlier conceptualization of mental retardation by the AAMR (Luckasson et al., 1992), we propose three purposes or functions of this construct: (1) to allow a common framework for further scientific understanding; (2) to qualify individuals for social services like special education or social security through the documentation of life limitations; and (3) to plan for the provision of supports for individuals with certain ability levels. Each of these conceptualizations evolves as new knowledge emerges. In addition, these purposes are not completely independent, so knowledge from one conceptualization of developmental disabilities may well inform other definitions or purposes.

Scientific Purpose: The Value of a Diagnosis

As noted, developmental disability is a summative descriptor for individuals that share common characteristics. While useful when speaking in generalities and for formation of some public policy (see H. R. Turnbull, Stowe, A. P. Turnbull, & Schrandt, Chapter 2, this volume), precise diagnostic definitions are important for identification of etiology, prediction of effects on development or behavior, design of intervention, and organization of scientific programs of study. Accurate diagnostic information is critical for some types of scientific research. In medical research, the determination of the effectiveness of a pharmacological treatment, the association of a certain set of chromosomes, or the reoccurrence of features on structural or functional brain images are made meaningful when individuals' characteristics or phenotypes are precisely defined. In behavioral research, developmental characteristics associated with diagnostic conditions may inform scientific knowledge about cognitive or social processes. Similarly, there is a strong emphasis in psychological and educational research on determining the features or characteristics of individuals with diagnosed developmental disabilities that may predict their response to treatment (see Odom, Rogers, McDougle, Hume, & McGee, Chapter 10, this volume).

Formal diagnostic classification may also be linked to medical treatment or educational decisions. For example, a diagnosis of phenylketonuria (PKU) leads to an immediate decision about nutrition in order to prevent developmental disabilities. Children diagnosed with Prader–Willi syndrome will require close supervision of their access to food. Most clinicians and educators agree that children diagnosed with autism require early and intensive instruction in communication and social interactions. Even for children with Down syndrome, in which cognitive and adaptive abilities vary substantially, monitoring for early congenital heart defects and sensory impairments is important (Batshaw, 2002).

Prominent diagnostic classification systems have been established that include specific developmental disabilities. These will be briefly described, but for a more in depth description, the readers are referred to an excellent review by Harris (2006). Several of these systems have emerged from the medical community. The most prominent international system, the *International Classification of Diseases* (ICD-10), was created by the World Health Organization (1992) to provide consistent diagnostic criteria for physical diseases, but it also includes classification for mental disorders. ICD-10 is a multiaxial system that specifies assessment related to the individual diagnostic disorder, as well as information about medical conditions, psychiatric conditions, psychosocial disability, and abnormal psychosocial conditions. ICD-10 does not have a single diagnostic classification for developmental disabilities, but it provides precise classification for mental retardation, autism, Asperger syndrome, and cerebral palsy.

In the United States, the *Diagnostic and Statistical Manual of Mental Disorders*, known as the DSM, was established by the American Psychiatric Association for purposes similar to the ICD. The manual is now in a revised form of its fourth edition, DSM-IV-TR (American Psychiatric Association, 2000). Like ICD-10, DSM-IV-TR is multiaxial, with five axes organized around clinical disorders (i.e., all disorders but mental retardation), underlying pervasive or personality disorders (e.g., mental retardation), general medical conditions, psychosocial and environmental functioning, and global assessment of functioning. Again, like ICD-10, DSM-IV-TR does not have a general classification for developmental disabilities, but does have specific criteria and guidelines for mental retardation and pervasive developmental disorder (PDD), the latter being a summary diagnosis that contains specific criteria for autistic disorder, Asperger syndrome, and pervasive developmental disorder-not otherwise specified (PD-NOS). In layperson terms, these PDD categories are now called autism spectrum disorders.

The American Association on Intellectual and Developmental Disabilities (AAIDD; formerly the AAMR) has a long history in establishing diagnostic criteria for mental retardation (MR). In 1959, AAIDD defined MR as "subaverage general intellectual functioning which originates during the developmental period and is associated with impairment in one or more of the following: (1) maturation, (2) learning, (3) social adjustment" (Heber, 1959, p. 3). By this definition, subaverage referred to an IQ score "less than one standard deviation (SD) below the population mean of the age group involved on measures of general intellectual functioning" (p. 3). In addition, impairments in maturation, learning, and/or social adjustment (later called adaptive behavior) and onset before the age of 16 were two other critical diagnostic features of the definition (Schalock, Luckasson, & Shogren, 2007). One of the best examples of the social construction of developmental disabilities and evolution of the construct occurred in 1973, when the seventh revision of the AAMR definition lowered the IQ diagnostic criteria for mental retardation from 85 to less than 70 (Grossman, 1973). With this change in criteria, the social construction of mental retardation was redefined to exclude individuals with IQs between approximately 85 and 70, which significantly reduced the official prevalence of mental retardation.

Current IQ criteria in the AAMR definitions remain essentially unchanged from 1973 until present (Schalock et al., 2007). During this same time period there also has been consistency in the two other defining criteria (i.e., that concurrent significant limitations exist in adaptive behavior/skills, and that the age of onset must occur before 18 years). These three AAMR diagnostic criteria influenced the criteria established in the ICD-10 and original DSM classifications.

Perhaps the most current change in the conceptualization of mental retardation is the recent decision to substitute the term "intellectual disability" for "mental retardation," with the definition and assumptions of intellectual disability/mental retardation remaining the same as those set forth by AAMR in 2002 (Luckasson et al., 2002). Schalock et al. (2007) make the case for intellectual disability belonging within the general construct of disability and being a preferred term to replace mental retardation. They argue that the term intellectual disability: "(a) reflects the changed construct of disability proposed by AAIDD and WHO; (b) aligns better with current professional practices that focus on functional behaviors and contextual factors; (c) provides a logical basis for individualized supports provision due to its basis in a social-ecological framework; (d) is less offensive to persons with disabilities; and (e) is more consistent with international terminology" (p. 12).

In summary, from a scientific/diagnostic perspective, our working conceptualization of developmental disabilities would enfold formal diagnostic classifications of mental retardation, autism and pervasive developmental disabilities, cerebral palsy, and more specifically identified syndromes that exhibit mental retardation and/or other behavioral manifestation (e.g., Down syndrome, Prader–Willi syndrome, Williams syndrome, Rett syndrome).

Eligibility for Services and Life Limitations

Society's response to developmental disabilities has often been to provide educational and social services that would prepare individuals to live as independently as possible; support the participation of individuals in community, home, and workplace; and provide the financial supports needed for medical and social services. To provide such support, social institutions and agencies must decide who is eligible for services, which again requires definitions and classification.

The educational system in the United States is a primary mechanism for providing training and preparation for independent functioning in society. Broadly construed, educational and multidisciplinary services may begin at the birth of a child with developmental disabilities (See Dunst, Chapter 8, this volume) and extend up to the individual's 22nd birthday. To qualify for special education services, the Individuals with Disabilities Education Improvement Act (IDEIA) in the United States has established eligibility criteria similar to the diagnostic criteria noted previously. The key feature distinguishing this set of criteria from others, such as the DSM or ICD systems, is that the identified disability must affect the child's or youth's educational performance. Several, but not all, of the disability classifications in IDEIA fall within our working definition of developmental disabilities. For example, for infants and toddlers who qualify under Part C of the law, the classification of "developmental delay" is admissible, and states now have the option to use the classification for older children as well. Other classifications used for children from 3 to 22 that could fit into a developmental disabilities classification are autism, deaf-blindness, mental retardation, multiple disabilities, orthopedic disabilities, and traumatic brain injury.

The Administration on Developmental Disabilities (ADD), within the U.S. Department of Health and Human Services, defines developmental disabilities as

> severe, life-long disabilities attributable to mental and/or physical impairments, manifested before age 22. Developmental disabilities result in substantial limitations in three or more areas of major life activities:
>
> - Capacity for Independent Living
> - Economic Self-sufficiency
> - Learning
> - Mobility
> - Receptive and Expressive Language
> - Self-Care
> - Self-Direction (Administration on Developmental Disabilities, 2007).

As the primary U.S. federal agency responsible for implementing legislation and policy that provides support for individuals with developmental disabilities (e.g., the Developmental Disabilities Assistance and Bill of Rights Act of 2000), the ADD definition serves as a guide for the development of eligibility criteria for state and local social service agencies. Notably, the current definition focuses on "substantial limitations of major life activities" and does not identify specific disabilities. This represents a shift in ADD definition, in that previous descriptions of developmental disabilities included specific disability designations such as mental retardation, autism, cerebral palsy, epilepsy, and traumatic brain injury, as well as the life limitations designation in the current definition.

The life limitation approaches employed by the U.S. federal government agencies provides a mechanism for setting criteria for children, youth, and adults with developmental disabilities who will receive resources through the educational and social service systems. It may also indicate the types of and extent of services provided. That is, individuals with more extensive life limitations may be in need of more services, although the specific social support or education plan is usually not based on this definition or these criteria. Rather, more specific information about the functional abilities of individuals and the quality of support needed provides the foundation for planning and implementing specific services. The necessity of this information underlies a third purpose of the construct of developmental disabilities and a different set of definitional criteria—those of functional abilities and support.

Functional Abilities and Life Support

A paradigmatic shift in the conceptualization of developmental disabilities occurred in the 1990s and, in retrospect, seems to be a natural evolution of the developmental disabilities construct. The diagnostic approach established developmental disabilities through behavioral or medical criteria. The life limitation approach expanded the conceptualization of developmental disabilities to recognize the impact of the disability on features of an individual's life, implicitly involving an individual's life circumstances in determining the limitations that exist for the individual. The shifting paradigm for the late 1990s and into the current century has established a greater emphasis on the match between the individual's abilities and the requirements of environmental context.

Rather than applying a deficits approach and documenting the things an individual cannot do, the functional abilities and life support perspective focuses on skills and abilities that an individual possesses and the types of supports needed for successful participation in the individual's specific environmental context (e.g., home, school, community). Although the importance of functional skills for individuals with developmental disabilities had long been recognized (Brown et al., 1979; Snell, 1978) and been used in developing educational and habilitation programs for individuals with disabilities, they were never part of the definitional portion of developmental disabilities.

The 1992 AAMR revision of the definitional and classification criteria for mental retardation (Luckasson et al., 1992) is a prime example of this shift. Rather than continuing with level of intellectual and adaptive abilities as the primary defining criteria for mental retardation, AAMR established "level of support" as the central feature of the organization's classification system. Level of support is the amount of assistance an individual needs to participate in normal life activities. AAMR identified four levels of support: (1) intermittent (i.e., provided on an "as needed" basis), (2) limited (i.e., time limited but provided consistently over time), (3) extensive (i.e., ongoing support provided regularly in some environments), (4) pervasive (i.e., provided throughout the day and across environments). The specific support provided and its intensity are based on the assessment of an individual's functional and adaptive abilities and their match with requirements of their environment. Environment, we maintain, should be construed broadly as different contexts in which an individual participates. Bronfenbrenner (1979) identified these as microsystems (e.g., home, class, community), as well as the culture or cultures in which an individual lives (e.g., Bronfenbrenner's macrosystem).

A similar shift has occurred in international classification. To describe the functional abilities and characteristics of individuals with health impairments and developmental disabilities, in 2000 the World Health Organization approved the *International Classification of Functioning, Disability, and Health* (ICF). The purpose of the ICF is to provide a common and international language across disciplines for communicating functional abilities and to serve as a clinical and educational tool for planning treatments. The ICF is a revision of the *International Classification of Impairments, Disabilities, and Handicaps* (ICIDH), which was published in 1980 but infrequently used. Although important at the time because it distinguished between disease (or disability) and its consequences, the ICIDH was limited in that it did not reference function and disability to requirements of the environment (Simeonsson et al., 2003). In their revision, the WHO shifted the conceptualization of their classification system from one of disease to one of health (or abilities) (World Health Organization, 2002). Assessment of individuals occurs in four domains: body function, body structure, activities of participation, and environmental factors. This broad set of information allows for examination of the dynamic relationship between abilities of an individual and the functioning of that individual in different environmental contexts.

In summary, the functional abilities and life support perspective moves the focus of developmental disabilities from that of the individual to the individual situated in several ecological contexts. It implies that assessment would include the individual, the environmental contexts, and the relationship between the two. In addition, as Simeonsson, Lolar, Hollowell and Adams (2000) and Bronfenbrenner and Morris (1998) remind us, such relationships also operate in a developmental and temporal context (i.e., the relationships are different for individuals with developmental disabilities and their families at different points of the lifespan).

FUTURE DIRECTIONS AND THE CONCEPTUALIZATION OF DEVELOPMENTAL DISABILITIES

As we look to the future two assumptions appear important. The first is that developmental disabilities will continue as a social construct understood in the context of broader societal trends. The second is that the construct will continue to evolve as science improves our understanding of the basic mechanisms and intervention strategies affecting disability. We argue here that our understanding of developmental disabilities as a social construct is important for effective science as well as for social change. How we define, understand, and respond to this construct affects family adjustment to disability, as well as the social roles, societal investment, and daily opportunities available to people with disabilities in our society. We see the following as trends worthy of consideration for all people concerned about individuals with developmental disabilities.

Social Trends Affecting Our Understanding of Developmental Disabilities

Among the greatest social shifts occurring world wide is the increasing heterogeneity of society (Friedman, 2006; Shinagawa & Jang, 1998). An array of global factors is transforming traditional monocultural communities into diverse sub-societies. Communities that were defined by a "majority" culture are being redefined, not just by "minorities" who become the new "majority," but by diversity itself (Hatton, 2004). This trend will affect the social construct of developmental disability. For example, there are discussions within both the autism spectrum disorders and the deaf communities about the cultures of autism (Mesibov, Shea, & Schopler, 2005) and deafness (Hyde & Power, 2006), respectively.

Increasing contact with social differences will likely bring both conflict and gradual recognition that "differences" are part of the long-term social fabric of society (Miles & Ahuja, 2007). We are optimistic in perceiving this trend as having the long-range effect of changing the perception that differences are inherently suspect. Developmental disabilities are handicaps when they create barriers to personal and social development of an individual within the expectations, constraints, and supports available. As perceptions of social "difference" shift, so will perceptions of developmental disabilities. Our message is not one of Pollyanna optimism, but a call to frame future science, technology, and social policy in the context of broader social themes. Research, and the use of research, occurs within social contexts. The application of research in developmental disabilities over the next 20 years will be affected by the social context in which that research is received.

Changing Terminology and the Risks for Individuals with Developmental Disabilities

Whenever a disability definition changes the individuals included under its umbrella may also change, potentially creating risks for these individuals. For example, in 1992, the AAMR definition of mental retardation was accompanied by several essential assumptions. One assumption stated that the life functioning of persons with mental retardation who were given "the appropriate supports over a sustained period" would generally improve (Luckasson, 1992, p. 5). Family members quickly expressed concern that such improvement in their children would disqualify them for the diagnosis and that supports and services would be removed by schools and adult agencies. The authors had not anticipated that this statement about the positive effect of supports would threaten ongoing supports and acted to clarify that "the use of supports can fluctuate" and "supports should not be withdrawn prematurely" (Schalock et al., 1994, p. 187).

In the wake of the Supreme Court's ruling in *Adkins v. Virginia* (2002), the AAMR's 2002 manual on definition and terminology has become a guide for determining "whether a criminal defendant should or should not be exempted from the death penalty on the grounds of having mental retardation" (Greenspan & Switzky, 2006, p. 283). State laws now must state an accepted definition of mental retardation and the steps for its diagnosis. Juries, lawyers, and judges play various roles in determining whether the death penalty can be considered or will be carried out. But on the horizon another change in terminology may create risks for individuals with this disability. Schalock and his coauthors (2007) argue that "intellectual disability" replace "mental retardation" and that this term covers "the same population of individuals who were diagnosed previously with mental retardation in number, kind, level, type, and duration of the disability" (Schalock et al., 2007, p. 120). While this change is applauded by many as being more respectful and consistent with international usage, there is also concern that it may pose new risks. In changing terminology, it is possible that judges and lawmakers may become confused and the protections in the law may be reduced. Similarly, concerns exist about whether the legal system can absorb this change without having people fall between definitional cracks.

Integrating Basic Research on Disabilities

The future of developmental disabilities will also be affected by our emerging understanding of the basic mechanisms affecting the etiology and structure of disabilities. As examples, our understanding of the genetics, physiology, and neurochemistry of autism spectrum disorders, Lesch–Nyhan disease, Down syndrome, and mental retardation is changing our perception of these disabilities, as well as our ability to both prevent and remediate core limitations (see Tartaglia, Hansen, & Hagerman, Chapter 6, this volume; Odom et al., Chapter 10, this volume; Sandman & Kemp, Chapter 7, this volume).

Research on the basic mechanisms of disabilities will continue to expand our understanding and dispel myths we have held dear. But this simple linear process has long been part of the field. In this changing context lies a tremendous challenge to integrate new knowledge from different arenas. The information now becoming available about the neurochemistry of self-injurious behavior (Sandman & Kemp, Chapter 7, this volume), learning (Pakulak & Neville, 2006), and pharmacology (Thompson, Moore, & Symons, Chapter 25, this volume) are exciting advances as individual programs of study. Understanding behavioral phenotypes (Dykens, Hodapp, & Finucane, 2000), aging (Bigby, Balandin, & Fyffe, 2004), and sleep disorders (Doran, Harvey & Horner, 2006) for individuals with disabilities will continue to be important. However, research agendas that will lead to the greatest gains will likely come from our ability to integrate these areas of knowledge. Effective integration will challenge both our current standards for research methods and our process for research collaboration (Parmenter, 2004).

Transforming Research Findings into Support Strategies

Research can make a difference. The knowledge from research findings helps us understand what is, what is not, and what might be. Research findings in developmental disabilities come to life, however, when they are transformed into strategies for how we should organize schools, work settings, medical supports, and social policy. Family contexts are also impacted by research, particularly when it affects the purchase of services to support families. Too often the gap between what is known and what is done is embarrassingly large (Carnine, 1997). Describing research findings is insufficient if we do not transform those findings into strategies that produce valued improvements in the lives of people with disabilities (Kame'enui & Carnine, 2002; Schalock, 2000; Schalock & Felce, 2004). For example, documenting the value of living in community settings is insufficient if we cannot weave the full fabric of supports for establishing, adapting, assessing, and improving community support options over time (see Felce & Perry, Chapter 20, and Stancliffe & Lakin, Chapter 21, this volume). Any developmental disabilities research agenda for the 21st century will need to include formal strategies for transforming advances in basic knowledge into efficient strategies for organizing and delivering support.

CONCLUSION: A PERSPECTIVE

We offer in this chapter a perspective on the current, past, and future meanings of developmental disabilities as a useful social construct. We hope this perspective may serve as a context in which to examine the following chapters. The goal in each chapter is to provide both a statement about the current knowledge related to a topic and a proposed research agenda aimed toward moving the field of developmental disabilities forward. We believe these chapters emerge from a rich social, scientific, and policy foundation. We further believe that the next 20 years hold potential for research advances that can be truly transformational. To achieve this vision, however, we will need highly credible and rigorous scholarship that is applied to practical, efficient, and effective systems of support.

REFERENCES

Administration on Developmental Disabilities. (2007). *What are developmental disabilities?* Washington, DC: Author. Retrieved January 26, 2007, from *www.acf.hhs.gov/programs/add/addaboutwhatis.html*

American Psychiatric Association. (2000). *Diagnostic and statistical manual of mental disorders* (4th ed., text rev.). Washington, DC: Author.

Asperger, H. (1944/1991). *Die "Autistischen Psychopathen" im Kindesalter* (Autistic psychopathology in childhood). *Archiv fur Psychiatrie und Nervenkrankheiten, 177,* 76–136. (Translated and annotated U. Frith (Ed.), (1991), *Autism and Asperger syndrome* (pp. 37–92). New York: Cambridge University Press.

Batshaw, M. L. (2002). *Children with disabilities* (5th ed.). Baltimore: Brookes.

Bettelheim, B. (1967). *The empty fortress: Infantile autism and the birth of self.* New York: Free Press.

Bigby, C., Balandin, S., & Fyffe, C. (2004). Retirement or just change of pace: An Australian national survey of disability day services used by older people with disabilities. *Journal of Intellectual and Developmental Disabilities, 29,* 239–254.

Bronfenbrenner, U. (1979). *The ecology of human development: Experiments by nature and design.* Cambridge, MA: Harvard University Press.

Bronfenbrenner, U., & Morris, P. A. (1998). The ecology of developmental process. In R. Lerner (Ed.), *Handbook of child psychology* (5th ed.): Vol 1. Theoretical models of human development (pp. 993–1028). New York: Wiley.

Brown, L., Branston, M. B., Hamre-Nietupski, S., Pumpian, I., Certo, N., & Gruenewald, L. (1979). A strategy for developing chronological-age-appropriate and functional curricular content for severely handicapped adolescents and young adults. *Journal of Special Education, 13,* 81–90.

Carnine, D. W. (1997). Bridging the research-to-practice gap. *Exceptional Children, 63,* 513–521.

Doran, S. M., Harvey, M. T., Horner, R. D. (2006). Sleep and developmental disabilities: Assessment, treatment, and outcome measures. *Mental Retardation, 44,* 13–27.

Dykens, E. M., Hodapp, R. M., & Finucane, B. M. (2000). *Genetics and mental retardation syndromes: A new look at behavior and interventions.* Baltimore: Brookes.

Friedman, T. (2006). *The world is flat: A brief history of the twenty first century.* New York: Farrar, Straus & Giroux.

Greenspan, S., & Switzky, H. N. (2006). Lessons from the Atkins decision for the next AAMR manual. In H. N. Switzky & S. Greenspan, S. (Eds.). *What is mental retardation?: Ideas for an evolving disability in the 21st century* (rev. ed., pp. 283–302). Washington, DC: American Association on Mental Retardation.

Grossman, H. J. (Ed.). (1973). *Manual on terminology in mental retardation* (1973 rev.). Washington, DC: American Association on Mental Deficiency.

Harris, J. C. (2006). *Intellectual disability: Understanding its development, causes, classification, evaluation, and treatment.* New York: Oxford University Press.

Hatton, C. (2004). Cultural Issues. In E. Emerson, C. Hatton, T. Thompson, & T. Parmenter (Eds.), *Applied research in intellectual disabilities* (pp. 41–60). West Sussex, UK: Wiley.

Heber, R. A. (1959). A manual on terminology and classification in mental retardation. *American Journal of Mental Deficiency, 64 (Monograph Supplement).*

Hyde, M., & Power, D. (2006). Some ethical dimensions of cochlear implantation for deaf children and their families. *Journal of Deaf Studies and Deaf Education, 11,* 102–111.

Kame'enui, E. J., & Carnine, D. W. (2002). *Effective teaching strategies that accommodate diverse learners* (2nd ed.). Upper Saddle River, NJ: Merrill.

Kanner, L. (1943). Autistic disturbances of affective contact. *Nervous Child, 2,* 217–405.

Luckasson, R., Borthwick-Duffy, S., Buntinx, W. H. E., Coulter, D. L., Craig, E. M., Reeve, A., et al. (2002). *Mental retardation: Definition, classification, and systems of supports* (10th ed.). Washington, DC: American Association on Mental Retardation.

Luckasson, R., Coulter, D. L., Polloway, E. A., Reiss, S., Schalock, R. L., Snell, M. E., et al. (1992). *Mental retardation: Definition, classification, and systems of supports* (9th ed.). Washington, DC: American Association on Mental Retardation.

Mesibov, G., Shea, V., & Schopler, E. (2005). *The TEACCH approach to autism spectrum disorders.* New York: Springer.

Miles, S., & Ahuja, A. (2007). Learning from differences: Sharing international experiences of development in inclusive education. In L. Florian (Ed.), *The SAGE handbook of special education* (pp. 131–145). Thousand Oaks, CA: Sage.

Pakulak, E. and Neville, H. (2006). Exploring the relationship between environment, proficiency, and brain organization for language in children from different socioeconomic backgrounds. *CUNY: Online Methods in Children's Language Processing.*

Parmenter, T. (2004). Historical overview of applied research in intellectual disabilities: The foundation years. In E. Emerson, C. Hatton, T. Thompson, & T. Parmenter (Eds.), *Applied research in intellectual disabilities* (pp. 3–40). West Sussex, UK: Wiley.

Schalock, R. (2000). Three decades of quality of life. In M. L. Wehmeyer & J. R. Patton (Eds.), *Mental retardation in the 21st century* (pp. 335–358). Austin TX: PRO-ED.

Schalock, R., & Felce, D. (2004). Quality of life and subjective well-being: Conceptual and measurement issues. In E. Emerson, C. Hatton, T. Thompson, & T. Parmenter (Eds.), *Applied research in intellectual disabilities* (pp. 262–280). West Sussex, UK: Wiley.

Schalock, R., Luckasson, R., & Shogren, K. (2007). The renaming of mental retardation: Understanding the change to the term intellectual disability. *Intellectual and Developmental Disabilities, 45,* 116–124.

Schalock, R. L., Stark, J. A., Snell, M. E., Coulter, D. L., Polloway, E. A., Luckasson, R., et al. (1994). The changing conception of mental retardation: Implications for the field. *Mental Retardation, 32,* 181–193.

Schmidt, B. D. (2006). *Sleep positions for young infants.* Ann Arbor, MI: McKesson Corporation. Retrieved January 15, 2007, from *www.med.umich.edu/1libr/pa/pa_infslpos_hhg.htm*

Shinagawa, L. H., & Jang, M. (1998). *Atlas of American diversity.* Walnut Creek, CA: AltaMira.

Simeonsson, R. J., Leonardi, M., Lollars, D., Bjorck-Akesson, E., & Hollenweger, J. (2003). Applying the international classification of functioning, disability, and health (ICF) to measure childhood disability. *Disability and Rehabilitation, 25,* 3–17.

Simeonsson, R. J., Lollar, D. J., Hollowell, J., & Adams, M. (2000). Revision of the international classification of impairments, disabilities, and handicaps: Developmental issues. *Journal of Clinical Epidemiology, 53,* 113–124.

Snell, M. E. (Ed.). (1978). *Systematic instruction of the moderately and severely handicapped.* Columbus, OH: Charles E. Merrill.

World Health Organization. (1992). *International classification of diseases: Diagnostic criteria for research* (10th ed.). Geneva, Switzerland: Author.

World Health Organization. (2002). *International classification of function, disability, and health.* Geneva, Switzerland: Author.

Public Policy and Developmental Disabilities

A 35-Year Retrospective and a 5-Year Prospective Based on the Core Concepts of Disability Policy

H. Rutherford Turnbull, III
Matthew J. Stowe
Ann P. Turnbull
Mary Suzanne Schrandt

THE CORE-CONCEPTS APPROACH

There are at least two tried-and-true ways to introduce a reader to public policy as it affects people with developmental disabilities (hereinafter, "DD policy"). One way is to trace the development of policy over time, beginning in the early 1970s, when the disability-rights revolution began. Another is to hone in on specific rights, such as rights to education, treatment, liberty, and equal opportunity. A chapter in a handbook published more than a decade ago would emphasize these approaches.

Today, the time-line approach simply does not hold water any longer. There was a "rights establishing" era. It began with the courts' decisions in some right-to-education cases (*PARC v. Commonwealth of Pennsylvania*, 1971, 1972; *Mills v. D.C. Board of Education*, 1972), right-to-treatment cases (*Wyatt v. Stickney*, 1971, 1974) and the accompanying right-to-refuse-treatment cases (*Mills v. Rogers*, 1982); cases of protection from harm in institutions (*Youngberg v. Romeo*, 1982); cases limiting compulsory sterilization (*NCARC v. North Carolina*, 1976; but see *In re Lee Ann Grady*, 1981); civil confinement cases (*Jackson v. Indiana*, 1972; *O'Connor v. Donaldson*, 1974); and parents'-rights limitation cases (*Parham v. J.R.*, 1979). (See Table 2.1 for more information about these cases.) It also began with the enactment of the anti-discrimination law now known as Section 504 of the Vocational Rehabilitation Act in 1973 and Public Law 94-142, the Education of All Handicapped Children Act, in 1975.

TABLE 2.1. Case References and Holdings

Board of Education v. Arline, 480 U.S. 273 (1987)	A person who has tuberculosis is a "handicapped individual" within the meaning of Sec. 504 of the Rehabilitation Act.
Board of Education v. Rowley, 458 U.S. 176 (1982)	The Individuals with Disabilities Education Act does not require that states "maximize the educational potential of handicapped children commensurate with the opportunity provided non-handicapped children," but rather provide an opportunity for a "free appropriate public education."
Bowen v. American Hospital Association, 476 U.S. 610 (1986)	Sec. 504 of the Rehabilitation Act did not give the Secretary of Health and Human Services authority to issue regulations relating to newborns with disabilities that have the effect of superseding parental decision making and commandeering state agencies.
Brown v. Board of Education, 347 U.S. 483 (1954)	In overturning *Plessy v. Ferguson,* the "separate but equal doctrine," the Court ordered schools to desegregate by race, with all due deliberate speed, in order to secure compliance with the 14th Amendment's equal-protection clause.
Cedar Rapids Community School District v. Garrett F., 526 U.S. 66 (1999)	The Individuals with Disabilities Education Act requires provision of the related services of a full-time nurse (which is not a medical service).
Chevron v. Echazabal, 536 U.S. 73 (2002)	The Americans with Disabilities Act allows employers to refuse to hire a person with a disability if the job would aggravate the person's existing disability.
City of Cleburne v. Cleburne Living Center, 473 U.S. 432 (1985)	Zoning discrimination targeted solely at persons with mental retardation and animated solely by invidious purposes violates the equal protection provisions of the 14th Amendment.
Cruzan v. Director, Missouri Department of Health, 497 U.S. 261 (1990)	A state may require a decision on withholding life-maintaining services to be protected by proof, at a clear and convincing level, that the decision is consistent with the wishes/consent of the person/patient.
DeShaney v. Winnebago County Department of Social Services, 489 U.S. 189 (1989)	A local government agency may not be held liable for damage to a child caused by the child's father when the child is in the foster-care system but not within the physical custody of the agency; liability under Section 1983 of the Civil Rights Act does not attach in the absence of physical custody by the state.
Elk Grove Unified School District v. Newdow, 124 S. Ct. 2301 (2004)	A noncustodial father lacks standing to sue a school district in federal court to secure a court order prohibiting the school from asking students to say the Pledge of Allegiance, including the words "under God," where the noncustodial father claimed the school's practice/policy violated the establishment and free exercise clauses of the 1st Amendment.
Honig v. Doe, 484 U.S. 305 (1988)	School authorities may not unilaterally exclude a child with a disability from the classroom during the pendency of proceedings concerning the child's education and dangerous or disruptive conduct growing out of the child's disabilities.

(continued)

TABLE 2.1. *(continued)*

In re Lee Ann Grady, 426 A.2d 467 (1981)	Parents of a legally incompetent woman, in their role as their daughter's guardians, are permitted to exercise their substituted judgment on behalf of their daughter on the subject of sterilization.
Irving Independent School District v. Tatro, 468 U.S. 883 (1984)	The Individuals with Disabilities Education Act authorizes related services that include clean intermittent catheterization.
Jackson v. Indiana, 406 U.S. 715 (1972)	A person's civil commitment violated the equal protection clause of the 14th Amendment because he was subjected to a more lenient commitment standard and a more stringent standard of release and was committed solely on account of his incompetency to stand trial.
Larry P. v. Riles, 793 F. 2d 969 (1984)	Standard intelligence tests used to place African American elementary school children into special classes violate Sec. 504, IDEA, and the Civil Rights Act because they disproportionately place these students into special education (relative to other students) and lack a scientific basis for a placement decision.
Mills v. D.C. Board of Education, 348 F. Supp. 866 (D.D.C. 1972)	A school district that did not provide publicly supported education to "exceptional" children when under an affirmative duty to do so violates the children's substantive due process rights under the 5th and 14th Amendments.
Mills v. Rogers, 457 U.S. 291 (1982)	The state may provide greater rights than the U.S. Constitution for involuntarily committed patients who wish to refuse antipsychotic drugs; there is a 1st Amendment (liberty–substantive due process) right to refuse treatment.
North Carolina Association for Retarded Children v. North Carolina, 420 F. Supp. 451 (1976)	A state's involuntary sterilization statute does not violate the 14th Amendment's equal protection guarantee because the statute has sufficient procedural safeguards and relies on the doctrine of the least restrictive/drastic means.
O'Connor v. Donaldson, 422 U.S. 563 (1974)	A state may not constitutionally confine in a mental hospital an individual who is not dangerous to him- or herself or others and who is capable of surviving safely in freedom by him- or herself or with the help of willing and responsible family members or friends.
Olmstead v. L.C., 527 U.S. 581 (1999)	Unwarranted placement in segregated facilities constitutes discrimination that is prohibited by the Americans with Disabilities Act; ADA compels the states to deinstitutionalize unless doing so creates an undue burden on the state's treasury or is unwanted by an individual or unsafe for an individual.
Oregon v. Gonzales, 126 S. Ct. 904 (2006)	The U.S. Attorney General lacks authority to determine that using controlled substances to assist suicide is an illegitimate medical practice under the federal Controlled Substances Act.
Parham v. J.R., 442 U.S. 584 (1979)	The 14th Amendment's substantive due process clause (liberty) requires a state to offer at least an independent review of a decision by a parent to admit a minor to a state institution; the admission decision may not be made solely by the parent and the institutional director.

(continued)

TABLE 2.1. *(continued)*

Pennhurst State School and Hospital v. Halderman (Pennhurst I), 451 U.S. 1 (1981)	The Developmental Disabilities Act does not create for persons with mental retardation any substantive rights, including treatment, services, habilitation, and the provision of those services in the least restrictive setting.
Pennsylvania Association for Retarded Children (PARC) v. Commonwealth of Pennsylvania, 334 F. Supp. 1257 (E.D. Pa. 1971); 343 F. Supp. 279 (E.D. Pa. 1972)	Schools may not exclude students with disabilities solely on the basis of their disabilities; exclusion violates the 14th Amendment's equal-protection guarantee.
PGA Tour, Inc. v. Martin, 121 S. Ct. 1879 (2001)	The PGA Tour is a "public accommodation," and the operators of the tour violate the Americans with Disabilities Act requirement of reasonable accommodation when, in insisting on the "walking requirements" that they apply to all tour competitors, they refuse to allow a professional golfer with a physical impairment to use a golf cart while competing; using the cart does not fundamentally alter the nature of the competition, the essence of which is hitting the golf ball into a hole with a golf club.
Santosky v. Kramer, 455 U.S. 745 (1982)	Before a state may sever completely and irrevocably the rights of parents with respect to their natural child, the 14th Amendment's substantive due-process guarantee requires the state to prove, by at least clear and convincing evidence, that the parent is unfit to raise the child.
In re Guardianship of Schiavo, 855 So. 2d 621 (Fla. 2003)	When families cannot agree, the best forum for this private, personal decision is a public courtroom, and the best decision maker is a judge with no prior knowledge of the person; the law provides no better solution that adequately protects the interests of promoting the value of life.
Southeastern Community College v. Davis, 442 U.S. 397 (1979)	The refusal of an institution of higher education to admit an individual with a hearing disability to the program leading to an RN degree does not violate Sec. 504 of the Rehabilitation Act because the admission would require the institution to make unreasonable accommodations to the person and run counter to the patient safety that the state's nursing licensing board is committed to protecting.
State of Tennessee v. Lane, 124 S. Ct. 1978 (2004)	A state is subject to the Americans with Disabilities Act and Congress may abrogate state immunity when there is a record of state discrimination against individuals in their exercise of the fundamental right to vote.
Strunk v. Strunk, 445 S.W.2d 145 (1969)	The courts have sufficient power to employ substituted judgment and to give or authorize parents to consent for an incompetent individual to undergo a medical procedure if the operation is deemed to be in the individual's best interest.
Superintendent v. Saikewicz, 373 Mass. 721 (1977)	Both the doctrine of informed consent and the 14th Amendment's right of privacy (deriving from the 1st Amendment and applicable to the states through the 14th) protect the right of a patient to refuse medical treatment in appropriate circumstances; in the case of an incompetent patient, the right may be asserted by a guardian.

(continued)

TABLE 2.1. *(continued)*

Sutton v. United Airlines, 527 U.S. 471 (1999)	The determination of whether an individual is disabled under the Americans with Disabilities Act must be made with reference to measures that mitigate the individual's impairment; if an individual has mitigated an impairment, the person is not protected by ADA.
Toyota v. Williams, 524 U.S. 184 (2002)	The proper standard for demonstrating "a substantial limitation in the major life activity of performing manual tasks" under the Americans with Disabilities Act is whether or not the impairment prevents or restricts a person from performing manual tasks that are "of central importance to most people's daily lives" and has "permanent or long-term" impact; being limited in performing a "class of manual activities" (i.e., activities affecting the ability to perform specific manual tasks at work) is an insufficient standard for meeting the ADA definition of a "qualified" individual with a disability.
Troxel v. Granville, 530 U.S. 57 (2000)	Fundamental liberty interests, protected under the 1st Amendment and applicable to the states through the 14th, include parents' rights to raise children and to make decisions concerning their care, custody, and control; a state statute that grants child-visitation rights to others than the parents, without identifying the basis on which those rights may be exercised, unduly interferes with parents' rights to raise their children.
University of Alabama v. Garrett, 531 U.S. 356 (2001)	The Americans with Disabilities Act may not abrogate the states' sovereign immunity and subject them to monetary damages when there is not a sufficient record of state discrimination in employment against individuals with disabilities to justify the abrogation.
US Airways v. Barnett, 535 U.S. 391 (2002)	Ordinarily, the Americans with Disabilities Act does not require an employer to assign an employee with a disability to a particular position as a "reasonable accommodation" if another employee is entitled to that position under the employees' established seniority system.
Vacco v. Quill, 521 U.S. 793 (1997)	It is consistent with the 14th Amendment for New York to treat assisted suicide and the refusal of lifesaving treatment differently.
Washington v. Glucksberg, 521 U.S. 702 (1997)	Washington's ban on assisted suicide is rationally related to a legitimate government interest and does not violate the due-process clause of the 14th Amendment.
Wyatt v. Stickney, 325 F. Supp. 781; 503 F.2d 1305 (1971, 1974)	To deprive any citizen of his or her liberty on the altruistic theory that the confinement is for humane, therapeutic reasons and then fail to provide adequate treatment violates the very fundamentals of substantive due process.
Youngberg v. Romeo, 457 U.S. 307 (1982)	An involuntarily committed person with mental retardation has 14th Amendment due-process liberty interests requiring the state to provide minimally adequate training to ensure safety and freedom from undue restraint.

Likewise, there was a "rights consolidation" era. It began before but is most manifest in the middle of the 1980s and is represented by decisions that interpret disability under Section 504 (*Southeastern Community College v. Davis*, 1979; *Board of Education v. Arline*, 1987); that favor community-based placements (*City of Cleburne v. Cleburne Living Center*, 1985; *Olmstead v. L.C.*, 1999); that protect the rights of those who cannot speak for themselves but who have otherwise indicated their desires (*Cruzan v. Director*, 1990) or who are incapable of doing so in any way (*Superintendent v. Saikewicz*, 1977); that interpret the Individuals with Disabilities Education Act (IDEA) as conferring a substantive benefit, not merely procedural protections (*Board of Education v. Rowley*, 1982); that interpret Public Law 94-142 (now, IDEA) to prohibit disability-based expulsion (*Honig v. Doe*, 1988) and to require health-related services to be provided by the public schools (*Irving Independent School District v. Tatro*, 1984); that limit the enforceability of the Developmental Disabilities Assistance and Bill of Rights Act (*Pennhurst State School and Hospital v. Halderman*, 1981), the states' child-protection laws, and the Civil Rights Act (*DeShaney v. Winnebago County Department of Social Services*, 1989); and that limit the enforceability of Section 504 (*Bowen v. American Hospital Association*, 1986). It also was represented by an amendment to the Social Security Act's Title XIX (Medicaid) that allowed federal funds to be used for home- and community-based services (1981); the enhancement of IDEA through the enactment of early-intervention and transition provisions, the Technology-Related Assistance for Individuals with Disabilities Act (2000), the Adoption Assistance and Child Welfare and Adoption and Safe Families Acts (1980, 1997); and, most significantly, the Americans with Disabilities Act (ADA, 1990).

Similarly, the "rights dilution" or "rights refinement" era is represented by a series of cases in the 1990s in which the Supreme Court narrowed ADA's scope and the power of individuals to enforce it against state agencies (*University of Alabama v. Garrett*, 2001; but see *PGA Tour v. Martin*, 2001 and *State of Tennessee v. Lane*, 2004) and employers (*Sutton v. United Airlines*, 1999; *Chevron v. Echazabel*, 2002; *Toyota v. Williams*, 2002; *US Airways* v. *Bennett*, 2002) largely on the basis that long-standing institutions of society should be allowed to make certain decisions (Stowe, Turnbull, & Sublet, 2006).

Nowadays, however, there is so much complexity in DD policy that it is hard to say, with any accuracy, that we are in one type of an era or another. Just as the Supreme Court reduces some rights, so Congress enlarges others; and just as Congress retrenches on some rights, the Court preserves still others (Stowe et al., 2006), largely in order to advance an individual's decision to choose how to live. Moreover, it is less appealing nowadays to describe public policy according to specific rights (such as rights to education, treatment, nondiscrimination, and services). Congress and the Court have already established so many of the fundamental rights of people with disabilities that the task they face currently is whether to expand or diminish existing rights.

So for these days and in the future, a more useful way to understand policy is to ask, Are there any core concepts that survive the test of time and also undergird the rights-specific approaches? The answer is yes, and the core-concepts approach (Turnbull, Beegle, & Stowe, 2001) is the one that we discuss here. Its benefit is that it is relatively timeless and does not limit one's understanding to only particular rights. It focuses on "core" and "concepts." It is a generalized analytical approach. The term "core" means central and foundational. The term "concept" means an abstract or generic idea generalized from particular instances. Thus a core concept is one that is utterly indispensable to the formation of public policy and to our understanding of policy. The core concepts apply generally to people with a variety of disabilities, not just to those with developmental disabilities. Disability policy is a generic, umbrella concept; DD policy is a specific, subsumed one.

THE CORE CONCEPTS: A 35-YEAR RETROSPECTIVE

We define the concept and then point out how Congress or the Supreme Court or other courts have established or interpreted it. We refer to only those court decisions that are "core" in the sense that they established the concept as a matter of constitutional law or set precedents in interpreting federal statutes. We point out instances in which the statute or decision applies specifically to people with a developmental disability.

Because there are so many core concepts, we have developed a taxonomy for organizing them (Turnbull & Stowe, 2001). The taxonomy sorts the core concepts into three constitutional principles (life, liberty, and equality); three ethical principles (dignity, family as foundation, and community); three health professional principles (beneficence, autonomy, and justice); and three administrative principles (capacity, individualization, and accountability) that implement the other principles. Figure 2.1 displays these 12 principles (designed as a ramp) and groups the core concepts under each. As is shown, many of the core concepts belong to more than one principle. For example, the core concept "protection from harm" is grouped with the ethical principles of dig-

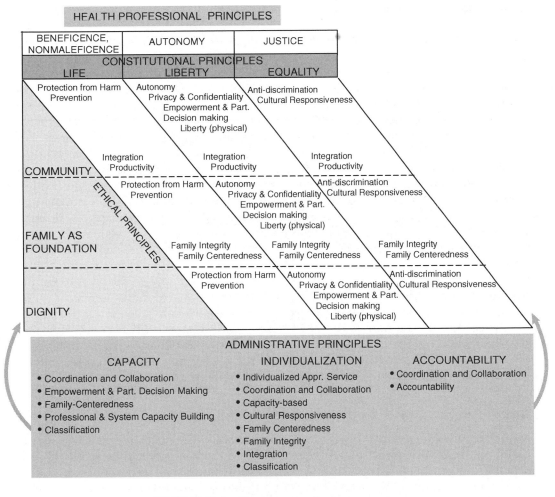

FIGURE 2.1. A taxonomy of core concepts.

nity, family as foundation, and community. Similarly, the core concept "integration" is grouped with the constitutional principles of life, liberty, and equality. For this reason, we have organized this chapter according to the core concepts, not the principles. Accordingly, we describe each one.

Anti-Discrimination

The right not to suffer discrimination because of one's unalterable trait (such as race, sex, or disability) derives from the 14th Amendment to the U.S. Constitution. The amendment provides that no state may deny anyone the equal protection of the laws. The amendment grants Congress authority to enforce the equal-guarantee provision, and Congress has done so by enacting two federal anti-discrimination statutes.

Section 504 of the Rehabilitation Act amendments of 1973 prohibits recipients of federal financial assistance from discriminating against an otherwise qualified person with a disability solely on the basis of the person's disability. The ADA (1990) provides for similar protection but covers entities that do not receive federal financial assistance, including state and local government agencies, private employers, private entities that offer their service to the general public ("public accommodations"), and the transportation and telecommunications media.

A person is otherwise qualified if the person can participate in a covered entity's activities with reasonable accommodations. Indeed, Section 504 and ADA both require a covered entity to offer reasonable accommodations to people with disabilities. If the accommodations do not make it possible for the person to participate, then the person is not "otherwise" qualified (the "otherwise" means "with reasonable accommodations"), and any action by the covered entity that is based on the person's disability is not illegal under Section 504 or ADA (*Southeastern Community College v. Davis*, 1979).

The Supreme Court applied the anti-discrimination core concept to people with developmental disabilities in two cases. In *City of Cleburne v. Cleburne Living Center* (1985), the Court held that a local zoning ordinance that prohibits people with mental retardation from living in a congregate setting, such as a group home, but allows other people with disabilities and all of those without disabilities to live in such a home in a residential zone violates the equal-protection clause. The only reason for the prohibition was to single out those with mental retardation; the bias was irrational (there was no reason to exclude those with mental retardation) and could be explained only by prejudice.

Cleburne led Congress to enact the ADA, and the Court applied the ADA to people with mental retardation in *Olmstead v. L.C.* (1999). There, it held that a state violates the ADA by failing to offer community-based care to those who are able to live in the community safely and who want to do so. The state's action in unjustifiably confining people with mental retardation and other disabilities in state facilities discriminates against them; they are "otherwise qualified" to live in the community safely if they receive the "reasonable accommodations" of community-based support and services.

Individualized and Appropriate Services

As the "reasonable accommodations" provisions make clear, a person with a disability is entitled to have individualized and appropriate services in order to benefit from the activities in which that person may participate with those services.

Section 504 and ADA provide for "reasonable accommodations." Other statutes provide for rights that are expressly tailored to the nature of the services that the law authorizes. For example, IDEA enacts a right to a free, appropriate, individualized, and beneficial education in the least restrictive environment (*Board of Education v. Rowley*, 1982; *Irving Independent School District v. Tatro*, 1984; *Cedar Rapids Community School District v. Garrett F.*, 1999).

Two court decisions reflect the core concept of individualized and appropriate services for people with mental retardation and related developmental disabilities. In *Wyatt v. Stickney* (1971, 1974), a federal court held that people with mental retardation who were confined involuntarily in a state institution are entitled to have individualized treatment plans and services; to confine them without offering them some benefit violates their right to substantive due process as guaranteed by the 14th Amendment. That amendment contains not only the equal-protection guarantee but also a guarantee that no state will deny anyone the "due process" of law. So a state may not deprive a person of liberty simply because the person is undesirable (on account of his or her disability). To do so without also providing some individualized benefit deprives the person of due process. In *Youngberg v. Romeo* (1982), the Supreme Court adopted a similar approach, holding that a minor with mental retardation who has been admitted to a state institution by a parent has a due-process liberty interest that requires the state to offer minimally adequate training to ensure safety and freedom from undue restraint.

Classification

People with disabilities often are determined to be eligible (or ineligible) to participate in various activities or to receive certain services simply because they have a disability or have a certain kind or extent of disability. Eligibility determination is an act of classifying a person. Sometimes, the classification—the denial of services or the placement into service categories that are inappropriate for the person—results from racial, ethnic, linguistic, socioeconomic, or other bias based on professionals' use of evaluations that were not validated for the purposes for which they were used or for their use with a certain person or group of persons. When classification is based on bias, it constitutes discrimination and results in the denial of individual and appropriate services. Accordingly, misclassification violates both the equal-protection and due-process assurances of the 14th Amendment. Nondiscriminatory classification—fair classification—is ensured when the professionals who make eligibility determinations use processes (means) and standards (criteria) that do not discriminate and that yield an accurate assessment of the person's abilities and disabilities.

In 1975, a federal court, in *Larry P. v. Riles* (1984), held that standardized IQ tests, when applied by California schools to students from racial minority groups (African Americans), were biased against these students on the basis of race and that the students' resulting placement into special education programs for students with mental retardation was not justified. That case influenced Congress to enact the nondiscriminatory evaluation requirements that have been part of IDEA ever since 1975. IDEA provides that state and local education agencies must conduct nondiscriminatory evaluations in order to determine whether a student has a disability and, if disability is present, to determine the consequences of that finding for the student's individualized and appropriate program of special education and the student's placement in or out of the general curriculum (the least restrictive alternative).

In addition, Congress has amended the Social Security Act so that children and adults may receive Supplemental Security Income (SSI) benefits if they have severe disabilities, including developmental disabilities. Severity of disability, then, is part of the core concept of classification. There is more to classification than a professionally defensible, unbiased finding that a person has a disability; often, the extent or severity of the disability is the fact that makes a person eligible or ineligible for individual and appropriate services (such as special education) or benefits (such as SSI).

Capacity-Based Services

Classification procedures and standards determine whether a person is eligible to participate in certain services or receive certain benefits. Invariably, classification seeks to know whether a person has a disability, and, if so, how extensive the disability is. In this respect, classification is "pathology" based; it seeks to determine a person's needs, deficits, disabilities, and limitations.

Accordingly, classification procedures and standards often have failed to focus on the person's strengths and capacities. In that respect, classification procedures and standards fail to regard the whole person; they produce only a limited picture of the person and thus also fail to identify the ways in which the person can function and participate in various activities with or without reasonable accommodations or individual and appropriate services.

Congress has responded to the focus on pathology by requiring educators (under IDEA), rehabilitation specialists (under the Rehabilitation Act), and early-intervention specialists (under the Maternal and Child Health Act) to determine the strengths and capacities of people with disabilities and to develop individual and appropriate service delivery plans not just on the basis of their needs but also on the basis of their capacities. The Developmental Disabilities and Bill of Rights Act ("DD Act"; 2000) is crystal clear about the core concept of capacity-based services, declaring that individuals with developmental disabilities have "competencies, capacities, and personal goals that should be recognized, supported, and encouraged" and that assistance to an individual should be provided "consistent with the unique strengths, resources, priorities, concerns, abilities, and capabilities" of people with developmental disabilities (DD Act § 15001[c][2], 2000).

Empowerment and Participatory Decision Making

Once a person has been protected against discrimination and been assured the benefit of individual and appropriate services based on fair classification procedures and standards that take into account the person's strengths, as well as needs, the next issue is how the person participates with a service provider agency or professional in receiving the services to which the person has a right or entitlement.

The core concept of empowerment and participatory decision making involves the means by which a person secures what he or she wants from a service provider system. If the person has such an extensive developmental disability that the person is unable to participate with the professional in making service delivery decisions or if the person is a minor, a surrogate (typically, a parent or a court-appointed guardian) will represent the person in decision making with a professional.

Empowerment and participatory decision making occur through the person's or surrogate's participation with the professional or the service delivery system in consenting to certain services or otherwise deciding how the services will be designed (planned), delivered, implemented, and evaluated. The concept of empowerment and participatory decision making applies to decisions at the individual level (such as special education programs and placement under IDEA) or at a system level (such as statewide services for people with developmental disabilities under the DD Act). The DD

Act is explicit about empowerment and participatory decision making and requires all activities funded under the act to involve people with developmental disabilities and their families in a variety of decision-making roles (DD Act § 15001, [c][2][3], 2000). IDEA also carries out this core concept by providing that a student's parents and the student, when appropriate, may participate in the development of an individualized education program (IDEA, § 1414).

Service Coordination and Collaboration

Among the issues that a person with a disability and the person's surrogate will discuss with a service professional is how to secure individual and appropriate services not only from that professional's agency but also from the agencies in which other services are available and for which the person is eligible.

The core concept of service coordination and collaboration recognizes that people with developmental disabilities have "horizontal needs"—their intellectual, developmental, physical, and emotional and behavioral needs interact with one another. The core concept also recognizes that service systems are designed on a "vertical basis"—there are separate service systems with separate funding streams, separate individual and appropriate services, separate classification and eligibility procedures and standards, and separate professional capacities and qualifications. Accordingly, statutes such as the DD Act, IDEA, and the Technology-Related Assistance for Persons with Disabilities Act (2000) provide for intra-agency and interagency coordination and collaboration.

Intra-agency collaboration refers to collaboration among professionals in the same service systems, such as among general and special educators under IDEA and the No Child Left Behind Act (NCLB; 2001). Agencies within an umbrella state or local education agency are aligned with each other to achieve certain policy outcomes (e.g., academic progress) and their professional staff members must therefore collaborate with each other.

Interagency collaboration refers, for example, to collaboration among agencies for people with developmental disabilities and mental health agencies when a person with a developmental disability also has emotional or behavioral disabilities ("co-occurring disabilities" or "dual diagnoses"). Likewise, assistive technologies that increase the ability of a person to function effectively may be available from vocational rehabilitation agencies, as well as from medical centers; federal laws authorize these agencies to coordinate and collaborate with each other, and the federal Technology-Related Assistance for Persons with Disabilities Act authorizes a state to create interagency systems for delivering that technology.

The core concepts that we have discussed so far—anti-discrimination, individual and appropriate services, classification, capacity-based services, empowerment and participatory decision making, and coordination and collaboration—all are concerned with who gets what. They address these issues: Is the person with a developmental disability entitled not to suffer discrimination and to receive reasonable accommodations in order not to experience discrimination? Is the person able to benefit from participation by reason of having individual and appropriate services based on unbiased classification procedures and standards, delivered with attention to the person's capacities, as well as his or her needs, planned and implemented through joint decision making, and coordinated among various agencies and their collaborating professionals?

These core concepts also proceed on the basis of "positive rights"—that is, they create rights that benefit individuals with developmental disabilities. The IDEA is a good example of a positive-rights approach in education; Section 504 of the Rehabilitation

Act and the ADA are good examples of laws that create a positive right, namely, the right to reasonable accommodations. Likewise, the DD Act creates rights for people with developmental disabilities to participate in the process whereby the state developmental disabilities planning council makes decisions about the state plan. These statutes are concerned with conferring a positive benefit, namely, services that are effective in the sense that they lead to predetermined outcomes.

None of these statutes, however, focuses on protecting a person from the negative consequences of being in a service delivery system or from being subject to state coercion. Three core concepts do address the issues of state coercion; they proceed on the basis of "negative rights"—that is, rights against state action. (Note that the core concept of anti-discrimination and its related statutes, Section 504 of the Rehabilitation Act and the ADA, are concerned with the negative right not to be subjected to state-based or private-sector discrimination; but the core concept itself and the statutes that implement it also involve the positive right to receive reasonable accommodations, which is why we discussed it under the "positive rights" core concepts.)

Liberty

The first of the three core concepts that proceed on the basis of negative rights is the core concept of liberty. That core concept holds that a person has a right to be free of unwarranted physical or other confinement by a government. The concept focuses on "unwarranted"; it acknowledges that there are two justifications for a state to deprive a person of liberty. One justification seeks public safety. A person who is imminently dangerous to others may be confined. The other seeks the safety of the person with a disability. When the person is unable to care for him- or herself and thus poses a danger to him- or herself, the state may confine the person in order to protect him or her and to provide services that assist the person in leaning how not to harm him- or herself.

As we noted earlier, *Wyatt v. Stickney* and *Youngberg v. Romeo* address the issue of liberty and individual and appropriate services during confinement. These are not the only cases on point. In *Pennhurst State School and Hospital v. Halderman* (1981), the Supreme Court held that the DD Act does not create any substantive rights for people with developmental disabilities to receive treatment, services, and habilitation outside of an institution.

That case disappointed advocates for people with disabilities, for they had expected the Court to follow its earlier decision in *O'Connor v. Donaldson* (1974), in which it held that a state may not constitutionally confine an individual in a mental hospital if the individual is not dangerous to others and is capable of living safely in the community by him- or herself or with support from others. Although *O'Connor* dealt with people with mental illness (or those who allegedly had mental illness), it clearly influenced Congress to enact the ADA, and it also was a precedent for the Court's decision in *Olmstead v. L.C.*

Congress has advanced the core concept of liberty by providing that state and local developmental disabilities agencies (under the DD Act), education agencies (under IDEA), and mental health agencies (under the Child Mental Health Act) may use federal funds to create community-based services. These services, delivered in the "least restrictive environment" of the community, make it possible for the agencies not to use the large institutions that were attacked unsuccessfully in the *Pennhurst* case and instead to create services that avoid confinement and ensure liberty.

Protection from Harm

Another one of the "negative rights" core concepts is protection from harm. This core concept proclaims that a person has the right not to be harmed while in the custody of the state and its agencies. IDEA advances this core concept by providing that a student's individualized education program team must consider whether the student needs positive behavioral supports and services and must provide for a functional behavioral assessment and a behavioral intervention plan for the student, which can include positive behavioral supports, when the student has been disciplined for longer than a 10-day period of time.

Further, the regulations implementing the federal Child Abuse Prevention and Treatment Act (2003) provide that, if an infant or other person with a disability is receiving medical care, there is a presumption in favor of continuing that care when the person is at the "edge" or "end" of life. Likewise, the Children's Mental Health Act (2000) and the Children's Health Act (2000) place limits on the power of state agencies to use restraints and seclusion. The Adoption Assistance and Child Welfare Act (1980) and its accompanying Adoption and Safe Families Act (1997) establish adoption and foster care programs that prevent "foster care drift" and seek to reunite the child with his or her biological parents in order to prevent any harm that separation from them might cause the child.

As we noted when discussing the core concept of individualized and appropriate services, the courts' decisions in *Wyatt v. Stickney* and the Supreme Court's decision in *Youngberg v. Romeo* seek not only those services but also, as a consequence of them, protection from the harm of neglect, abuse, or maltreatment when a person is in a state institution. Similarly, the Supreme Court has held, in *DeShaney v. Winnebago* (1989), that a person has a right not to be injured while in state care. That case raised the question of whether a child whose father so severely beat him as to cause brain damage and cognitive impairments may sue a local government foster care agency that returned the child to the father in spite of knowing that the father had a propensity to beat his child. The Court held that, unless the child is in the physical custody of the state and its agencies, the child may not sue the state; the father was acting as a private individual. Despite the outcome, *DeShaney* stands for the proposition that a person in state custody has the right not to be injured by state employees.

Autonomy

Whereas the core concepts of liberty and protection from harm relate to a state's physical custody over a person with a disability, the core concept of autonomy relates to the right of the person or the person's surrogate to consent, refuse to consent, or withdraw consent to what happens to him or her. This core concept acknowledges that a person has a claim to control what happens to him or her; the claim derives from the doctrine of due process in regard to liberty in the sense of freedom from state interference in the person's life, as expressed in the 5th and 14th Amendments to the Constitution. (The 5th Amendment applies to the federal government, and the 14th to state governments.) Congress upholds the core concept of autonomy when, for example, it provides in IDEA that a parent may give or withhold consent to his or her child's evaluation for special education services and when it stipulates that all federally funded researchers must obtain the prior consent of a person to be a research participant (Health and Human Services Policy for Protection of Human Research Subjects, 2005).

The Supreme Court has long recognized that parents have an autonomy right to raise their children as they see fit, free of state interference except to protect the public or the child (*Troxel v. Granville*, 2000; *Elk Grove Unified School District* v. *Newdow*, 2004). Parents exercise this right on their children's behalf, and surrogates for those who have intellectual or other disabilities exercise it for those people.

Among the Court's most important decisions is one that affected a person who was in a "persistent vegetative state" as a result of a lengthy loss of oxygen following an automobile accident. In *Cruzan v. Director, Missouri Department of Health* (1990), the Court held that a state may require parents who want to order the removal of life-sustaining food and water provided by tubes inserted into their adult child's body to prove, by clear and convincing evidence, that their adult child had expressed a desire not to be kept alive by these means.

Similarly, in *Superintendent v. Saikewicz* (1977), the Massachusetts Supreme Court held that the doctrine of informed consent and constitutional right of privacy protect the right of a person with significant intellectual disabilities to refuse, through a surrogate, medical care. The right to refuse treatment is embedded in the concept of autonomy; a person has a right to control what happens to his or her body. Even before *Cruzan* and *Saikewicz*, the Kentucky Supreme Court held in *Strunk v. Strunk* (1969) that a surrogate (parent) may consent to the removal of a kidney from a twin who has intellectual disability if the kidney is then transplanted into the twin who does not have a disability and on whom the donor twin relies for emotional support and comfort. Finally, the New Jersey Supreme Court has held, in *In re Lee Ann Grady* (1981), that a parent may consent to a tubal ligation for a minor daughter who has mental retardation in order to prevent the daughter from becoming pregnant and to facilitate her living in the community among members of the opposite sex.

Privacy and Confidentiality

The core concept of autonomy creates a general right against state interference in a person's life, and the core concepts of privacy and confidentiality particularize that core concept. "Privacy" refers to protection against unwarranted governmental interference in decision making that affects a person's private interests. It creates a "zone" of privacy around a person with respect to such matters as reproduction (abortion, in particular), as well as life-sustaining treatment (*Cruzan*). Although the Supreme Court has refused to recognize that a person has a federal constitutional right to assisted suicide (*Washington v. Glucksberg*, 1997, and *Vacco v. Quill*, 1997), the Court has held that the Attorney General of the United States has no standing under the federal Controlled Substances Act to challenge a state law that authorizes a person to request and receive medical assistance in dying (*Oregon v. Gonzales*, 2006). State legislatures are free to acknowledge the autonomy rights of state citizens with respect to end-of-life decision making.

Confidentiality refers to the right to control information about oneself that professionals possess and use. It includes access to the information, the opportunity to correct or expunge information, and the opportunity to determine who may have access to it other than the professionals to whom the information was given in the first place. Congress has recognized the privacy and confidentiality core concept by enacting the Family Education Rights and Privacy Act (FERPA, 1974). That law regulates who has access, and for what purposes, to a student's education records (infant and toddler through graduate school). IDEA specifically incorporates FERPA rights.

Integration

Although the core concepts of liberty, protection from harm, autonomy, and privacy and confidentiality reflect "negative rights" (rights against government interference), they do not explicitly announce any particular outcomes for people with mental retardation or related developmental disabilities. Other core concepts, however, are explicitly outcome driven, and principal among them is the core concept of integration. This concept recognizes that people with disabilities have been subjected to various types of segregation (as, for example, in institutions or in separate and traditionally inadequate special education schools, programs, or classes) and that although the core concepts of anti-discrimination and liberty will blunt unjustified confinement, they do not drive policy toward integration.

Accordingly, Congress has enacted several laws that favor integration over segregation. These laws proclaim that a person should be served in the least restrictive environment. IDEA provides that a student with a disability shall, to the maximum extent appropriate for the student, be educated with students who do not have disabilities and that that student may not be removed from such an education unless he or she cannot be educated there successfully even with related services and supplementary aids and services. The DD Act itself has the purpose of assisting states in developing services that are based in the community and that promote integration and inclusion in all facets of community life.

Arguably, the Social Security Act's Medicaid program (Title XIX) and its provisions related to home- and community-based services (HCBS) is the most important federal statute related to the core concept of integration. The reason is that it carries with it the greatest amount of funding to reimburse community-based health care providers for serving people with developmental disabilities in their communities.

Given that IDEA provides for integration in education, the DD Act authorizes a variety of state and local government activities that are community based, and the HCBS authority reimburses community-based health care services. Given the Supreme Court's decisions in the *O'Connor, Cleburne,* and *Olmstead* cases, it is clear that segregation is highly disfavored and that integration (sometimes called "inclusion") is highly favored.

Productivity and Contribution

Integration is a goal in and of itself; that is the reason that it is a separate core concept. But integration also is a means to an end, and that end is expressed in the core concept called productivity and contribution. As the DD Act makes clear, productivity (sometimes called "economic self-sufficiency") refers to engagement in income-producing work, and contribution refers to unpaid work that benefits a household or community.

The Vocational Rehabilitation Act (1974) authorizes state and local agencies to provide training and educational opportunities for people with disabilities. Among the most important of those opportunities for people with developmental disabilities are supported employment and community college or technical school training. The Ticket to Work and Work Incentives Improvement Act of 1999 advances the core concept of productivity and contribution by eliminating economic disincentives to work; those disincentives required a person to surrender some other benefits if his or her earned income exceeded certain limits.

Family Integrity and Unity

The family is the core unit of society, and so public policy presumes in favor of preserving and strengthening the families of people with disabilities. There are many reasons that policy seeks to preserve families' integrity and unity and to strengthen families to care for their members with disabilities. Among them are that children begin their lives in families; that families have legal and other duties to raise children, and families often provide care to adults with disabilities or assist others to do so; that family members often are the surrogate decision makers for or collaborators in making decisions with the member who has a disability; that families perform child-raising functions better and less expensively than state agencies do; and that families that are strong and self-determined usually produce adults with disabilities who also are strong and self-determined.

The DD Act itself contains a separate title (Title II) that authorizes the federal Administration on Developmental Disabilities to sponsor or to help states to sponsor family support programs. These programs consist of a variety of services that have the purpose of strengthening the family's role as a primary care provider, preventing inappropriate out-of-home placement of the member who has a developmental disability and thereby maintaining the family's unity, and reuniting families with members who have been placed out of their family homes. Further, the Adoption Assistance and Child Welfare Act (1980), as amended by the Adoption and Safe Families Act (1997), expresses the policy of family integrity and unity. Similarly, the Family and Medical Leave Act (1993) obliges employers to grant leave to their employees for medical reasons, including the birth of a child or to provide care to a child who has a serious health condition.

Further, the Supreme Court has long recognized that families have the rights to raise their children and make decisions about their care, custody, and control; its most recent cases, *Troxel v. Granville* (2000) and *Elk Grove Unified School District v. Newdow* (2004), simply restate the point (though they do not concern children with disabilities). In addition, the Court, in *Santosky v. Kramer* (1982), required state child welfare agencies to prove, by clear and convincing evidence, that a parent is abusive before a court may sever the parent–child bond. All of these decisions stand for the proposition that families have a due-process (liberty) right to raise their children and that family integrity and unity are valued as a means for implementing that right.

Family-Centered Services

The core concept of family-centered services acknowledges that when a family benefits, the member with a disability also benefits, and vice versa. It codifies the family systems theory: What happens to one member of a family affects all. To preserve families' integrity and keep them intact, services should be family centered.

Accordingly, the DD Act declares that family members can play an important role in enhancing the lives of their members with developmental disabilities if they have the necessary community services and other supports to do so. Although the DD Act does not explicitly authorize family-centered services, it is undoubtedly the case that the family support services that it does authorize do, indeed, provide for family-centered service delivery. Likewise, IDEA (particularly Part C, authorizing services for infants and toddlers and their families), and the Maternal and Child Health Act authorize federal funding of state and local programs that are family centered (sometimes called "family directed"). No court cases expressly advance this core concept.

Culturally Responsive Services

Just as family-centered services are a core concept and also a means to advancing another core concept, so too is the core concept that services should respond to the beliefs, values, interpersonal styles, attitudes, values, and cultural, ethnic, linguistic, and other socioeconomic traits of the person or family. Not surprisingly, the statutes that advance family-centered services also advance culturally responsive services. The DD Act itself provides that services funded under it must be culturally competent, and the federal Civil Rights Act of 1964 prohibits discrimination on the basis of race, color, or national origin.

Accountability

The core concept of accountability ensures that the foregoing concepts have real meaning in the lives of people with disabilities and their families. Among the accountability techniques are those embodied in IDEA and the Rehabilitation Act related to procedural safeguards (notice, consent, and joint decision making), administrative "due process" hearings and appeals to courts, recovery of attorneys' fees by the prevailing party in a lawsuit, programmatic monitoring and technical assistance, fiscal accountability by the local agencies to state agencies and by the state agencies to federal agencies, and provisions for participation by people with disabilities or their representatives on state or local policy-making boards and commissions.

In addition, the ADA and Section 504 of the Rehabilitation Act provide for recovery of money damages in the event that a covered entity violates the rights of a beneficiary, and both also authorize a court to issue an injunction requiring a covered entity to take or not take certain action consistent with the statute. Regrettably, the DD Act itself does not provide that an individual has a right to sue to enforce its broad policy statements and purposes (*Pennhurst*, 1977, 1981).

Among the most significant Supreme Court cases related to accountability is one that involved the parents of children with mental retardation. In *Parham v. J.R.* (1979), the Supreme Court held that a parent may not commit a minor child to a state institution and that the state may not admit the minor to the institution until a prior independent review of the appropriateness of the commitment has been conducted by an administrative tribunal or a court. The independent review is a means of ensuring accountability by the parents to the child and by the state to the parents and, especially, to the child.

Personal and Professional and System Capacity Development

This core concept seeks to develop the capacity of the person with a disability and the person's family. The core concepts of anti-discrimination, individual and appropriate services, coordination and collaboration, integration, productivity and contribution, family unity and integrity, and family-centered services are all designed to increase the capacity of the person and family to function in today's world.

But if a service system itself is not able to deliver appropriate services in the most integrated setting, those core concepts will have little effect. That is the reason that this core concept also focuses on the service systems and the development of a sufficient number of properly trained professionals to carry out the other core concepts and the various federal laws that authorize federal, state, and local government activities. For example, the DD Act authorizes university-based centers of excellence in research and training and state planning councils. The centers and councils assist in developing state and local capacity to carry out the DD Act. Similarly, Part D of IDEA authorizes personnel development, technical assistance, research and development, and various state and local education agency improvement activities.

Prevention

Finally, public policy seeks to prevent disabilities in three ways. Primary prevention, such as by fetal surgery, seeks to "cure" or prevent a disability before it occurs but after diagnosis signals that a disability might occur. Secondary prevention seeks to eliminate a condition that is known to cause disability; phenylketonuria (PKU) screening and treatment just after a baby is born exemplifies this kind of prevention. Finally, vocational rehabilitation and special education are forms of tertiary prevention because they seek to mitigate the effects of a disability.

THE CORE CONCEPTS: A 5-YEAR PROSPECTIVE VIEW OF POLICY

When we wrote that we would not use a time-line approach to describing policy, we justified our decision by arguing that, whereas some core concepts and rights are expanding, others are shrinking. We did not explain our argument out of consideration for the length of this chapter. But the fact that the Supreme Court expands personal rights, such as the right and core concept of autonomy, while simultaneously limiting the scope of ADA in employment cases and undercutting the core concept of anti-discrimination, makes the case for us (Stowe et al., 2006). And the fact that Congress in 2004 tightened up IDEA with respect to the core concept of accountability, making it more difficult than before for students to hold state and local agencies accountable for their actions while also imposing new accountability standards and procedures on federal, state, and local education agencies, also makes our case (Turnbull, Stowe, & Huerta, 2007).

Further, issues that were, at best, only dimly perceived during the past 35 years now have become hot issues. Although it is true, for example, that the core concepts of protection from harm and autonomy intersected in the *Cruzan* case (involving the state's interest in preserving life and a family's right to decide when a comatose member would have wanted to withdraw life-sustaining supports), few people then could have foreseen the Terri Schiavo case (*In re Guardianship of Schiavo,* 2003) and the policy debates that it has sparked.

Likewise, although the core concept of prevention could easily subsume such interventions as fetal surgery, PKU evaluations and treatment, and outcome-based special education and vocational rehabilitation services, it is only recently that the Human Genome Project has resulted in the identification and mapping of the entire human genome DNA. And it is only recently that brain research has begun to reveal how developmental delays are linked to neurological and protein-based factors.

Further, the development of such interventions as positive behavioral support and services, the use of universally designed facilities and curricula, the development of off-the-shelf assistive technologies that require little if any adaptations for people with developmental disabilities, and the insistence on outcome-based policies and measurable results in education (under IDEA and the NCLB) and in other federal services (under the Government Performance and Results Act) are transforming how professionals deliver services and how policy makers craft laws.

Moreover, the now-ascendant neoconservatism and now-descendant traditional liberalism have dramatically changed the ways in which policy makers and the public look at disability policy. Whereas the rights and entitlement perspective was once dominant under the liberal/liberating theories of the 1970s through the early 1990s, there is now a repeated insistence, in policy, on personal responsibilities and system-based accountability. The NCLB (2002) and the IDEA amendments of 2004 exemplify those changes and simply mirror the welfare law changes that Congress enacted in 1996 through the Personal Responsibilities and Work Opportunity Reform Act (Turnbull, 2005, 2006).

Finally, our country's economic condition has changed dramatically during the past decade. It has become globalized and thus dependent on world and regional economic conditions to a much greater degree than ever before. Tax and fiscal policies have contributed to significant federal and state budget deficits, and other economic policies have contributed to ever-escalating trade deficits. Our economic future is much less subject to our own control than ever before.

All of these changes make it extremely hazardous to project the future of public policy affecting individuals with developmental disabilities. What seems clear, however, is that each of these developments will cause changes in policy and that our ability to understand the changes will be better if we have a framework within which to accommodate them.

That is the ultimate value of the core-concepts approach we have described here. The core concepts have been part of the disability rights movement from the very beginning in the early 1970s. Many of them are fundamental in all policies that affect all people. Anti-discrimination emanated from the Supreme Court's interpretation of the 14th Amendment's equal-protection clause in the 1954 school desegregation decision, *Brown v. Board of Education* (1954). Liberty, autonomy, and protection from harm are constitutional doctrines established long ago, before any rights revolutions based on traits such as race, sex, or disability. Family integrity is fundamental because, in our country, families are the core unit of society. Accountability is also an anciently established doctrine and is embodied in the Bill of Rights (1st through 10th Amendments) and in the 14th Amendment, a post–Civil War amendment.

CONCLUSION

In this chapter, we described the 18 core concepts of disability policy and their sources, and we organized them into a taxonomy (Figure 2.1). We have not tried to predict how various factors will affect disability policy, although we have noted the most obvious recent ones. Instead, we have presented two frameworks that help students and analysts sort and classify changes in policy according to the core concepts and the taxonomy. Without frameworks, understanding of policy often is scant; with them, understanding and influence in policy arenas often is powerful. Knowledge, after all, is power.

REFERENCES

Stowe, M. J., Turnbull, H. R., & Sublet, C. (2006). The Supreme Court, "Our Town," and disability policy: Boardrooms and bedrooms, courtrooms and cloakrooms. *Mental Retardation, 44*(2), 83–99.

Turnbull, H. R. (2005). Individuals with Disabilities Education Act Reauthorization: Accountability and personal responsibility. *Remedial and Special Education, 26*(6), 320–326.

Turnbull, H. R. (2006). A response to Professor Vitello. *Remedial and Special Education, 27*(6), 69–71.

Turnbull, H. R., Beegle, G., & Stowe, M. S. (2001). The core concepts of disability policy affecting families who have children with disabilities. *Journal of Disability Policy Studies, 12*(3), 133–143.

Turnbull, H. R., & Stowe, M. J. (2001). A taxonomy for organizing the core concepts according to their underlying principles. *Journal of Disability Policy Studies, 23*(3), 177–197.

Turnbull, H. R., Stowe, M. J., & Huerta, N. E. (2007). *Free appropriate public education* (7th ed.). Denver: Love.

STATUTES CITED

Adoption Assistance and Child Welfare Act, 42 U.S.C. 620 (1980), amended by the Adoption and Safe Families Act, Public Law 105-89, 42 U.S.C. § 629 (1997).

Americans With Disabilities Act of 1990, 42 U.S.C.A. § 12101 *et seq.*

Child Abuse Prevention and Treatment Act, 42 U.S.C. § 5101, *et seq.* 45 C.F.R. § 1340.1 *et seq.* (2003).

Children's Health Act, U.S.C. § 290ii (2000).

Children's Mental Health Act, 42 U.S.C. § 290ff and 290jj (2000).

Civil Rights Act of 1964, 42 U.S.C. § 1971; of 1991, 42 U.S.C. § 1981 (1964).

Developmental Disabilities and Bill of Rights Act, 42 U.S.C. § 15001, *et seq.* (2000).

Education of All Handicapped Children Act, Public Law 94-142; Individuals with Disabilities Education Act, 20 U.S.C. § 1400, *et seq.* (2004).

Family and Medical Leave Act, 29 U.S.C. § 2601 (1993).

Family Educational Rights and Privacy Act, 20 U.S.C. § 1232g (1974).

Health and Human Services Policy for Protection of Human Research Subjects, 45 C.F.R., Part 46 (2005).

Home and Community-Based Services Amendments to Medicaid, Sec. 1915 of the Social Security Act, 42 U.S.C. 1396n (1987).

Maternal and Child Health Act, 42 U.S.C. § 701, *et seq.* (2000).

No Child Left Behind, Public Law 107-110 (2002).

Technology-Related Assistance for Individuals with Disabilities Act, 129 U.S.C. § 3001 (2000).

Ticket to Work and Work Incentives Improvement Act of 1999, 42 U.S.C. § 1320b-19 (1999).

Title XIX of the Social Security Act, Medicaid, 42 U.S.C. § 1396 (1981).

Vocational Rehabilitation Act, 29 U.S.C. § 794, Sec. 504 (1974).

3

Disability Research Methodology
Current Issues and Future Challenges

Zolinda Stoneman

For over a century, researchers have been working to understand disability and effective practices for supporting individuals with disabilities. The American Association on Intellectual and Developmental Disability, established in 1876, provided the first forum for researchers to discuss disability issues and to foster the development of services (Scheerenberger, 1983). In 1906, Henry Herbert Goddard developed the first research program exclusively for the study of people with intellectual disabilities at New Jersey's Vineland Training School (Scheerenberger, 1983). Although disability research has a rich history, methodological issues continue to challenge the research community. This chapter highlights some of these issues. The chapter begins with a discussion of research participants, followed by decisions concerning research settings, data collection methods and instrumentation, and research design. The final sections examine social influences on disability research methods and questions that research can and cannot answer.

SELECTION OF RESEARCH PARTICIPANTS
The Importance of Definitions: Who Are People with Developmental Disabilities?

One of the first tasks that disability researchers face is to define the group of people selected for study. This volume focuses on people with developmental disabilities. The term "developmental disability" was introduced in the Developmental Disabilities Services and Facilities Construction Amendments of 1970 (DD Act, Public Law 91-517). As used in this act, the term was defined as referring to mental retardation, cerebral palsy, epilepsy, and other neurological conditions. In subsequent reauthorizations, a functional definition evolved, focusing on the inability of an individual to perform certain activities. The 2000 DD Act (Public Law 106-402) defined "developmental disability" as a severe, chronic disability, attributable to a mental or physical impairment, manifesting before age 22, likely to continue indefinitely, and resulting from limitations in three of seven life activities: self-care, language, learning, mobility, self-direction, capacity for independent living, and economic self-sufficiency. The definition for young children focuses on the existence of, or conditions with a high probability of resulting in, a developmental delay.

As researchers attempt to use this federal definition, it becomes clear that major components are fraught with ambiguity. For example, no consensus exists on how substantial a functional limitation must be in order to trigger the definition. There are few instruments to measure key constructs such as capacity for economic self-sufficiency. An individual who experiences a brain injury at age 21 has a developmental disability; a person who sustains a similar injury at age 22 does not. There is no theoretical or empirically derived rationale for believing that this 1-year time span is scientifically meaningful. The "childhood" definition of "developmental disability" is not scientifically useful without further operationalization of key terms.

In the face of scientific pitfalls in the functional definition, most researchers have chosen to fall back on defining "developmental disability" in terms of diagnostic conditions. Unfortunately, this approach is also imprecise. Intellectual disability provides an illustrative example. People with intellectual disabilities compose the largest group considered to have developmental disabilities (Larson et al., 2000). In 1989, Landesman and Ramey wrote, "What is well accepted within the field of mental retardation, but often viewed as surprising to those outside it, is that mental retardation is an arbitrarily defined diagnostic category, which has changed frequently and substantively over the years . . . practices used to identify children with mental retardation vary dramatically across states and school districts" (p. 409). Intelligence and adaptive behavior exist along a continuum; the point at which these capabilities are low enough to be considered as an intellectual disability is subjective and inconsistent across time and settings (Fujiura, 2003).

Prevalence studies using the same national data set define disability differently, use different clusters of questions, and therefore yield discrepant estimates (Bernell, 2003). Questions on data sets such as the National Health Interview Survey (NHIS) change over time, creating variations in prevalence estimates (i.e., Hendershot, Larson, Lakin, & Doljanac, 2005). Using a functional definition, estimates drawn from the 1994 Disability Supplement to the NHIS found that 1.18% of the noninstitutionalized adult population had a developmental disability (Larson et al., 2000). More recent, shorter versions of the NHIS-D produced smaller estimates (Hendershot et al., 2005). Researchers from the Centers for Disease Control and Prevention (CDC) estimated developmental disability prevalence by tracking five conditions: intellectual disability, autism, cerebral palsy, hearing loss, and vision impairment (Bhasin, Brocksen, Avchen, & Braun, 2006). CDC estimates include mild disabilities not usually included in estimates based on a functional definition. Definitional problems caused Fujiura (2003) to conclude that the search for the *true* number of persons with developmental disabilities is a largely futile effort.

In addition to affecting prevalence estimates, definitional issues affect research in other ways. There is the very real possibility that failure to replicate findings across studies occurs because researchers use similar terms to describe participants with different characteristics. Many researchers draw participants from schools or service systems. Eligibility criteria vary across states and districts and even across programs in the same community (Bernell, 2003). This situation can result in the selection of research participants who are quite different depending on the geographic location of the study and the services being utilized. In addition, there are concerns related to methodologies that rely on the reports of family members or on self-identification to determine disability status. Accuracy of these data is questionable (Bernell, 2003). Few researchers have the resources to independently validate the diagnoses of study participants, although this would be ideal.

International differences in terminology are another important caveat (Fernald, 1995). The British, for example, use the term "learning disability" to describe below-average intelligence. "Learning disability" has a different meaning in the United States. There is an international move to replace the term "mental retardation" with "intellectual disability." It is important that researchers agree on terminology for use in the scientific study of disability so that meaningful comparisons across and within different countries are possible.

Etiology-Specific Research

In 1969, Ellis wrote, "I have faith that ultimately, with refined techniques, a physiological basis for all behavioral deviation may be found" (p. 560). Each year, the field comes closer to Ellis's vision. Biomedical research has resulted in identification of a myriad of new syndromes and conditions. With the Human Genome Project, discovery of previously unidentified syndromes can be expected to accelerate. For decades, researchers were influenced by the work of Stein and Jessop (1982) and others who proposed a noncategorical approach to understanding the effects of disability. This model was based on the belief that individuals with different disabilities and their families face similar life experiences because of generic characteristics that exist across syndromes and conditions. Hodapp and Dykens (2004) refute that approach, arguing that etiology groups are associated with specific patterns of skills and behaviors and should be studied individually. They describe a *quiet revolution* in which associations between genetic syndromes and behavior are influencing research methods and the selection of participants.

Identifying the optimal level of inquiry is an ongoing challenge. The ideal approach is to follow the guidance of the theory sponsoring the research. In the absence of theory, Burack, Hodapp, and Zigler (1988) suggested a bottom-up strategy in which researchers start at a more differentiated level and then combine groups if no etiological differences are found. This approach allows the researcher to examine processes and outcomes that are specific to a certain etiology, such as Down syndrome or autism, as well as those that occur across disabilities.

Availability of People to Study

A mundane but powerful force guiding research inquiry is the ability of researchers to find people to study. The most sophisticated research methodology is useless if the researcher is not able to identify and recruit members of the population of interest. Disability research has historically relied on small samples. Cheng and Powell (2005) noted that researchers interested in low-incidence populations are often required to answer questions using the best data that they have while being wary of distortions and lack of power that result from small samples.

Ironically, positive societal advances in creating inclusive schools, workplaces, and communities have made the researcher's task more difficult. Recruiting participants was easier when people with disabilities were grouped together. Warren, Brady, and Fey (2004) noted that research is more expensive now that potential participants must be reached in their homes or schools rather than in centralized settings. They suggest that one reason for the small number of studies focusing on certain questions may be the inability of researchers to recruit sufficiently large samples to ask these questions.

Another challenge is the frequent necessity of recruiting research participants through "gatekeepers," who often have little commitment to the study and face numerous competing demands (Becker, Roberts, Morrison, & Silver, 2004). Due to the confidential nature of services, researchers operating outside of the service system usually do not have direct access to these individuals or to their families. The researcher must convince an intermediary party (or, usually, many intermediary parties) of the importance of the research and motivate that person to recruit participants or, at minimum, to distribute information to potential participants. Although this practice is often unavoidable, it does introduce bias. Magaña (2000) noted that using gatekeepers is particularly problematic when it comes to recruiting minorities. Our experience has been that intermediaries often screen families and inform only those families whom they consider to be *good* participants who are likely to agree to take part in the research. We have found that families headed by single parents, low-income families, minority families, and families not actively involved with the service agency are less likely to be informed about the opportunity to participate in research.

Other methodological biases occur because of the population from which participants are recruited. When researchers recruit from the service system, individuals and families who are not receiving services are excluded. Participants recruited from advocacy groups tend to be more involved, savvy, and motivated. Snowball sampling can include people who are not receiving services, but it underrepresents those without extensive social networks. There is no perfect solution to recruitment dilemmas. The best that researchers can do is to be conscious of the compromises that have been made and communicate potential biases when disseminating research findings.

The Dominance of Comparison-Group Studies

In 1967, Baumeister noted that the typical research study of the day compared the performances of individuals with and without intellectual disabilities on a standard task. Not surprisingly, individuals with disabilities learned more slowly and performed less well. A classic series of articles in the late 1960s and early 1970s provides the clearest discussion of the use of comparison groups in disability research (i.e., Baumeister, 1967; Ellis, 1969; Heal, 1970). A decade later, Haywood (1976) called for a moratorium on these studies, arguing that they wasted effort by asking such questions as "Do poor learners learn poorly?" (p. 315). However, eliminating comparison groups is not a panacea. Early research on families of individuals with disabilities often lacked comparison groups (Stoneman, 1989). In essence, families were compared with the researcher's vision of an "ideal" family. Shortcomings or deviations from the researcher's subjective ideal were attributed to the disability of a family member.

The use of comparison groups in disability research suffers from the fallacies that have plagued research on ethnic and racial minorities. There is an unfortunate history of European American researchers labeling other groups as being deficient when they were found to differ from white, middle-class norms. These researchers incorrectly interpreted differences as being deficits. They also succumbed to another flaw—attributing group differences to the factor being studied even though the groups also differed on numerous other characteristics. In classic experimental design, the aim is to hold all factors constant except the variable(s) under study so that confounds and alternate explanations are minimized. Unfortunately, in disability research, groups have almost always differed on variables other than disability status. Group differences, when found, have usually been attributed solely to disability (Stoneman, 1989).

Some of the most difficult groups to equate on demographic characteristics are those that compare groups of people with different disabilities. When a group with one disability is compared with the general population, it is plausible that the population is sufficiently large and diverse that an appropriate comparison group can be identified. Equating two or more low-incidence groups is substantially more difficult. For example, frequently implemented comparisons, such as between Down syndrome and autism, often result in groups that are dissimilar on gender (individuals with autism are more likely to be male) and maternal age (mothers of children with Down syndrome tend to be older). Comparing children with Down syndrome and a heterogeneous group of children with intellectual disabilities almost always yields groups that differ on socioeconomic status (SES). Heal (1970) stressed the importance of using statistical controls, in addition to sampling controls. Most often, groups differ on multiple factors, making statistical controls difficult to use.

There are two ways to address these problems: Either develop more careful comparison studies or use other research methods. Some research questions are best addressed by comparison-group designs. These designs, however, are probably overused. Many of the most interesting questions involve the examination of within-group processes and outcomes.

RESEARCH SETTINGS

Historical Influences

Until relatively recently, most researchers worked in institutional and other congregate settings. In the United States, institutions for people with disabilities and mental illness date from 1773 (Scheerenberger, 1983). The first institutions were designed to provide education, primarily for children. By the late 1800s, the institution had developed into what Scheerenberger described as a "large, overpopulated, underfinanced multipurpose facility that would typify institutions for generations to come" (p. 123). For many years, the demands and constraints of institutional environments defined the research agenda. As public education for children with disabilities became more available, researchers shifted to conducting research in schools. By the 1980s, institutions were being downsized or closed, and researchers examined effects of community living on former residents (i.e., Larson & Lakin, 1989). More recently, as community inclusion has grown, researchers have broadened their research settings to include family homes, the workplace, child care centers, and other community locations (Nisbet, 1992).

Researchers have frequently compared settings. Comparisons across physical settings (self-contained vs. inclusive class, etc.) are compromised by many of the same issues as other comparison research. Unless individuals are randomly assigned to settings, participants in different settings usually differ from each other in important ways. Bronfenbrenner (1979) referred to cross-setting research as taking a *social address* perspective on understanding environments and recommended an alternative approach: examining important processes as they operate within different environments.

Conducting Research in Laboratory versus Naturalistic Settings

House, in 1977, made an elegant argument for collecting data in laboratory settings, noting that in everyday settings a myriad of irrelevant factors can influence research findings. This position began to be questioned as researchers noted the limited generalizability of laboratory findings. Disability research was influenced by the work of Bronfenbrenner, reflected in the publication of *The Ecology of Human Development* in 1979. Bronfenbrenner described existing laboratory research as "the science of the strange behavior of children in strange situations with strange adults for the briefest possible periods of time" (p. 19). He argued for conducting research in natural settings, using variations across individuals, families, and settings as the focus for understanding complex interactions between behavior and context.

Most disability researchers now work in naturalistic settings. The work is difficult. Smylie and Kahne (1997) described classrooms as "a swarming dynamic system of interrelated phenomena" (p. 363). Tracking the numerous influences on behavior present in a single setting is a Herculean task, intensified by the involvement of most individuals in multiple settings. Koroloff and Friesen (1997) challenged researchers to "find ways to identify and track all services that the family receives, both formal and informal, and weigh the contributions of each to outcomes" (p. 135). This seems ideal, but creating methodologies that accomplish this goal will require going far beyond current practices. There is still much that we do not know about how to conduct research amid the ongoing stream of everyday life (Berliner, 2002).

DATA COLLECTION METHODS AND INSTRUMENTS
In the Eye of the Beholder

The disability researcher uses numerous sources of information. An initial question to be answered is whether to obtain data by observing people or by asking questions of participants (or both). Olson (1977) noted that observation and self-report methods "tap different aspects of reality" (p. 127). He argued that both methods are valid and important, although they often yield discrepant data. Observation is often considered to be the more objective method, less influenced by the biases and subjective perceptions of individuals. Observation allows examination of contextual variations and identification of processes not understood by participants in the setting. With individuals with limited language, observation can reveal information that the person is unable to directly communicate. It is important to remember, however, that observations, even extensive observations across time, are only samples of behavior. Observational methods have limitations. Behaviors observed may or may not reflect behaviors not observed. Low-frequency behaviors are difficult to observe, although they may have a dramatic impact. Quantifying interactions in social groups larger than dyads is complex. The presence of observers or of a video camera can distort behavior, depressing occurrence of certain behaviors and escalating others.

For certain research questions, the subjective perceptions of research participants are the focus of study, rather than a method bias to be overcome. Questionnaires or interviews offer a window into subjective reality that is unobtainable through observation. As with all research methods, self-reports have limitations. Self-reports often require the respondent to generalize across contexts or to compare their experiences with those of "average" individuals, which can be difficult. Mood states, stress, and fatigue can influence responses. Multiple questionnaires completed by the same person tend to be correlated, producing spurious findings.

Finlay and Lyons (2001) reviewed research examining the self-report responses of individuals with intellectual disabilities. Challenges in obtaining valid data include acquiescence (i.e., the tendency to say yes to questions regardless of their content) and other response biases, problems in understanding multiple-choice and Likert-type questions, and questions about what usually happens or about general feelings. They note that limited life experiences also can skew responses. Interviewers working with individuals with intellectual disabilities often paraphrase questions in order to increase understandability and prompt a response (Finlay & Lyons, 2001). The effects of these alterations in interview protocol are unknown.

The challenges of obtaining research information from people with intellectual disabilities has often led to the use of proxy respondents, people who know the target person well and can provide information about his or her life. Subjective self-ratings and ratings made by outside observers often do not agree, however (Olson, 1977). Perry and Felce (2002) found low agreement on a quality-of-life measure between proxy responses and first-person responses of people with intellectual disabilities. Olson suggested behavioral self-report data (i.e., asking questions about observable behavior) as a way to increase agreement. Consistent with this premise, Perry and Felce (2002) found that agreement between people with disabilities and their proxies was higher when the measure was more objective and observable. The limited communication skills of many individuals leave the researcher no choice but to rely on the reports of those who know the person. It is important that researchers carefully consider the possible biases of designated informants.

Advances in Measurement: Moving Away from the Lamppost

Like the proverbial intoxicated man looking for his keys under the lamppost because that is where the light is, we as researchers study what we can measure, even if it is not what we really want to study. Scientific inquiry can advance only as far as scientific measurement allows. "Thus, before a scientific analysis can discover what caused what, it must define and measure both of the *whats*" (Holburn, 2002, p. 255). New tools have been developed, including the Family Quality of Life Scale (Summers et al., 2005) and the Supports Intensity Scale (Thompson et al., 2004). However, many important constructs have not yet yielded to empirical assessment.

As early as the 1970s, scholars called for research on interactions between disability and the environmental contexts in which behavior occurs (Brooks & Baumeister, 1977; Haywood, 1976). More recently, social construction theorists have stressed the role of the environment in creating disability (Gross & Hahn, 2004). Limitations in our ability to assess environments are holding back research on person–setting interactions (Baumeister, 1997; Carr, Innis, Blakeley-Smith, & Vasdev, 2004; Gross & Hahn, 2004; Stancliffe, Emerson, & Lakin, 2004). Friendship and social connectedness are important outcomes for children and adults with disabilities. A few scales exist to measure these constructs, but more work is needed (Kennedy, 2004). Koroloff and Friesen (1997) noted that many important outcomes of family-centered interventions have yet to be successfully measured.

A debate exists about the ability and advisability of quantifying certain constructs, such as the processes and outcomes of person-centered planning (Holburn, 2002; O'Brien, 2002). In the past, researchers have evaluated complex interventions using narrow instruments that clearly were not up to the task (e.g., using increases in children's IQ scores as the singular outcome of early intervention). Is it possible to quantify all outcomes that are important? At present, the answer is clearly no. In the future, creative approaches that combine qualitative and quantitative inquiry hold promise (Johnson & Onwuegbuzie, 2004), but we will never reach the point at which it is possible, or preferable, to reduce all human dimensions to quantifiable data.

Cultural Considerations: Going Beyond Language Translation

Weisner (1993) posed an important question: "What is the single most important thing to know about a child with a disability and his or her siblings in order to understand the course of their lives together?" (p. 51). His answer was their *cultural place*: shared beliefs, practices, values, and physical settings. In the United States, minorities are overrepresented among people with disabilities. "Disability, poverty, and minority status are linked" (Fujiura & Yamaki, 1997, p. 293). Yet most disability research has focused on white, middle-class individuals and families.

Conducting research in a culturally competent fashion requires more than just translating questionnaires. Magaña (2000) cautions that using instruments and procedures developed for the majority culture may bias results. Response items can have different meanings across cultures. Culture is constantly changing, and it does not influence each individual or family in the same way; all members of a culture do not subscribe to the same values or beliefs. Magaña argues for the importance of within-group analyses rather than comparisons with a mainstream sample. The latter carry the risk of equating difference with dysfunction. These issues highlight the importance of involving the community in the conceptualization and interpretation of research.

The Emerging Discipline of Disability Studies: Power, Oppression, and Finding a Voice

The emergence of disability studies as a scholarly discipline is having a strong effect on disability research methodology. Following in the traditions of feminist and minority studies, research inspired by a disability-studies perspective examines the life experiences of people with disabilities with a focus on power, oppression, exclusion, and civil rights. In traditional research, the researcher sets the agenda, and participants are disengaged from the research process. Disability-studies scholars assert that people with disabilities should be considered experts on their own lives and call for researchers to create nonhierarchical relationships between researchers and research participants (Davis, 2000; Lloyd, Preston-Shoot, Temple, & Wuu, 1996; Sample, 1996). These scholars recommend that researchers take a participatory action research (PAR) approach, involving people with disabilities in defining the research question, devising the research strategy, analyzing data, and interpreting and disseminating results.

Booth and Booth (1996) describe the *storytelling movement*, in which personal narratives and life histories are used to understand life experiences. They stress the importance of listening to individuals with intellectual disabilities, whose stories have been overlooked in the research literature. Dennis (2002) cautioned that it is easier to call for inclusion of people with substantial disabilities in research than it is to successfully collect research information from these individuals. Social isolation, learned compliance, memory problems, and social oppression affect responses (Booth & Booth, 1996). When individuals are unable to produce detailed life narratives, researchers may feel pressed to fill in the gaps by emphasizing their own beliefs and biases (Goodley, 1996). To collect meaningful information, researchers must be willing to spend substantial time getting to know the person and learning to communicate (Booth & Booth, 1996).

RESEARCH DESIGN: ARE WE MAKING A DIFFERENCE?

Macrosystem and Policy Research Methods: Asking the Big Questions

Bronfenbrenner (1979) argued for the importance of studying macrosystem effects, such as changes brought about by fundamental societal shifts. He posited that these changes result in alterations in all levels of the social system, filtering down to the individual. In the past decades, there have been massive macrosystem changes relating to people with disabilities. For example, Public Law 94-142, the Education for All Handicapped Children Act of 1975, mandated that all children with disabilities were entitled to an appropriate, free public education. In 1986, Public Law 99-457, Part H, provided incentives for states to serve children from birth through age 2. Section 504 of the Rehabilitation Act of 1973, followed by the Americans with Disabilities Act (ADA) of 1990, protected individuals with disabilities against discrimination in work, school, transportation, and other settings. In *Olmstead v. L.C., & E.W.* (119 S.Ct. 2176, 1999), the U.S. Supreme Court decided that unnecessary segregation and institutionalization constitute discrimination against people with disabilities and violate the ADA. Also, medical advances have extended the lifespan of people with disabilities, and the Human Genome Project is identifying the functions of human genes.

Parmenter (2004) called for disability researchers to focus more on macrolevel systems. Unfortunately, research methodologies are often not up to the task of tackling these important questions. Answering straightforward questions, such as how many people with disabilities are employed or what proportion of eligible families are enrolled in early intervention services, is very difficult. Estimates derived from different data sources often do not agree (Silverstein, Julnes, & Nolan, 2005). One of the most ambitious and continuous efforts of macrosystem benchmarking is the work of Braddock and colleagues, who have recently completed the eighth nationwide survey of state services and funding for individuals with developmental disabilities (Braddock et al., 2005). These efforts, representing 25 years of data collection, allow state-by-state examination of the effects of important societal events, such as the U.S. Supreme Court's Olmstead decision. Although data are affected by state differences in eligibility definitions, as well as by imprecision and inconsistencies in state data collection practices, the information allows an unparalleled examination of national trends across multiple years.

Attempting to draw conclusions about processes linking macrosystem shifts to resulting effects on people with disabilities highlights macrolevel research complexities. For example, there is clear evidence that moving to the community from an institution has positive outcomes for people with disabilities and their families (Stancliffe et al.,

2004). In the United States, community residential support is more cost-effective (Lakin & Stancliffe, 2005). The Olmstead decision declared unnecessary institutionalization to be a violation of civil rights. Why are so many individuals still living in institutions? Why do families protest institutional closings? In the United States, nine states have successfully eliminated institutions. What is different about these states? How did they develop the will to close institutions? These questions hold the key to improved quality of life for persons with disabilities, but so far they have escaped empirically based explanations.

Although clear data support the effectiveness of exemplary early-intervention programs in achieving positive outcomes for children and families, we know little about the results of interventions as they are implemented on a national scale (Harbin, Rous, & McLean, 2005). State variations in service delivery and differences in eligibility provide natural experiments with which to examine early intervention effectiveness (Harbin et al., 2005). As federal and state governments demand increased accountability, researchers, such as those involved with the Early Childhood Outcomes Center, are beginning to tackle these complex issues and to define nationally relevant outcomes for children and families receiving early intervention services (Hebbeler, 2005).

Outcome indicators for adults with developmental disabilities have also been developed. The Council on Quality and Leadership in Supports for People with Disabilities has designed the Personal Outcome Measure to evaluate adult services using a defined set of individualized outcomes (Gardner & Carran, 2005). Their database of more than 3,600 interviews is allowing examination of relationships between outcomes and individual and programmatic variables. More recently, the Core Indicators Project has developed a set of outcomes for services delivered to people with developmental disabilities. Adopted by 25 states, this measure allows states to benchmark their progress over time (Human Services Research Institute, 2005).

Evaluation Research and Evidence-Based Practice

The passage of the federal No Child Left Behind Act of 2001, which requires that schools use practices that have been demonstrated to be effective by rigorous scientific research, has stimulated a national debate on criteria for deeming a practice to be scientifically validated (i.e., Odom et al., 2005; Yell, Drasgow, & Lowrey, 2005). Numerous authors have noted that there are no clear, widely accepted criteria for determining which research evidence is of high enough quality to guide service delivery (i.e., National Center for the Dissemination of Disability Research, 2005; Odom et al., 2005; Silverstein et al., 2005).

The National Center for the Dissemination of Disability Research (2005) differentiates between *research* and *evidence*. A body of research informs evidence-based practice. The important factors are research quality and the quality of synthesis across studies. Meta-analysis, which analyzes effect-size values across studies, is often used to synthesize knowledge in a specific area. As Weisz, Sandler, Durlak, and Anton (2005) note, effect sizes are not always ideal metrics. Small effect sizes may hold major importance if they address a significant or prevalent issue. In the introductory article to a special issue of *Exceptional Children* focusing on quality indicators in special education research, Odom et al. (2005) move the debate forward by providing an informed discussion of key issues involved in research synthesis and in identifying evidence-based practices. Other articles in this issue provide quality indicators for experimental, quasi-experimental, single-subject, correlational, and qualitative research designs.

Recent federal funding priorities, in part stimulated by the No Child Left Behind Act, have set in motion funding preferences for randomized clinical trials (RCT), which have long been accepted by many disciplines as the gold standard of evaluation research. As with any research design, clinical trials have both strengths and limitations (Silverstein et al., 2005). Low-incidence populations are difficult to randomize. RCT disability research usually must span multiple states and intervention sites, making these studies very expensive. For this and other reasons, disability researchers usually have selected other designs. Quasi-experimental designs are probably the most common. Unfortunately, these designs are vulnerable to confounds. Individuals self-select into certain interventions. Programs prioritize some potential recipients over others. Individuals on waiting lists differ from those receiving services. The list of potential confounds seems almost endless; these biases cannot be remedied by equating groups on sex, age, or similar variables.

One of the most elegant and frequently overlooked intervention designs is single-subject research. These strategies use precise operational definitions combined with tightly controlled intervention and data collection techniques to conduct experiments that allow inferences about causal relationships. Single-subject research is usually conducted in natural environments and provides opportunities to examine intervention effectiveness across settings and persons and to track multiple outcomes (Carr et al., 2004). Single-subject researchers have demonstrated leadership in examining the effects of multicomponent interventions (Carr et al., 2004). Horner et al. (2005) provide guidelines for identifying quality single-subject studies.

Determining and defining desired outcomes for a practice or intervention is an often-overlooked problem. Some intervention research focuses on narrowly defined outcomes, such as the increase or decrease of a certain behavior or learning a specific skill. Other interventions target broad outcomes, such as improved quality of life or success in an inclusive classroom. An important question for the researcher to ask is whether the targeted outcome would make a meaningful difference if it were successfully achieved. In the past, countless hours were devoted to using sophisticated task analyses and educational strategies to teach children with disabilities to tie shoelaces. A few strips of Velcro have replaced all of this research and programmatic effort. The interventions were effective, the designs were elegant, but the outcome was trivial.

Many evaluators ask recipients to rate their satisfaction with services. Across studies, individuals with and without disabilities report high satisfaction with the services they receive, but that satisfaction often is not related to objective measures of service quality (Stancliffe et al., 2004). Koroloff and Friesen (1997) question what it means when outcomes and satisfaction are discrepant. They provide an example of parents who are highly satisfied with an intervention that produces no objectively measured changes in child or family outcomes. Terminating a program with high customer satisfaction that has not produced important objective outcomes can result in a strong outcry from program recipients. Also, satisfaction ratings of families often differ from those of individuals with disabilities; ratings of different audiences are not interchangeable and should be examined separately (Stancliffe et al., 2004).

Effectiveness cannot be understood by simply analyzing outcome differences between those who do and those who do not receive an intervention. To truly understand intervention effects, it is necessary to examine the processes of change. Through what mechanisms or pathways are the outcomes achieved? Numerous authors (i.e., Carr et al., 2004; Warren et al., 2004) have noted the importance of longitudinal designs that track intervention effects across time. In addition, certain factors serve as moderators, changing the nature of intervention outcomes when they are present. For example, research on syndrome-specific interventions holds promise (Dykens & Hodapp, 2001). There are cultural differences in whether or not an intervention is accepted and effective. Ceci and Papierno (2005) express caution about a frequently occurring multiplier effect. When all children receive an intervention, higher functioning children tend to benefit more than lower functioning children; performance gaps actually increase. These more sophisticated evaluation questions are usually asked within the group of participants receiving the intervention, often through structural modeling techniques, rather than solely by making comparisons across groups.

Individualization of Interventions and Research Methods

Current intervention models emphasize individualization of strategies and outcomes. For example, person-centered planning approaches work with individuals to identify their desired futures and to develop strategies to support the person in moving toward those desired outcomes. Family support programs identify families' priority needs and then plan together to address those needs. Strategies and outcomes are often changed or refined over time (Koroloff & Friesen, 1997). Some interventions are designed to be easy to test experimentally (DeAngelis, 2005). Others rely on the ability to choose and tailor treatments to an individual's changing situation.

How can researchers examine effectiveness of an intervention when no two individuals receive the same intervention? Individualized approaches conflict with the researcher's desire for the clear operationalization of a standard set of intervention procedures, for outcome measurement using psychometrically sound instruments, and for minimal intervention *drift* over time (Holburn, 2002; Koroloff & Friesen, 1997). The challenge is "to find or develop standardized measures that allow for generalizability of the results and at the same time to adopt some measures that capture individualized outcomes" (Koroloff & Friesen, p. 134). Individual outcomes often have been addressed by tracking progress on individualized goals (goal attainment scaling; Kiresuk, Smith, & Cardillo, 1994), but numerous issues compromise the usefulness of these designs. For certain interventions, such as those designed to decrease challenging behavior, single-subject designs are most appropriate (Carr et al., 2004). Single-subject designs in the behavioral tradition do not fit the evaluation of interventions such as family support or person-centered planning. Progress in evaluating individualized interventions will require innovative methodological advancements.

SOCIAL INFLUENCES ON DISABILITY RESEARCH METHODS
Advocates, Research Methods, and Evidence-Based Practice

Shakespeare (1996) described a complex relationship between research and disability politics. There are often dramatic tensions between advocates, who base decisions on values and civil rights, and scientists, who are often removed from the values debate and call for more data (Ramey, 1990). Halle and Lowrey (2002) suggested that the divide between advocates and researchers is often so entrenched that neither can see merit in the other's perspective. Although journal editors and grant proposal reviewers frequently force researchers to consider the applied implications of their work, all too often the reasons for asking certain questions and the usefulness of the resulting data are not apparent to those outside academia. Researchers are sometimes viewed as asking irrelevant questions, whereas questions important to advocates remain unaddressed (Koroloff & Friesen, 1997). More than 30 years ago, Haywood (1976) warned of "siren songs" that threatened empirical advancement. These included "If we spent our time and money putting into practice what we already know, there would be no need for further research" and "With limited funds, it is immoral to spend money on research when we need so many services" (p. 313). These same siren songs exist today, perhaps stronger than they were in the 1970s.

It is important that disability researchers address these issues. The first step is for us as researchers to choose research questions and measure outcomes that are important to advocates (Koroloff & Friesen, 1997). In part, this involves communicating with advocates the importance of research currently being conducted. It also involves being sensitive to issues important to advocates, such as the desire of people with disabilities to avoid negative labels. Many positive changes for people with disabilities have stemmed from advocacy initiatives rather than from research advances (Baumeister, 1997; Parmenter, 2004). Recognizing and respecting the important role of advocates in systems change can help bridge the research–advocacy divide.

Pressures Related to Evaluation Research

An often-invisible influence on researchers is the pressure for positive findings. Kytle and Millman (1986) describe service providers who feared evaluation results that could be used to close programs "which *everyone* knew worked" (p. 171). No program directors consent to having their efforts evaluated in order to document that they are ineffective. There can be ramifications for the researcher from a negative evaluation report. Undesired findings can undermine the relationship between program personnel and the researcher and can compromise future funding. At the very least, negative findings are usually not disseminated. There are few journal outlets for insignificant or negative evaluation findings. Multiple forces line up to reward good news.

It is impossible to know the extent to which unpublished data, residing in filing cabinets and storage boxes around the world, could inform us about the conditions that are associated with a lack of positive intervention outcomes. If a hypothetical intervention has been demonstrated effective in four quality studies, it would also be important to know that 20 researchers have documented situations in which the intervention was not effective. Negative findings that do receive attention often are those that relate to popular or controversial programs. The debate over facilitated communication is an example. Multiple quantitative studies document that it is the facilitator, not the person with a disability, who is generating the communication (Jacobson, Mulick, & Schwartz, 1995). Yet those who use qualitative data continue to assert the effectiveness of facilitated communication (e.g., Niemi & Kärnä-Lin, 2003). When faculty members from different universities disagree, how are service providers, educators, and families to make informed decisions?

Political and Funding Influences on Disability Research Methods

Disability research takes place in a social and political context (Emerson, Hatton, Thompson, & Parmenter, 2004; H. R. Turnbull, Stowe, A. P. Turnbull, & Schrandt, Chapter 2, this volume). Zigler, Hodapp, and Edison (1990) noted, "issues and solutions emphasized at any particular time often represent the swinging of the historical pendulum, whose path and speed are directed not only by the findings of scientific researchers, but also by political, economic, and social forces that often do not result in the clearest view of the problem under consideration" (p. 1). Across the years, disability research has paralleled societal swings from optimism to pessimism about the lives of people with disabilities (Scheerenberger, 1983).

Political pressures influence research through government funding priorities. Baumeister (1997) stated the issue the most directly when he wrote, "The engine that drives research may be intellectual, but the fuel is money" (p. 35). Appealing to different funding sources can require researchers to shift how they conduct studies. A recent example is the shift in educational funding in favor of randomized clinical trials. Researchers adapt to the political realities of research funding (Odom et al., 2005; Yell et al., 2005). Some influences of funding priorities are subtler. Boudah and Lenz (2000) note, for example, that funding agencies tend not to support replication studies or those that examine relatively small variations in intervention strategies. Journal editors also shape the methodologies used by disability researchers. In the past, qualitative studies were difficult to publish, so their numbers were few. Unfortunately, few scholars have focused on documenting the political and ethical dilemmas encountered in social research or the effects of these forces on our knowledge (Kytle & Millman, 1986).

Turning Research Findings into Widespread, Sustained Practice

Applied researchers hope that their intervention methods will achieve widespread adoption and that they will be implemented in a manner that remains true to the validated protocol. Boudah and Lenz (2000) noted that research seldom directly results in change in practices. "We must lament the sad fact that practices are seldom based on empirically proven methods. . . . Historically, best practice has been influenced somewhat by empirical findings, more by ideology, but mostly by the conviction of practitioners" (Heal, 1990, pp. 18–19). Three interrelated issues warrant attention: adoption, sustainability, and implementation drift.

The first issue, adoption, concerns translation of research findings into practice. Service providers make numerous decisions about methods and programs to use in their daily work. Researchers often express frustration that these choices seem to be unrelated to scientific evidence of effectiveness. We know very little about how adoption choices are made. Vaughn, Klingner, and Hughes (2000) pondered about why teachers often choose less effective techniques over more effective ones, suggesting that the answer to this question involves aspects of the school setting, the nature of the intervention, and characteristics of the students and teachers.

Disability service providers are bombarded by a competing array of catalogs, exhibitors, testimonials, consultants, and e-mail and Web-based announcements seeking to influence adoption decisions. "The words 'research says' introduce so many statements about practices, programs, and materials, that most of us are compelled to reply 'What research?' " (Vaughn et al., 2000, p. 164). Ascertaining which products really are empirically based requires investigation. In the midst of this deluge of information, scholarly journal articles are unexciting and difficult to access. Few researchers are adept at reaching out to grab the attention of educators and providers.

Boudah and Lenz (2000) suggest that researchers often send an implied message, "I did the research; now you go put it into practice" (p. 158). Weisz et al. (2005) present a *deployment-focused* model of intervention designed to maximize adoption, which pro-

poses that interventions should be developed and tested in everyday settings with participants who will be the ultimate targets of the intervention and with providers who will
be responsible for implementing the intervention. The focus is on creating and validating interventions in real-world settings. Thus there is no need to translate the intervention to real-world settings at a later time.

After adoption, the second challenge is to sustain implementation of the intervention over time (Vaughn et al., 2000). Most applied researchers can point to examples of
interventions that were discontinued or that faded away with time. A recent study by
Sindelar, Shearer, Yendol-Hoppey, and Liebert (2006) tracks factors leading to the lack
of sustainability of an inclusion model in a middle school. More studies of this type are
needed.

When innovative programs are put into widespread practice, there is often a gradual deterioration of program quality, and important program components and practices are lost or distorted. This third challenge, intervention drift, is critical. Drift can
occur within programs, as intervention procedures lose focus and become ineffectual
over time, or across programs, as new agencies adopt the intervention and implement it
in a weakened or distorted fashion. Providers who adopt multicomponent interventions
often use only parts rather than the whole package. Medical research has an accepted
phased sequence for evaluating effectiveness of drugs or other interventions as they
move from small, controlled studies (I) to larger groups of participants (II) to large
groups (III) to widespread use (IV). Effectiveness is tracked, as are possible unintended
side effects. Behavioral scientists do not routinely utilize a similar phased protocol. It is
common for behavioral and educational interventions to be demonstrated effective in a
small, controlled setting and then widely disseminated without further research.

Disability researchers have seldom studied the processes through which interventions are adopted, the forces that affect sustainability, or the mechanisms underlying
intervention drift. Halle and Lowrey (2002) note that we do not even have research documenting whether adoption decisions made with supporting empirical data yield better
outcomes than those made in the absence of data. This is true, in part, because the
research methods for studying systems-level changes are complex, expensive, and in
need of additional innovation. Few researchers are prepared to tackle these important
questions, and few funding sources are willing to support this research.

Questions Research Can and Cannot Answer: The Boundaries of Methodological Advancement

Evans (2002) posed an important question: If you could not demonstrate measurable
outcomes, "would you really abandon the values of fairness, natural justice, and respect,
and revert to some former approach?" (p. 265). Obviously, the answer is no. Focusing
on person-centered planning, Evans goes on to write, "Some questions, I would argue,
are simply not scientific questions, in that they are not amenable to being answered by
standard scientific method. As with apple pie, parking spaces for individuals with handicaps, or academic freedom, the principles of person-centered planning are based on
values that feel right and that fit our cultural beliefs at a given point in societal development" (p. 265). Even with the most advanced research methods, certain questions will
never be answered through data. Conversely, certain research findings will never guide
practice because they contradict key societal values.

Baumeister (1981) suggested that the role of research is to provide information
about how to best accomplish certain aims but that decisions about desired aims must

be decided based on values and ethical principles. "Science does not reveal truth: it sometimes reveals facts in certain restricted domains. Truth is ultimately a moral test, the outcome of the confrontation of values; truth does not depend on scientific methods" (p. 451). Community inclusion, closing institutions, supporting families, and ending employment discrimination, for example, are directions that we want to move in as a society based on our beliefs about who we are as a people. Researchers support these goals by identifying effective (and ineffective) ways of moving toward those goals. It is important that as a society, as advocates, and as researchers we are clear about the outcomes that we value and about the limited but important role of research in achieving those outcomes.

SUMMARY AND CONCLUDING THOUGHTS

A century has passed since Goddard set up his research program to study people with intellectual disabilities. The past century has been busy and productive for disability researchers. Research publications devoted to the study of developmental disabilities fill countless shelves in academic libraries across the world. This chapter celebrates important advances that have occurred in disability research. In the midst of celebration, however, lie concern and some disappointment. Many people with developmental disabilities remain excluded from society, spending meaningless days in large residential facilities that strayed from their enlightened purpose shortly after they were developed. In the community, people with substantial disabilities are all too often lonely, poor, and powerless. Too many children begin a lifetime of segregation in special preschools, culminating in high school transitions to endless waiting lists for adult services. Although we have made great progress, much work remains to be done.

Issues of research methodology, such as the definition of developmental disability and the operationalization of intervention outcomes, may seem esoteric and trivial in light of the daily struggles of people with disabilities and their families. The underlying premise of this chapter is that researchers have an important role to play in creating better lives for people with disabilities. Research does not solve societal problems, but high-quality research can be part of the solution. Continuing to improve our research methods, approaches, and designs will enable the results of our efforts to be more useful and to have greater impact. That aim is neither esoteric nor trivial.

Years ago, I came to believe in a perverse law of research: *The importance of any research question is inversely related to the ease of designing and implementing research to address the question* (Stoneman, 1993). Meaningful research tends to be the most difficult. Boudah and Lenz (2000) bring to mind an interesting question: What if the contingencies were changed and research success were defined by the extent to which our work makes a difference rather than by the number of publications that we generate or the research grants that we receive? If this were the case, how would it change disability research? It is an interesting question to ponder.

REFERENCES

Baumeister, A. A. (1967). Problems in comparative studies of mental retardates and normals. *American Journal of Mental Deficiency, 71*, 869–875.
Baumeister, A. A. (1981). Mental retardation policy and research: The unfulfilled promise. *American Journal of Mental Deficiency, 85*, 449–456.

Baumeister, A. A. (1997). Behavioral research: Boom or bust? In W. E. MacLean, Jr. (Ed.), *Ellis' handbook of mental deficiency, psychological theory and research* (3rd ed., pp. 3–45). Mahwah, NJ: Erlbaum.

Becker, H., Roberts, G., Morrison, H., & Silver, J. (2004). Recruiting people with disabilities as research participants. *Mental Retardation, 42*, 471–475.

Berliner, D. C. (2002). Educational research: The hardest science of all. *Educational Researcher, 31*, 18–20.

Bernell, S. L. (2003). Theoretical and applied issues in defining disability in labor market research. *Journal of Disability Policy Studies, 14*, 36–45.

Bhasin, T. K., Brocksen, S., Avchen, R. N., & Braun, K. V. N. (2006, January). Prevalence of four developmental disabilities among children aged 8 years: Metropolitan Atlanta Developmental Disabilities Surveillance Program, 1996 and 2000. *MMWR Surveillance Summaries, 55*(SS01), 1–9.

Booth, T., & Booth, W. (1996). Sounds of silence: Narrative research with inarticulate subjects. *Disability and Society, 11*, 55–69.

Boudah, D. J., & Lenz, B. K. (2000). And now the rest of the story: The research process as intervention in experimental and qualitative studies. *Learning Disabilities Research and Practice, 15*(3), 149–160.

Braddock, D., Hemp, R., Rizzolo, M. C., Coulter, D., Haffer, L., & Thompson, M. (2005). *The state of the states in developmental disabilities.* Boulder: University of Colorado Press.

Bronfenbrenner, U. (1979). *The ecology of human development.* Cambridge, MA: Harvard University Press.

Brooks, P. H., & Baumeister, A. A. (1977). A plea for consideration of ecological validity in the experimental psychology of mental retardation: A guest editorial. *American Journal of Mental Deficiency, 81*, 407–416.

Burack, J. A., Hodapp, R. M., & Zigler, E. (1988). Issues in the classification of mental retardation: Differentiating among organic etiologies. *Journal of Clinical Psychology and Psychiatry, 29*, 765–779.

Carr, E. G., Innis, J., Blakeley-Smith, A., & Vasdev, S. (2004). Challenging behavior: Research design and measurement issues. In E. Emerson, C. Hatton, T. Thompson, & T. R. Parmenter (Eds.), *The international handbook of applied research in intellectual disabilities* (pp. 423–458). West Sussex, UK: Wiley.

Ceci, S. J., & Papierno, P. B. (2005). The rhetoric and reality of gap closing: When the "have-nots" gain but the "haves" gain even more. *American Psychologist, 60*, 149–160.

Cheng, S., & Powell, B. (2005). Small samples, big challenges: Studying atypical family forms. *Journal of Marriage and Family, 67*, 926–935.

Davis, J. M. (2000). Disability studies as ethnographic research and text: Research strategies and roles for promoting social change? *Disability and Society, 15*, 191–206.

DeAngelis, T. (2005). Shaping evidence-based practice. *Monitor on Psychology, 26*(3), 26–31.

Dennis, R. (2002). Nonverbal narratives: Listening to people with severe intellectual disability. *Research and Practice for Persons with Severe Disabilities, 27*, 239–249.

Dykens, E. M., & Hodapp, R. M. (2001). Research in mental retardation: Toward an etiologic approach. *Journal of Child Psychology and Psychiatry, 42*, 49–71.

Ellis, N. R. (1969). A behavioral research strategy in mental retardation: Defense and critique. *American Journal of Mental Deficiency, 73*, 557–566.

Emerson, E., Hatton, C., Thompson, T., & Parmenter, T. R. (2004). Preface. In E. Emerson, C. Hatton, T. Thompson, & T. R. Parmenter (Eds.), *The international handbook of applied research in intellectual disabilities* (pp. xv–xvi). West Sussex, UK: Wiley.

Evans, I. M. (2002). Trying to make apple pie an independent variable: Comment on "How science can evaluate and enhance person-centered planning." *Research and Practice for Persons with Severe Disabilities, 27*, 265–267.

Fernald, C. D. (1995). When in London . . . : Differences in disability language preferences among English-speaking countries. *Mental Retardation, 33*, 99–103.

Finlay, W. M. L., & Lyons, E. (2001). Methodological issues in interviewing and using self-report questionnaires with people with mental retardation. *Psychological Assessment, 13*, 319–335.

Fujiura, G. T. (2003). Continuum of intellectual disability: Demographic evidence for the "forgotten generation." *Mental Retardation, 41*, 420–429.

Fujiura, G. T., & Yamaki, K. (1997). Analysis of ethnic variations in developmental disability prevalence and household economic status. *Mental Retardation, 35*, 286–294.

Gardner, J. F., & Carran, D. T. (2005). Attainment of personal outcomes by people with developmental disabilities. *Mental Retardation, 43*, 157–174.

Goodley, D. (1996). Tales of hidden lives: A critical examination of life history research with people who have learning difficulties. *Disability and Society, 11*, 333–348.

Gross, B. H., & Hahn, H. (2004). Developing issues in the classification of mental and physical disabilities. *Journal of Disability Policy Studies, 15*, 130–134.

Halle, J. W., & Lowrey, K. A. (2002). Can person-centered planning be empirically analyzed to the satisfaction of all stakeholders? *Research and Practice for Persons with Severe Disabilities, 27*, 268–271.

Harbin, G., Rous, B., & McLean, M. (2005). Issues in designing state accountability systems. *Journal of Early Intervention, 27*, 137–164.

Haywood, H. C. (1976). The ethics of doing research . . . and of not doing it. *American Journal of Mental Retardation, 81*, 311–317.

Heal, L. W. (1970). Research strategies and research goals in the scientific study of the mentally subnormal. *American Journal of Mental Deficiency, 75*, 10–15.

Heal, L. W. (1990). Bold relief or bold re-leaf? *American Journal on Mental Retardation, 95*, 17–19.

Hebbeler, K. (2005). Aligning outcomes across multiple systems, attribution, and the fear factor. *Journal of Early Intervention, 27*, 165–166.

Hendershot, G. E., Larson, S. A., Lakin, K. C., & Doljanac, R. (2005, June). Problems in defining mental retardation and developmental disability: Using the National Health Interview Survey. *DD Data Brief, 7(1)*, 1–9.

Hodapp, R. M., & Dykens, E. M. (2004). Studying behavioral phenotypes: Issues, benefits, challenges. In E. Emerson, C. Hatton, T. Thompson, & T. R. Parmenter (Eds.), *The international handbook of applied research in intellectual disabilities* (pp. 203–220). West Sussex, UK: Wiley.

Holburn, S. (2002). How science can evaluate and enhance person-centered planning. *Research and Practice for Persons with Severe Disabilities, 27*, 250–260.

Horner, R. H., Carr, E. G., Halle, J., McGee, G., Odom, S., & Wolery, M. (2005). The use of single-subject research to identify evidence-based practice in special education. *Exceptional Children, 71*, 165–179.

House, B. J. (1977). Scientific explanation and ecological validity: A reply to Brooks and Baumeister. *American Journal of Mental Deficiency, 81*, 534–542.

Human Services Research Institute. (2006). *National Core Indicators Project*. Retrieved February 2007, from *www.hsri.org/nci*.

Jacobson, J. W., Mulick, J. A., & Schwartz, A. A. (1995). A history of facilitated communication: Science, pseudoscience, and antiscience. *American Psychologist, 50*, 750–765.

Johnson, R. B., & Onwuegbuzie, A. J. (2004). Mixed methods research: A research paradigm whose time has come. *Educational Researcher, 33*, 14–26.

Kennedy, C. H. (2004). Research on social relationships. In E. Emerson, C. Hatton, T. Thompson, & T. R. Parmenter (Eds.), *The international handbook of applied research in intellectual disabilities* (pp. 297–310). West Sussex, UK: Wiley.

Kiresuk, T. J., Smith, A., & Cardillo, J. E. (1994). *Goal attainment scaling*. Hillsdale NJ: Erlbaum.

Koroloff, N. M., & Friesen, B. J. (1997). Challenges in conducting family-centered mental health services research. *Journal of Emotional and Behavioral Disorders, 5(3)*, 130–136.

Kytle, J., & Millman, E. J. (1986). Confessions of two applied researchers in search of principles. *Evaluation and Program Planning, 9*, 167–177.

Lakin, K. C., & Stancliffe, R. J. (2005). Expenditures and outcomes. In R. J. Stancliffe & K. C. Lakin (Eds.), *Costs and outcomes of community services for people with intellectual disabilities* (pp. 313–337). Baltimore: Brookes.

Landesman, S., & Ramey, C. (1989). Developmental psychology and mental retardation. *American Psychologist, 44*, 409–415.

Larson, S., & Lakin, C. (1989). Deinstitutionalization of persons with mental retardation: Behavioral outcomes. *Journal of the Association for Persons with Severe Handicaps, 14*, 324–332.

Larson, S., Lakin, C., Anderson, L., Kwak, N., Lee, J. H., & Anderson, D. (2000, April). Prevalence of mental retardation and/or developmental disabilities: Analysis of the 1994/1995 NHIS-D. *MR/DD Data Brief, 2(1)*, 1–11.

Lloyd, M., Preston-Shoot, M., Temple, B., & Wuu, R. (1996). Whose project is it anyway? Sharing and shaping the research agenda. *Disability and Society, 11,* 301–315.

Magaña, S. M. (2000). Mental retardation research methods in Latino communities. *Mental Retardation, 38,* 303–315.

National Center for the Dissemination of Disability Research. (2005). What are the standards for quality research? *Focus: A Technical Brief, 9.*

Niemi, J., & Kärnä-Lin, E. (2003). Four vantage points to the language performance and capacity of human beings: Response to Saloviita and Sariola. *Mental Retardation, 41,* 380–385.

Nisbet, J. (Ed.). (1992). *Natural supports in school, at work, and in the community for people with severe disabilities.* Baltimore: Brookes.

O'Brien, J. (2002). Person-centered planning as a contributing factor in organizational and social change. *Research and Practice for Persons with Severe Disabilities, 27,* 261–274.

Odom, S. L., Brantlinger, E., Gersten, R., Horner, R. H., Thompson, B., & Harris, K. R. (2005). Research in special education: Scientific methods and evidence-based practices. *Exceptional Children, 71,* 137–148.

Olson, D. H. (1977). Insiders' and outsiders' views of relationships: Research studies. In G. Levinger & H. L. Raush (Eds.), *Perspectives on the meaning of intimacy* (pp. 115–135). Amherst: University of Massachusetts Press.

Parmenter, T. R. (2004). Historical overview of applied research in intellectual disabilities: The foundation years. In E. Emerson, C. Hatton, T. Thompson, & T. R. Parmenter (Eds.), *The international handbook of applied research in intellectual disabilities* (pp. 3–40). West Sussex, UK: Wiley.

Perry, J., & Felce, D. (2002). Subjective and objective quality of life assessment: Responsiveness, response bias, and resident:proxy concordance. *Mental Retardation, 40,* 445–456.

Ramey, S. L. (1990). Staging (and re-staging) the trio of services, evaluation, and research. *American Journal on Mental Retardation, 95,* 26–29.

Sample, P. L. (1996). Beginnings: Participatory action research and adults with developmental disabilities. *Disability and Society, 11,* 317–332.

Scheerenberger, R. C. (1983). *A history of mental retardation.* Baltimore: Brookes.

Shakespeare, T. (1996). Rules of engagement. *Disability and Society, 11,* 115–119.

Silverstein, R., Julnes, G., & Nolan, R. (2005). What policymakers need and must demand from research regarding the employment rate of persons with disabilities. *Behavioral Sciences and the Law, 23,* 399–448.

Sindelar, P. T., Shearer, D. K., Yendol-Hoppey, D., & Liebert, T. W. (2006). The sustainability of inclusive school reform. *Exceptional Children, 72,* 317–331.

Smylie, M. A., & Kahne, J. (1997). Why what works doesn(t in teacher education. *Educational and Urban Society, 29,* 355–372.

Stancliffe, R. J., Emerson, E., & Lakin, K. C. (2004). Residential supports. In E. Emerson, C. Hatton, T. Thompson, & T. R. Parmenter (Eds.), *The international handbook of applied research in intellectual disabilities* (pp. 459–478). West Sussex, UK: Wiley.

Stein, R. E. K., & Jessop, D. J. (1982). A noncategorical approach to chronic childhood illness. *Public Health Reports, 97,* 354–362.

Stoneman, Z. (1989). Comparison groups in research on families with mentally retarded members: A methodological and conceptual review. *American Journal on Mental Retardation, 94,* 195–215.

Stoneman, Z. (1993). Common themes and divergent paths. In Z. Stoneman & P. W. Berman (Eds.), *The effects of mental retardation, disability, and illness on sibling relationships* (pp. 355–365). Baltimore: Brookes.

Summers, J. A., Poston, D. J., Turnbull, A. P., Marquis, J., Hoffman, L., Mannan, H., et al. (2005). Conceptualizing and measuring family quality of life. *Journal of Intellectual Disability Research, 49,* 777–783.

Thompson, J. R., Bryant, B. R., Campbell, E. M., Craig, E. M., Hughes, C. M., Rotholz, D. A., et al. (2004). *Supports Intensity Scale Users Manual.* Washington DC: American Association on Mental Retardation.

Vaughn, S., Klingner, L., & Hughes, M. (2000). Sustainability of research-based practices. *Exceptional Children, 66,* 163–171.

Warren, S. F., Brady, N. C., & Fey, M. E. (2004). Communication and language: Research design and measurement issues. In E. Emerson, C. Hatton, T. Thompson, & T. R. Parmenter (Eds.), *The international handbook of applied research in intellectual disabilities* (pp. 383–405). West Sussex, UK: Wiley.

Weisner, T. S. (1993). Ethnographic and ecocultural perspectives on sibling relationships. In Z. Stoneman & P. W. Berman (Eds.), *The effects of mental retardation, disability, and illness on sibling relationships* (pp. 51–83). Baltimore: Brookes.

Weisz, J. R., Sandler, I. N., Durlak, J. A., & Anton, B. S. (2005). Promoting and protecting youth mental health through evidence-based prevention and treatment. *American Psychologist, 60*, 628–648.

Yell, M. L., Drasgow, E., & Lowrey, K. A. (2005). No Child Left Behind and students with autism spectrum disorders. *Focus on Autism and Other Developmental Disabilities, 20*, 130–139.

Zigler, E., Hodapp, R. M., & Edison, M. R. (1990). From theory to practice in the care and education of mentally retarded individuals. *American Journal on Mental Retardation, 95*, 1–12.

4

Race, Culture,
and Developmental Disabilities

Janette K. Klingner
Wanda J. Blanchett
Beth Harry

Our nation's school-age population is becoming culturally and linguistically diverse at an unprecedented rate. Wealth and economic opportunity have increased for some, but disparities by race persist, and poverty levels have remained relatively constant (e.g., roughly between 35 and 40% for Hispanic children and 40 and 45% for African American children). Children of color and poor children are increasingly concentrated in urban areas in which schools were constructed decades earlier and are in disrepair (Kozol, 2005). This context provides the backdrop for our discussions of race, culture, and developmental disabilities in this chapter.

Despite a wealth of information published in the professional literature regarding developmental disabilities in general, it is rare for research to articulate how issues of race, culture, class, and language affect children and families with developmental disabilities. Few studies offer suggestions for assisting individuals of color with developmental disabilities and their families in gaining access to appropriate services.[1] Similarly, few resources are available to assist educators and service providers in tailoring their service delivery models and interventions to meet the diverse needs of people of color with developmental disabilities and their families. Researchers have given inadequate attention to determining how existing identification processes and procedures,

---

[1]We prefer to use the term "people of color" rather than "culturally and linguistically diverse" or "minority." The latter term we avoid because in many geographic areas "minority" populations are actually in the majority. Also, the term "minority" appears to diminish the importance of a group and has become associated with issues of power that result in the devaluing of racial, cultural, or linguistic features of the group.

assessment tools, and interventions might be made more culturally and linguistically responsive. Even though students of color with developmental disabilities are very much a part of our increasingly diverse society, special education has yet to sufficiently address issues of race, culture, class, and language as they relate to this segment of the student body. Though there have been some notable attempts to address these issues, challenges continue.

Given that more than 3.8 million Americans have been identified as having developmental disabilities and that more than 25% of these individuals are African Americans and other people of color, these findings are surprising. Further, because issues of race, culture, and class seems to play an important role in determining the risk ratio of African Americans, Hispanics, Native Americans, and Asian Americans for developmental disabilities, it is important that attention be given to these issues. For the purpose of this chapter, the term "developmental disabilities" includes individuals identified as having mental retardation and developmental delay, including autism. Culturally and linguistically responsive services are defined here as those services that recognize, value, and infuse the ethnic, cultural, and linguistic knowledge of individuals of color with developmental disabilities to inform pedagogical and service delivery practices and to employ that knowledge to design instructional strategies, communication strategies, assessment tools, and service delivery models.

Existing research documents a number of factors that may place people of color at increased risk of experiencing developmental disabilities. Being a person of color in and of itself does not cause developmental disabilities, but people of color experience social and economic disparities in the form of high levels of unemployment or underemployment, decreased earnings, economic instability, and decreased distribution of income and wealth that increase their risk ratio for developmental disabilities. Among the social and economic factors most commonly cited as contributing to the greater risk of people of color for developmental disabilities are inadequate access to appropriate health care, high incidence of low birthweight, limited access to prenatal care, greater risk of exposure to trauma due to illness or injury, greater exposure to environmental toxins, and higher instances of infectious diseases (Fujiura & Yamaki, 1997).

With the exception of a very small number of teacher educators and researchers (e.g., Harry, 1992; Correa, 1989), few have acknowledged that issues of race, culture, social class, and language should also be prominent in discussions regarding teacher preparation, inclusion, and access to appropriate instruction and/or services for students with developmental disabilities. Often the diagnosis of "developmental disability" trumps all other aspects of one's life—and little relevance is noted in other, more defining influences such as culture, race, and poverty (Ford, Blanchett, & Brown, 2006). Harry and colleagues (Harry, Kalyanpur, & Day, 1999) remind us that issues of race, culture, social-class standing, religion, and gender greatly affect families and shape their views of disability, their plans for their children, and their approach to schools and services. As researchers and teacher educators examine best practices in the area of developmental disabilities, it is important to (1) understand the continuing impact of white privilege and discrimination; (2) understand how one's cultural stance affects interactions with families; (3) appreciate and be responsive to the ethnic, racial, cultural, and linguistic backgrounds of students and their families; and (4) see "cultural responsiveness" as relevant for students with developmental disabilities, too.

Failure to place issues of race, class, culture, and language at the center of educational considerations and decision making assumes that the special education and community and human service systems are neutral on these issues. More important, the absence of a dialogue about issues of race, class, culture, and language reinforces the misperception that these issues have no impact on individuals of color with developmental disabilities and their families' pursuit of equitable educational programming and service delivery (Ford et al., 2006). Although the research on individuals of color with developmental disabilities and their families is sparse, the available research clearly indicates that they experience a number of service delivery barriers that their white-majority peers do not encounter (Gammon, 2000).

WHAT DOES CULTURE HAVE TO DO WITH DEVELOPMENTAL DISABILITIES?

On first thought, one might wonder, "What does culture have to do with developmental disabilities?" In response to this question, Kalyanpur and Harry (1999) would say not only that culture has everything to do with developmental disabilities and how the term was constructed but also that culture influenced and gave birth to the social constructs of "special education" and "disability." Given that cultural values, beliefs, and practices are the underpinnings of special education, it is impossible to view either the American special education system as a whole or the area of developmental disabilities in particular as culturally neutral. In fact, Kalyanpur and Harry (1999) refer to special education as a cultural institution and go on to discuss what it means to have membership in the culture of special education. To do this, they speak of special education as a subsystem within the larger social–cultural system of the American educational system. They conclude that the special education system reflects "the 'beliefs, values, and ideas' regarding both the ends and the means of education, which, in turn, reflect those of the national macroculture" (p. 5), or larger society. It stands to reason, then, that a special education system that was formed by embedding majority "American" core beliefs, values, and ideas might present challenges for microcultures, including individuals of color with significant disabilities and their families, as they try to navigate such a system that may or may not reflect their cultural perspectives, beliefs, values, ideas, and language. The same is also true for individuals and their families who are adversely affected by social class and/or the intersection of race, class, culture, and language as they try to access services that are primarily geared toward the beliefs, values, ideas, and language of the macroculture, or the middle-class white English-speaking majority.

The meanings constructed for both cognitive and physical disabilities are tremendously affected by culture. Different cultures vary in their perceptions about what is considered a "disability." For example, in a Navajo community in which a congenital hip deformity was common, the condition was not seen as a disability because it was compatible with horse riding (Locust, 1988). Among the Hmong, neither clubfoot nor epilepsy (Fadiman, 1997) was interpreted as a handicap or illness. Various cultures also differ in their views of intelligence. In a Zambian community (Serpell, Mariga, & Harvey, 1993), perceptions of intelligence focused on moral and interpersonal abilities more than on one's ability to complete cognitive tasks. And in the United States, Bogdan (1992) studied community members' views of a farmer accused of murder. He found that the community's definition of normalcy had much more to do with the ability of a member to abide by the community's norms of hard work and "minding one's business" than with higher level thinking abilities. In sum, as Gallego, Cole, and The Laboratory of Human Cognition (2002) note, psychological theories of learning tend to assume that culture is irrelevant to the process of knowledge acquisition. This assumption is particularly disturbing when we consider the culturally specific tasks on which "assessments" of IQ and other developmental abilities are constructed.

PROBLEMATIC ASSESSMENT ASSUMPTIONS AND PRACTICES WITH STUDENTS OF COLOR

For decades, experts have expressed concerns about using standardized tests with students of color (Laosa, 1977). Thus procedural safeguards for conducting nondiscriminatory assessments were included in the original passage of the Education of All Children with Handicaps Act in 1975 and have been part of each reauthorization since. Nondiscriminatory assessment is defined as "reducing the chance that a child might be incorrectly placed in special classes and increasing the use of intervention programs which facilitate his [her] physical, social, emotional, and academic development" (Tucker, 1977, p. 109).

Cognitive tests are based on several questionable assumptions when used with students of color. One enduring belief is that a cognitive test is capable of measuring an individual's actual level of competence. For years, researchers considered cognitive testing procedures to be context and culture-free. In other words, it was thought possible to accurately assess an individual's cognitive abilities through the presentation of arbitrary preselected, discrete tasks in a controlled situation without considering life experiences (Rogoff, 2003). It appears that insufficient attention is given to the extent to which value systems and cultural norms are built into the procedures and interpretation of tests. Any test performance is the result of a complex interaction between the task characteristics and the constraints inherent in the testing situation. Numerous situational factors can complicate the task of inferring competence from performance.

Cultural Influences on Test Performance

Variance across cultural groups in test performance may be due to different interpretations of the nature of the task, of the problem being solved, and of how to go about reaching a solution (Goodnow, 1976). Rogoff (2003) proposed that cognitive tests rely on particular conversation forms that may be unfamiliar to some children. The child who is familiar with these forms is more likely to appear confident and to respond in ways expected by the examiner, whereas the child who is unfamiliar with them is more likely to appear wary. For example, the test taker may interpret the situation as one that calls for showing respect by remaining silent, or the test taker might be unaccustomed to "known answer questions" and be unsure how to respond (Heath, 1983). Also, some children learn by observing and how to are socialized to believe that displaying a skill before it has been fully learned is improper (Cazden & John, 1971). In addition, the extent to which speed of completion is esteemed varies across cultures as well. Although speed is highly valued in Western cultures, in some other cultures intelligence is associated with such characteristics as "slow" and "careful" (Wober, 1972). García and Pearson (1994) noted that test performance by children from some cultures may be affected by the speed of their responses.

An individual's performance on cognitive tasks is affected by the extent to which he or she is familiar with the content of the test and the context in which the testing occurs. For example, Serpell (1994) compared Zambian and British children's ability to build structures using familiar and unfamiliar materials, such as blocks, wire, and clay, and found that the Zambian children were superior when building with wire, the British children were superior with blocks, and both groups performed similarly with clay. Serpell (1994) concluded that their participants did much better when using materials they knew well. In a similar study, Guatemalan Mayan children performed at least as well as middle-class Salt Lake City children on a task involving objects with which they were familiar (Rogoff & Waddell, 1982). Cole, Gay, Glick, and Sharp (1971) investigated cultural differences in memory skills and found that, although Liberian rice farmers initially appeared to be quite deficient in comparison with U.S. white middle-class individuals, their performance improved substantially when the tasks were adapted to make them more culturally relevant (see also Cole, 1996; Greenfield & Childs, 1977). These research studies are important because they demonstrate that intelligence tests can underestimate potential when they include tasks and materials with which the test taker is not familiar and that are culturally irrelevant.

Similarly, another faulty assumption when using standardized tests with students of color is that of content validity, or the extent to which those taking the test have been exposed to and are familiar with the universe of information from which test items are drawn (Samuda, 1989). In many cases, students of color have not been exposed to this information and thus are placed at a disadvantage (Hilliard, 1977; Williams, 1974). It is natural that tests reflect the abilities, skills, and language valued by the U.S. "core culture" (Mercer, 1973, p. 13), and yet this reality is not often taken into account when assessing the potential or achievement of students from backgrounds other than the mainstream.

Test taking is also affected by other cultural variables. For instance, in sorting a group of disparate objects, Western thinking would expect a classification based on taxonomic categories (such as grouping food, animals, or implements into separate categories), whereas in some cultures the items would be sorted by their functions (e.g., "putting a hoe with a potato because it is used to dig up a potato" (Rogoff & Chavajay, 1995, p. 861). Performance on Western cognitive tasks by people from a variety of cultures reveals the cultural basis of cognitive development.

Although poor performance does not necessarily reflect lack of competence, and although the results of any test should be interpreted with caution, it would be unjustified to conclude that poor performance has no relevance whatsoever (Cole & Bruner, 1971). The challenge is to determine just what can and cannot be concluded from assessment results and what a score on a given test means. Cognitive activity does not take place in a vacuum but must be understood in terms of the social, cultural, and historical processes that influence the contexts within which activities occur. Cultural variation is due more to differences in the situations in which dissimilar cultural groups apply their skills than to differences in the actual skills (Cole & Bruner, 1971). Assessment, particularly of students of color, must be attentive to situational and cultural variables.

Linguistic Influences on Test Performance

Much has been written about the potential for linguistic bias on cognitive tests (Rogoff, 2003; Valdés & Figueroa, 1994). Test performance can be affected by misinterpretations of questions, lack of knowledge of vocabulary, limited English-language proficiency, and issues of language dominance. The majority of bilingual groups exhibit the same low verbal IQ, higher nonverbal IQ profile on intelligence tests. Unfortunately, this profile has led many researchers to erroneously conclude that bilingualism retards verbal intelligence, despite evidence to the contrary (August & Hakuta, 1997). Diagnosticians and educators have misconstrued students' lack of full proficiency in English as a second language as a widespread intelligence deficit (Oller, 1991) or as a language or learning disability (Langdon, 1989). Misdiagnoses can occur when a student is tested in English before he or she has acquired full proficiency. Determining when a child has acquired full cognitive academic English proficiency and is ready to be assessed in English continues to be a challenge (Cummins, 1984). Even students who appear to be fluent in English based on oral language measures may not be ready to be assessed at higher cognitive levels in English.

Despite good intentions and written guidelines designed to prevent biased assessment procedures, in practice: (1) language proficiency is not always taken into account; (2) testing is done primarily in English; (3) factors related to second-language acquisition are misinterpreted as performance deficits; (4) home data are ignored; and (5) the same few tests are used with most children (e.g., Figueroa, 1989; Ochoa, Rivera, & Powell, 1997). Ochoa and colleagues surveyed 859 members of the National Association of School Psychologists who were located in eight states and who had prior experience conducting bilingual psychoeducational assessments. They found that psychologists failed to consider students' native language and the number of years of English instruction they had received (Ochoa et al., 1997). Although over half of these psychologists used interpreters, only about a third of the interpreters had received any formal training (Ochoa, Powell, & Robles-Piña, 1996).

Harry and Klingner (2006) examined factors that affected the assessment process and the decision to identify a student as qualifying for special education in culturally and linguistically diverse schools. Although school personnel expressed confidence in the accuracy of the assessment process to discern who truly met eligibility criteria and who did not, the researchers found that assessors tended to overrely on the results of English-language testing, to exclude native-language test results, and to give inadequate attention to language acquisition issues or classroom context as possible explanations for students' struggles.

Predictive Validity

Many intelligence tests possess strong psychometric qualities for certain groups of students but tend to underestimate the potential of students of color (Rueda, 1997), thus weakening their predictive validity. A longitudinal study of 60% of the 2,100 students from the triethnic norming sample for the System of Multicultural Pluralistic Assessment (SOMPA) provides a clear example (Figueroa & Sassenrath, 1989). The researchers compared students' scores on the 1972 Full Scale Wechsler Intelligence Scale for Children—Revised (WISC-R) with their grade-point averages (GPAs), standardized reading scores, and standardized math scores in 1982. They considered students who achieved at higher levels than predicted by their IQ scores to be "overachievers" and students who achieved at lower levels than predicted to be "underachievers." Latino students who in 1972 had scored at or below the mean on the WISC-R were more likely than their mainstream counterparts to obtain higher-than-expected school grades, thus placing them in the overachiever category. These findings demonstrated that the WISC-R lacked predictive validity for the Latino students and underestimated their potential.

Adaptive Behavior

Another dilemma in the assessment and classification of individuals having mental retardation (MR) is the requirement for a test of adaptive functioning (American Association on Mental Retardation, 2002; Reschly, Myers, & Hartel, 2002). This dimension is an attempt to verify that the child's delays are general and are exhibited in all phases of the child's daily living rather than limited to academic achievement. However, assessments are controversial precisely because they test domains that are very different from those for which a child is usually referred, because adaptive behavior is culturally specific, and because the processes for obtaining assessment information differ (e.g., direct observation, third-party report). Further, there is no agreement as to what cutoff points should be used on the adaptive scales.

Perhaps of greatest concern when using adaptive behavior scales with students of color is that behavior considered appropriate at any given age varies appreciably by culture, as well as by socioeconomic status. For example, one section of adaptive behavior scales focuses on self-care activities, such as getting dressed, brushing one's teeth, or eating without help. The age at which children are expected to perform these tasks on their own varies a great deal by culture. Although independence is greatly valued in U.S. American culture, it is not necessarily as valued in other cultures around the world.

An additional issue regarding adaptive behavior scales is that they are not always included in assessment batteries before qualifying students for special education. This was the case in Harry and Klingner's (2006) research on the disproportionate representation of students of color in special education. They found that psychologists did not always use these measures, even though the district's written guidelines stipulated that they do so. Instead, they based their decision on an intelligence test score and clinical judgment, as with one fourth-grade Hispanic girl who spoke Spanish as her home language but was tested only in English with the WISC-III and was then determined to have MR when her Full Scale IQ was found to be 51.

PUBLIC SCHOOLING AND RACE IN THE UNITED STATES: SORTING, STRATIFYING, AND EXCLUDING

Race has figured prominently in the evolution of public schooling in the United States since its inception. The latter half of the 20th century was marked by a struggle for equity within general and special education (Bullivant, 1993). The arguments regarding the role of schooling as a means of social reproduction (Bowles & Gintis, 1976; Oakes, 1985) rather than as a vehicle for social mobility (Blau & Duncan, 1967, Sewell, Haller, & Portes, 1969) are well known, and we do not detail them here. Suffice it to say that although schooling has provided a certain degree of social mobility for some, its structure, content, and methods of inculcating knowledge are readily recognized as being developed to suit the goals of the majority white American society, and, until the civil rights movement of the 1960s, the social mobility of students of color was not a goal of American education.

Special Education: Equity and Efficiency in Conflict

Progress toward universal schooling for children regardless of handicapping condition was fueled by the civil rights movement and deeply influenced by its rhetoric of equality and solidarity. Although they were envisioned as parallel movements, it is not far-fetched to say that the special education and civil rights movements were actually on a collision course (Harry & Klingner, 2006). Special education became a way to provide separate services for some students, a disproportionate percentage of whom were students of color. The advocates for the right of all children with disabilities to a public education framed special education as one of the answers to the inequities of eras past. For the parent groups and other advocates who lobbied for the passage of a federal mandate for these programs, this was the purpose and vision of special education. Indeed, the establishment of the Bureau of Education for the Handicapped in the 1960s and the passage of the Education for All Handicapped Children Act (EHA) in 1975 followed in the wake of the civil rights movement. There is no doubt that, for the thousands of children for whom there was no available schooling prior to 1975, the EHA represented the achievement of the society's goal of equity.

The issue of placement of nonwhite children in classes for students perceived as "slow" or mildly retarded came to public attention after the *Brown v. Board of Education* (1954) desegregation decision. The reluctance of many states to comply with the *Brown* ruling led to the first official allegations of the use of special classes to continue covert forms of racial segregation. Prasse and Reschly (1986) noted that such allegations were reported in San Francisco as early as 1965 and that the first legal suit on the subject was *Johnson v. San Francisco Unified School District* (1971), which charged that the district was "dumping" African American children in classes for the "mildly retarded." The landmark *Larry P. v. Riles* (1972) case was filed just months after Johnson (1972), charging that biased IQ tests resulted in gross overrepresentation of African American students in MR programs. The argument was based on the fact that, whereas African American students composed 28.5% of the total student body in the school district, they composed 66% of all students in classes for MR. The courts supported the plaintiffs' charge that the IQ tests being used to place children in the MR category were biased against African American children and declared that the disproportionate representation of African American students in programs for students with mild mental retardation was discriminatory. They banned the use of IQ tests with African American students and ordered the elimination of overrepresentation of African American students in MR programs. Around the same time, similar charges were brought by Mercer (1973) regarding the high rates of placement of Hispanic children in MR programs in California. The most influential cases on this topic centered on the language of testing, with *Diana v. State Board of Education* (1970) in California arguing that Hispanic children were being inappropriately tested in English even when they only spoke Spanish and *Guadalupe Organization v. Tempe Elementary School District No. 3* (1972) in Arizona making similar charges regarding both Hispanic and Native American children. In both of these cases the plaintiffs were supported by the courts. These landmark court cases of the 1970s provided impetus for the mandate for nondiscriminatory assessment procedures in the civil rights legislation of Section 504 of the Rehabilitation Act of 1973 that laid the groundwork for the requirements for nondiscriminatory testing and the due-process safeguards against misclassification in the passage of the EHA (Jacob-Timm & Hartshorne, 1998).

Prior to 1969, the American Association on Mental Deficiency (AAMD) used a cutoff score of 1 standard deviation from the mean (i.e., an IQ of 85). This definition was changed by the AAMD in 1969 to 2 standard deviations from the mean (i.e., an IQ of 70). Mercer (1973) pointed out the irony in this change, noting that it brought about a "swift cure" for many who had previously been determined to be retarded. Since then, many states have used a variable guideline of a score between 70 and 75 on an IQ test. This, however, has only compounded charges of subjectivity and ambiguity, as a leeway of just 5 points actually results in large differences in the percentages of students who qualify (MacMillan & Reschly, 1998). Such debates highlight the arbitrariness of placement decisions and the social construction of disability (i.e., decisions about who has and who does not have a disability).[2]

With the passage of the EHA in 1975, the special education and desegregation movements officially collided (Harry & Klingner, 2006). The concept of deficit had become a well-established part of the educational belief system and would become the driving force behind decisions about how to educate those who appeared different from the mainstream. Students of color who had once been excluded from schools with whites would now be placed in special education at rates greater than their percentages in the overall school-age population.

The Overrepresentation of Students of Color in Special Education Programs

When the disproportionate representation of ethnically and linguistically diverse students in high-incidence special education programs (mental retardation, learning disabilities, and emotional disturbance) was first brought to the nation's attention by Dunn in 1968 and studied by a National Academy of Sciences panel (Heller, Holtzman, & Messick, 1982), the focus was on the overrepresentation of African American, Hispanic, and high-poverty students in MR programs.[3] Between 1948 and 1966 there had been a 400% increase in the number of students identified as mentally retarded, and in 1975, when the Education for All Handicapped Children Act was passed, MR had the highest count of any exceptional child diagnosis. Although the MR category has, historically, been the source of most controversy regarding ethnic disproportionality, it is now used much less frequently than in the past. Whereas the numbers in the LD category have increased almost sixfold over the past two decades, the rates of placement for all ethnicities in MR have been reduced by almost half. Nonetheless, among those students who are designated as mentally retarded, African Americans are more than twice as likely as students of other ethnicities to be identified (Donovan & Cross, 2002). Thus, although MR rates have declined overall, we still see significant overrepresentation of students of color in this category.

Disproportionate Representation by Ethnic Group

Although disproportionate representation is most apparent among African American students when nationally aggregated data are the focus, there are marked differences across states and notable instances of overrepresentation among other ethnic and linguistic groups when data are disaggregated and population subgroups are examined (Artiles, Rueda, Salazar, & Higareda, 2005; Oswald, Coutinho, Best, & Singh, 1999). Compared with all other groups combined, African American students are 2.99 times more likely to be classified as having MR, 1.17 times more likely to be classified as having autism, and 1.65 times more likely to be identified as having developmental delay. In contrast, Hispanic students are about half as likely to be classified as having MR and/or developmental delay (U.S. Department of Education, 2003).

---

[2]For further discussion of the social construction of disabilities, see Gergen (1994) and Reid and Knight (2006).
[3]Mental retardation (MR), learning disabilities (LD), and emotional disturbance (ED) are the labels used by Donovan and Cross (2002).

As the disability rights movement has taken hold, overall more students with disabilities are being included in general education classrooms. But this is not the case for students of color. Unlike their white peers, students of color are often excluded from inclusive education programs and the general education curriculum (Fierros & Conroy, 2002; LeRoy & Kulik, 2003). Instead, they tend to spend 60% or more of their school day in segregated special education placements (i.e., in separate classrooms or separate schools from those attended by their nondisabled peers; U.S. Department of Education, 2002). They are also more likely to have uncertified or provisionally licensed teachers and to graduate with a certificate of attendance or completion versus a high school diploma (Chamberlain, 2005). Once students of color exit special education, most commonly by dropping out or receiving a certificate of attendance, they experience high unemployment rates, a lack of preparation for the workforce, and difficulty gaining access into postsecondary education (Ferri & Connor, 2005; Losen & Orfield, 2002).

Assumptions about the Causes of Disproportionate Representation

Disproportionate representation is a complex phenomenon that cannot be explained by simplistic views that focus narrowly on the role of poverty or on students' presumed lack of intelligence or other deficits and that pay too little attention to the role of context and other factors external to the child (Klingner et al., 2005), including but not limited to institutionalized white privilege and racism (Blanchett, 2006). By context we mean the various nested systems that influence a child's experiences, as well as how the child is perceived, from the classroom to the school to the local community to the larger society, much as with Bronfenbrenner's (1977) ecological systems model.

Assumptions about the Role of Poverty

We question the notion that students of color are overrepresented in the MR category because they are more likely to have a disability because of an impoverished environment. In other words, although poverty and associated risk factors, such as low birthweight, exposure to alcohol during pregnancy, tobacco and drug use, malnourishment, and exposure to lead, are often described as causal factors in the development of language or cognitive deficits or maladaptive behaviors (Donovan & Cross, 2002), poverty itself does not automatically result in low learning potential, as evidenced by the significant number of children and schools who "beat the odds" (Donovan & Cross, 2002; O'Connor, 2002). O'Connor argued that there is nothing about poverty in and of itself that places poor children at academic risk but that, rather, it is how structures of opportunity and constraint come to bear on their likelihood for achieving competitive educational outcomes. O'Connor and Fernandez (2006) noted that a focus on poverty as the explanation for the overrepresentation of African Americans in MR programs oversimplifies the concept of "development" and consequently underanalyzes how the normative culture of society and thus schools (i.e., of the white middle and upper classes) situate minority youth as academically and behaviorally deficient in comparison. They assert that it is the culture and organization of schools (and not poverty) that places minority students at heightened risk for special education placement. Skiba, Poloni-Staudinger, Simmons, Feggins, and Chung (2005) made a similar argument based on their research in school districts in Indiana.

Assumptions about Intelligence

One of the most lasting legacies of Western racism is a deep-seated belief in the inferior intelligence of individuals of color. Consider, for example, the impact of the best-selling book, *The Bell Curve* (Herrnstein & Murray, 1994), which, despite its numerous flaws (e.g., Fraser, 1995), was taken seriously by a large segment of the mainstream population. Although many scholars have pointed out the arbitrariness of race and the fallacies inherent in attributing presumed variations in intelligence to racial differences (e.g., Gould, 1981), beliefs about inferior intelligence have been institutionalized in the policies and practices of our public schools (Steele, Perry, & Hilliard, 2004). Much has been written about drawbacks when using intelligence tests with nonmajority populations (a point on which we elaborate elsewhere in this chapter), yet most school districts continue to classify students as mentally retarded based on IQ test scores. IQ tests reflect the cultural, social, and linguistic knowledge of the mainstream (e.g., Hilliard, 1994; Samuda, 1998), and thus, in comparison, students of color are more likely to appear deficient when, in fact, they are not. Because of concerns about the biased nature of IQ tests, numerous scholars have recommended the elimination or reduction of IQ testing. Hilliard (1995) contended that we need "either a paradigm shift or no mental measurement" (p. 6). The National Research Council (Donovan & Cross, 2002) emphasized that cutoff points for "disability" or "giftedness" are "artificial and variable" (p. 26) and called for an end to the requirement for IQ tests as a "primary criterion" for eligibility for special education (p. 313). They stated:

> IQ tests are measures of what individuals have learned—that is, it is useful to think of them as tests of general achievement, reflecting broad culturally rooted ways of thinking and problem solving. These tests are only indirect measures of success with the school curriculum and imperfect predictors of school achievement. (pp. 284–285)

Assumptions about the Importance of Contextual Issues

Students of color are at greater risk of being identified for special education when too much emphasis is placed on finding within-child deficits through a decontextualized assessment process that does not account for their opportunity to learn. Donovan and Cross (2002) emphasized that context matters. They discussed the significance of classroom context in terms of teacher effectiveness:

> The same child can perform very differently depending on the level of teacher support. . . . In practice, it can be quite difficult to distinguish internal child traits that require the ongoing support of special education from inadequate opportunity or contextual support for learning and behavior. (p. 3)

Students of color are disproportionately educated in inner-city schools that lack the resources of schools in wealthier neighborhoods. Teachers' degrees, qualifications, and licensing or certification status in affluent communities are impressive and increasingly improving, whereas teachers in high-poverty schools are underprepared and know too little about teaching culturally and linguistically diverse learners (Villegas & Lucas, 2002). In their investigation of the disproportionate representation of students of color in special education in a large, diverse school district, Harry and Klingner (2006) found that teachers in inner-city schools with predominantly African American populations had fewer advanced degrees, were less qualified, and were more likely to demonstrate weak instructional and classroom management skills than teachers in other schools in their sample. Kozol (e.g., 1991, 2005) focused the nation's attention on the failure of U.S. schools to improve the status of education for children of color from low socioeconomic backgrounds. This substantial inequality in practice actually serves to perpetuate the status quo (Gutierrez, Asato, Santos, & Gotanda, 2002).

Developmental Disabilities as Points on the Continuum of Learning and Behavior

The recent National Academy of Sciences panel (Donovan & Cross, 2002) and Harry and Klingner (2006) emphasized that being placed in special education in high-incidence-disabilities categories cannot be assumed to represent actual intrinsic deficits in children. Although disabilities have been conceptualized as distinct categories into which a child either fits or does not, in fact, dimensions of cognitive, academic, and behavioral proficiency fall along a continuum. The designation of a student as having a disability reflects a complex series of events and judgments that affect where a student falls along the spectrum of normal to disabled. The NAS report noted:

> In terms of cognitive and behavioral competence, students fall along a continuum . . . ; there is no black and white distinction between those who have disabilities or gifts and those who do not. At the far ends of the continuum there is little dispute about a children's need for something different. . . . But as one moves away from the extremes, where the line should be drawn between students who do and do not require special supports is unclear. . . . Perhaps of greater concern, however, are factors that affect where a student falls along the continuum. For students having difficulty in school that do not have a medically diagnosed disability, key aspects of the context of schooling itself . . . may contribute to their identification as having a disability and may contribute to the disproportionately high or low placements of minorities. The complexity of issues of culture and context in schools makes it nearly impossible to tease out the precise variables that affect patterns of special education placement. (Donovan & Cross, 2002, pp. 26–27)

In other words, the process of determining children's eligibility for special education is an arbitrary decision that is the result of various interrelated social forces that work together to create an identity of "dis-abled" for children whom the general education system considers too challenging to teach. At some point, a level of failure raises a red flag regarding a child's needs for the specialized services of special education.

Our position is not that disabilities do not exist but that the decisions by which students are determined to have a disability are dependent on clinical judgment and socially constructed arbitrary cutoff points along a continuum (Mercer, 1973) rather than on the empirical measurement of biological anomalies. As an example, we referred earlier to the well-known history of changeable definitions regarding MR. Although special educators have come to think of disabilities as categorical (i.e., either a child has the disability or does not) and believe that there are fail-safe assessment procedures that can "find" disabilities, challenges to the notion that disabilities are intrinsic and culture-free indicate the vulnerable nature of disability categories. Harry and Klingner (2006) studied factors that affected assessment procedures and the decision to identify a student as qualifying for special education in 12 schools. Although school personnel conveyed confidence in the power of psychological testing to distinguish between those who met eligibility criteria and those who did not, the researchers found multiple external factors that influenced the identification process: (1) teachers' informal diagnoses; (2) school personnel's negative impressions of the family; (3) pressure to identify students as having a disability by teachers and administrators (e.g., so that their scores on high-stakes tests would not count against the school); (4) the exclusion of information on classroom ecology; (5) inconsistencies in the selection of assessment instruments; (6) placement decisions based on factors other than whether or not the child was found to have a disability (e.g., to get him or her more individualized attention); (7) a disregard for established identification criteria; (8) a preference for some labels over others; and (9) inadequate attention to language acquisition issues.

Similarly, in their 5-year ethnographic study of special education placement decisions, Mehan, Hertwick, and Meihls (1986) found that the determination of special education eligibility was essentially a ratification of actions taken earlier as a "culmination, a formalization, of a lengthy process that originates in the classroom . . . when the teacher makes the first referral" (p. 165). Mehan et al. (1986) noted that the identification of a disability reflected much more than a student's measured abilities or background characteristics. Rather, eligibility decisions were the result of social processes that must be understood at both microlevel and macrolevel, taking into account the entire institutional context within which decisions about individual children's identities are made.

Even though research suggests that children are placed in special education for a variety of reasons, some of which are internal to the child and others external, it is not surprising that the cornerstone of special education, the belief in intrinsic deficits, is so pervasive and enduring. Hacking (1999) described the *idea* of disability as "interactive"; that is, by interacting with conditions, actions, and individuals, such ideas can affect people's behaviors. He explained that classifications can change the ways in which individuals experience themselves and may even cause their feelings and behaviors to evolve in part because they are so classified.

The danger in this is that when an ambiguous idea, in this case a disability label, becomes treated as a concrete reality, it colors both the individual's self-perception and others' perceptions, and it can become the overarching characterization of the individual, overshadowing the person's many other qualities and capabilities (Bogdan & Knoll, 1988; Goffman, 1963). Goffman noted that labels or classifications can become the "master status" by which the person is then defined. Labels are developed for a variety of reasons and have been applied not only to portray disabilities but also to represent other features of identity, such as race. Whereas racial classifications were developed with the intention of separating and "othering"[4] (Ferrante & Brown, 1998; Rosenblum & Travis, 2000), other categorizations, such as disability labels, have been conceptualized as a way of singling out those in need for the purpose of providing them with assistance. Yet it appears that when racial labels and disability labels are joined, the result, at least in many cases, is to cause greater harm than good. Disability labels can stigmatize students as inferior, separate them from their peers, result in lowered expectations by their teachers and others, restrict their access to educational programs, and lead to poor educational and life outcomes (Patton, 1998). For the child with the label, "to be labeled by mental deficit terminology is . . . to face a potential lifetime of self-doubt" (Gergen, 1994, p. 151).

---

[4]"Othering" is a way of delineating one's own positive identity through the illusory stigmatization and denigration of an "other." The markers of social differentiation that form the meaning of "us" and "them" can be racial, cultural, economic, geographic, or ideological.

In conclusion, even though the National Research Council acknowledges that disability categories represent "artificial and variable" cutoff points on a continuum of ability (Donovan & Cross, 2002, p. 26), it appears that few in society share this understanding. For most teachers and others, a child so labeled "has a disability" or "is retarded," in the same way that, according to one of the participants in Harry and Klingner's research (2006, p. 14), "some children have blue eyes."

ACCESS ISSUES AND BARRIERS FOR DIVERSE INDIVIDUALS AND FAMILIES

Next we portray service delivery access issues and barriers for diverse individuals with developmental disabilities and their families. These include, but are not limited to, differing cultural perspectives of disability, limited access and unfamiliarity with available service delivery options, service providers' lack of understanding of the impact of families' race, social class, cultural values and beliefs, experiences, and perspective of disabilities on service delivery, and families' lack of access to culturally and linguistically responsive curricula and services (e.g., Harry et al., 1999; Rueda, Monzo, Blacher, Shapiro, & Gonzalez, 2005).

Families' Cultural Beliefs and the Institutional Culture of Special Education Disconnection

Because families' cultural beliefs and cultural frames of reference influence their understanding, acceptance, and perspectives of disability, it is important that educators and service providers understand how issues of culture influence families' perceptions of disability and ultimately their experiences in securing services for their loved ones with developmental disabilities. Research has clearly documented that parents' culture, values, and beliefs influence how they perceive and respond to their child with a disability (e.g., Harris, 1996; Harry, 1992). Most families go through a process of grieving over the birth of a child with significant disabilities and eventually move through various stages toward acceptance of the reality that their child has a disability that may alter their child's life as well as their dreams for their child. Yet parents' adaptation to and acceptance of their child's condition varies. For example, in research comparing the attitudes of mothers toward the birth of a child with a developmental disability, Mary (1990) found that Hispanic mothers were more likely than white or African American mothers to adopt an attitude of "self-sacrifice toward their young child with a disability." Similarly, in her research with African American parents and Hispanic parents, Harry (1992) found that these mothers were more likely to see the birth of their child with a developmental disability as a "gift from God" and, as such, believed that it was their responsibility to care for their children, not the responsibility of external caregivers.

Parents' cultural perspectives of disability also affect the extent to which they seek out relevant services. Parents' cultural perspectives also play a role in how they experience the American special education system. For example, according to Kalyanpur and Harry (1999), special education is grounded in three core American macrocultural values that are major tenets of the Individuals with Disabilities Education Act of 1990 (IDEA): individualism, equity, and choice. In providing an explanation of how these core macrocultural values affect special education, they indicated that, "the value of individualism underlies the principles of due process and individualized, appropriate education, whereas the principles of parent participation and the least restrictive environment are grounded in the right to freedom of choice. Similarly, the value of equity is embedded in the principles of zero reject, nondiscriminatory assessment, and parental participation" (p. 20). To work effectively with ethnically, culturally, and linguistically diverse individuals with developmental disabilities and their families, educators and service providers must be aware that special education is a cultural institution that may or may not reflect the values, belief, and cultural perspectives of all parents. This is particularly true for parents of color, as well as parents who are not native English speakers. Hence, it is critically important that educators and service providers engage in dialogue that will allow parents to share their perspectives on developmental disabilities in a nonthreatening manner and to have those perspectives respected and included in the provision of service delivery options afforded them.

Limited Access and Unfamiliarity with Available Services

The professional literature is replete with documentation of the limited access to or unfamiliarity with available special education, community, and human services that afflicts individuals of color with developmental disabilities and their families. Although people of color with developmental disabilities across all socioeconomic levels experience access issues, access to appropriate services and unfamiliarity with available services seems to be further compounded by lower socioeconomic status and by living in either rural or urban areas (Gammon, 2000; Reichard, Sacco, & Turnbull, 2004). This is especially true for families who are caring for adults with MR or developmental disabilities, because they tend to be more isolated, less supported, and more in need of comprehensive services than parents of younger individuals with MR or developmental disabilities (Black, Cohn, Smull, & Crites, 1985; Hayden & DePaepe, 1994). Additionally, once individuals of color with developmental disabilities exit the public school system, their families and caregivers encounter even greater hardships and more access difficulties because available services are severely limited, especially in rural areas (Gammon, 2000).

Families of color experience greater difficulties in access and utilization of social services, and as such they are less likely than majority families to receive innovative or best-practices services such as "family support system" and "supported employment" (e.g., Traustadottir, Lutfiyya, & Shoultz, 1994). The barriers to access for individuals of color with developmental disabilities and their families often are issues related to poverty, racism, and a lack of culturally relevant services. As a result of not receiving access to innovative services, individuals of color and their families with developmental disabilities must continue to rely on the traditional supports of Supplemental Security Income (SSI) checks and health insurance in the form of Medicaid (Children's Defense Fund, 1974). African Americans with developmental disabilities and their families may tend to rely heavily on the traditional supports of SSI and Medicaid because families are often so consumed with the struggle for survival as they deal with the realities of living in poverty while serving as caregivers that they just do not have the energy or time to pursue special programs and services (Harry, 1992).

Another issue that affects families of color in their pursuit of appropriate services for their children with developmental disabilities is the availability of health care providers who accept Medicaid and who are also adequately trained to treat individuals with developmental disabilities (Donovan & Cross, 2002; Reichard et al., 2004).

Although this is a problem for many families, regardless of their race, families of color are disproportionately poor, and, when they also live in rural areas, it is difficult for them to identify physicians and dentists who are both trained and willing to treat patients with developmental disabilities because of the additional time involved in treating these patients and the often limited means of communication. Even when individuals of color with developmental disabilities and their families have access to needed special education and relevant social, community, and adult services, these services are often not culturally and linguistically sensitive; even more rarely are they culturally and linguistically responsive (Harry, 1992; Gammon, 2000).

Traditional versus Culturally and Linguistically Responsive Service Delivery

Traditional service delivery models have tended to approach developmental disabilities from the perspective that race, class, cultural beliefs and values, and language do not influence service delivery options and the quality of the services ultimately provided to individuals with developmental disabilities and their families (Ford et al., 2006). In recent years, researchers (e.g., Ford et al., 2006; Harry et al., 1999; Reichard et al., 2004) have emphasized the need to reexamine assessments, educational and social service practices, and interventions to ensure that they are culturally sensitive and better targeted toward diverse individuals and their families. However, despite numerous calls (e.g., Gammon, 2000) for the curricula, assessments, and services used with students with developmental disabilities to be culturally responsive and tailored to students' learning styles, family values, and cultural and linguistic frames of reference, they continue to be largely monocultural.

To ensure that the values, beliefs, and perspectives of diverse individuals with developmental disabilities and their families are considered when conducting assessments and developing and implementing services, it is important for service providers to be knowledgeable about what it means to provide culturally and linguistically responsive services. As stated earlier, culturally and linguistically responsive services are those services that recognize, value, and infuse the ethnic, cultural, and linguistic knowledge of individuals of color with developmental disabilities to inform pedagogical and service delivery practices and to employ that knowledge to design instructional strategies, communication strategies, assessment tools, and service delivery models. Service providers who provide culturally and linguistically relevant services acknowledge that the American special education system is grounded in American macrocultural values regarding communication and language and that, as such, it disproportionately favors parents who speak English as a first language and those who speak and comprehend the "official" language. The term "official" language is used here to refer to the professional jargon that is most commonly used by teachers and professionals in the special education system that draws heavily on white middle-class communication and language patterns and styles.

Implications for Working Effectively with Diverse Students and Families

In response to the many issues and challenges we have described, we offer several suggestions for working with students of color with disabilities and their families.

1. Recognize the impact of issues of race, class, culture, language, and social class on families' access to relevant special education and social and community services. For example, educators and service providers who work with diverse students and families need to be educated about how race, class, culture, language, and social class may serve as barriers and thereby result in diverse families having limited access to relevant special education and human and community services.

2. Acknowledge that special education and related service provisions are based on white, middle-class, English-speaking cultural norms and values and may not reflect the cultural beliefs and values of diverse families, especially those who live in poverty and for whom English is not their first language.

3. Communicate with students and families in their native language using a professional interpreter rather than a family member.

4. Communicate using lay and cultural terminology and avoid overreliance on professional jargon.

5. When meeting with families, ask about their hopes and dreams for their child, and recognize that these may be different from those typical of mainstream culture (but just as valid).

6. Make sure that printed materials are prepared in the native language.

7. Learn about and respect cultural, communication, and language norms and mores.

8. Be familiar with and acknowledge within-group ethnic, cultural, linguistic, and social-class differences. For example, educators and service providers must recognize that even though diverse families might be members of a larger ethnic, culture, racial, or linguistic group, they are individuals and should be treated as such.

9. Whenever possible, provide services to ethnically, culturally, and linguistically diverse families within the context of relevant community or cultural centers.

10. Involve individuals of color in the development of appropriate individualized education plans (IEPs) and individualized family-service plans (IFSPs) that reflect their values and priorities.

CONCLUSION

In summary, in this chapter we attempted to illuminate the complex intersections of race, culture, language, social class, and disability and how these play out in U.S. schools, currently as well as from a historical perspective. We emphasized the central role of culture in shaping notions of normalcy and disability. We challenged acultural and monocultural views of intelligence and describe problematic testing procedures. We discussed the alarming overrepresentation of students of color, particularly African American students, in programs for students with mental retardation and disputed simplistic views of this phenomenon. We tried to raise awareness about the challenges students of color with developmental disabilities and their families face when trying to access appropriate services. Our hope is that the reader will be concerned about how limited conceptualizations of culture can further marginalize students of color and their families. More important, we would like to encourage researchers to keep culture in mind when conducting research and to recognize that race, language, and social class are also critically important contextual variables that must be included and continuously examined in today's educational research.

REFERENCES

American Association on Mental Retardation. (2002). *Mental retardation: Definition classification and systems of supports* (10th ed.). Washington, DC: Author.

Artiles, A. J., Rueda, R., Salazar, J., & Higareda, I. (2005). Within-group diversity in minority disproportionate representation: English language learners in urban school districts. *Exceptional Children, 71,* 283–300.

August, D., & Hakuta, K. (1997). *Improving schooling for language minority children: A research agenda.* Washington, DC: National Academy Press.

Black, M. M., Cohn, J. F., Smull, M. W., & Crites, L. S. (1985). Individual and family factors associated with risk of institutionalization of mentally retarded adults. *American Journal of Mental Deficiency, 90*(3), 271–276.

Blanchett, W. J. (2006). Disproportionate representation of African Americans in special education: Acknowledging the role of White privilege and racism. *Educational Researcher, 35*(6), 24–28.

Blau, P., & Duncan, O. D. (1967). *The American occupational structure.* New York: Wiley.

Bogdan, R. (1992). A "simple" farmer accused of murder: Community acceptance and the meaning of deviance. *Disability, Handicap and Society, 7,* 303–320.

Bogdan, R., & Knoll, J. (1988). The sociology of disability. In E. L. Meyen & T. M. Skrtic (Eds.), *Exceptional children and youth* (3rd ed., pp. 449–477). Denver, CO: Love.

Bowles, S., & Gintis, H. (1976) *Schooling in capitalist America.* New York: Basic Books.

Bronfenbrenner, U. (1977). Toward an experimental ecology of human development. *American Psychologist, 32,* 513–531.

Brown v. Board of Education, 347 U.S. 483 (1954). Available at *www.nps.gov/brub/pages/decisions54. htm*

Bullivant, B. M. (1993). Culture: Its nature and meaning for educators. In J. A. Banks & A. M. Banks (Eds.), *Multi-cultural education: Issues and perspectives* (pp. 27–46). Boston: Allyn & Bacon.

Cazden, C. B., & John, V. P. (1971). Learning in American Indian children. In M. L. Wax, S. Diamond, & F. O. Gearing (Eds.), *Anthropological perspectives in education* (pp. 252–272). New York: Basic Books.

Chamberlain, S. P. (2005). Issues of overrepresentation and educational equity for culturally and linguistically diverse students. *Intervention in School and Clinic, 41*(2), 110–113.

Children's Defense Fund. (1974). *Children out of school in America.* Washington, DC: Author.

Cole, M. (1996). *Cultural psychology: A once and future discipline.* Cambridge, MA: Harvard University Press.

Cole, M., & Bruner, J. (1971). Cultural differences and inferences about psychological processes. *American Psychologist, 26,* 867–876.

Cole, M., Gay, J., Glick, J, & Sharp, D. W. (1971). *The cultural context of learning and thinking.* New York: Basic Books.

Correa, V. I. (1989) Involving culturally diverse families in the educational process. In S. H. Fradd & M. J. Weismantel (Eds.), *Meeting the needs of culturally and linguistically different students* (pp. 130–144). Boston: College Hill Press.

Cummins, J. (1984). *Bilingualism and special education: Issues in assessment and pedagogy.* San Diego, CA: College Hill.

Diana v. State Board of Education, CA 70 RFT (N.D. Cal. 1970).

Donovan, S., & Cross, C. (2002). *Minority students in special and gifted education.* Washington, DC: National Academies Press.

Dunn, L. (1968). Special education for the mildly retarded: Is much of it justifiable? *Exceptional Children, 35,* 5–22.

Fadiman, A. (1997). *The spirit catches you and you fall down: A Hmong child, her American doctors, and the collision of two cultures.* New York: Farrar, Straus & Giroux.

Ferrante, J., & Brown, P. (1998). Classifying people by race. In J. Ferrante & P. Brown (Eds.), *The social construction of race and ethnicity in the United States* (pp. 109–119). New York: Longman.

Ferri, B. A., & Connor, D. (2005). Tools of exclusion: Race, disability and (re)segregated education. *Teachers College Record, 107,* 453–474.

Fierros, E. G., & Conroy, J. W. (2002). Double jeopardy: An exploration of restrictiveness and race in special education. In D. Losen & G. Orfield (Eds.), *Racial inequity in special education* (pp. 39–70). Cambridge, MA: Harvard Education Press.

Figueroa, R. A. (1989). Psychological testing of linguistic-minority students: Knowledge gaps and regulations. *Exceptional Children, 56,* 145–152.

Figueroa, R. A., & Sassenrath, J. M. (1989). A longitudinal study of the predictive validity of the system of multicultural pluralistic assessment. *Psychology in the Schools, 26,* 5–19.

Ford, A., Blanchett, W., & Brown, L. (2006). *Teacher education and students with significant disabilities: Revisiting essential elements* (COPSSE Document No. 1B–11). Gainesville: University of Florida, Center on Personnel Studies in Special Education.

Fraser, S. (Ed.). (1995). *The bell curve wars: Race, intelligence, and the future of America.* New York: Basic Books.

Fujiura, G. T., & Yamaki, K. (1997). Analysis of ethnic variations in developmental disability prevalence and household economic status. *Mental Retardation, 35,* 286–294.

Gallego, M. A., Cole, M., & The Laboratory of Human Cognition. (2002). Classroom cultures and cultures in classrooms. In V. Richardson (Ed.), *Handbook of research on teaching* (4th ed., pp. 951–997). Washington, DC: American Educational Research Association.

Gammon, E. (2000). Examining the needs of culturally diverse rural caregivers who have adults with severe developmental disabilities living with them. *Families in Society, 81,* 174–185.

Garcia, G. E., & Pearson, P. D. (1994). Assessment and diversity. In L. Darling-Hammond (Ed.), *Review of research in education* (Vol. 20, pp. 337–391). Washington, DC: American Educational Research Association.

Gergen, K. J. (1994). *Realities and relationships: Soundings in social construction.* Cambridge, MA: Harvard University Press.

Goffman, E. (1963). *Stigma: Notes on the management of spoiled identity.* Englewood Cliffs, NJ: Prentice-Hall.

Goodnow, J. J. (1976). The nature of intelligent behavior: Questions raised by cross-cultural studies. In L. B. Resnick (Ed.), *The nature of intelligence* (pp. 168–188). Hillsdale, NJ: Erlbaum.

Gould, S. J. (1981). *The mismeasure of man.* New York: Norton.

Greenfield, P. M., & Childs, C. P. (1977). Weaving, color terms and pattern representation: Cultural influences and cognitive development among the Zinancantecos of Southern Mexico. *Inter-American Journal of Psychology, 11,* 23–48.

Guadalupe Organization v. Tempe Elementary School District No. 3, 71-435 (1973). U.S. Dist. Court, District of Arizona.

Gutierrez, K. D., Asato, J., Santos, M., & Gotanda, N. (2002). Backlash pedagogy: Language and culture and the politics of reform. *Review of Education, Pedagogy, and Cultural Studies, 24,* 335–351.

Hacking, I. (1999). *The social construction of what?* Cambridge, MA: Harvard University Press.

Harris, S. L. (1996). Serving families of children with developmental disabilities: Reaching diverse populations. *Special Services, 12,* 79–86.

Harry, B. (1992). Restructuring the participation of African American parents in special education. *Exceptional Children, 59,* 123–131.

Harry, B., Kalyanpur, M., & Day, M. (1999). *Building cultural reciprocity with families: Case studies in special education.* Baltimore: Brookes.

Harry, B., & Klingner, J. K. (2006). *Why are so many minority students in special education? Understanding race and disability in schools.* New York: Teachers College Press.

Hayden, M., & DePaepe, P. (1994). Waiting for community services: The impact on persons with mental retardation and other developmental disabilities. In M. Hayden & B. Abery (Eds.), *Challenges for a service system in transition: Ensuring quality, community experiences for persons with developmental disabilities* (pp. 173–206). Baltimore: Brookes.

Heath, S. B. (1983). *Ways with words: Language, life, and work in communities and classrooms.* New York: Cambridge University Press.

Heller, K. A., Holtzman, W. H., & Messick, S. (Eds.). (1982). *Placing children in special education: A strategy for equity.* Washington, DC: National Academy Press.

Herrnstein, R., & Murray, C. (1994). *The bell curve: Intelligence and class structure in American life.* New York: Free Press.

Hilliard, A. G. (1977). The predictive validity of norm-referenced standardized tests: Piaget or Binet? *Negro Educational Review, 25,* 189–201.

Hilliard, A. G., III. (1994). What good is this thing called intelligence and why bother to measure it? *Journal of Black Psychology, 20,* 430–444.

Hilliard, A. G., III. (1995). Either a paradigm shift or no mental measurement: The non-science and nonsense of *The Bell Curve*. *Psych Discourse, 76*(10), 6–20.

Jacob-Timm, S., & Hartshorne, T. S. (1998). *Ethics and law for school psychologists.* New York: Wiley.

Johnson v. San Francisco Unified School District, 339 F. Supp. 1315 (N.D. Cal. 1971).

Kalyanpur, M., & Harry, B. (1999). *Culture in special education: Building reciprocal family-professional relationships.* Baltimore: Brookes.

Klingner, J. K., Artiles, A. J., Kozleski, E., Harry, B., Zion, S., Tate, W., et al. (2005). Addressing the disproportionate representation of culturally and linguistically diverse students in special education through culturally responsive educational systems. *Education Policy Analysis Archives, 13*(38), 1–39.

Kozol, J. (1991) *Savage inequalities: Children in America's schools.* New York: Crown.

Kozol, J. (2005). *The shame of the nation: The restoration of apartheid schooling in America.* New York: Crown.

Langdon, H. W. (1989). Language disorder or language difference? Assessing the language skills of Hispanic students. *Exceptional Children, 56,* 160–167.

Laosa, L. M. (1977). Nonbiased assessment of children's abilities: Historical antecedents and current issues. In T. Oakland (Ed.), *Psychological and educational assessment of minority children* (pp. 1–20). New York: Brunner/Mazel.

Larry P. v. Riles, 343 F, Supp 1308 (N.D. Cal. 1972). Preliminary injunction.

LeRoy, B., & Kulik, N. (2003). *The demography of inclusive education.* Detroit, MI: Developmental Disabilities Institute.

Locust, C. (1988). Wounding the spirit: Discrimination and traditional American Indian belief systems. *Harvard Educational Review, 58,* 315–330.

Losen, D. J., & Orfield, G. (Eds.). (2002). *Racial inequity in special education.* Cambridge, MA: Harvard University Press.

MacMillan, D. L., & Reschly, D. L. (1998). Overrepresentation of minority students: The case for greater specificity or reconsideration of the variables examined. *Journal of Special Education, 32,* 15–24.

Mary, N. L. (1990). Reactions of black, hispanic, and white mothers to having a child with handicaps. *Mental Retardation, 28,* 1–5.

Mehan, H., Hertwick, A., & Meihls, J. L. (1986). *Handicapping the handicapped: Decision-making in students' educational careers.* Stanford, CA: Stanford University Press.

Mercer, J. (1973). *Labeling the mentally retarded.* Berkeley: University of California Press.

Oakes, J. (1985). *Keeping track: How schools structure inequality.* New Haven, CT: Yale University Press.

Ochoa, S. H., Powell, M. P., & Robles-Piña, R. (1996). School psychologists' assessment practices with bilingual and limited-English-proficient students. *Journal of Psychoeducational Assessment, 14,* 250–275.

Ochoa, S. H., Rivera, B. D., & Powell, M. P. (1997). Factors used to comply with the exclusionary clause with bilingual and limited-English-proficient pupils: Initial guidelines. *Learning Disabilities Research and Practice, 12,* 161–167.

O'Connor, C. (2002). Black women beating the odds from one generation to the next: How the changing dynamics of constraint and opportunity affect the process of educational resilience. *American Educational Research Journal, 39,* 855–903.

O'Connor, C., & Fernandez, S. D. (2006). Race, class, and disproportionality: Reevaluating the relationship between poverty and special education placement. *Educational Researcher, 35*(6), 6–11.

Oller, J. W., Jr. (1991). *Language and bilingualism.* Cranbury, NJ: Bucknell University Press.

Oswald, D. P., Coutinho, M. J., Best, A. M., & Singh, N. (1999). Ethnic representation in special education: The influence of school-related economic and demographic variables. *Journal of Special Education, 32,* 194–206.

Patton, J. M. (1998). The disproportionate representation of African-Americans in special education: Looking behind the curtain for understanding and solutions. *Journal of Special Education, 32,* 25–31.

Prasse, D., & Reschly, D. (1986). Larry P.: A case of segregation, testing, or program efficacy? *Exceptional Children, 52,* 333–346.

Reichard, A., Sacco, T. M., & Turnbull, R. (2004). Access to health care for individuals with developmental disabilities from minority backgrounds. *Mental Retardation, 42,* 459–470.

Reid, D. K., & Knight, M. G. (2006). Disability justifies exclusion of minority students: A critical history grounded in disability studies. *Educational Researcher, 35*(6), 18–23.

Reschly, D. J., Myers, T. G., & Hartel, C. R. (Eds.). (2002). *Mental retardation: Determining eligibility for Social Security benefits.* Washington, DC: National Academy Press.

Rogoff, B. (2003). *The cultural nature of human development.* New York: Oxford University Press.

Rogoff, B., & Chavajay, P. (1995). What's become of research on the cultural basis of cognitive development? *American Psychologist, 50,* 859–877.

Rogoff, B., & Waddell, K. J. (1982). Memory for information organized in a scene by children from two cultures. *Child Development, 53,* 1224–1228.

Rosenblum, K. E., & Travis, T. C. (2000). *The meaning of difference: American constructions of race, sex and gender, social class, and sexual orientation.* New York: McGraw–Hill.

Rueda, R. (1997). Changing the context of assessment: The move to portfolios and authentic assessment. In A. J. Artiles & G. Zamora-Duran (Eds.), *Reducing the disproportionate representation of culturally diverse students in special and gifted education* (pp. 7–25). Reston, VA: Council for Exceptional Children.

Rueda, R., Monzo, L., Blacher, J., Shapiro, J., & Gonzalez, J. (2005). Cultural models and practices regarding transition: A view from Latina mothers of young adults with developmental disabilities. *Exceptional Children, 71,* 401–414.

Samuda, R. J. (1989). Psychometric factors in the appraisal of intelligence. In R. J. Samuda & S. L. Kong (Eds.), *Assessment and placement of minority students* (pp. 25–40). Toronto, Ontario, Canada: Hogrefe.

Samuda, R. J. (1998). *Psychological testing of American minorities: Issues and consequences* (2nd ed.). Thousand Oaks, CA: Sage.

Serpell, R. (1994). The cultural construction of intelligence. In W. J. Lonner & R. S. Malpass (Eds.), *Readings in psychology and culture* (pp. 157–163). Boston: Allyn & Bacon.

Serpell, R., Mariga, L., & Harvey, K. (1993). Mental retardation in African countries: Conceptualization, services, and research. *International Review of Research in Mental Retardation, 19,* 1–39.

Sewell, W. H., Haller, A. O., & Portes, A. (1969). The educational and early occupational attainment process. *American Sociological Review, 34,* 82–92.

Skiba, R. J., Poloni-Staudinger, L., Simmons, A. B., Feggins, L. R., & Chung, C. G. (2005). Unproven links: Can poverty explain ethnic disproportionality in special education? *Journal of Special Education, 39*(3), 130–144.

Steele, C., Perry, T., & Hilliard, A., III. (2004). *Young, gifted, and Black: Promoting high achievement among African American students.* Boston: Beacon Press.

Traustadottir, R., Lutfiyya, Z. M., & Shoultz, B. (1994). Community living: A multicultural perspective. In M. Hayden & B. Abery (Eds.), *Challenges for a service system in transition: Ensuring quality community experiences for persons with developmental disabilities* (pp. 405–426). Baltimore: Brookes.

Tucker, J. A. (1977). Operationalizing the diagnostic-intervention process. In T. Oakland (Ed.), *Psychological and educational assessment of minority children* (pp. 91–111). New York: Brunner/Mazel.

U.S. Department of Education. (2002). *24th annual report to Congress.* Washington, DC: Author.

U.S. Department of Education, Office of Special Education Programs. (2003). *25th annual report to Congress.* Washington, DC: Author.

Valdés, G., & Figueroa, R. A. (1994). *Bilingualism and testing: A special case of bias.* Norwood, NJ: Ablex.

Villegas, A. M., & Lucas, T. (2002). Preparing culturally responsive teachers: Rethinking the curriculum. *Journal of Teacher Education; 53*(1), 20–32.

Williams, R. L. (1974). The problem of match and mis-match in testing Black children. In L. P. Miller (Ed.), *The testing of Black students: A symposium* (pp. 17–30). Englewood Cliffs, NJ: Prentice-Hall.

Wober, M. (1972). Culture and the concept of intelligence: A case in Uganda. *Journal of Cross-Cultural Psychology, 3,* 327–328.

CURRENT ISSUES IN HEALTH, NEUROSCIENCE, AND GENETICS

Without trying to sound hyperbolic, the chapters in this section underscore how far we have come since the United States first put a man on the moon. Certainly, we never would have anticipated the current advances in neuroscience or genetics, today's concerns for basic health issues, and the focus on the "whole person" with developmental disabilities. Together, the following three chapters build stronger linkages among genetics, cognition, behavior, and environment. The new information in these chapters challenges the proverbial nature vs. nurture debate by requiring more targeted strategies for intervention and teaching.

Almost in defiance of the old saying, "You can't take it with you," these chapters emphasize the opposite. Nehring and Betz provide a comprehensive overview of general health issues for persons with developmental disabilities. Certainly, this population has rarely had equal access to quality health services, and with full inclusion of individuals with serious health/medical conditions, the availability of high standards of care in community settings becomes even more crucial. Equity issues go beyond access, according to Nehring and Betz, and include affordability and maintenance across the life course. All too often, even if persons with developmental disabilities have health care, there is no guarantee that they will always have it. At some point, they may find themselves uninsured, or at the very least, underinsured. Thus, they "can take it with them" only if they have affordable, accessible health care to begin with!

One thing we can—and do—take with us from conception is our genes. The advances in genetics detailed in the chapter by Tartaglia, Hansen, and Hagerman, underscore the role that genes play in the development of cognition, learning, and behavior. In addition, these authors weave together different strands of research, from the identification of gene abnormalities to behavioral phenotyping of genetic syndromes. Although the authors note that there is no "cure" for genetic disorders at this time, they do provide examples of treatment recommendations and educational interventions for some specific syndromes, and speculate upon future medical interventions that may reduce or eliminate cognitive and behavioral problems.

One of the most significant changes taking place in the field of developmental disabilities in general is recent knowledge of "the nature" of disabilities. Certainly developments in neuroscience have contributed to a better understanding of the relationship between biological markers and behavior. The chapter by Sandman and Kemp provides an intensive overview of the neuroscience of developmental disorders, with a targeted presentation of neuroimaging and its capabilities for identifying and defining brain structures within and between phenotypes. Rather than leaving the reader with a sense that neurodevelopment is preordained and unalterable, the authors highlight exciting new developments in the field that point to future possibilities for repair of the nervous system.

Together, the chapters in this section provide both a bold reality of the challenges of developmental disabilities and an optimistic view of future possibilities.

5

General Health

Wendy M. Nehring
Cecily L. Betz

The health of persons with intellectual disabilities has been a topic of discussion for several hundreds of years, but even today, in the early years of the 21st century, we are still discussing the principle that every person, regardless of disability and ethnicity, deserves access to affordable, quality health care. We have learned much about conditions that cause intellectual disabilities over the years through research at the cellular level, on patterns of inheritance, on the influence of and interaction between an individual genotype and the environment, and on medications and immunizations that can help prevent the onset of intellectual disabilities. We have also made many accomplishments in the field of health and medical sciences, from the evolution of the practice of obstetrical and gynecological care to the invention of machines that can help in diagnosis and treatment and that can enhance survival. Yet further conditions are emerging, such as environmental neurotoxicants, that will result in continual incidences of intellectual disabilities or an increase in secondary conditions. The health status and health disparities that exist for persons with intellectual disabilities has come to the attention of the current and past surgeon generals, and it is time to address the disparities that exist so that all people can experience improved outcomes that result from appropriate and adequate health care. In this chapter, we address the issues that have arisen across time for health care professionals, provide a summary of relevant and current research and accomplishments in health care, discuss emerging conditions and research that will influence the next generation, and conclude with implications for practitioners, policy makers, and researchers.

RELEVANT DEFINITIONS

Over the years, health care professionals have defined and classified persons with intellectual disabilities. In 1877, William W. Ireland wrote *On Idiocy and Imbecility*, in which he defined 12 subclassifications of what we now term "mental retardation." For the first time, the focus was on disease. Subsequent classifications were based on the etiologies that were thought to cause mental retardation at that time. For example, in the late 1800s, George Shuttleworth, Issac Kerlin, and Harvey B. Wilbur, all physicians, thought that mental retardation was caused by congenital factors or by accident (Whitney, 1950). In 1903, members of the Association of Medical Officers of American Institutions for Idiotic and Feebleminded Persons (now the American Association on Intellectual and Developmental Disabilities [AAIDD]) developed a classification scheme based on etiology. This early knowledge is compared with our understanding of the various etiologies today in Table 5.1.

The 10th edition of the AAIDD definition and classification text was published in 2002 (Luckasson et al., 2002) and is based on an environmental support model. Although the definition has not varied much in several years, the classification model has radically changed. Since the ninth edition in 1992, the categories of mild, moderate, severe, and profound were replaced with levels of support. In other words, a person is assessed by the levels of support that are needed to live at an optimal level. The 1992 edition also introduced categories of risk: biomedical, social, behavioral, and educational (Luckasson et al., 1992). The American Psychological Association has retained the four categories of functioning in its classification system, which is based on psychological assessment (Jacobson & Mulick, 1996).

Another important classification system that has international appeal is the one developed by the World Health Organization titled *International Classification of Functioning, Disability, and Health* (ICIDH-2; 2001). This recently developed classification system is designed to describe the health and health-related features of well-being. The classification system uses a biopsychosocial framework and recognizes the complexity of living with a disability in terms of the impact on bodily functions and structure and level of functioning as denoted by activities and participation. Environmental factors are identified in terms of their effect on the individual's bodily functions, level of activities, and societal participation.

Across time, it is important to note that these definitions and classifications have served professionals in their efforts to provide treatment and seek funding for programs. These definitions and classifications have evolved as a result of changes in societal view; feedback from individuals with intellectual disabilities and their families; the work of advocates and professionals; and changing budgets and governmental emphases. These issues were discussed in Chapter 1, this volume.

HEALTH-RELATED ISSUES AFFECTING HEALTH PROFESSIONALS ACROSS TIME

A number of health-related issues have affected health professionals across the past century. These issues include segregation, sterilization, deinstitutionalization, delivery systems of care, and stigma. Although other issues exist, these issues are highlighted in this chapter.

TABLE 5.1. A Comparison of the Etiologies of Mental Retardation, 1903 and 2005

Scheme for etiological study—1903[a]	Etiologies of mental retardation—2005[b]

A. Before labor
  1. Hereditary
  2. Health of parents
    a. Syphilis
    b. Tuberculosis
  3. Alcohol
  4. Health and condition of father at the time of conception
  5. Injury to mother during pregnancy
  6. Worry, anxiety, and grief to mother during pregnancy
  7. Uterine or placental disease
  8. Imperfected cerebral development—origin undetected
  9. Sporadic cretinism
B. During labor—trauma
  1. Instrumental
  2. Noninstrumental
C. After labor
  1. Trauma
  2. Disease
	A. Prenatal causes
	  1. Genetic abnormalities, including chromosomal abnormalities (e.g., trisomies, X-chromosomal, micro-deletions, and subtelomeric rearrangements), single-gene disorders (e.g., X-linked recessive conditions), multifactorial/polygenic conditions (e.g., spina bifida), and unknown genetic etiologies
	  2. Congenital infections (e.g., rubella)
	  3. Alcohol and other drug exposure
	  4. Other teratogens
	  5. Disorders in the pregnant woman (e.g., maternal diabetes mellitus)
	B. Perinatal causes
	  1. Placental complications
	  2. Pre-eclampsia and eclampsia
	  3. Birth trauma
	  4. Metabolic abnormalities (e.g., hypoglycemia and hyperbilirubinemia)
	  5. Complications of prematurity (e.g., hypoxia and ischemia)
	  6. Infections (e.g., bacterial meningitis)
	  7. Intracerebral hemorrhage
	C. Postnatal causes
	  1. Infections (e.g., *Haemophilus influenzae* type B, *Streptococcus pneumoniae*)
	  2. Trauma
	    a. Accidental
	    b. Nonaccidental
	  3. Environmental pollutants/neurotoxicants
	  4. Environmental deprivation
	  5. Malnutrition
	  6. Inborn errors of metabolism
	  7. Multifactorial and familial
	D. Unknown causes

[a]Data from Sloan and Stevens (1976).
[b]Data from Lashley (2005) and Handmaker (2005).

Segregation

During the early years of the 1900s, eugenics was the norm as society strove to cast off anyone who did not meet the expected behavior or appearance. Society feared persons with intellectual disabilities and, as a result, institutions, asylums, and poorhouses arose so that such individuals could be separated from society (Crane, 1907). The depression years further hampered some families' efforts to keep their family members with intellectual disabilities at home; often because of financial problems, they had to institutionalize their family members (Trent, 1994). Even into the 1960s, when a child was born with intellectual disabilities, physicians told the father that the child should be committed to an institution while telling the mother that the child had died. Other families were assured that committing their child to an institution would be in the "best interest" of the child and family as a means of alleviating caretaker burden and lack of available resources in the community. Some families were advised that their child's prognosis implied a shortened lifespan, extending into adolescence at best, and a level of functioning that was extremely limited.

Sterilization

Laughlin (1926) wrote that the state in which he lived had two specific duties in thwarting the problem of "feeblemindedness": segregation and sterilization. The first sterilization law was passed in 1907 in Indiana; this movement did not wane until after World War II (Devine, 1983), although the legal debate continued on until the 1970s (Trent, 1994).

Deinstitutionalization

Deinstitutionalization, occurring largely in the late 1960s and 1970s, radically altered residential care of persons with intellectual disabilities. This movement took place because society witnessed, through books and television, the many horrible conditions that existed in these places (Blatt & Kaplan, 1966; Edgerton, 1967). But the move into the community has not been without problems. At first, many communities did not want to accept group homes in their neighborhoods. Differences in the standards of care became obvious between settings, and this continues to be a problem today. Additionally, many families, accustomed to the level of care and protection provided by large congregate facilities on self-contained and segregated campuses, were resistant to having their children relocated into inclusive community settings.

Delivery Systems of Care

Medical care in the institutions was led by physicians. This was a unidimensional model of care and was focused on a diagnosis of illness and subsequent needed treatments. By the 1940s, another delivery system of care emerged—the multidisciplinary team. The physician remained the leader of the team, but assessments and plans for care were deliberated among the different professionals who saw the individual with intellectual disabilities. It was the physician who summarized the results and shared them with the individual and his or her family (Foley, 1990).

Twenty years later, President John F. Kennedy instituted overarching changes in the care of persons with mental illness and mental retardation by establishing the President's Panel on Mental Retardation (1962). One of the recommendations of this presidential panel called for using a new and innovative model of care, the interdisciplinary team. Services offered included prevention, early case finding, care, and follow-up provided by an interdisciplinary team of professionals. Still viewed today as the model of choice, this form of delivery includes the individual with intellectual disabilities and his or her family members as core members of the team. In this model, professionals and consumers alike are seated around the table and are equal participants in assessment and deliberations to determine what the plan of care will be for that individual. Unlike the models of the past, the team leader of an interdisciplinary team is usually the professional, regardless of discipline, whose expertise is most needed by the individual.

The transdisciplinary model developed during the 1980s was used most often in early intervention programs. In this model, the professionals share in the delivery of care; it is not necessarily divided by discipline. For example, an occupational therapist could assist with the physical therapy for an individual. This model has not worked successfully due to territorial issues (Robinson, 1997).

It should be noted that these models of care have largely been used in segregated settings, such as institutions, group homes, clinics, and early-intervention programs, in which health care professionals care for persons with intellectual disabilities. Now, in the time of deinstitutionalization, health care professionals have debated about whether health care is best given in these segregated settings or in the primary health care settings in the community. This debate continues today, and we mention it again later in discussing the reports from the current and past surgeon generals.

Stigma

Stigma and prejudice constitute the final overarching health issue seen across time. As can be seen from the discussion of segregation, society has not viewed differentness as an acceptable trait. We continue to see this generalized view as we examine cultural differences today. The culture of disability is another form of culture. There is indeed a stigma and prejudice associated with this population. Although advances have been made in promoting improved quality of life for individuals with intellectual disabilities, as evidenced by their living and working in inclusive communities, there is considerable progress yet to be achieved. Some individuals with intellectual disability have obtained roles as actors on television and in the movies, but this is rare, as members of the general public still want to see "perfection" in their role models.

There is further stigma for the professionals who care for this population. For example, as nurses, we did not see this specialty recognized by the American Nurses Association until 1997 (Nehring, 1999). At that time, the letter that granted this recognition had a postscript that asked, "What is the difference between developmental disabilities and physical disabilities?" Health care professionals may respond in a prejudicial manner with unwillingness to provide care to individuals with intellectual disabilities due to beliefs that they are of impaired value and worth as human beings.

Some of the issues presented in this section have reached an end, and it is hoped that they will not become active issues again (e.g., segregation in some places and mandatory sterilization), but other issues remain active (e.g., stigma and segregation). Although the delivery of care is not a negative issue, it is an evolving issue of how best to provide accessible yet affordable health care to individuals with intellectual disabilities. We must also examine this issue globally in the future (Ouellette-Kuntz et al., 2005).

SIGNIFICANT HEALTH-RELATED RESEARCH

The most significant health-related research that has directly affected the lives of persons with intellectual disabilities has occurred in the past century. Table 5.2 lists these areas of research. It is amazing that the discovery of the double-helix model for DNA in 1953 led to the Human Genome Project (1990–2003), which resulted in the mapping of and the complete identification of all genes in the human genome. Earlier, physicians and researchers began to identify and describe the etiologies of a number of conditions that resulted in intellectual disabilities. Table 5.1 clearly indicates the evolution of our knowledge in this area. Our understanding of genetics has also led to the identification and description of genetic inheritance patterns that have, in turn, facilitated the development of new technologies. In recent years we have given more attention to the identification and description of environmentally induced conditions that result in intellectual disabilities, such as fetal alcohol syndrome disorder and lead and mercury poisoning. The discovery of phenylketonuria (PKU) by Asbjorn Folling in 1934 and the test to screen for it was the first step in preventing a condition that caused many people to have intellectual disabilities (Kanner, 1967). We have also identified the etiology and treatment of Rh incompatibility, resulting in the prevention of many birth defects. More recently, researchers have identified and described the broader aspects of autism spectrum disorders, discovered the use of folic acid to prevent neural tube defects, and developed maternal serum screens for chromosomal abnormalities. Perhaps most controversial now is the discovery of how and when to clone. Cloning is a current and emerging health issue with ramifications as yet unknown. Although it raises serious ethical and legal implications, it is likely that much good will be generated from this new knowledge and technology.

SIGNIFICANT HEALTH-RELATED ACCOMPLISHMENTS

Although many of the significant health-related accomplishments that have affected persons with intellectual disabilities in the past century have come about as a result of research, it is important to additionally mention significant health-related accomplishments in the areas of practice, science, and technology. The list of these accomplishments is found in Table 5.3.

TABLE 5.2. Significant Health-Related Research

- Birth defect prevention
- Cloning
- Discovery of double-helix model for DNA
- Discovery of maternal serum screen for chromosome abnormalities
- Discovery of phenylketonuria (PKU) and screening test
- Discovery of the etiologies for a number of conditions that result in intellectual disabilities
- Discovery of the use of folic acid to prevent neural tube defects
- Identification and description of autism spectrum disorders
- Identification and description of environmentally induced conditions that result in intellectual disabilities (e.g., fetal alcohol spectrum disorder [FASD], lead, mercury)
- Identification and description of genetic inheritance patterns
- Identification of Rh incompatibility
- Mapping of the human genome

TABLE 5.3. Significant Health-Related Accomplishments

Practice

- AAIDD environmental initiative
- Advancements in prenatal and postnatal care
- Attention to the need for dental care
- Birth delivery techniques
- Dual diagnosis and avoidance of "diagnostic overshadowing"
- Health programs by Special Olympics
- Identification and treatment of secondary conditions
- Prenatal treatment
- Recognition of legal and ethical issues
- Surgeon general's reports and 2001 conference
- Treatment of prematurity

Science

- Dietary supplements (e.g., folic acid)
- Discovery of new medications, specifically penicillin, sulfa, and psychopharmaceutical agents
- Fetal surgery
- Genetic engineering
- Gene therapy
- Immunizations
- Newborn screening techniques, including tandem mass spectrometry

Technology

- Equipment accommodations
- Invention of EEG and neuroimaging machines, including CT, PET, and MRI scans

Practice

The majority of practice accomplishments in the past century have revolved around obstetrics. Prenatal treatments, treatment of prematurity, advances in prenatal and postnatal care, and birth delivery techniques have all greatly affected infant morbidity and mortality. Health care professionals have argued that such changes have also resulted in the survival of very-low-birthweight and low-birthweight infants who live with intellectual and physical disabilities. Although this is true, many infants are born without disabilities who would not have survived in the past. The increase in the survival rate of premature infants has certainly raised legal and ethical issues and ongoing discussion of how best to practice.

Knowledge and Management of Intellectual Disabilities

In recent years our knowledge of conditions that result in intellectual disabilities and their health management has greatly affected the care of specific subgroups, in particular older adults and women. We also know more about secondary conditions and mental and dental health needs. We discuss each in more detail.

The age of the population of individuals with intellectual disabilities is increasing, and this fact will have significant health care implications, including increased prevalence of secondary conditions. Current and future projections estimate that the number of individuals over 60 years of age with intellectual disabilities will increase from approximately 1 million to several million by 2030. Currently, the average life expectancy for these individuals is 66 years (Fisher & Kettl, 2005; Horwitz, Kerker, Owens, & Zigler, 2000; Janicki, Dalton, Henderson, & Davidson, 1999). As individuals with intellectual disabilities age, their risk for mental and physical problems increases (Ailey, 2005). Other secondary problems associated with aging that occur with increased incidence in individuals with intellectual disabilities are visual impairments, thyroid problems, cardiovascular disease, and dementia (Fisher & Kettl, 2005).

Women with intellectual disabilities may be at greater risk for developing osteoporosis due to activity limitations, medication side effects, and early menopause (Massachusetts Department of Mental Retardation, University of Massachusetts Medical School Center for Developmental Disabilities Evaluation and Research, 2003). Other problems typically associated with aging, such as changes in visual acuity, early menopause, and urinary incontinence, may be more problematic for individuals with intellectual disabilities due to limited access to health care services, difficulty communicating symptoms to health care providers, and negative attitudes of health care providers that result in the provision of suboptimal care (Hahn & Service, 2005).

Health care professionals have also identified and described secondary conditions that may occur in individuals with intellectual disabilities. For example, children with Down syndrome have higher incidences of heart defects, intestinal problems, and upper respiratory conditions. On the other hand, they have fewer instances of myocardial infarction and stroke in later years (Cohen, 1999). The knowledge of these conditions is important in the lifespan health care management of individuals with intellectual disabilities.

Dual diagnosis of intellectual disability and psychiatric impairment persists as a clinical challenge today, although the phenomenon of "diagnostic overshadowing," or the attribution of behavioral manifestations of a mental health problem to the primary diagnosis of intellectual disability was recognized in the 1980s (Reiss, Levitan, & Szyszko, 1982). Individuals with the dual diagnosis of intellectual disability and a mental health problem continue to be misdiagnosed and fail to receive appropriate treatment. Recently, there has been increased attention to the need for more and better dental and psychological care for persons with intellectual disabilities. There is a paucity of qualified dentists and mental health professionals who are knowledgeable in the care of this population (Corbin & Fenton, 2005; U.S. Public Health Service, 2002). The attention and recognition of this need is a significant accomplishment at this time.

Models of Care and Best Practices

How we deliver care to persons with intellectual disabilities has changed dramatically over time. We discuss this history and highlight examples of best practice.

Current health care efforts directed to individuals with intellectual disabilities have shifted from the medical model of care that emphasizes the diagnosis and treatment of illness to a model of care that focuses on health promotion based on a biopsychosocial model. This shift in philosophical focus has highlighted the issue of health disparities for individuals with intellectual disabilities (Agency for Healthcare Research and Quality [AHRQ], 2005a). In response, national efforts have been directed to addressing this public health dilemma (Lollar, 2002). The development of the National Center for Birth Defects and Developmental Disabilities (NCBDDD) in the Centers for Disease Control and Prevention (CDC) was an important step by the federal government. A number of health programs have also been initiated by Special Olympics, AAIDD's environmental initiative, and the conferences, focus groups, and reports issued by the current and past surgeon generals about the need to eliminate the disparity of health care for persons with intellectual disabilities (U.S. Public Health Service, 2002) and the need to provide appropriate and accessible health care to all persons with intellectual disabilities (Coulter, 2005; U.S. Department of Health and Human Services, 2005). Each is detailed here.

Special Olympics, Inc., has initiated several programs to address the lack of ongoing preventive health care that their athletes receive. These programs include Fit Feet, FUNfitness, Health Promotion, Healthy Hearing, Opening Eyes, and Special Smiles. At many of their events, a MedFest is held at which screening and physical exams are conducted at clinics set up at the event. Findings of health screenings conducted on more than 3,500 athletes who participated in the 2003 Special Olympics World Summer Games revealed that these athletes demonstrated a myriad of serious health problems at a rate greater than was found in the general population. Forty-eight percent of athletes had hearing impairments, 41% had visual acuity problems (30% were nearsighted; 18% were farsighted), 36% had obvious dental decay, and 50% had foot disease. Twenty-nine percent of males and 13% of females (average age 24.7 years) had below-normal bone mineral density (BMD), a condition found in women 65 years old and older. Thirty percent of the athletes were obese, and 23% were overweight (Special Olympics, 2005). (For more information on these programs see the Special Olympics website, *www.specialolympics.org*).

AAIDD received funding in 2002 to address environmental conditions and neurotoxicants, such as lead, alcohol, toluene, and pesticides, which can cause and exacerbate existing intellectual disabilities. They have sponsored a national invitational conference, met with legislators, and sponsored many audio conferences led by national leaders in environmental health. These efforts have helped to bring attention to the effects that the environment has on the primary and secondary health of individuals with intellectual disabilities.

The former Surgeon General of the United States, Dr. David Satcher, answered the call from health care professionals and self-advocates to address the public health concerns of health disparities and sponsored an invitational conference in 2001. This resulted in the landmark document *Closing the Gap: A National Blueprint for Improving the Health of Individuals with Mental Retardation. Report of the Surgeon General's Conference on Health Disparities and Mental Retardation* (U.S. Public Health Service, 2002), in which six goals were identified:

1. Integrate health promotion into community environments of people with mental retardation.
2. Increase knowledge and understanding of health and mental retardation, ensuring that knowledge is made practical and easy to use.
3. Improve the quality of health care for people with mental retardation.
4. Train health care providers in the care of adults and children with mental retardation.
5. Ensure that health care financing produces good health outcomes for adults and children with mental retardation.
6. Increase sources of health care services for adults, adolescents, and children with mental retardation, ensuring that health care is easily accessible for them. (pp. 3, 5, 7, 9, 10, 12)

This effort, along with the chapter on disabilities in *Healthy People 2010* (U.S. Department of Health and Human Services, 2000) and President Bush's (2001) *New Freedom Initiative*, fueled the national interest in the health care and health status of persons of all ages with intellectual disabilities. Different organizations have responded to this document through initiatives to address one or more of these goals. Two examples are the Arc of the United States 2003 national goals conference, which set a national research agenda and resulted in a book (Lakin & Turnbull, 2005) that includes a chapter on health (Coulter, 2005), and the AAIDD health promotion conference in 2004, which also resulted in a book, *Health Promotion for Persons with Intellectual and Developmental Disabilities* (Nehring, 2005).

In 2005, the current surgeon general, Dr. Richard Carmona, renewed the call for health care professionals and society to maintain their attention to the health disparities in persons with intellectual disabilities in *The Surgeon General's Call to Action to Improve the Health and Wellness of Persons with Disabilities* (U.S. Department of Health and Human Services, 2005). This document addressed the following four issues:

1. People nationwide understand that persons with disabilities can lead long, healthy, productive lives.
2. Health care providers have the knowledge and tools to screen, diagnose, and treat the whole person with a disability with dignity.
3. Persons with disabilities can promote their own good health by developing and maintaining healthy lifestyles.
4. Accessible health care and support services promote independence for persons with disabilities (U.S. Department of Health and Human Services, 2005, p. 21).

This document informs us that health promotion efforts must be a part of any primary care visit and that individuals with intellectual disabilities need to be informed and educated on ways that they can lead healthier lives. Ideally, these efforts should be determined by an interdisciplinary team that includes the individual with intellectual disabilities and his or her family.

Science

Several scientific developments over the past century have affected morbidity and mortality for persons with intellectual disabilities. The development of new medications across the years, such as penicillin, aspirin, sulfa, and psychopharmaceutical agents, has revolutionized how primary care providers can practice in order to affect morbidity and mortality rates. The development of immunizations and dietary supplements has also had a major effect on morbidity and mortality. Although recent controversy has focused on the possibility that certain immunizations might cause autism spectrum disorders, there has been no research that fully supports this idea (Wing & Potter, 2002). Genetic engineering, gene therapy, and newborn screening techniques, including tandem mass spectrometry, have greatly increased our ability to identify and treat early many conditions that cause intellectual disabilities and that we did not know about only a few years ago. The list of 29 conditions that have been recommended for screening by a national panel (Health Resources and Services Administration, 2005) are listed in Table 5.4. A final health accomplishment of science has been the development of techniques by which fetal surgery can be performed prior to birth, thus preventing disabling conditions.

TABLE 5.4. Twenty-Nine Core Conditions That Should Be Screened in Each Newborn

- 3-Methylcrotonyl-CoA carboxylase deficiency (3MCC)
- 3-OH 3-CH$_3$ glutaric aciduria (HMG)
- Argininosuccinic academia (ASA)
- Beta-ketothiolase deficiency (BKT)
- Biotinidase deficiency (BIOT)
- Carnitine uptake defect (CUD)
- Citrullinemia (CIT)
- Congenital adrenal hyperplasia (CAH)
- Congenital hypothyroidism (HYPOTH)
- Cystic fibrosis (CF)
- Galactosemia (GALT)
- Glutaric academia type 1 (GA1)
- Hb S/beta-thalassemia (Hb S/Th)
- Hb S/C disease (HB S/C)
- Hearing deficiency

- Homocystinuria (HCY)
- Isovaleric academia (IVA)
- Long-chain L-3-OH acyl-CoA dehydrogenase deficiency (LCHAD)
- Maple syrup urine disease (MSUD)
- Medium chain acyl-CoA dehydrogenase deficiency (MCAD)
- Methylmalonic academia (Cbl A,B)
- Methylmalonic academia (mutase deficiency) (MUT)
- Multiple carboxylase deficiency (MCD)
- Phenylketonuria (PKU)
- Propiionic academia (PROP)
- Sickle cell anemia (SCA)
- Trifunctional protein deficiency (TFP)
- Tyrosinemia type 1 (TYR 1)
- Very-long-chain acyl-CoA dehydrogenase deficiency (VLCAD)

Note. Data from Health Resources and Services Administration (2005).

Technology

Technological advancements have influenced how health professionals are able to diagnose and manage the health care of persons with intellectual disabilities, resulting in the extension of life expectancies. The increased survival rates have created the need to focus more attention on health promotion efforts as a means of enhancing the quality of life of individuals with intellectual disabilities. This technology includes the invention of electroencephalographic (EEG) machines and neuroimaging equipment, such as positron emission tomography (PET) scans, magnetic resonance imaging (MRI), and computerized tomography (CT) scans. The invention of equipment that allows for necessary accommodations for the delivery of health care or that enhances the ability of persons with intellectual disabilities to live to their optimal level are also significant. For example, the ability to adapt the examining table in a clinic office so that needed diagnostic and screening tests, such as Pap smears, can be conducted has enabled primary care providers to do a more thorough and accurate examination. Likewise, the evolving development of wheelchairs and other mobility aids has greatly expanded the environment and enhanced the quality of life for persons who are in need of this equipment.

All of these accomplishments have made a significant impact, but the documents by the Surgeon Generals and other health professionals alert us that much still needs to be done.

EMERGING HEALTH AREAS

We have listed what we feel are emerging areas of health, and we believe that they can be divided into three categories: influencing agents, emerging areas of knowledge, and practice issues. These are listed in Table 5.5. Although there may be overlap among categories, each item is listed in only one category.

TABLE 5.5. Emerging Health Areas

Influencing agents

- Aging and chronic childhood conditions/intellectual disabilities
- Changes in health care delivery system, including roles and responsibilities of health care professionals, settings for care, insurance, and Medicaid
- Environmental neurotoxicants

Emerging areas of knowledge

- Changing terminology (e.g., "mental retardation" to "intellectual disabilities")
- Cloning
- Cultural and ethical differences
- Eugenics
- Mapping of human genome
- Pharmacogenetics
- Proteomics
- Stem-cell research
- Understanding the trajectory of childhood chronic conditions, including intellectual and developmental disabilities, across the lifespan

Practice

- Accessibility of health care
- Alternative and complementary medicine
- Evidence-based practice (medicine)
- Health disparities
- Health promotion and assessment of health concerns across the lifespan that occurs across the general population (e.g., arthritis, hypertension)
- Service coordination
- Family/youth/individual-centered care
- International collaboration efforts
- Standardized care for specific conditions resulting in intellectual and developmental disabilities
- Transition issues

Influencing Agents

The first category is influencing agents. As discussed earlier, the area of environmental neurotoxicants and their influences on persons with intellectual disabilities is an emerging science. We have knowledge of the effects of lead, alcohol, smoking, and mercury, for example, but we do not know about the adverse effects of hundreds of additional chemicals. We know that such conditions as asthma are on the rise in school-age children (e.g., Liu, Spahn, & Leung, 2004) and that some suggest a link to environmental toxins (Graff, Murphy, Ekvall, & Gagnon, 2006). Graff and colleagues (2006) have indicated that persons with intellectual disabilities may be predisposed to adverse effects "due to (a) behaviors persisting past a developmentally appropriate age, (b) communication skills, (c) motor skills, (d) nutrition issues, and (e) health problems related to intellectual disabilities" (p. 596) that make it difficult to identify and/or interpret signs and symptoms of neurotoxicity. They also speak to the need for primary care providers to conduct environmental histories, to routinely assess this population for effects of neurotoxins during primary care visits, and to have a basic awareness of neurotoxins and how they can be prevented and/or treated if harmful effects are present. The CDC (2005) publishes a national report on a regular basis on human exposure to chemicals in the environment.

Another influencing agent is the need to study conditions that cause intellectual disabilities across the lifespan (Blacher, 2005) so that we might understand the influences of normal chronic conditions that occur with aging, such as arthritis and diabetes, and their influences on persons with intellectual disabilities. We need to understand not only how these conditions influence each other physiologically but also how we should best treat short- and long-term conditions in which the treatments may contraindicate each other (Boyd et al., 2005). As the life expectancy of individuals with intellectual disabilities increases, experts are learning more about the aging process and about the emergence of secondary conditions later in life.

A final influencing agent is the dynamic change taking place in our health care delivery system. Such change involves the roles and responsibilities of all health care professionals about decisions regarding access to the most appropriate settings for care, access to affordable health insurance, and stemming the rising cost of health care. Medicare and Medicaid changes also can dramatically influence the population of persons with intellectual disabilities (Coulter, 2005; National Council on Disability, 2005). As the cost of and demand for health care continues to increase, innovative, cost-effective, and time-efficient service approaches will be developed and tested. These innovations include the use of highly educated and clinically competent (yet less costly) health care practitioners. Personnel replacements for physicians include nurse practitioners, physician assistants, nurse anesthetists, pharmacologists, physical and occupational therapists, social workers, and psychologists. Costly delivery settings of care are being replaced by low-tech settings such as community clinics and specialized satellite hubs for diagnostic testing (endoscopies) and outpatient surgeries.

Emerging Areas of Knowledge

Numerous emerging areas of knowledge will continue to evolve for many years and will require health care professionals to peruse pertinent websites almost daily for up-to-date information on diagnosis, etiology, and management. This list includes proteomics, further mapping of the human genome, pharmacogenetics, understanding the trajectory of childhood chronic conditions across the lifespan, cultural and ethical differences, and, as our genetic knowledge increases, eugenics, stem-cell research, and cloning. Although "cultural and ethnic differences" and "eugenics" are not new terms in this field, our expanding knowledge of increasing numbers of cultures and ethnicities in our world and of genetics demands renewed attention. For example, the annual *National Healthcare Disparities Reports* from AHRQ remind of us continued healthcare disparities for persons with intellectual disabilities, and even more so for minorities (AHRQ, 2005a). The knowledge in the field has increased exponentially in recent years, and health care professionals must have avenues for finding the pertinent information.

Practice

The final category of emerging health issues comprises items that influence practice. These include discussions that need to take place to determine whether standards of care for the general population should include information on intellectual disabilities or whether there should be separate guidelines specific to conditions, such as Down syndrome and fragile X syndrome. Other practice issues include accessibility to afford-able health care, increased health promotion efforts, progression to person-centered care, elimination of health disparities, evidence-based practice, care coordination needs, alternative and complementary medicine, transition issues, and international collaborative efforts.

The identification of relevant and significant health advances leads to the need to discuss implications for health care professionals, families, policy makers, and research-ers. Each is discussed separately.

IMPLICATIONS FOR PRACTITIONERS

Health care for individuals with intellectual disabilities is in the process of a major ser-vice reorganization. The traditional medical model is considered to be an outdated approach in providing care to individuals with intellectual disabilities. Comprehensive interdisciplinary care, including the components of early identification, service coordi-nation, and health promotion, is considered to be the "best practice" service delivery model. The health care literature on the care of individuals with intellectual disabilities is replete with topics on the principles of care, including the medical home (American Academy of Pediatrics, Medical Home Initiatives for Children with Special Needs Pro-ject Advisory Committee, 2004). The principles of care include a consumer-oriented approach that encourages self-determination and the development of self-management skills to enable the consumer to function as independently as possible in the commu-nity of his or her choice.

There is also a growing body of clinical guidelines that are condition specific and primarily constructed for the pediatric age range (e.g., American Academy of Pediat-rics, Committee on Genetics, 1995, 1996, 2001), as well as a few guidelines across the lifespan (e.g., Cohen, 1999). Other clinical guidelines are specific to pediatric health care practices in, for example, care coordination, choosing complementary and alterna-tive medicine, and developmental surveillance and screening (American Academy of Pediatrics, Committee on Children with Disabilities, 1999, 2001a, b) and evidence reports in relation to the medical care and treatment of cerebral palsy (American Acad-emy for Cerebral Palsy and Developmental Medicine, 2005). Standards of care are also available for out-of-home child care programs for children with intellectual disabilities (American Academy of Pediatrics, American Public Health Association, & National Resource Center for Health and Safety in Child Care, 2002) and for screening and pre-ventive services (U.S. Preventive Services Task Force, 1996). Finally, Internet websites provide health care professionals with databases for such clinical guidelines (e.g., Agency for Healthcare Research and Quality, 2005b; The Cochrane Collaboration, 2005).

Nursing is the only discipline that has developed standards of care. Two standards are available: Intellectual and Developmental Disabilities Nursing: Scope and Standards of Practice (Nehring et al., 2004; copublished by the American Nurses Association and the American Association on Mental Retardation) and the standards of practice pub-lished by the Developmental Disabilities Nurses Association (Aggen et al., 2004). The first part of the Nehring et al. (2004) document provides a discussion of the definition of the nurse in this specialty—roles and responsibilities of the basic, advanced, and spe-cialty nurse when caring for a person with intellectual and developmental disabilities; practice settings; and trends and issues. The second section includes the standards of practice, which are divided into standards of practice and standards of professional performance.

There is also the need to help the individual with intellectual disabilities to learn the skills and knowledge needed to function as independently as possible, ideally beginning with diagnosis, whether at birth or later when the child reaches the age of majority and thus becomes able to make health decisions. Nurses are in an ideal position to support the youth and his or her family in learning more about his or her condition and self-care skills. Nurses can support patients through consumer education efforts, beginning in childhood, that focus on instructing the consumer to learn self management skills. Such skills include (1) learning about the pathophysiology and symptomology of the disability and understanding the triggers that cause untoward reactions, such as the aura preceding a seizure; (2) learning to manage the treatment regimen as independently as possible, from knowing when to call the health care provider to ordering refills of medication; and (3) learning healthy behaviors such as not smoking, eating a healthy and well-balanced diet, and engaging in an ongoing exercise program in an effort to control weight, promote cardiovascular functioning, prevent osteoporosis, and strengthen the musculoskeletal system.

The challenge in forming health partnerships with consumers to promote healthy lifestyles is the lack of incentives within the health care system to do so. Public and private health insurance plans have been slow to reimburse health promotion programs. However, a promising development is the recent announcement by both Kaiser Permanente, a major health maintenance organization, and Medicare that the monthly cost of belonging to Curves, a national fitness chain for women, will be covered as a health promotion benefit. Hopefully, other health insurance plans will extend benefits for fitness membership costs to covered individuals. Additionally, health care providers are not generally reimbursed for health education activities held for consumers or their circle of support. Most health education activities are conducted in haphazard fashion, with very little information provided. Community outreach training on health-related topics for community providers—such as those who serve as attendants, job coaches, and case managers—is not reimbursable by health insurance plans, making it difficult for health care providers to conduct cross-training. Cross-training has been promoted as a strategy to foster improved knowledge and understanding of the ongoing health-related needs of individuals with intellectual disabilities, leading to improved health outcomes.

IMPLICATIONS FOR POLICY MAKERS

The surgeon generals' reports (U.S. Public Health Service, 2002; U.S. Department of Health and Human Services, 2005) bring to our attention the fact that individuals with intellectual disabilities deserve quality health care that is accessible and affordable. Such care, which should be provided across the individual's lifespan, includes health promotion, the prevention of disease, and the prevention of secondary conditions specific to the primary condition that resulted in intellectual disabilities. Changes in a person's health are due to both genetic and environmental factors, and each has to be assessed when diagnosing and treating any presenting symptomatology. Attention must be given to accessible and affordable quality care, but often affordable care is least likely to be discussed by policy makers. Very often the allowable reimbursement rates for health care services are so low as to be a disincentive to health care professionals to participate as service providers.

This situation is regrettable, as many persons with intellectual disabilities are uninsured or underinsured or living in poverty. Their health care needs are not adequately addressed because the costs of health care and treatment are not adequately reimbursed due to their low socioeconomic status (Rubin & Nehring, 2002).

Policy makers must also determine whether health care for persons with intellectual disabilities is best delivered in integrated health care settings in the community, in segregated clinics, or in health care settings specific to persons with intellectual disabilities. It is known that such individuals need subspecialty care and specialized therapies, as well as coordination of their services, at different times in their lives, but such services are best provided in the community, not in large institutional settings. There is also a dearth of psychologists, psychiatrists, and dentists who are proficient in the care of persons with intellectual disabilities, and this scarcity affects the availability of health care services to provide the optimal care needed (Perrin, 2002). Finally, the recent changes in Medicaid have the potential to adversely affect drug coverage to persons with intellectual disabilities.

IMPLICATIONS FOR RESEARCHERS

Research accomplishments have moved this field forward in many positive directions, as discussed earlier, but there is much to be done to promote the optimal quality of life and health status for persons with intellectual disabilities. The field of genetics and proteomics will greatly enhance our knowledge of the causes of conditions that result in intellectual disabilities. The emergence of new epidemics will create chronic conditions that may become disabling. We must understand the trajectory of chronic childhood conditions that result in intellectual disabilities to understand how disabilities and health change across time, to determine whether symptoms and secondary conditions can be predicted, and to identify which services are most beneficial at different periods of life. Research studies must also be conducted to identify, once and for all, what makes for successful transitions to adulthood health care services (Perrin, 2002). National surveys, such as the National Survey of Children with Special Health Care Needs, the State and Local Integrated Telephone Survey for Children with Special Health Care Needs, and the National Health Interview Survey will assist individuals with intellectual disabilities, their families, health care professionals, policy makers, and researchers to better understand the experience of having an intellectual disability (Allen, 2004; McPherson et al., 2004; Strickland et al., 2004). Adequate funding of the National Children's Study will further assist research efforts to foster better understanding of intellectual disabilities, among other conditions. Finally, research is needed to identify desired health outcomes across the lifespan for persons with intellectual disabilities (Jette & Keysor, 2002).

SUMMARY

In this chapter, issues pertaining to the health needs of individuals with intellectual disabilities were reviewed. A summary of the relevant and current research and health care achievements pertaining to individuals with intellectual disabilities was discussed. Emerging areas of practice and research in health care were examined with implications for practice, research, and policy making. As has been discussed throughout this chapter, the advances in health care have and will continue to have significant impact on the lives of individuals with intellectual disabilities. The challenge is to ensure that this disenfranchised population has affordable access to health care that embodies best practices and evidence-based care.

REFERENCES

Agency for Healthcare Research and Quality. (2005a). *2005 national healthcare disparities report.* Retrieved January 10, 2006, from *www.ahrq.gov/qual/nhqr05/nhqr05.htm.*

Agency for Healthcare Research and Quality. (2005b). *National guideline clearinghouse.* Retrieved December 1, 2005, from *www.guidelines.gov.*

Aggen, R. L., DeGennaro, M. D., Fox, L., Hahn, J. E., Logan, B. A., VonFumetti, L., et al. (2004). *Standards of developmental disabilities nursing practice.* Eugene, OR: Developmental Disabilities Nurses Association.

Ailey, S. H. (2005). Behavior management and mental health. In W. Nehring (Ed.), *Core curriculum for specializing in intellectual and developmental disability: A resource for nurses and other health care professionals* (pp. 291–304). Boston: Jones & Bartlett.

Allen, P. L. J. (2004). Children with special health care needs: National survey of prevalence and health care needs. *Pediatric Nursing, 30,* 307–314.

American Academy for Cerebral Palsy and Developmental Medicine. (2005). *AACPDM database of evidence reports.* Retrieved November 4, 2005, from *www.aacpdm.org/index?service-page/outcomeStudies-Resources.*

American Academy of Pediatrics, American Public Health Association, & National Resource Center for Health and Safety in Child Care. (2002). *Caring for our children. National health and safety performance standards: Guidelines for out-of-home child care programs* (2nd ed.). Bethesda, MD: Maternal Child Health Bureau, Health Resources and Services Administration, and Department of Health and Human Services.

American Academy of Pediatrics, Committee on Children with Disabilities. (1999). Care coordination: Integrating health and related systems of care for children with special health care needs. *Pediatrics, 104,* 978–981.

American Academy of Pediatrics, Committee on Children with Disabilities. (2001a). Counseling families who choose complementary and alternative medicine for their child with chronic illness or disability. *Pediatrics, 107,* 598–601.

American Academy of Pediatrics, Committee on Children with Disabilities. (2001b). Developmental surveillance and screening of infants and young children. *Pediatrics, 108,* 192–195.

American Academy of Pediatrics, Committee on Genetics. (1995). Health supervision for children with achondroplasia. *Pediatrics, 95,* 443–451.

American Academy of Pediatrics, Committee on Genetics. (1996). Health supervision for children with fragile X syndrome. *Pediatrics, 96,* 297–300.

American Academy of Pediatrics, Committee on Genetics. (2001). Health supervision for children with Down syndrome. *Pediatrics, 107,* 442–449.

American Academy of Pediatrics, Medical Home Initiatives for Children with Special Needs Project Advisory Committee. (2004). The medical home. *Pediatrics, 113,* 1545–1547.

Blacher, J. (2005). Widening the lens on intellectual disabilities: An emerging focus on genetics, the lifespan and evidence-based practice. *Current Opinion in Psychiatry, 18*(5), 467–468.

Blatt, B., & Kaplan, F. (1966). *Christmas in purgatory.* Boston: Allyn & Bacon.

Boyd, C. M., Darer, J., Boult, C., Fried, L. P., Boult, L., & Wu, A. W. (2005). Clinical practice guidelines and quality of care for older patients with multiple comorbid diseases. *Journal of the American Medical Association, 294,* 716–724.

Bush, G. W. (2001). *New freedom initiative.* Retrieved December 5, 2005, from *www.hhs.gov/newfreedom.*

Centers for Disease Control and Prevention. (2005). *Third national report on human exposure to environmental chemicals: Executive summary.* Atlanta, GA: Author.

Cochrane Collaboration. (2005). *Abstracts of new and updated Cochrane reviews.* Retrieved December 1, 2005, from *www.cochrane.org.*

Cohen, W. I. (1999). Health care guidelines for individuals with Down syndrome (rev. ed.). *Down Syndrome Quarterly, 4*, 1–16.

Corbin, S., & Fenton, S. J. (2005). Oral health. In W. Nehring (Ed.), *Core curriculum for specializing in intellectual and developmental disability: A resource for nurses and other health care professionals* (pp. 361–377). Boston: Jones & Bartlett.

Coulter, D. L. (2005). Comprehensive health supports and health promotion. In K. C. Lakin & A. Turnbull (Eds.), *National goals and research for people with intellectual and developmental disabilities* (pp. 109–124). Washington, DC: American Association on Mental Retardation.

Crane, C. B. (1907). Almshouse nursing: The human need; the professional opportunity. *American Journal of Nursing, 7*, 872–881.

Devine, P. (1983). Mental retardation: An early subspecialty in psychiatric nursing. *Journal of Psychiatric Nursing and Mental Health Services, 21*, 21–30.

Edgerton, R. (1967). *The cloak of competence.* Berkeley: University of California Press.

Fisher, K., & Kettl, P. (2005). Aging with mental retardation: Increasing population of older adults with mental retardation require health interventions and prevention strategies. *Geriatrics, 60*(4), 26–29.

Foley, G. M. (1990). Portrait of the ARENA evaluation: Assessment in the transdisciplinary approach. In E. D. Gibbs & D. M. Teti (Eds.), *Interdisciplinary assessment of infants: A guide for early intervention professionals* (pp. 271–286). Baltimore: Brookes.

Graff, J. C., Murphy, L., Ekvall, S., & Gagnon, M. (2006). In-home toxic chemical exposures and children with intellectual and developmental disabilities. *Pediatric Nursing, 32*, 596–603.

Hahn, J. E., & Service, K. P. (2005). Older adults. In W. M. Nehring (Ed.), *Core curriculum for specializing in intellectual and developmental disability: A resource for nurses and other health care professionals* (pp. 207–230). Boston: Jones & Bartlett.

Handmaker, S. D. (2005). Etiology of intellectual and developmental disabilities. In W. M. Nehring (Ed.), *Core curriculum for specializing in intellectual and developmental disability: A resource for nurses and other health care professionals* (pp. 33–46). Boston: Jones & Bartlett.

Health Resources and Services Administration. (2005). *Newborn screening: Toward a uniform screening panel and system: Draft report.* Washington, DC: Author.

Horwitz, S. M., Kerker, B. D., Owens, P. L., & Zigler, E. (2000). *The health status and needs of individuals with mental retardation.* New Haven, CT: Yale University School of Medicine, Department of Epidemiology and Public Health and Department of Psychology.

Ireland, W. W. (1877). *On idiocy and imbecility.* London: Churchill.

Jacobson, J. W., & Mulick, J. A. (Eds.). (1996). *Manual of diagnosis and professional practice in mental retardation.* Hyattsville, MD: American Psychological Association.

Janicki, M. P., Dalton, A. J., Henderson, C. M., & Davidson, P. W. (1999). Mortality and morbidity among older adults with intellectual disability: Health services considerations. *Disability and Rehabilitation, 21*, 284–294.

Jette, A. M., & Keysor, J. J. (2002). Uses of evidence in disability outcomes and effectiveness research. *Milbank Quarterly, 80*, 325–345.

Kanner, L. (1967). Medicine in the history of mental retardation 1800–1965. *American Journal of Mental Deficiency, 72*, 165–189.

Lakin, K. C., & Turnbull, A. P. (2005). *National goals and research for people with intellectual and developmental disabilities.* Washington, DC: American Association on Mental Retardation.

Lashley, F. R. (2005). *Clinical genetics in nursing practice* (3rd ed.). New York: Springer.

Laughlin, H. H. (1926). The eugenical sterilization of the feeble-minded. *American Journal of Psycho-Esthetics, 31*, 210–218.

Liu, A. H., Spahn, J. D., & Leung, D. Y. M. (2004). Childhood asthma. In R. E. Behrman, R. M. Kliegman, & H. B. Jenson (Eds.), *Nelson textbook of pediatrics* (17th ed., pp. 760–774). St. Louis, MO: Elsevier.

Lollar, D. J. (2002). Public health and disability: Emerging opportunities. *Public Health Reports, 117*, 131–136.

Luckasson, R., Borthwick-Duffy, S., Buntinx, W. H. E., Coulter, D. L., Craig, E. M., Reeve, A., et al. (2002). *Mental retardation: Definition, classification, and systems of supports* (10th ed.). Washington, DC: American Association on Mental Retardation.

Massachusetts Department of Mental Retardation, University of Massachusetts Medical School Center for Developmental Disabilities Evaluation and Research. (2003). *Preventive health recommendations for adults with mental retardation.* Boston: Author.

McPherson, M., Weissman, G., Strickland, B. B., vanDyck, P. C., Blumberg, S. J., & Newachek, P. W. (2004). Implementing community-based systems of services for children and youths with special health care needs: How well are we doing? *Pediatrics, 113,* 1538–1544.

National Council on Disability. (2005). *The state of 21st-century long-term services and supports: Financing and systems reform for Americans with disabilities.* Washington, DC: Author.

Nehring, W. M. (1999). *A history of nursing in the field of mental retardation and developmental disabilities.* Washington, DC: American Association on Mental Retardation.

Nehring, W. M. (Ed.). (2005). *Health promotion for persons with intellectual and developmental disabilities.* Washington, DC: American Association on Mental Retardation.

Nehring, W. M., Roth, S. P., Natvig, D., Betz, C. L., Savage, T., & Krajicek, M. (2004). *Intellectual and developmental disabilities nursing: Scope and standards of practice.* Washington, DC: American Nurses Association and American Association on Mental Retardation.

Ouellette-Kuntz, H., Garcin, N., Lewis, M. E. S., Minnes, P., Martin, C., & Holden, J. J. A. (2005). Addressing health disparities through promoting equity for individuals with intellectual disability. *Canadian Journal of Public Health, 96*(Suppl. 2), S8–S22.

Perrin, J. M. (2002). Health services research for children with disabilities. *Milbank Quarterly, 80,* 303–324.

President's Panel on Mental Retardation. (1962). *A proposed program for national action to combat mental retardation.* Washington, DC: Author.

Reiss, S., Levitan, G. W., & Szyszko, J. (1982). Emotional disturbance and mental retardation: Diagnostic overshadowing. *American Journal of Mental Deficiency, 87,* 567–574.

Robinson, C. (1997). Team organization and function. In H. M. Wallace, J. C. MacQueen, R. F. Biehl, & J. A. Blackman (Eds.), *Mosby's resource guide to children with disabilities and chronic illness* (pp. 268–280). St. Louis, MO: Mosby.

Rubin, L., & Nehring, W. M. (2002). From medical model to integrated health care delivery: AAMR medicine and nursing initiatives from 1975–1999. In R. L. Schalock, P. C. Baker, & M. D. Croser (Eds.), *Embarking on a new century: Mental retardation at the end of the 20th century* (pp. 167–184). Washington, DC: American Association on Mental Retardation.

Sloan, W., & Stevens, H. A. (1976). *A century of concern: A history of the American Association on Mental Deficiency, 1876–1976.* Washington, DC: American Association on Mental Deficiency.

Special Olympics. (2005). *Healthy athletes.* Retrieved August 29, 2005, from *www.specialolympics.org.*

Strickland, B., McPherson, M., Weissman, G., vanDyck, P., Huang, Z. J., & Newachek, P. (2004). Access to the medical home: Results of the National Survey of Children with Special Health Care Needs. *Pediatrics, 113,* 1485–1492.

Trent, J. W. (1994). *Inventing the feeble mind: A history of mental retardation in the United States.* Los Angeles: University of California Press.

U.S. Department of Health and Human Services. (2000). *Healthy people 2010* (2nd ed.). Washington, DC: U.S. Government Printing Office.

U.S. Department of Health and Human Services. (2005). *The Surgeon General's call to action to improve the health and wellness of persons with disabilities.* Washington, DC: Author.

U.S. Preventive Services Task Force. (1996). *Guide to clinical preventive services* (2nd ed.). Washington, DC: Author.

U.S. Public Health Service. (2002). *Closing the gap: A national blueprint for improving the health of individuals with mental retardation: Report of the Surgeon General's conference on health disparities and mental retardation.* Washington, DC: Author.

Whitney, E. A. (1950). Mental deficiency in the 1880s and 1940s: A brief review of 60 years' progress. *American Journal of Mental Deficiency, 54,* 151–154.

Wing, L., & Potter, D. (2002). The epidemiology of autistic spectrum disorders: Is the prevalence rising? *Mental Retardation and Developmental Disabilities Research Reviews, 8,* 151–161.

World Health Organization. (2001). *International classification of functioning, disability, and health (ICIDH-2).* Retrieved February 5, 2007, from *www.who.int/icf/icftemplate.cfm.*

6

Advances in Genetics

Nicole R. Tartaglia
Robin L. Hansen
Randi J. Hagerman

Over the past two decades, the Human Genome Project and genetic research have led to dramatic advances in our understanding of the role of genetics in cognition and development. The final sequence of the human genome was completed in 2003, 50 years after the discovery of the double-helix structure of DNA by Watson and Crick (Valle, 2004). These advances have furthered our understanding of the role of genetics in human variation in learning, and they have begun to influence interventions and teaching techniques.

Many types of learning disabilities (LD) and mental retardation (MR) are now understood to arise from genetic abnormalities. We now know that approximately 30,000 genes make up the human genome, and more than 1,000 different genetic causes of MR have been identified. Genetic disorders now account for approximately 55% of cases of moderate to severe MR (IQ < 50) and 10–15% of cases of mild MR (IQ 50–70), and these percentages continue to increase with advances in the field of genetics and the use of new molecular techniques to identify genetic disorders (Chelly, Khelfaoui, Francis, Cherif, & Bienvenu, 2006; Flint & Knight, 2003). Some genetic disorders result from mutations in a single gene, such as fragile X syndrome (FXS) and Rett syndrome, which result in the absence of a single protein (FMRP or MECP2) critical for normal brain development. Other disorders, such as Smith–Magenis syndrome or velocardiofacial syndrome (also known as 22q11.2 deletion syndrome), are called microdeletion syndromes and result from the deletion of multiple genes. Disorders such as Down syndrome (trisomy 21) and the X and Y chromosome aneuploidies

(47,XXY/Klinefelter syndrome, 47,XYY syndrome, 45,X/Turner syndrome) are characterized by the addition or absence of entire chromosomes, leading to overexpression or imbalance of many genes and subsequent neurodevelopmental abnormalities.

The X chromosome alone contains more than 200 genes related to the development of the human brain. Approximately 25% more males have mental retardation than females because males are uniquely vulnerable to genetic mutations on the X chromosome, as they have only one X chromosome. X chromosome mutations that cause mental retardation in males may cause only learning disabilities in females because the female's second, normal X chromosome can compensate, such as in Coffin–Lowry syndrome or fragile X syndrome (FXS). In addition, milder forms of mutations in genes known to be linked to mental retardation can lead to LD, such as mild mutations in the *MECP2* gene associated with Rett syndrome. Advances in understanding common learning problems such as dyslexia have also revealed new genes associated with phonological processing (Meng et al., 2005). In cases of environmental neurotoxicity, such as fetal alcohol syndrome (FAS), a genetic component exists in the mother that affects the vulnerability of the developing fetus. The rate at which mothers metabolize alcohol is genetically based and influences the toxic effect on the fetus and the severity of FAS. Collaboration between the fields of neuroscience, psychology, and genetics has furthered our understanding of the structural and functional changes that occur in the developing brain and that lead to problems with cognition and behavior.

Collaborative research over the past 20 years has led to better characterization of hundreds of genetic syndromes, resulting in the emergence of the field of behavioral phenotypes. In this field, the characteristic behavioral and cognitive profiles of many genetic neurodevelopmental disorders are systematically quantified and compared (Hodapp & Dykens, 2005; O'Brien, 2002). Many of the genetic disorders described in this chapter have unique cognitive and behavioral profiles that have been well characterized and linked to the specific genotype (genetic makeup of an individual) of each disorder (Hagerman, 1999). Behavioral phenotyping of genetic syndromes has been on the cutting edge of research that is helping to gain a better understanding of the relationship of specific genes and cognitive-behavioral development. Additionally, advances in neuroimaging have also allowed scientists to identify structural and functional differences in the brains of individuals with various genetic disorders.

As a result of this new research, educational interventions are being developed that are tailored to the unique cognitive profiles that are typical for specific genetic disorders. It is anticipated that further collaborative research in genetics, neuroscience, psychology, and education will lead to the development of new and effective interventions for complex genetic disorders such as autism and the individual genetic disorders described later in this chapter.

ADVANCES IN GENETIC DIAGNOSTIC TECHNIQUES

The medical evaluation of a child or adult with mental retardation or severe learning disability has increasingly focused on genetic diagnostic techniques. These evaluations have improved remarkably over the past two decades with advances in molecular biology. Beginning in the 1970s, techniques in the field of cytogenetics became more consistently available and allowed geneticists to use blood samples to count the number of chromosomes and to recognize missing or extra elements from the normal 46 human chromosomes. A technique called G-banding led to recognizable banding patterns for each chromosome, and such studies became routinely ordered for any individual presenting with mental retardation of unknown etiology.

In the 1990s fluorescent *in situ* hybridization (FISH) techniques were developed that utilize a fluorescent DNA probe with the normal sequence for critical areas in the genome. The DNA probe is mixed with the patient's DNA from a blood sample to detect any missing or duplicated sequences that are too small to be seen under the standard light microscope. Clinicians were encouraged to order FISH testing or "go FISHing" for a specific genetic diagnosis, particularly when features of a specific syndrome were present physically or behaviorally. The search to find a specific diagnosis is important for guiding medical and educational interventions, providing prognostic information, and often has genetic counseling implications for the extended family, as well.

The past few years have led to an escalation of new diagnostic techniques, some of which are beginning to have more widespread use in clinical practice. High-resolution chromosome testing is regularly used for detecting small deletions or duplications and it is routinely enhanced with FISH testing. Multilocus FISH testing allows clinicians to test for multiple common abnormalities at once, and it is becoming more common because the assessment of individuals with developmental delays without features of a specific genetic syndrome has yielded a significant number with cryptic deletions or duplications. Specific gene testing can be carried out using techniques such as Southern blot analysis and a polymerase chain reaction (PCR) study when a repetitive sequence of base pairs in the DNA is involved, as in FXS, which has a trinucleotide (CGG) repeat sequence in the front end of the gene that prevents production of normal levels of FMRP protein.

A new technique called comparative genomic hybridization (CGH) allows for detailed evaluation of the whole genome (all of the chromosomes and genes) in one test. In this technology, DNA from normal individuals is compared with the patient's DNA from a blood sample to identify any differences in the DNA sequence. This allows researchers to detect DNA sequence abnormalities that may not be associated with a known genetic syndrome or that may be too small to identify by standard techniques. In addition, another new technology called the expression microarray can detect differences in the level of expression of specific gene(s), which can be measured by looking at the levels of messenger RNA (mRNA). Expression microarrays can profile the levels of thousands of mRNA transcripts in a given patient sample, although these levels can change depending on tissue type or timing of the sample in development (Levitt, 2005).

Sometimes a structural change in one single gene can affect the expression of many genes. For instance, the gene that is defective in Rett syndrome, *MECP2*, controls the transcription process (the reading of the gene to make mRNA) for many genes important in the development of the brain. When *MECP2* is mutated, the expression of many genes will change, leading to the behavioral and cognitive phenotype of Rett syndrome or related phenotypes.

Genomic CGH arrays will also give us information about DNA sequence, and allows a more thorough evaluation of the whole genome at once, in contrast to conventional cytogenetics and even FISH testing. For example, genomic CGH microarrays are able to detect abnormalities in the telomeres, or the ends of chromosomes. Approximately 5–10% of nonsyndromic mental retardation cases can be attributed to submicroscopic, subtelomeric deletions (De Vries, Winter, Schinzel, & van Ravenswaaij-Arts, 2003). Although specific telomeric deletions can also be detected by FISH testing, the behavioral phenotypes in these disorders have not been studied sufficiently to identify individual telomere deletion syndromes clinically. The use of these new tools to evaluate patients with developmental disabilities is becoming more widespread and will greatly enhance the identification of genetic abnormalities in these patients. These new genetic techniques will also result in the discovery of many new genes involved in brain development and learning.

EXAMPLES OF ADVANCES IN IDENTIFICATION AND TREATMENT OF GENETIC SYNDROMES

In the following sections we present some examples of genetic syndromes and the syndrome-specific treatment recommendations and educational interventions that have resulted from recent research. It is recommended that educators, school psychologists, and other professionals working with children with developmental disabilities become familiar with the cognitive and behavioral features of common genetic disorders so that they can incorporate syndrome-specific intervention strategies into educational plans.

Fragile X Syndrome

FXS is the most common inherited cause of mental retardation; it was initially described in 1969. FXS is caused by a mutation in a single gene, called the fragile X mental retardation1 (*FMR1*) gene, located on the X chromosome, which was discovered in 1991. Approximately 2–3% of individuals with MR and 2–6% of individuals with autism have FXS (Reddy, 2005). The *FMR1* gene mutation comes in two forms: the premutation with 55–200 CGG repeats on the front end of the gene and the full mutation with greater than 200 CGG repeats.

The premutation is also called the "carrier state," and it occurs in approximately 1 in 130 females and 1 in 800 males in the general population (Beckett, Yu, & Long, 2005). Individuals with the fragile X premutation tend to be unaffected intellectually in childhood and early adulthood, although problems with attention-deficit/hyperactivity disorder (ADHD) and social relatedness are common, and some individuals have autism spectrum disorders (Farzin et al., 2006). In older male carriers and in some female carriers (> 50 years), problems with tremor and ataxia can develop, associated with cognitive decline (Hagerman & Hagerman, 2004). This aging problem, called the fragile X–associated tremor/ataxia syndrome (FXTAS), was first described in 2001 and occurs in about 40% of premutation males as they age (Jacquemont et al., 2004). FXTAS is caused by a toxic effect of elevated *FMR1* mRNA that occurs in carriers, leading to the formation of inclusions in the neurons and astrocytes in the brain (Greco et al., 2006). Carriers may also show enhancement of verbal comprehension skills (Loesch, Huggins, Bui, Taylor, & Hagerman, 2003), combined with a drive for learning related to obsessive–compulsive behavior (Hessl et al., 2005), that can make them exceptional students. In our research, we have found that 45% of carrier males have advanced degrees (e.g., M.S., M.D., Ph.D.), and it is possible that the elevated levels of *FMR1* mRNA have a beneficial effect on learning before FXTAS develops.

Individuals with the full mutation have fragile X syndrome (FXS), and the *FMR1* gene is turned off through methylation, which leads to little or no production of *FMR1* mRNA. Without the presence of *FMR1* mRNA, little or no *FMR1* protein (FMRP) is produced. It is the deficiency or absence of FMRP that causes FXS. The typical physical features of FXS are prominent ears, a long face, flat feet, and hyperextensible finger joints (Hagerman, 2002b; see Figure 6.1). As infants, individuals with FXS have low muscle tone with mild motor delays and prominent speech delays. They are usually diagnosed just before 3 years of age because of the significant language delays (Mirrett, Bailey, Roberts, & Hatton, 2004), and approximately 10% of children with FXS are non-verbal at 5 years of age. Approximately 30% of young children with FXS also have autism, with a behavioral profile that is indistinguishable from that of a child with autism without FXS (Rogers, Wehner, & Hagerman, 2001). Currently, a DNA test for FXS that includes Southern blot and PCR testing is available and recommended for any individual with mental retardation or autism of unknown etiology.

Approximately 85% of boys and 25% of girls with FXS have MR, and those without MR have learning disabilities. Therefore, many children with FXS, particularly girls, will present as learning disabled instead of mentally retarded and will require special education services. The IQ level in FXS directly correlates with the level of FMRP, with higher protein levels associated with higher IQ (Loesch, Huggins, & Hagerman, 2004). Parental IQ and the quality of the environment are also related to the child's developmental level and behavior (Hessl et al., 2001).

Longitudinal studies demonstrate that some children with FXS can experience an IQ decline over time, stimulating further research into whether the IQ decline is due to regression of cognitive functioning or to failure to maintain the expected rate of cognitive development. Results have shown that the IQ decline in children with FXS relates to molecular variables, including FMRP levels (Wright-Talamante et al., 1996). Additional follow-up studies looking at nonverbal IQ scores using the Leiter International Performance Scale—Revised (Leiter-R) showed a small but linear increase in cognitive skills despite declining IQ scores. These studies suggest that the decline in IQ is the result of steady but suboptimal intellectual growth rather than a true deterioration in overall intellectual functioning. Children with FXS and autism were also more likely to show a decline in IQ (Skinner et al., 2005). Comprehensive medical and educational interventions are recommended to optimize intellectual growth for these children and to prevent the decline in IQ over time.

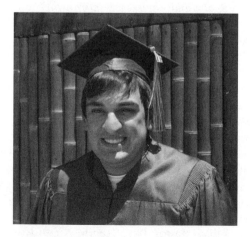

FIGURE 6.1. Eighteen-year-old male with fragile X syndrome on his high school graduation day. Notice his mildly long face and prominent jaw, but his ears are not prominent as in many children with FXS.

Children with FXS have a variety of other behavioral and emotional difficulties that affect development and education. Many have significant overreactivity to sensory stimuli, which can lead to tantrum behavior, hyperactivity, and impulsivity (Hagerman, 2002a; Roberts, Boccia, Bailey, Hatton, & Skinner, 2001). The sympathetic nervous system overreacts to all types of sensory stimuli, and habituation to repetitive stimuli typically does not occur. This can manifest as anxiety or behavioral difficulties in noisy environments, tactile defensiveness, and difficulty with transitions from one environment to another. Almost all children with FXS have significant executive function deficits, as well (Bennetto & Pennington, 2002). Approximately 80% of males and 30% of females with FXS meet criteria for ADHD, with a short attention span, hyperactivity, and impulsivity. Anxiety is another common problem in FXS. On occasion, the anxiety can be so severe that children refuse to speak (called selective mutism), particularly at school (Hagerman, Hills, Scharfenaker, & Lewis, 1999). Multidisciplinary treatments for the cognitive, speech, behavioral, and emotional problems of children with FXS are recommended for optimal outcomes.

Recent Research in FXS

Active research in the field of FXS is ongoing across multiple disciplines, including basic molecular research on the *FMR1* gene and FMRP, neuroimaging, and clinical research on FXTAS, autism, and treatments for FXS. Research on individuals and families affected by FXS since the mid-1990s has revealed a variety of medical and developmental problems related to the premutation carrier state in both children and adults. Prior to this time, it was recognized that individuals with the full mutation were affected with FXS, but individuals with the premutation were considered unaffected. Recent studies have found that children with the premutation (especially males) commonly have problems with ADHD and social relatedness, with some individuals meeting criteria for a diagnosis of autism spectrum disorder (Farzin et al., 2006). The cause of these attention difficulties or social deficits in some school-age carriers is unknown, because levels of FMRP are usually normal, but a developmental effect of the elevated *FMR1* mRNA is currently being investigated. Women with the premutation are more likely to have emotional problems, including anxiety, social phobia, and obsessive–compulsive behaviors (Franke et al., 1998; Hessl et al., 2005), and to suffer from premature ovarian failure as well (Welt, Smith, & Taylor, 2004). In the past 5 years, FXTAS has also been discovered in aging individuals with the premutation, and it is now estimated to account for approximately 4–5% of adult cases of ataxia (Macpherson, Waghorn, Hammans, & Jacobs, 2003). Due to the discovery of these new medical and developmental problems associated with the carrier state, making a diagnosis of FXS is important not only for improving treatments for children with FXS but also to give information to the family members regarding genetic counseling and cascade testing of extended family members (McConkie-Rosell et al., 2005).

Advances in our understanding of the neurobiology of FXS in animal models, such as the fragile-X mouse and fruit fly models, have led to targeted treatment endeavors that may eventually reverse the neurodevelopmental abnormalities. It has recently been discovered that low levels of the FMRP protein in FXS enhances activity of a cellular signaling pathway in the brain, called the mGluR5 pathway, which may be related to a number of clinical features of FXS, including MR, seizures, and social deficits (Bear, Huber, & Warren, 2004). This discovery is extremely important because medications have been developed that can regulate activity of the mGluR5 pathway, including lith-ium and mGluR5 antagonists (Hagerman, 2006). Trials of these agents are currently under way in animal models with promising results, and the use of lithium in patients with FXS is being studied with hopes that it will improve cognitive and behavioral out-comes in these patients.

Recent research on the visual pathways in the brains of children with FXS has sup-ported the development of specific educational strategies for children with FXS. The M and P pathways are two anatomically separate pathways that process visual information in the brain. The magnocellular (M) pathway is important for visual processing of action or object motion, and the parvocellular (P) pathway is important for form per-ception and object recognition. The absence of FMRP in FXS has a dramatic impact on the M visual pathway, but not the P visual pathway, of the brain (Kogan et al., 2004). The intact functioning of the P visual pathway in FXS supports the effectiveness of edu-cational interventions that utilize strengths in visual object recognition, such as the Logo Reading Program described in the following section. Other, similar projects incorporating neuropsychological research results into educational interventions for children with FXS are under way.

Treatment Recommendations in FXS

Multidisciplinary evaluation and individualized treatment programs are strongly rec-ommended for all children with FXS. Children with the premutation generally do not require such intensive treatments, but they should have a full psychological and educa-tional assessment if there are any concerns to determine whether interventions are needed. The problems in carriers are typically less difficult to treat medically, such as through use of stimulant medications for attention problems or ADHD, or through a social skills group for their social deficits. Special education or individual tutoring for the LD sometimes associated with the premutation is also often required.

Effective treatment plans for children with FXS should include developmental, cog-nitive, emotional, and behavioral considerations. Due to the language delays that are almost universal in FXS, early speech and language therapy is important. For children with FXS who have very little or no expressive language, more intensive language inter-vention techniques are recommended, including sign language, the Picture Exchange Communication System (PECS), and other augmentative communication techniques. The combination of speech and language therapy with occupational therapy, so that movement and rhythms can be utilized to enhance language expression, has been use-ful in anecdotal cases (Scharfenaker, O'Connor, Stackhouse, & Noble, 2002).

All children with FXS should be evaluated and treated for ADHD symptoms. The majority of these children respond well to stimulant medication (Hagerman, 2002a). In addition to medication treatments, it is also important for teachers to use strategies in the classroom to improve attention, including sitting in front of the classroom, repeat-ing and reinforcing instructions with visual input, and preparing children for transi-tions. Because of these children's increased sensory reactivity, transitions can often be overwhelming, and visual schedules can help to prepare the children for what will come next (Braden, 2002; Scharfenaker et al., 2002). Physical calming techniques can also be used in the classroom, and an occupational therapist can share these skills with teachers as well as parents so that consistent strategies are used across contexts. Weekly speech and language therapy and occupational therapy are essential for the special education program for a child with FXS.

Anxiety symptoms are also important to identify and treat in FXS. Most individuals will benefit from medical treatment with selective serotonin reuptake inhibitors (SSRIs). If severe anxiety or selective mutism is present, a combination of treatments consisting of speech and language therapy, psychotherapy, and an SSRI are recommended (Hagerman, 2004). Behavioral problems can result from the sensory reactivity, anxiety, and mood instability common in FXS, and work with a behavioral specialist to develop an appropriate behavior plan that can be used in both the school and home settings is often a very important component of treatment. Children with FXS and autism also need typical autism interventions, including applied behavior analysis (ABA) and structured learning environments with strong visual schedules to reinforce routines such as emphasized by the Treatment and Education of Autistic and Related Communication-Handicapped Children (TEAACH) programs (Braden, 2000, 2002; Ozonoff, Rogers, & Hendren, 2003).

Children with FXS have a number of cognitive strengths and weaknesses that are reflected in their academic achievement. Although the boys typically have weaknesses in all academic areas, their strengths are seen in general knowledge because they have an ability to integrate experiential information (Roberts et al., 2005). Because of these abilities and their strengths in object recognition, Braden (2002) developed a technique called Logo Reading that utilizes "logos," or easily recognized photo representations of objects or actions, paired with words to teach children with FXS reading skills. As the children with FXS learn to identify the words, the logo is gradually extinguished. This technique has been effective in teaching children with FXS to read.

Although children with FXS do well with object recognition, they have significant problems with visual–motor coordination, which affects their drawing and handwriting skills (Cornish, Munir, & Cross, 1999). Programs such as Handwriting Without Tears can be helpful for these problems. Another area of strength is their interest in and ability with computers. Thus programs that enhance written language, such as Writing with Symbols, and word-prediction programs, such as Write: Out Loud and Co: Writer, can be helpful for enhancing writing skills when at least a first-grade reading level is present.

In summary, children with FXS need intensive, multidisciplinary treatment programs that focus on the strengths of the individual child. Programs that include medical intervention to help with attention, anxiety, and mood instability; behavioral interventions to help with aggression, impulsivity, and social deficits; and speech and language and occupational therapy to work with the language and motor deficits can lead to significant developmental and academic progress for most children with FXS.

22q11.2 Deletion Syndrome/Velocardiofacial Syndrome

22q11.2 deletion syndrome (DS22q11.2) results from a deletion in a small piece of the long arm of chromosome 22. Individuals with a deletion in this region can have a variety of problems, including congenital heart disease, immunodeficiency, hypoparathyroidism, abnormalities of the palate, characteristic facial features, and cognitive deficits. Prior to the early 1990s, when microdeletions in the 22q11.2 region were first reported, a variety of syndromes were identified that described overlapping features of this disorder. For example, DiGeorge syndrome was defined as being composed of immune deficits, characteristic facial features, hypoparathyroidism, and cardiac defects, whereas Shprintzen syndrome (later renamed velocardiofacial syndrome [VCFS]) included patients with characteristic facial features and cardiac anomalies but also included those with learning abnormalities, cleft palate, and velopharyngeal abnormalities. Other syndromes with overlapping features included conotruncal anomaly face syndrome (CTAFS), and Cayler cardiofacial syndrome.

In 1981, the first report of a visible deletion at chromosome region 22q11 was reported in patients with DiGeorge syndrome (de la Chapelle, Herva, Koivisto, & Aula, 1981), and then from 1991 to 1993 microdeletions at chromosome region 22q11 were detected using molecular probes in patients with DiGeorge syndrome, Shprintzen/velocardiofacial syndrome, and CTAFS in separate studies (Burn et al., 1993; Scambler et al., 1991; Scambler et al., 1992). Since that time, it has been increasingly recognized that deletions in this chromosome region can vary in length and can produce many combinations of the characteristic features. Due to the common etiology, and to avoid confusion from all the previous names, individuals with these disorders are now usually referred to by the most inclusive name, 22q11.2 deletion syndrome, although VCFS and DiGeorge syndrome are still frequently used. Recent population-based studies have estimated that 22q11.2 deletions occur in approximately 1 in 4,000 individuals (Botto et al., 2003).

More than 180 clinical features, both physical and developmental/behavioral, have been reported to be associated with DS22q11.2 (Goldberg, Motzkin, Marion, Scambler, & Shprintzen, 1993). Although none of the features occurs with 100% frequency, the most common features include developmental delays or learning disabilities in 85–90% and cardiac abnormalities in 80% of children with this disorder. Characteristic facial features include mildly wide-set eyes (hypertelorism), narrow palpebral fissures and hooded upper eyelids, small ears with an overfolded helix, and a prominent nasal bridge with a bulbous nasal tip. Overt cleft palates are present in 18%, but more commonly the palatal abnormalities are submucous or occult clefts that are not able to be seen on examination. Clefs and palatal dysfunction lead to problems with speech articulation and a hypernasal voice. (See Figure 6.2.)

The common developmental features include early speech and motor delays and cognitive impairments. Speech and language impairment in DS22q11.2 starts in infancy (Scherer, D'Antonio, & Kalbfleisch, 1999), and impairments in expressive language are significantly greater compared with receptive language scores in young children (Moss et al., 1999). Expressive language typically improves around 4–5 years of age, and in adolescence expressive language scores may surpass receptive language scores. This "flip" is likely due to the increased demand on abstraction and language comprehension skills when testing receptive language in older children (Solot et al., 2001).

The specific psychological and cognitive profile in DS22q11.2 has been well studied. Only 40–50% of children with DS22q11.2 have mild to moderate mental retardation; however, almost all have some degree of learning disability, even when their IQs are in the normal range (Swillen et al., 1997). Verbal IQ is typically significantly higher than performance IQ, although this is not universal (Moss et al., 1999). The classic neuropsychological profile includes problems with abstract reasoning, visual–spatial reasoning, math, and higher order language. Early learning of concrete information is often adequate and comparable to that of their peers (including letter and word recognition, counting, and spelling); however, problems with reasoning and application of concepts become evident in the early grade school years and persist through school. These difficulties with higher order comprehension, abstract verbal understanding, and language formulation often manifest as "immature and concrete thought"

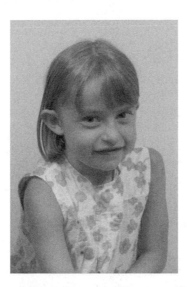

FIGURE 6.2. Seven-year-old female with 22q11.2 deletion syndrome. Notice her small, prominent ears and slightly bulbous nasal tip. She also had congenital heart disease and a hypernasal voice. She currently receives speech therapy and resource help for mild learning problems in reading, writing, and math.

(Golding-Kushner, Weller, & Shprintzen, 1985). Although rote reading, word recognition, rote memory, and spelling can be relative strengths, reading comprehension and complex memory (e.g., for stories) are especially difficult.

The visual–spatial impairments in DS22q11.2 include poor memory for spatial reasoning (relative locations of objects), visuomotor construction (putting together patterns and puzzles), or any other task that requires mentally or physically manipulating objects and spatial relationships. Because these deficits typically manifest with performance IQ scores lower than verbal IQ scores, the term "nonverbal learning disability" (NVLD) has been used to describe the profile in DS22q11.2 (Moss et al., 1999; Swillen et al., 1999). This classification has been controversial in DS22q11.2 because these children also have higher order language comprehension deficits and other neuropsychological impairments.

DS22q11.2 is also associated with neurodevelopmental and psychiatric disorders. Forty to sixty percent of children with DS22q11.2 meet diagnostic criteria for ADHD. Approximately 50% of adolescents and young adults develop mood disorders, including anxiety, depression, or bipolar disorder, and 20–30% of individuals develop schizophrenia or other psychotic disorders (Bassett et al., 2003).

Recent Research in DS22q11.2

Genetic research over the past 15 years has better characterized the deleted region of chromosome 22 and has identified some genes in this region that play a role in the features of DS22q11.2. The size of the deleted region varies between individuals, with anywhere from 25 to 30 genes deleted. The length of the deletion has not been found to correlate with the physical or developmental phenotype, but a few specific genes within the deleted region have been identified that are implicated in various features of the syndrome. For example, the *TBX1* gene is located in the deleted region, and lower expression levels of this gene have been shown to correlate with the severity of heart defects found in DS22q11.2 (Liao et al., 2004). Another gene, the *COMT* gene, has been reported to be associated with the developmental and psychiatric phenotype in DS22q11.2 (Lachman et al., 1996). The *COMT* gene codes for the enzyme catechol-O-methyltransferase that breaks down the neurotransmitters dopamine and norepinephrine in the synapses between neurons. In typical individuals it is expressed from both copies of chromosome 22, but with a *COMT* deletion in DS22q11.2, only one chromosome actively expresses the enzyme. The *COMT* gene comes in two variations (polymorphisms), and one variation (*Met*) results in an enzyme with an activity level 3–4 times lower than the other variant (*Val*), resulting in decreased degradation (and higher levels) of dopamine and norepinephrine in the synapse (see Simon, Burg, & Gothelf, 2007, for a review). Recent research has found a strong association between the low-activity *COMT Met* variation and the development of psychotic symptoms, declining verbal IQs, and decreased size of the prefrontal areas of the brain in adolescent patients with DS22q11.2 followed over many years (Gothelf, Furfaro, Penniman, Glover, & Reiss, 2005). Another study has found that executive function and behavioral problems are more common in patients with DS22q11.2 and the *Val* allele (Bearden et al., 2004). Although not all individuals with DS22q11.2 with the *Met* allele develop schizophrenia, and although other genetic influences are actively being investigated, this research will definitely have implications for this population in the future by allowing early identification of individuals with DS22q11.2 at high risk for developing schizophrenia or psychotic symptoms. Future research will be directed at developing early psychological and medical interventions that target abnormalities in this genetic pathway to prevent these outcomes.

Other interesting studies in DS22q11.2 have focused on the etiology and transmission of the deletion. The deletion is passed from a parent to a child in only 10–15% of cases, whereas most cases are *de novo* deletions of a small part of chromosome 22 found only in the child. In general, children who inherit the deletion are typically more affected cognitively than the group with the *de novo* deletions (Moss et al., 1999; Ryan et al., 1997). Also, children with a deletion from the maternal chromosome have more impaired language abilities than those with a paternal deletion (Glaser et al., 2002), suggesting that genes in the 22q-deleted region involved in language development may be imprinted, a genetic mechanism by which gene expression differs depending on the parental origin of the chromosome on which the gene is located. Neuroimaging studies in DS22q11.2 have also found that overall brain gray matter is reduced in children with maternal origin of the deletion (Eliez & Blasey, 2001). Ongoing research in this area will determine whether imprinting does indeed play a role in the DS22q11.2 phenotype.

More recently, sophisticated cognitive experimentation studies designed specifically to identify the neural circuits involved in the deficits in DS22q11.2 have shown the existence of dysfunction in a neural network called the frontoparietal network, a neural system connecting the parietal and frontal lobes of the brain that is known to be involved in visual–spatial attention, enumeration (identifying the number of objects), magnitude judgment (judgment of how long or how much), and the ability to inhibit irrelevant information or inappropriate responses. Children with DS22q11.2 perform poorly on all of these tasks compared with controls (Simon et al., 2005). These studies are critical because they deconstruct the general problems known to be present in DS22q11.2 (such as visuospatial skills or math) and identify very specific deficits at the basic level, and this knowledge can then be translated into the development of specific educational interventions. Other active research on the role of the deleted 22q11.2 genes in neurodevelopment will continue to lead to specific medical and educational interventions for this group of children.

Treatment Recommendations in DS22q11.2 (VCFS)

The treatment plan for children with DS22q11.2 should involve a combination of medical follow-up and psychological and educational interventions. A complete evaluation should be completed by a medical team to address the various medical problems associated with the syndrome. Evaluation by a medical craniofacial team that includes an experienced speech therapist is essential for all children with DS22q11.2 due to the high rate of submucous cleft palate and palatal dysfunction, and strong speech therapy interventions are recommended to start within the first 2 years of life and continue through the school years. Surgical intervention is sometimes necessary and helpful for speech production and to improve hypernasality. Hearing testing is also very important due to frequent ear infections with hearing loss that may interfere with speech development. Hearing screens every year until at least 8 years of age are recommended (Shprintzen, 2005). When early expressive language problems are severe, augmentative communication interventions, such as sign language and other communication devices, can be helpful, although almost all children with DS22q11.2 will outgrow the need for these as their speech improves.

Although rote reading, word recognition, rote memory, and spelling can be relative strengths in children with DS22q11.2, reading comprehension and complex memory (e.g., for stories) is especially difficult. Because early reading can often be mastered through their strengths in word recognition and rote memory, it is important for educators to recognize that comprehension is often lacking despite relative strengths in word recognition and spelling. These deficits often become more evident when academic demands shift to more complex tasks during the early grade school years. Many of the learning problems in DS22q11.2 are related to deficiencies in abstract reasoning, so educational techniques that use concrete examples and divide complex problems into simple components are recommended (Shprintzen, 2005).

Although there is some controversy regarding the diagnosis of nonverbal learning disability (NVLD) in children with DS22q11.2 due to the complexity of their language deficits and neuropsychological impairments, many educational strategies for children with nonverbal developmental dysfunction can be successfully applied to children with DS22q11.2. These include techniques such as presenting information in clear verbal terms without use of figurative speech or slang, encouraging active verbalization of each step of a task or multistep problem, simplifying answer-sheet or work-sheet layouts, providing occupational therapy to help with motor skills and dexterity, using word processing programs for written assignments, understanding that visual–spatial assignments (maps, graphs, etc.) may require assistance, and providing speech therapy interventions that focus on pragmatic and nonverbal language skills.

Interventions using educational computer programs have also been shown to be helpful for a small group of children with VCFS, improving both math and reading skills (specifically phonemic awareness, sight-word recognition, reading decoding, and fluency) and also improving self-esteem (Kok & Solman, 1995). Many children with DS22q11.2 seem to have a strong affinity for computers, and other educational computer programs can be incorporated into their educational plans as well.

Identification and treatment of ADHD symptoms is also important in the treatment plan for children with DS22q11.2. A study of methylphenidate treatment for ADHD symptoms in DS22q11.2 showed a good response and no significant side effects in a 1-month trial (Gothelf et al., 2003). Concerns about the use of stimulant medications in patients with DS22q11.2 have been raised due to their action at the synapse, increasing neurotransmitter levels (i.e., dopamine) that require degradation by an enzyme (*COMT*) that is found in the deleted region of chromosome 22. Some reports have linked the use of stimulant medications for ADHD treatment to the development of psychotic symptoms (Lachman et al., 1996), although with up to 60% of DS22q11.2 patients having ADHD and up to 20% developing psychosis, it is difficult to prove this association based on case reports. Long-term, controlled studies that look at medication treatment and the development of psychiatric symptoms are needed to answer this question. Nonstimulant ADHD medications such as atomoxetine in DS22q11.2 are currently being investigated. Behavioral interventions for ADHD symptoms are also recommended for use in children with DS22q11.2, including structured learning and home environments, preferential seating with limited distractions in the classroom, daily planners, positive reinforcement techniques, and cognitive techniques for improving impulsivity and inattention, such as the Think Aloud program (Bloomquist, 1996).

Mood stabilizer and antipsychotic medications are less controversial and are recommended if mood instability, aggression, mania, depression, or psychosis develop (Hagerman, 1999; McElroy & Weller, 1997), although controlled trials of these medications in DS22q11.2 have not yet been completed. Parents and teachers should be educated about the early signs of mood disorders or psychotic symptoms so that appropriate treatments can be initiated. Ongoing prospective research studies hope to find genetic markers, brain imaging abnormalities, or other clinical symptoms that can identify the children with DS22q11.2 who are at higher risk for these more severe mental health problems.

In summary, children with DS22q11.2 require strong early medical evaluations, as well as early speech and language therapies; complete psychoeducational evaluation for educational planning, with an emphasis on their neuropsychological strengths and weaknesses; and ongoing evaluation and treatment (behavioral and medical) for ADHD and other psychiatric disorders.

Smith–Magenis Syndrome

Smith–Magenis syndrome (SMS) is a genetic disorder characterized by developmental delays, mental retardation, and behavioral disturbances that occurs in 1 out of 15,000–25,000 births (Greenberg et al., 1991). SMS was first described in 1982, at which time cytogenetic studies showed that it was caused by deleted genetic material on chromosome 17p11.2. SMS is considered to be a contiguous gene syndrome, which by definition suggests that the deletion of multiple, functionally unrelated genes located in close proximity on chromosome 17 is responsible for the phenotype. Since its initial description in 1982 (Smith, McGavran, & Waldstein, 1982), specific FISH testing for this deletion has been developed, and the vast majority of all cases of SMS have been identified by the FISH technique in the past 10 years.

Children with SMS have a characteristic facial appearance that includes broad, square-shaped faces with prominent foreheads, deep-set and upslanting eyes, eyebrows that meet in the middle (synophrys), a broad nasal bridge, and a "tented" appearance to the mouth. Laryngeal anomalies are common, including abnormal vocal cord structure, polyps, nodules, or partial vocal cord paralysis that can lead to a hoarse voice in 80% of patients. Hearing is affected in many children with SMS due to recurrent ear infections and conductive hearing loss, as well as frequent sensorineural hearing loss. Hearing loss can also contribute to the speech delays commonly seen in SMS children. Stature is usually below the normal range for age, and high cholesterol is present in up to 60% of children with SMS (Smith et al., 2002; Smith, Magenis, & Elsea, 2005).

The majority of individuals with SMS function in the mild to moderate range of mental retardation, with IQ scores between 40 and 55 (Greenberg et al., 1996). Speech delays occur in up to 90% of children with SMS, and expressive language abilities are more impaired than receptive language abilities, likely partially related to structural abnormalities of the larynx/palate and oral-sensory-motor dysfunction. Although IQs are usually in the MR range, there are relative strengths in long-term memory, computer skills, and perceptual skills, with weaknesses in sequential processing and short-term memory (Dykens, Finucane, & Gayley, 1997).

Behavioral characteristics in SMS change from infancy through childhood. Infants with SMS tend to have feeding difficulties, poor growth, and low muscle tone. They have prolonged sleep periods and frequently need to be awakened for feedings. By 18 months, inattention, hyperactivity, temper tantrums, impulsivity, aggression, and self-injurious behaviors begin to emerge, and later in childhood up to 80% of children with SMS meet criteria for ADHD. Expressive language difficulties are likely to contribute to many of these behavioral problems (Greenberg et al., 1996). Two characteristic stereotypic behaviors that appear to be specific to SMS include the "self-hug" (spasmodic upper-body squeeze) and "lick and flip" (hand licking and page flipping). Other stereotypic behaviors include mouthing of their hands or other objects, teeth grinding, rocking, and spinning objects. Self-injurious behaviors become more prevalent during adolescence and can be very difficult to manage. These include self-hitting, biting, and skin picking, insertion of objects into body orifices (polyemoilokomania), and pulling out fingernails or toenails (onchyotillomania). Day–night wakefulness is also disturbed and represents a major issue for caretakers. With increasing age, the number and frequency of naps increases, and total sleep time at night decreases. Diminished REM sleep has been documented (Greenberg et al., 1996; Potocki et al., 2000). Research has shown that aberrant melatonin synthesis and/or degradation is the underlying cause of the sleep disturbance (De Leersnyder et al., 2001; Potocki et al., 2000).

Recent Research in SMS

As with 22q11.2 deletion syndrome described earlier, there is considerable research interest in the genes located within the deleted region of chromosome 17 in SMS and the role these genes may play in the psychological and physical phenotypes. The deleted "critical region" in SMS contains approximately 25 genes (Lucas, Vlangos, Das, Patel, & Elsea, 2001), and a recent study has shown that individuals with larger deletions had lower levels of cognition (in the severe-to-profound range of MR) and adaptive functioning compared with individuals with small deletions (Madduri et al., 2006).

The specific genes within the deleted region responsible for the major features of SMS have also started to be identified. Recent research has focused on the *RAI1* gene (retinoic-acid-induced-1), which codes for a protein thought to be involved in the transcription of other genes involved in neuronal differentiation. This gene was discovered by studying a small group of individuals with the characteristic physical and behavioral phenotype of SMS but who tested negative for SMS on standard FISH testing. Although these individuals did not have the classic deletion at 17p11.2, further genetic testing using CGH array and DNA sequencing discovered that they all had small mutations in the *RAI1* gene, which had not been identified using the standard FISH test for SMS (Schoumans et al., 2005; Slager, Newton, Vlangos, Finucane, & Elsea, 2003). These findings show that deletion of this single gene in the 17p11.2 critical region may be responsible for the majority of the neurobehavioral features of SMS. Research on other genes in the SMS critical region has identified genes that may be responsible for some of the more variable features of SMS, such as the *MYO15* gene involved in sensorineural hearing loss, the *COP9* gene related to sleep dysregulation, and the *SREBF1* gene involved in cholesterol homeostasis.

Treatment Recommendations in SMS

Although SMS was described only in 1982, active research has led to the development of comprehensive medical and developmental treatment recommendations for patients with SMS. Medical issues that need to be followed carefully include management of ear and sinus infections, hearing assessments, testing of thyroid function, lipid and cholesterol profiles, urine analysis for kidney problems, and monitoring for scoliosis.

It is recommended that all children with SMS have an individualized educational program developed following a complete multidisciplinary assessment, including cognitive, physical, occupational, and speech therapy evaluations. Functional behavioral assessments and behavioral plans are also an important part of educational programming for individuals with SMS due to their behavioral difficulties and self-injurious behaviors. Early and intensive work with speech and language services is important, and the use of sign language and total communication programs are felt to improve communication skills and behavior (Smith & Gropman, 2005).

Educational techniques that recognize the inherent weaknesses in sequential processing (counting, math tasks, multistep tasks) and short-term memory while taking advantage of relative strengths in long-term memory and visual reasoning are most effective. Use of pictures, computers, and other visual learning techniques are recommended in the school setting (Smith & Gropman, 2005).

Research on the use of medications to help with the behavioral features of SMS is under way. Stimulant medication can sometimes be helpful in increasing attention and decreasing hyperactivity (Smith & Gropman, 2005), whereas treatment with atypical neuroleptics such as risperidone have been reported to help behavioral problems and aggression (Hagerman, 1999). Managing the sleep disturbance is a challenge, and reports of therapeutic benefit from melatonin are encouraging (Wheeler, Taylor, Simonsen, & Reith, 2005). Low doses of melatonin at bedtime have resulted in general improvement in sleep and few adverse side effects. Ongoing studies are investigating other medications to try to improve sleep patterns (De Leersnyder et al., 2003). Growth hormone treatment may also help with sleep problems (Itoh, Hayashi, Hasegawa, Shimohira, & Kohyama, 2004). A comprehensive treatment plan that includes close medical follow-up, speech therapy, occupational therapy, behavioral management, and an educational plan that recognizes the specific neurocognitive strengths and weaknesses caused by the 17p11.2 deletion will improve outcomes for children with SMS.

X and Y Chromosome Aneuploidies

Individuals with X and Y chromosome aneuploidies have an atypical number of X and/or Y chromosomes. Typical males have a 46,XY sex chromosome constitution, whereas typical females have 46,XX sex chromosomes. Differences from these normal sex chromosome pairs can occur in many forms and include males with 47,XXY (Klinefelter syndrome), 47,XYY, or 48,XXYY, and females with 45,X (Turner syndrome) and 47,XXX (trisomy X). Many other, rarer forms of X and Y chromosome aneuploidy occur as well, with variations in males such as 48,XXXY, 48,XYYY and 49,XXXXY and variations in females such as 48,XXXX (tetrasomy X) and 49,XXXXX (pentasomy X). The most common variations are the trisomies (XXY, XYY, XXX), which commonly result in learning disabilities and very rarely fall in the MR range. As additional X and Y chromosomes are added, the physical and cognitive problems generally increase in severity, and the percentage of children with cognitive functioning in the MR range increases, although MR is not universal.

Overall, X and Y chromosome aneuploidies are the most common chromosomal abnormalities in humans, and newborn screening studies have shown that as a group they occur in approximately 1 in 400 births (Nielsen, 1990). Although this is a very high prevalence, significant variability exists in the physical, cognitive, and behavioral manifestations of these disorders; and although many individuals are significantly affected, many others go undiagnosed due to very mild clinical symptoms. Recent estimates suggest that medical professionals diagnose only 25% of all cases of 47,XXY/Klinefelter syndrome (Bojesen, Juul, & Gravholt, 2003) and 10% of 47,XYY syndrome (Abramsky & Chapple, 1997). The others remain undiagnosed for two main reasons: (1) lack of professional recognition of the cognitive-behavioral phenotype, physical, and medical manifestations of these disorders and (2) very mild expression of characteristic symptoms of the disorders in individual patients.

A large amount of research on the most common forms of X and Y chromosome aneuploidies was done in the 1970s and 1980s, when multiple cohorts of patients around the United States, Canada, and Europe with XXY, XXX, and XYY were identified by newborn screening tests. These infants were followed prospectively into young adulthood, with data collected on physical and cognitive development and on psychological and psychosocial characteristics. Results from these prospective studies form the base of our knowledge on the natural history of X and Y chromosome aneuploidies, and current research is building on this base to better understand the molecular and brain abnormalities in these disorders in order to develop individual treatments. Research on less common forms of the X and Y chromosome aneuploidies, such as 48,XXYY, 49,XXXXY, and tetrasomy and pentasomy X, is scarce, although active research is under way to better characterize these disorders. Following are examples of recent advances in research and interventions for two common X and Y chromosome variations—47,XXY/Klinefelter syndrome and 45,X/Turner syndrome.

47,XXY/Klinefelter Syndrome

Klinefelter syndrome was first reported in 1942, when Dr. Harry Klinefelter described a group of adult males with tall stature, testosterone deficiency, and infertility; in 1956 it was discovered that Klinefelter syndrome resulted from an additional X chromosome in males. Physical and medical features of Klinefelter syndrome include tall stature, narrow shoulders, long legs, low muscle tone, hypogonadism (small testicles and testosterone deficiency), and infertility. There are no characteristic facial features, and low muscle tone, speech delays, and motor delays can be present in infancy (Visootsak, Aylstock, & Graham, 2001).

Prospective newborn screening studies in the 1970s and 1980s described the cognitive and behavioral phenotypes of males with 47,XXY and showed that most XXY males have IQs in the normal range, although their IQs are commonly approximately 10 points lower than those of their siblings and they have significant problems with verbal skills and language-based tasks (Robinson, Bender, Borelli, & Winter, 1986). Visual–spatial skills and performance IQ are preserved (Rovet, Netley, Keenan, Bailey, & Stewart, 1996), and verbal IQ is often significantly lower than performance IQ. Evaluations for reading disabilities show that 40–50% of XXY males have dyslexia and that up to 80% require reading interventions in school (Bender, Puck, Salbenblatt, & Robinson, 1986; Pennington, Bender, Puck, Salbenblatt, & Robinson, 1982). Significant difficulties with word retrieval affect expressive language skills. Math is also an academic weakness (Rovet et al., 1996). Frontal-executive dysfunction (Geschwind, Boone, Miller, & Swerdloff, 2000) manifests as problems with inhibitory skills and attentional difficulties. Approximately 35% of children with 47,XXY meet criteria for a clinical diagnosis of ADHD (Tartaglia, Reynolds, Davis, Hansen, & Hagerman, 2006), with symptoms of inattention and distractibility more common than hyperactivity. Auditory processing is also affected and, combined with language deficits and attentional problems, can make processing of verbally presented information very difficult. Salbenblatt and colleagues also described deficits in both gross and fine motor skills (Salbenblatt, Meyers, Bender, Linden, & Robinson, 1989). Fine motor skills can be further affected by hand tremors that are present in a large percentage of males with XXY.

Behavioral problems in early childhood, such as tantrums and withdrawal, are also common, and school-age and adolescent males with 47,XXY are at increased risk for poor self-esteem, mood disorders such as anxiety and depression, and social deficits (Bender, Harmon, Linden, & Robinson, 1995). The significant variability of developmental and psychological symptoms in individuals with 47,XXY must again be emphasized, with some children showing few of the aforementioned problems whereas others are more significantly affected.

The most important aspect of medical follow-up is assessment of the need for testosterone replacement therapy in adolescence. Puberty in 47,XXY boys typically begins at a normal age, although in some boys it is slightly delayed. During adolescence testosterone production in 47,XXY decreases due to fibrosis of the testicular tissue, and testosterone replacement therapy is important to ensure normal pubertal development and secondary sex characteristics (body hair, muscle bulk), as well as to improve stamina. The severity of testosterone deficiency varies between 47,XXY individuals, with a small percentage of individuals falling within the low-normal range without requiring additional testosterone treatment.

RECENT RESEARCH IN 47,XXY SYNDROME

Although previous research has better characterized the behavioral and cognitive phenotype of 47,XXY males, there has been little progress until very recently in identifying the genetic basis of the phenotypic variability in 47,XXY. Recent research has focused on genes on the X chromosome that escape X-inactivation, the process by which genes on one copy of the X chromosome are inactivated in females to maintain a balance of gene expression between males and females. It is now known that up to 20% of genes on the X chromosome escape inactivation and continue to be expressed from both X chromosomes in typical 46,XX females (Willard, 1996). Because males with 47,XXY have two X chromosomes, these genes that escape X-inactivation are postulated to play a role in the phenotype of 47,XXY, as they would be actively expressed from both X chromosomes in these males (Simpson et al., 2003). A majority of X chromosome genes that escape X-inactivation are found in newly identified regions of the X and Y chromosomes called the pseudoautosomal regions (PAR), which are located near the telomeres of the X and Y chromosomes and contain homologous (identical) genes on the X and Y. DNA microarray technology is currently being used to investigate large numbers of genes in the PAR that may be over- or underexpressed in males with XXY syndrome (Geschwind et al., 1998). The results of these types of large-scale molecular studies promise to identify multiple X and Y chromosome genes responsible for the variability in the phenotype of XXY and the other X and Y chromosome aneuploidies.

The androgen receptor (AR) gene on the X chromosome escapes X-inactivation and has recently been found to correlate with both physical appearance and psychosocial functioning in XXY males (Zinn et al., 2005; Zitzmann, Depenbusch, Gromoll, & Nieschlag, 2004). This gene codes for the receptor for androgen (testosterone hormone) and contains a CAG-repeat segment that varies between individuals and influences the responsiveness of the receptor to testosterone. In adult males with XXY, those with a lower number of CAG repeats have fewer physical characteristics of Klinefelter syndrome (shorter stature, less gynecomastia, and larger testicles) than those with the larger number of CAG repeats in the AR gene. The males with the shorter CAG repeat length were also more likely to have successful relationships and professional jobs, showing that variations in this gene may be involved in brain and social development in 47,XXY genotype–phenotype as well (Zitzmann et al., 2004). It is known that the AR gene is expressed in multiple areas of the brain in both males and females, and more specific studies that look at cognitive functioning in relation to the AR CAG repeat length are under way. This is the first specific gene described that shows a genotype–phenotype correlation for XXY syndrome, and it is an example of the types of ongoing molecular research that are working to explain the phenotypic variability of the X and Y chromosome aneuploidies.

Recent research has also challenged the classic view that testosterone levels are normal in 47,XXY males until adolescence and has suggested that signs of testosterone deficiency may be present in the first 2 years of life, with lower testosterone levels contributing to the smaller penis size and low muscle tone compared with typical 46,XY infants (Ross et al., 2005). The role of testosterone treatment in cognitive functioning and behavior is also under investigation. Many parents and adult males have reported improvements in speech and attention abilities and fewer mood and behavioral symptoms once starting testosterone treatment (Mandoki & Sumner, 1991), although this has not been studied in controlled trials. Active research that looks at the neurodevelopmental, motor, and behavioral effects of testosterone treatment in early childhood and adolescence is under way, and results of these studies may significantly change standard treatment for males with 47,XXY.

Other advances in neuroimaging and animal models of XXY have also added to our understanding of children with 47,XXY syndrome. Recent results from neuroimaging projects have begun to identify the structural brain abnormalities underlying the language deficits of 47,XXY individuals. MRI studies have shown that the volume of the left temporal lobe involved in language processing and production is smaller in males with XXY (Giedd et al., 2006; Patwardhan, Eliez, Bender, Linden, & Reiss, 2000) and that the smaller left temporal lobe volumes correlate with more significant deficits in language scores and verbal processing speed in XXY males (Itti et al., 2006). Other brain regions linked to cognition and emotional regulation, including the left hippocampus, insula, and medial limbic system, have also been found to be smaller in children with XXY (Giedd et al., 2006). A mouse model for XXY has also been developed that shows characteristic features of Klinefelter syndrome, including the development of hypogonadism and infertility, as well as learning deficits (Lue et al., 2005). Further studies on the XXY mouse model will allow new research on the cellular pathways involved in the medical and psychological features and also provide great opportunity for treatment trials that may translate to human treatments for infertility and neurodevelopmental abnormalities in 47,XXY/Klinefelter syndrome. Active research across many disciplines investigating genotype–phenotype relationships, together with clinical studies on neurodevelopmental disorders and treatments, will continue to shape intervention recommendations for children with 47,XXY/Klinefelter syndrome.

TREATMENT RECOMMENDATIONS FOR 47,XXY SYNDROME

Treatment recommendations for 47,XXY have been compiled (Rovet et al., 1996; Simpson, Graham, Samango-Sprouse, & Swerdloff, 2005; Visootsak et al., 2001; Hagerman, 1999) based on clinical experience and the aforementioned research findings. In infancy and early childhood, close developmental monitoring for developmental delays and early intervention that includes speech, physical, and occupational therapy is important for early speech and motor delays.

Specific recommendations for teachers have been published by Rovet et al. (1996) and emphasize techniques that recognize the verbal learning disability and strengths in visuospatial skills. Instruction using slow and clear speech in short concrete sentences is recommended, as well as other techniques, such as strategies to enhance memory, continuous checks during reading instruction, and providing extra support for word problems in math. Speech and language therapy that stresses vocabulary development, sentence understanding, reading comprehension, pragmatic language skills, phonemic awareness, and word finding is also recommended. Because research on reading problems in 80% of 47,XXY children shows neurocognitive features similar to those of children with idiopathic dyslexia, intensive treatments designed for dyslexia with emphasis on phonological processing are recommended (Geschwind & Dykens, 2004), such as the Lindamood–Bell learning program or the SpellRead PAT (Phonological Auditory Training) system.

Motor coordination problems and handwriting problems are also very common in 47,XXY males, and ongoing interventions in the school years through occupational therapy and handwriting programs are also sometimes helpful with both gross motor and fine motor challenges. As with other children with fine motor deficits, keyboarding and word processing programs are recommended to ease frustrations and fatigue with handwriting. Occupational therapy can also be very helpful for the sensory processing problems that are common in children with XXY syndrome.

Identification and treatment of associated neurodevelopmental and emotional disorders such as ADHD or anxiety are also very important for these children. Classroom modifications and accommodations for attention and organization problems, such as reduction of ambient noise, short instruction sessions, consistent use of daily planners or homework notebooks, picture schedules, and other ADHD behavioral interventions are often helpful. Psychopharmacological medication treatment with stimulant medications has been reported to be effective for treatment of ADHD symptoms (Hagerman, 1999; Tartaglia et al., 2006) and other behavioral problems (Mandoki & Sumner, 1991), although placebo-controlled trials are still needed in both of these areas. Treatments for anxiety and mood symptoms with behavioral, psychological, and pharmacological interventions are also important for some children with XXY, although controlled trials are needed for these symptoms as well.

In early adolescence, a medical endocrinological evaluation is important to determine whether testosterone deficiency is present and the timing of testosterone replacement therapy. Testosterone treatment can have a positive effect on physical development, including muscle strength and endurance; can improve symptoms of fatigue; and can have positive effects on mood and self-esteem. Research is under way to determine whether testosterone therapy may also improve attention, executive function, motor coordination, or cognition (Ross, Stefanatos, Phil, & Roeltgen, 2007).

Because significant variability exists in the learning problems and emotional and behavioral features of children with 47,XXY syndrome, individualized assessments and interventions are important for all children. Because these children often present with milder cognitive problems rather than with MR, they are more likely to be in a mainstream classroom setting, and their educational and developmental needs are often undertreated. It is important for schools and educators to recognize that the language impairments, reading problems, ADHD, behavioral symptoms, and executive dysfunction are features of their genetic syndrome that require specific interventions that should be incorporated into individualized education plans to support these children.

Although this section of the chapter has focused on 47,XXY syndrome, many of the same recommendations for educational interventions apply to children with other variations of X and Y chromosomes, such as in males with XXYY, XYY, XXXY, or XXXXY syndromes and in females with trisomy X (XXX syndrome), tetrasomy X (XXXX syndrome) and pentasomy X (XXXXX syndrome). These children also suffer from various degrees of language deficits, verbal learning disabilities, motor coordination problems, ADHD symptoms, and behavioral symptoms. Individualized comprehensive treatment plans are also recommended for these children. (See Figure 6.3.)

Turner Syndrome

The clinical features of Turner syndrome (TS) were first described in the 1930s in girls with short stature, congenital webbed neck, and pubertal delays, and in 1959 it was discovered to be due to the absence of one X chromosome. Since then, many additional X-chromosome abnormalities have been identified that give rise to the Turner syndrome phenotype, with approximately 50% being due to a 45,X karyotype and the other 50% associated with isochromosomes, chromosome rings, deletions, and mosaicism (Jacobs et al., 1997). Turner syndrome occurs in approximately 1 in 3,000 female births, and the physical features have been further characterized to include short stature, webbed neck, increased carrying angle of the elbows (cubitus valgus), congenital heart malformations, kidney malformations, and ovarian failure.

A characteristic neurodevelopmental and behavioral profile has also been described in females with TS. Studies have shown that females with TS have deficits in visual–spatial and perceptual abilities and nonverbal memory functions, although their

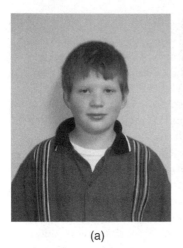
(a)

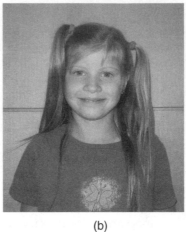
(b)

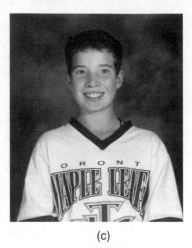
(c)

FIGURE 6.3. Children with X and Y chromosome aneuploidy. (a) Eight-year-old boy with XXY syndrome. Notice the slightly narrow shoulders and normal facial features, except for mild hypertelorism (wide-spaced eyes). He was at the 95th percentile for height. He began having educational problems in second grade and was diagnosed with a reading disorder and ADHD. He also received occupational therapy to help with fine motor skills and motor coordination. (b) Seven-year-old girl with trisomy X (XXX syndrome). Notice her lack of dysmorphic features. She received speech therapy in school for mild speech delays and currently is in mainstream classes doing very well and being followed closely for learning problems. (c) Ten-year-old boy with XXYY syndrome. Notice the mild hypertelorism (wide-spaced eyes). He is in a special education classroom for learning disabilities and is also receiving treatment for ADHD symptoms and anxiety and occupational therapy for fine motor skills and sensory processing problems.

language development is typically normal (Rovet, 2004). The mean IQ of more than 200 girls with TS was 94.6, compared with 103.9 in controls (Rovet, 1995), and a significantly higher verbal than performance IQ has been found in multiple studies (Mazzocco, 2001; Pennington et al., 1985). These deficits in visual–spatial skills are evident as early as 4 years of age and persist into adulthood. Math difficulties are present in up to 75% of girls with TS; detailed studies dissecting the basic deficits underlying math problems (dyscalculia) in girls with TS have shown strengths in learning math facts but difficulties with manipulating numbers for simple calculations (see Rovet, 2004, for a review). Executive function deficits and ADHD have been found in multiple studies as well, with a recent study showing a clinical diagnosis of ADHD in 25% of girls with TS (Russell et al., 2006). Girls with TS can also have psychosocial difficulties, including immaturity relative to peers and social skills deficits. The cognitive profile in TS is similar to the patterns found in children with nonverbal learning disability (NVLD; Rovet, 1995), and many girls with TS are diagnosed with NVLD. The TS cognitive phenotype is an interesting contrast to the opposite profile of individuals with extra X and Y chromosomes who typically have good visual–spatial skills and language-based learning disabilities, as described for 47,XXY/Klinefelter syndrome earlier.

The effects of TS on the reproductive system include ovarian dysgenesis, with resulting infertility and low levels of the sex hormones, including estrogen and androgens, in almost all patients. Treatments for the estrogen deficiency in TS have been shown to be effective in improving some domains of cognitive functioning in girls with

TS, including memory skills, processing speed, and motor functioning (Ross, Roeltgen, Feuillan, Kushner, & Cutler, 2000), whereas visual–spatial and perceptual problems do not seem to be responsive to estrogen treatment (Ross et al., 2002). A trial of androgen replacement with oxandrolone in girls with TS showed improvements in working memory in a controlled trial but no improvements in spatial cognition or executive function (Ross et al., 2003). Growth hormone (GH) replacement is also important in the treatment plan to help improve short stature, with GH treatment resulting in increased mean adult height in TS from 4'7" to 5'0". Girls with TS treated with GH showed improved self-esteem, fewer emotional problems, better overall quality of life, and improvements in math skills compared with untreated girls with TS (Bannink, Raat, Mulder, & de Muinck Keizer-Schrama, 2006; Siegel, Clopper, & Stabler, 1998).

RECENT RESEARCH IN TS

As in the case for 47,XXY males discussed earlier, significant variability occurs in the severity of the physical and neurodevelopmental manifestations between individuals with TS. Recent research has focused on identifying the neuroanatomical and genetic basis for the phenotype and its variability. Studies comparing the karyotypes of girls with TS have shown that the ring karyotype and the 45,X group were more severely affected physically and cognitively than the mosaic group or controls (Ross, Kushner, & Zinn, 1997). Recent imaging studies in TS have shown that brain regions involved in visual–spatial processing in the parieto–occipital cortex are smaller in women with TS than in controls (Cutter et al., 2006).

There have been conflicting studies correlating the parent-of-origin (imprinting) of the X chromosome in girls with TS with X-chromosome monosomy to their behavioral phenotypes. One study found that patients with TS who have maternally inherited X chromosomes are more likely to have cognitive problems and social disabilities than girls with TS who have paternally inherited X chromosomes (Skuse et al., 1997). Another found that facial recognition was more impaired in a group of girls with TS who had maternally inherited X chromosomes. Other studies have not replicated the parent-of-origin effects on cognitive or psychosocial measures in large groups of patients with TS (Ross, Roeltgen, Kushner, Wei, & Zinn, 2000). Recent research on ADHD in TS also shows no evidence of imprinting (Russell et al., 2006). Further research in this area is needed to determine whether imprinting may play a role in the TS phenotype.

In TS, it is also postulated that there is a deficiency of gene expression (haplo-insufficiency) in the X-chromosome genes that escape inactivation and that are typically expressed from both X chromosomes in normal 46,XX females. Decreased expression from these genes in females with TS is thought to result in the characteristic phenotype, and, in fact, haploinsufficiency of the *SHOX* gene (short homeobox gene) at the chromosome region Xp22 is related to the short stature in girls with TS (Clement-Jones et al., 2000). Using a combination of molecular mapping and neurocognitive profiling in a large group of females with TS, the visual–spatial deficits have also mapped to the pseudoautosomal region (PAR1) of the short arm of the X chromosome (Xp22.33), in which there are less than 10 identified genes (Ross, Roeltgen, Kushner, et al., 2000). Although there may be more than one gene in this region involved in the neurocognitive profile of TS, further research into these specific genes and their roles in neurodevelopment will provide important information about TS specifically but also about the role of these genes in visual–spatial development and functioning in all individuals.

Guidelines for ongoing medical care for children with Turner syndrome have been established by the American Academy of Pediatrics (Frias & Davenport, 2003) and further detail the recommendations for evaluation and monitoring of medical problems associated with TS, including heart and kidney problems, hearing loss, thyroid problems, musculoskeletal abnormalities, and other medical issues. The recent research on hormone replacement therapy in TS described earlier has shown benefits for final adult stature, self-esteem, and emotional well-being and beneficial effects on neurodevelopment. Thus standard-of-care medical treatment guidelines now include GH treatment starting in early childhood, with the addition of androgen, estrogen, and progesterone later in childhood or early adolescence on an individual basis (Frias & Davenport, 2003; Sybert, 2005).

Infants and toddlers with TS should have early developmental assessments that target all domains of development, including motor skills, speech and language, and socioemotional development. Early intervention services with physical, occupational, or speech therapy should be initiated at the first sign of delays. Because it is recognized that adolescent girls with TS often have emotional difficulties and poor self-esteem, interventions and activities that build self-esteem and social relationships in early childhood should be encouraged by families and school systems.

Research on the cognitive phenotype and the visual–spatial deficits in girls with TS has also led to the development of specific instructional recommendations for school-age girls that include methods to improve visual–spatial organizational skills and to use verbal skills to compensate for nonverbal learning deficits. Because IQ falls in the normal range for most girls with TS and because verbal skills are usually relative strengths, learning disabilities in these patients are often missed. A full psychoeducational evaluation is recommended for any girl with a diagnosis of TS. Individual tutoring, study-skills training, allowing extra time on tests and calculators for math classes, and using computer-based learning programs are all part of the educational strategies recommended for girls with TS (Rosenfeld, Tesch, Rodriguez, & McCauley, 1994). Other important interventions include specific training in social skills and social communication and occupational or physical therapy for motor-skills deficits. Medication treatments for ADHD and executive function deficits have not yet been studied specifically for TS, but case reports have shown good responses with stimulant medications (Hagerman, 1999; Russell et al., 2006), and standard treatments for ADHD are recommended, with careful evaluation and follow-up (Sybert, 2005).

CONCLUSIONS

Genetic disorders are present in up to 50% of individuals with MR or developmental disabilities, and with today's rapid biotechnological advances, new discoveries about genetic disorders are being made daily. Multidisciplinary research on effective treatments for individual genetic syndromes is providing information that will greatly affect families, educators, and other professionals working with these children. The descriptions of the genetic syndromes in this chapter have emphasized the variability in physical and cognitive-behavioral characteristics within individuals with the same genetic mutation. Although many genetic disorders are associated with obvious facial dysmorphology and MR, others are much less obvious and may be associated with only mild learning disabilities. Educators, psychologists, speech therapists, occupational therapists, and physical therapists are very likely to find individuals with these and many other genetic disorders in their classrooms and clinics, and they can aid in the diagnostic process by recognizing the physical, medical, and psychological characteristics of common genetic disorders. Recognition of these problems will enhance targeted educational interventions.

Although we have presented just a few examples of specific genetic disorders and recent research advances in this chapter, more than 1,000 genetic disorders leading to developmental disabilities have been identified, many with active research across multiple disciplines. A genetic diagnosis should be considered for all individuals with developmental disabilities. We recommend consultation with a clinical geneticist or a developmental–behavioral pediatrician for all individuals with motor or speech delays, LD, MR, severe behavioral problems, or autism spectrum disorders so that appropriate genetic testing can be performed (Moeschler, Shevell, & AAP Committee on Genetics, 2006). Educators and other professionals working with children or adults with developmental disabilities should inquire whether a medical evaluation of the cause of the individual's disabilities has been completed and should suggest further evaluation given the recent advances in techniques to identify genetic abnormalities that lead to developmental disabilities. Older adolescents or adults with DD or MR of unknown etiology should also be reevaluated for genetic problems by a medical team, because new diagnostic tools and techniques now exist that were not available 15 or 20 years ago, when they were first evaluated.

Although there is no cure for these genetic disorders at this time, identification of a genetic disorder is important for many reasons. First, diagnosis-specific recommendations and interventions have been developed for many disorders, including therapy techniques, educational strategies, and effective medication treatments. Schools and educators will benefit when a specific genetic syndrome is identified because the diagnosis provides a profile of cognitive, emotional, and behavioral features common in each syndrome that can help in designing the educational plan. Also, evaluation for medical problems related to the various syndromes and genetic counseling for the individual and other family members is also important when a specific genetic diagnosis is identified. Receiving a specific diagnosis for their child's problems can also provide peace of mind to many parents, who can then act as better advocates for their child's needs. Local and national organizations have been created to provide support for coping with hundreds of specific genetic syndromes. These organizations can act as important resources for families, educators, and other professionals involved in treating children and adults with various genetic disorders. Most of these organizations now have Internet websites with links to literature developed for school psychologists, therapists, and educators that can significantly aid in the development of individualized educational plans by providing instructional strategies and recommendations for management of behavioral difficulties specific to the child's genetic syndrome. Research in the upcoming years also promises evidence-based intervention programs and targeted medical treatments for these disorders, decreasing or preventing the cognitive and behavioral problems in these individuals.

ACKNOWLEDGMENTS

This work was supported by the M.I.N.D. Institute; the XXYY Project; the Bonfils–Stanton Foundation; Klinefelter Syndrome and Associates; National Institutes of Health Grant Nos. HD36071, R0142974HD, HD02274, and HD42974; National Institutes of Health Pediatric Research Loan Repayment Program for Nicole R. Tartaglia, and Centers for Disease Control and Prevention Grant No. U10/CCU92513.

REFERENCES

Abramsky, L., & Chapple, J. (1997). 47,XXY (Klinefelter syndrome) and 47,XYY: Estimated rates of and indication for postnatal diagnosis with implications for prenatal counselling. *Prenatal Diagnosis, 17*(4), 363–368.

Bannink, E. M., Raat, H., Mulder, P. G., & de Muinck Keizer-Schrama, S. M. (2006). Quality of life after growth hormone therapy and induced puberty in women with Turner syndrome. *Journal of Pediatrics, 148*(1), 95–101.

Bassett, A. S., Chow, E. W., AbdelMalik, P., Gheorghiu, M., Husted, J., & Weksberg, R. (2003). The schizophrenia phenotype in 22q11 deletion syndrome. *American Journal of Psychiatry, 160*(9), 1580–1586.

Bear, M. F., Huber, K. M., & Warren, S. T. (2004). The mGluR theory of fragile X mental retardation. *Trends in Neurosciences, 27*(7), 370–377.

Bearden, C. E., van Erp, T. G., Monterosso, J. R., Simon, T. J., Glahn, D. C., Saleh, P. A., et al. (2004). Regional brain abnormalities in 22q11.2 deletion syndrome: Association with cognitive abilities and behavioral symptoms. *Neurocase, 10*(3), 198–206.

Beckett, L., Yu, Q., & Long, A. N. (2005). *The impact of fragile X: Prevalence, numbers affected, and economic impact.* Paper presented at the National Fragile X Awareness Day Research Seminar, Sacramento, CA.

Bender, B. G., Harmon, R. J., Linden, M. G., & Robinson, A. (1995). Psychosocial adaptation of 39 adolescents with sex chromosome abnormalities. *Pediatrics, 96*(2, Pt. 1), 302–308.

Bender, B. G., Puck, M. H., Salbenblatt, J. A., & Robinson, A. (1986). Dyslexia in 47,XXY boys identified at birth. *Behavior Genetics, 16*(3), 343–354.

Bennetto, L., & Pennington, B. F. (2002). Neuropsychology. In R. J. Hagerman & P. J. Hagerman (Eds.), *Fragile X syndrome: Diagnosis, treatment, and research* (3rd ed., pp. 206–248). Baltimore: Johns Hopkins University Press.

Bloomquist, M. (1996). *Skills training for children with behavioral disorders: A parent and therapist guidebook.* New York: Guilford Press.

Bojesen, A., Juul, S., & Gravholt, C. H. (2003). Prenatal and postnatal prevalence of Klinefelter syndrome: A national registry study. *Journal of Clinical Endocrinology and Metabolism, 88*(2), 622–626.

Botto, L. D., May, K., Fernhoff, P. M., Correa, A., Coleman, K., Rasmussen, S. A., et al. (2003). A population-based study of the 22q11.2 deletion: Phenotype, incidence, and contribution to major birth defects in the population. *Pediatrics, 112*(1, Pt. 1), 101–107.

Braden, M. L. (2000). *Fragile, handle with care: More about Fragile X syndrome, adolescents and adults.* Dillon, CO: Spectra.

Braden, M. (2002). Academic interventions in fragile X. In R. J. Hagerman & P. J. Hagerman (Eds.), *Fragile X syndrome: Diagnosis, treatment and research* (3rd ed., pp. 428–464). Baltimore: Johns Hopkins University Press.

Burn, J., Takao, A., Wilson, D., Cross, I., Momma, K., Wadey, R., et al. (1993). Conotruncal anomaly face syndrome is associated with a deletion within chromosome 22q11. *Journal of Medical Genetics, 30*(10), 822–824.

Chelly, J., Khelfaoui, M., Francis, F., Cherif, B., & Bienvenu, T. (2006). Genetics and pathophysiology of mental retardation. *European Journal of Human Genetics, 14*, 701–713.

Clement-Jones, M., Schiller, S., Rao, E., Blaschke, R., Zuniga, A., Zeller, R., et al. (2000). The short stature homeobox gene SHOX is involved in skeletal abnormalities in Turner syndrome. *Human Molecular Genetics, 9*(5), 695–702.

Cornish, K. M., Munir, F., & Cross, G. (1999). Spatial cognition in males with fragile-X syndrome: Evidence for a neuropsychological phenotype. *Cortex, 35*(2), 263–271.

Cutter, W. J., Daly, E. M., Robertson, D. M., Chitnis, X. A., van Amelsvoort, T. A., Simmons, A., et al. (2006). Influence of X chromosome and hormones on human brain development: A magnetic resonance imaging and proton magnetic resonance spectroscopy study of Turner syndrome. *Biological Psychiatry, 59*(3), 273–283.

de la Chapelle, A., Herva, R., Koivisto, M., & Aula, P. (1981). A deletion in chromosome 22 can cause DiGeorge syndrome. *Human Genetics, 57*(3), 253–256.

De Leersnyder, H., Bresson, J. L., de Blois, M. C., Souberbielle, J. C., Mogenet, A., Delhotal-Landes, B., et al. (2003). Beta 1-adrenergic antagonists and melatonin reset the clock and restore sleep in a circadian disorder, Smith–Magenis syndrome. *Journal of Medical Genetics, 40*(1), 74–78.

De Leersnyder, H., De Blois, M. C., Claustrat, B., Romana, S., Albrecht, U., Von Kleist-Retzow, J. C., et al. (2001). Inversion of the circadian rhythm of melatonin in the Smith–Magenis syndrome. *Journal of Pediatrics, 139*(1), 111–116.

De Vries, B. B., Winter, R., Schinzel, A., & van Ravenswaaij-Arts, C. (2003). Telomeres: A diagnosis at the end of the chromosomes. *Journal of Medical Genetics, 40*(6), 385–398.

Dykens, E. M., Finucane, B. M., & Gayley, C. (1997). Brief report: Cognitive and behavioral profiles in persons with Smith–Magenis syndrome. *Journal of Autism and Developmental Disorders, 27*(2), 203–211.

Eliez, S., & Blasey, C. M. (2001). Chromosome 22q11 deletion and brain structure. *British Journal of Psychiatry, 179*, 270.

Farzin, F., Perry, H., Bacalman, S., Gane, L., Hessl, D., Loesch, D., et al. (2006). Autism spectrum disorders and attention deficit/hyperactivity disorder in boys with the fragile X premutation. *Journal of Developmental and Behavioral Pediatrics, 27*(2), S137–S144.

Flint, J., & Knight, S. (2003). The use of telomere probes to investigate submicroscopic rearrangements associated with mental retardation. *Current Opinion in Genetics and Development, 13*, 310–316.

Franke, P., Leboyer, M., Gansicke, M., Weiffenbach, O., Biancalana, V., Cornillet-Lefebre, P., et al. (1998). Genotype–phenotype relationship in female carriers of the premutation and full mutation of FMR-1. *Psychiatry Research, 80*(2), 113–127.

Frias, J. L., & Davenport, M. L. (2003). Health supervision for children with Turner syndrome. *Pediatrics, 111*(3), 692–702.

Geschwind, D. H., Boone, K. B., Miller, B. L., & Swerdloff, R. S. (2000). Neurobehavioral phenotype of Klinefelter syndrome. *Mental Retardation and Developmental Disabilities Research Reviews, 6*(2), 107–116.

Geschwind, D., & Dykens, E. (2004). Neurobehavioral and psychosocial issues in Klinefelter syndrome. *Learning Disabilities Research and Practice, 19*(3), 166–173.

Geschwind, D. H., Gregg, J., Boone, K., Karrim, J., Pawlikowska-Haddal, A., Rao, E., et al. (1998). Klinefelter's syndrome as a model of anomalous cerebral laterality: Testing gene dosage in the X chromosome pseudoautosomal region using a DNA microarray. *Developmental Genetics, 23*(3), 215–229.

Giedd, J., Clasen, L., Lenroot, R., Greenstein, D., Wallace, G., Ordaz, S., et al. (2006). Puberty-related influences on brain development. *Molecular and Cellular Endocrinology, 254–255*, 154–162.

Glaser, B., Mumme, D. L., Blasey, C., Morris, M. A., Dahoun, S. P., Antonarakis, S. E., et al. (2002). Language skills in children with velocardiofacial syndrome (deletion 22q11.2). *Journal of Pediatrics, 140*(6), 753–758.

Goldberg, R., Motzkin, B., Marion, R., Scambler, P. J., & Shprintzen, R. J. (1993). Velo-cardio-facial syndrome: A review of 120 patients. *American Journal of Medical Genetics, 45*(3), 313–319.

Golding-Kushner, K. J., Weller, G., & Shprintzen, R. J. (1985). Velo-cardio-facial syndrome: Language and psychological profiles. *Journal of Craniofacial Genetics and Developmental Biology, 5*(3), 259–266.

Gothelf, D., Furfaro, J. A., Penniman, L. C., Glover, G. H., & Reiss, A. L. (2005). The contribution of novel brain imaging techniques to understanding the neurobiology of mental retardation and developmental disabilities. *Mental Retardation and Developmental Disabilities Research Reviews, 11*(4), 331–339.

Gothelf, D., Gruber, R., Presburger, G., Dotan, I., Brand-Gothelf, A., Burg, M., et al. (2003). Methylphenidate treatment for attention-deficit/hyperactivity disorder in children and adolescents with velocardiofacial syndrome: An open-label study. *Journal of Clinical Psychiatry, 64*(10), 1163–1169.

Greco, C., Berman, R. F., Martin, R. M., Tassone, F., Schwartz, P. H., Chang, A., et al. (2006). Neuropathology of fragile X-associated tremor/ataxia syndrome (FXTAS). *Brain, 129*, 243–255.

Greenberg, F., Guzzetta, V., Montes de Oca-Luna, R., Magenis, R. E., Smith, A. C., Richter, S. F., et al. (1991). Molecular analysis of the Smith–Magenis syndrome: A possible contiguous-gene syndrome associated with del(17)(p11.2). *American Journal of Human Genetics, 49*(6), 1207–1218.

Greenberg, F., Lewis, R. A., Potocki, L., Glaze, D., Parke, J., Killian, J., et al. (1996). Multidisciplinary clinical study of Smith–Magenis syndrome (deletion 17p11.2). *American Journal of Medical Genetics, 62*(3), 247–254.

Hagerman, P. J., & Hagerman, R. J. (2004). The fragile-X premutation: A maturing perspective. *American Journal of Human Genetics, 74*(5), 805–816.

Hagerman, R. J. (1999). *Neurodevelopmental disorders: Diagnosis and treatment.* New York: Oxford University Press.

Hagerman, R. J. (2002a). Medical follow-up and pharmacotherapy. In R. J. Hagerman & P. J. Hagerman (Eds.), *Fragile X syndrome: Diagnosis, treatment and research* (3rd ed., pp. 287–338). Baltimore: Johns Hopkins University Press.

Hagerman, R. J. (2002b). Physical and behavioral phenotype. In R. J. Hagerman & P. J. Hagerman (Eds.), *Fragile X syndrome: Diagnosis, treatment and research* (3rd ed., pp. 3–109). Baltimore: Johns Hopkins University Press.

Hagerman, R. J. (2004). Fragile X syndrome. In P. Allen Jackson & J. A. Vessey (Eds.), *Primary care of the child with a chronic condition* (4th ed., pp. 498–510). St. Louis, MO: Mosby.

Hagerman, R. J. (2006). Lessons from fragile X regarding neurobiology, autism, and neurodegeneration. *Journal of Developmental and Behavioral Pediatrics, 27*(1), 63–74.

Hagerman, R. J., Hills, J., Scharfenaker, S., & Lewis, H. (1999). Fragile X syndrome and selective mutism. *American Journal of Medical Genetics, 83*, 313–317.

Hessl, D., Dyer-Friedman, J., Glaser, B., Wisbeck, J., Barajas, R. G., Taylor, A., et al. (2001). The influence of environmental and genetic factors on behavior problems and autistic symptoms in boys and girls with fragile X syndrome [Electronic version]. *Pediatrics, 108*(5), e88.

Hessl, D., Tassone, F., Loesch, D. Z., Berry-Kravis, E., Leehey, M. A., Gane, L. W., et al. (2005). Abnormal elevation of FMR1 mRNA is associated with psychological symptoms in individuals with the fragile X premutation. *American Journal of Medical Genetics: Part B. Neuropsychiatric Genetics, 139*(1), 115–121.

Hodapp, R. M., & Dykens, E. M. (2005). Measuring behavior in genetic disorders of mental retardation. *Mental Retardation and Developmental Disabilities Research Reviews, 11*(4), 340–346.

Itoh, M., Hayashi, M., Hasegawa, T., Shimohira, M., & Kohyama, J. (2004). Systemic growth hormone corrects sleep disturbance in Smith–Magenis syndrome. *Brain and Development, 26*(7), 484–486.

Itti, E., Gaw Gonzalo, I. T., Pawlikowska-Haddal, A., Boone, K. B., Mlikotic, A., Itti, L., et al. (2006). The structural brain correlates of cognitive deficits in adults with Klinefelter's syndrome. *Journal of Clinical Endocrinology and Metabolism, 91*(4), 1423–1427.

Jacobs, P., Dalton, P., James, R., Mosse, K., Power, M., Robinson, D., et al. (1997). Turner syndrome: A cytogenetic and molecular study. *Annals of Human Genetics, 61*(Pt. 6), 471–483.

Jacquemont, S., Hagerman, R. J., Leehey, M. A., Hall, D. A., Levine, R. A., Brunberg, J. A., et al. (2004). Penetrance of the fragile X-associated tremor/ataxia syndrome in a premutation carrier population. *Journal of the American Medical Association, 291*(4), 460–469.

Kogan, C. S., Boutet, I., Cornish, K., Zangenehpour, S., Mullen, K. T., Holden, J. J., et al. (2004). Differential impact of the FMR1 gene on visual processing in fragile X syndrome. *Brain, 127*(Pt. 3), 591–601.

Kok, L. L., & Solman, R. T. (1995). Velocardiofacial syndrome: Learning difficulties and intervention. *Journal of Medical Genetics, 32*(8), 612–618.

Lachman, H. M., Morrow, B., Shprintzen, R., Veit, S., Parsia, S. S., Faedda, G., et al. (1996). Association of codon 108/158 catechol-O-methyltransferase gene polymorphism with the psychiatric manifestations of velo-cardio-facial syndrome. *American Journal of Medical Genetics, 67*(5), 468–472.

Levitt, P. (2005). New technical approaches to developmental disability research: An introduction. *Mental Retardation and Developmental Disabilities Research Reviews, 11*(4), 277–278.

Liao, J., Kochilas, L., Nowotschin, S., Arnold, J. S., Aggarwal, V. S., Epstein, J. A., et al. (2004). Full spectrum of malformations in velo-cardio-facial syndrome/DiGeorge syndrome mouse models by altering Tbx1 dosage. *Human Molecular Genetics, 13*(15), 1577–1585.

Loesch, D., Huggins, R., Bui, Q. M., Taylor, A., & Hagerman, R. J. (2003). Effect of the fragile X status categories and FMRP deficits on cognitive profiles estimated by robust pedigree analysis. *American Journal of Medical Genetics, 122A*(1), 12–23.

Loesch, D. Z., Huggins, R. M., & Hagerman, R. J. (2004). Phenotypic variation and FMRP levels in fragile X. *Mental Retardation and Developmental Disabilities Research Reviews, 10*(1), 31–41.

Lucas, R. E., Vlangos, C. N., Das, P., Patel, P. I., & Elsea, S. H. (2001). Genomic organisation of the approximately 1.5 Mb Smith–Magenis syndrome critical interval: Transcription map, genomic contig, and candidate gene analysis. *European Journal of Human Genetics, 9*(12), 892–902.

Lue, Y., Jentsch, J. D., Wang, C., Rao, P. N., Hikim, A. P., Salameh, W., et al. (2005). XXY mice exhibit gonadal and behavioral phenotypes similar to Klinefelter syndrome. *Endocrinology, 146*(9), 4148–4154.

Macpherson, J., Waghorn, A., Hammans, S., & Jacobs, P. (2003). Observation of an excess of fragile-X premutations in a population of males referred with spinocerebellar ataxia. *Human Genetics, 112*(5–6), 619–620.

Madduri, N., Peters, S., Voigt, R., Llorente, A., Lupski, J., & Potocki, L. (2006). Cognitive and Adaptive Behavior Profiles in Smith–Magenis Syndrome. *Developmental and Behavioral Pediatrics, 27*(3), 188–192.

Mandoki, M. W., & Sumner, G. S. (1991). Klinefelter syndrome: The need for early identification and treatment. *Clinical Pediatrics, 30*(3), 161–164.

Mazzocco, M. M. (2001). Math learning disability and math LD subtypes: Evidence from studies of Turner syndrome, fragile X syndrome, and neurofibromatosis type 1. *Journal of Learning Disabilities, 34*(6), 520–533.

McConkie-Rosell, A., Finucane, B. M., Cronister, A. C., Abrams, L., Bennett, R. L., & Pettersen, B. J. (2005). Genetic counseling for fragile X syndrome: Updated recommendations of the National Society of Genetic Counselors. *Journal of Genetic Counseling, 14*(4), 249–270.

McElroy, S., & Weller, E. (1997). Psychopharmacological treatment of bipolar disorder across the life span. In S. McElroy (Ed.), *Psychopharmacology across the lifespan* (pp. 31–85). Washington, DC: American Psychiatric Press.

Meng, H., Smith, S. D., Hager, K., Held, M., Liu, J., Olson, R. K., et al. (2005). DCDC2 is associated with reading disability and modulates neuronal development in the brain. *Proceedings of the National Academy of Sciences of the USA, 102*(47), 17053–17058.

Mirrett, P. L., Bailey, D. B., Jr., Roberts, J. E., & Hatton, D. D. (2004). Developmental screening and detection of developmental delays in infants and toddlers with fragile X syndrome. *Journal of Developmental and Behavioral Pediatrics, 25*(1), 21–27.

Moeschler, J., Shevell, M., & AAP Committee on Genetics. (2006). Clinical genetic evaluation of the child with mental retardation or developmental delays. *Pediatrics, 117*, 2304–2316.

Moss, E. M., Batshaw, M. L., Solot, C. B., Gerdes, M., McDonald-McGinn, D. M., Driscoll, D. A., et al. (1999). Psychoeducational profile of the 22q11.2 microdeletion: A complex pattern. *Journal of Pediatrics, 134*(2), 193–198.

Nielsen, J. (1990). Sex chromosome abnormalities found among 34,910 newborn children: Results from a 13-year incidence study in Arhus, Denmark. *Birth Defects Original Article Series, 26*(4), 209–223.

O'Brien, G. (Ed.). (2002). *Behavioral phenotypes in clinical practice.* London: McKeith Press.

Ozonoff, S., Rogers, S. J., & Hendren, R. L. (2003). *Autism spectrum disorders: A research review for practitioners.* Washington, DC: American Psychiatric.

Patwardhan, A. J., Eliez, S., Bender, B., Linden, M. G., & Reiss, A. L. (2000). Brain morphology in Klinefelter syndrome: Extra X chromosome and testosterone supplementation. *Neurology, 54*(12), 2218–2223.

Pennington, B. F., Bender, B., Puck, M., Salbenblatt, J., & Robinson, A. (1982). Learning disabilities in children with sex chromosome anomalies. *Child Development, 53*(5), 1182–1192.

Pennington, B. F., Heaton, R. K., Karzmark, P., Pendleton, M. G., Lehman, R., & Shucard, D. W. (1985). The neuropsychological phenotype in Turner syndrome. *Cortex, 21*(3), 391–404.

Potocki, L., Glaze, D., Tan, D. X., Park, S. S., Kashork, C. D., Shaffer, L. G., et al. (2000). Circadian rhythm abnormalities of melatonin in Smith–Magenis syndrome. *Journal of Medical Genetics, 37*(6), 428–433.

Reddy, K. S. (2005). Cytogenetic abnormalities and fragile-X syndrome in autism spectrum disorder. *BMC Medical Genetics, 6*(1), 3.

Roberts, J. E., Boccia, M. L., Bailey, D. B., Hatton, D., & Skinner, M. (2001). Cardiovascular indices of physiological arousal in boys with fragile X syndrome. *Developmental Psychobiology, 39*(2), 107–123.

Roberts, J. E., Schaaf, J. M., Skinner, M., Wheeler, A., Hooper, S., Hatton, D. D., et al. (2005). Academic skills of boys with fragile X syndrome: Profiles and predictors. *American Journal of Mental Retardation, 110*(2), 107–120.

Robinson, A., Bender, B., Borelli, J., & Winter, J. (1986). Sex chromosome aneuploidy, prospective and longitudinal studies. In S. Ratcliffe & N. Paul (Eds.), *Prospective studies on children with sex chromosome aneuploidy: March of Dimes birth defects original article series: Vol. 22, No. 3* (pp. 23–71). New York: Liss.

Rogers, S. J., Wehner, E. A., & Hagerman, R. J. (2001). The behavioral phenotype in fragile X: Symptoms of autism in very young children with fragile X syndrome, idiopathic autism, and other developmental disorders. *Journal of Developmental and Behavioral Pediatrics, 22*(6), 409–417.

Rosenfeld, R., Tesch, L., Rodriguez, L., & McCauley, E. (1994). Recommendations for diagnosis, treatment, and management of individuals with Turner syndrome. *Endocrinologist, 4*, 351–358.

Ross, J. L., Kushner, H., & Zinn, A. R. (1997). Discriminant analysis of the Ullrich–Turner syndrome neurocognitive profile. *American Journal of Medical Genetics, 72*(3), 275–280.

Ross, J. L., Roeltgen, D., Feuillan, P., Kushner, H., & Cutler, G. B., Jr. (2000). Use of estrogen in young girls with Turner syndrome: Effects on memory. *Neurology, 54*(1), 164–170.

Ross, J. L., Roeltgen, D., Kushner, H., Wei, F., & Zinn, A. R. (2000). The Turner syndrome-associated neurocognitive phenotype maps to distal Xp. *American Journal of Human Genetics, 67*(3), 672–681.

Ross, J. L., Roeltgen, D., Stefanatos, G. A., Feuillan, P., Kushner, H., Bondy, C., et al. (2003). Androgen-responsive aspects of cognition in girls with Turner syndrome. *Journal of Clinical Endocrinology and Metabolism, 88*(1), 292–296.

Ross, J. L., Samango-Sprouse, C., Lahlou, N., Kowal, K., Elder, F. F., & Zinn, A. (2005). Early androgen deficiency in infants and young boys with 47,XXY Klinefelter syndrome. *Hormone Research, 64*(1), 39–45.

Ross, J. L., Stefanatos, G. A., Kushner, H., Zinn, A., Bondy, C., & Roeltgen, D. (2002). Persistent cognitive deficits in adult women with Turner syndrome. *Neurology, 58*(2), 218–225.

Ross, J., Stefanatos, G., Phil, D., & Roeltgen, D. (2007). Klinefelter syndrome. In M. Mazzocco & J. Ross (Eds.), *Neurogenetic developmental disorders: Variation of manifestation in childhood* (pp. 47–72). Cambridge, MA: MIT Press.

Rovet, J. (1995). Turner syndrome. In B. P. Rourke (Ed.), *Syndrome of nonverbal learning disabilities: Neurodevelopmental manifestations* (pp. 351–371). New York: Guilford Press.

Rovet, J. (2004). Turner syndrome: Genetic and hormonal factors contributing to a specific learning disability profile. *Learning Disabilities Research and Practice, 19*(3), 133–145.

Rovet, J., Netley, C., Keenan, M., Bailey, J., & Stewart, D. (1996). The psychoeducational profile of boys with Klinefelter syndrome. *Journal of Learning Disabilities, 29*(2), 180–196.

Russell, H. F., Wallis, D., Mazzocco, M. M., Moshang, T., Zackai, E., Zinn, A. R., et al. (2006). Increased prevalence of ADHD in Turner syndrome with no evidence of imprinting effects. *Journal of Pediatric Psychology, 31*(9), 945–955.

Ryan, A. K., Goodship, J. A., Wilson, D. I., Philip, N., Levy, A., Seidel, H., et al. (1997). Spectrum of clinical features associated with interstitial chromosome 22q11 deletions: A European collaborative study. *Journal of Medical Genetics, 34*(10), 798–804.

Salbenblatt, J. A., Meyers, D. C., Bender, B. G., Linden, M. G., & Robinson, A. (1989). Gross and fine motor development in 45,X and 47,XXX girls. *Pediatrics, 84*(4), 678–682.

Scambler, P. J., Carey, A. H., Wyse, R. K., Roach, S., Dumanski, J. P., Nordenskjold, M., et al. (1991). Microdeletions within 22q11 associated with sporadic and familial DiGeorge syndrome. *Genomics, 10*(1), 201–206.

Scambler, P. J., Kelly, D., Lindsay, E., Williamson, R., Goldberg, R., Shprintzen, R., et al. (1992). Velo-cardio-facial syndrome associated with chromosome 22 deletions encompassing the DiGeorge locus. *Lancet, 339*(8802), 1138–1139.

Scharfenaker, S., O'Connor, R., Stackhouse, T., & Noble, L. (2002). An integrated approach to intervention. In R. J. Hagerman & P. J. Hagerman (Eds.), *Fragile X syndrome: Diagnosis, treatment and research* (3rd ed., pp. 363–427). Baltimore: Johns Hopkins University Press.

Scherer, N. J., D'Antonio, L. L., & Kalbfleisch, J. H. (1999). Early speech and language development in children with velocardiofacial syndrome. *American Journal of Medical Genetics, 88*(6), 714–723.

Schoumans, J., Staaf, J., Jonsson, G., Rantala, J., Zimmer, K. S., Borg, A., et al. (2005). Detection and delineation of an unusual 17p11.2 deletion by array-CGH and refinement of the Smith–Magenis syndrome minimum deletion to approximately 650 kb. *European Journal of Medical Genetics, 48*(3), 290–300.

Shprintzen, R. (2005). Velo-cardio-facial syndrome. In S. Cassidy & J. Allanson (Eds.), *Management of genetic syndromes* (2nd ed., pp. 615–632). Hoboken, NJ: Wiley.

Siegel, P. T., Clopper, R., & Stabler, B. (1998). The psychological consequences of Turner syndrome and review of the National Cooperative Growth Study psychological substudy. *Pediatrics, 102*(2, Pt. 3), 488–491.

Simon, T. J., Bish, J. P., Bearden, C. E., Ding, L., Ferrante, S., Nguyen, V., et al. (2005). A multilevel analysis of cognitive dysfunction and psychopathology associated with chromosome 22q11.2 deletion syndrome in children. *Development and Psychopathology, 17*(3), 753–784.

Simon, T. J., Burg, M., & Gothelf, D. (2007). Cognitive and behavioral characteristics of children with chromosome 22q11.2 deletion. In M. Mazzocco & J. Ross (Eds.), *Neurogenetic developmental disorders: Variation of manifestation in childhood* (pp. 163–198). Cambridge, MA: MIT Press.

Simpson, J. L., de la Cruz, F., Swerdloff, R. S., Samango-Sprouse, C., Skakkebaek, N. E., Graham, J. M., Jr., et al. (2003). Klinefelter syndrome: Expanding the phenotype and identifying new research directions. *Genetics in Medicine, 5*(6), 460–468.

Simpson, J. L., Graham, J. M., Jr., Samango-Sprouse, C., & Swerdloff, R. (2005). Klinefelter syndrome. In S. Cassidy & J. Allanson (Eds.), *Management of genetic syndromes* (2nd ed., pp. 323–333). Hoboken, NJ: Wiley.

Skinner, M., Hooper, S., Hatton, D. D., Roberts, J., Mirrett, P., Schaaf, J., et al. (2005). Mapping nonverbal IQ in young boys with fragile X syndrome. *American Journal of Medical Genetics A, 132*(1), 25–32.

Skuse, D., James, R., Bishop, D., Coppin, B., Dalton, P., Aamodt-Leeper, G., et al. (1997). Evidence from Turner's syndrome of an imprinted X-linked locus affecting cognitive function. *Nature, 387*, 705–708.

Slager, R. E., Newton, T. L., Vlangos, C. N., Finucane, B., & Elsea, S. H. (2003). Mutations in RAI1 associated with Smith–Magenis syndrome. *Nature Genetics, 33*(4), 466–468.

Smith, A., & Gropman, A. (2005). Smith–Magenis syndrome. In S. Cassidy & J. Allanson (Eds.), *Management of genetic syndromes* (2nd ed., pp. 507–526). Hoboken, NJ: Wiley.

Smith, A. C., Gropman, A. L., Bailey-Wilson, J. E., Goker-Alpan, O., Elsea, S. H., Blancato, J., et al. (2002). Hypercholesterolemia in children with Smith–Magenis syndrome: Del (17) (p11.2p11.2). *Genetics in Medicine, 4*(3), 118–125.

Smith, A. C., Magenis, R. E., & Elsea, S. H. (2005). Overview of Smith–Magenis syndrome. *Journal of the Association of Genetic Technologists, 31*(4), 163–167.

Smith, A., McGavran, L., & Waldstein, G. (1982). Deletion of the 17 short arm in two patients with facial clefts. *American Journal of Human Genetics, 34*(Suppl.), A410.

Solot, C. B., Gerdes, M., Kirschner, R. E., McDonald-McGinn, D. M., Moss, E., Woodin, M., et al. (2001). Communication issues in 22q11.2 deletion syndrome: Children at risk. *Genetics in Medicine, 3*(1), 67–71.

Swillen, A., Devriendt, K., Legius, E., Eyskens, B., Dumoulin, M., Gewillig, M., et al. (1997). Intelligence and psychosocial adjustment in velocardiofacial syndrome: A study of 37 children and adolescents with VCFS. *Journal of Medical Genetics, 34*(6), 453–458.

Swillen, A., Vandeputte, L., Cracco, J., Maes, B., Ghesquiere, P., Devriendt, K., et al. (1999). Neuropsychological, learning and psychosocial profile of primary school-aged children with the velocardio-facial syndrome (22q11 deletion): Evidence for a nonverbal learning disability? *Child Neuropsychology, 5*(4), 230–241.

Sybert, V. P. (2005). Turner syndrome. In S. Cassidy & J. Allanson (Eds.), *Management of genetic syndromes* (2nd ed., pp. 589–605). Hoboken, NJ: Wiley.

Tartaglia, N., Reynolds, A., Davis, S., Hansen, R., & Hagerman, R. J. (2006). Comparison of ADHD and ODD in XXY and XXYY syndromes. *Journal of Investigative Medicine, 54*(1), S80.

Valle, D. (2004). Genetics, individuality, and medicine in the 21st century. *American Journal of Human Genetics, 74*(3), 374–381.

Visootsak, J., Aylstock, M., & Graham, J. M., Jr. (2001). Klinefelter syndrome and its variants: An update and review for the primary pediatrician. *Clinical Pediatrics, 40*(12), 639–651.

Welt, C. K., Smith, P. C., & Taylor, A. E. (2004). Evidence of early ovarian aging in fragile X premutation carriers. *Journal of Clinical Endocrinology and Metabolism, 89*(9), 4569–4574.

Wheeler, B., Taylor, B., Simonsen, K., & Reith, D. M. (2005). Melatonin treatment in Smith–Magenis syndrome. *Sleep, 28*(12), 1609–1610.

Willard, H. F. (1996). X chromosome inactivation and X-linked mental retardation. *American Journal of Medical Genetics, 64*(1), 21–26.

Wright-Talamante, C., Cheema, A., Riddle, J. E., Luckey, D. W., Taylor, A. K., & Hagerman, R. J. (1996). A controlled study of longitudinal IQ changes in females and males with fragile X syndrome. *American Journal of Medical Genetics, 64*(2), 350–355.

Zinn, A. R., Ramos, P., Elder, F. F., Kowal, K., Samango-Sprouse, C., & Ross, J. L. (2005). Androgen receptor CAGn repeat length influences phenotype of 47,XXY (Klinefelter) syndrome. *Journal of Clinical Endocrinology and Metabolism, 90*(9), 5041–5046.

Zitzmann, M., Depenbusch, M., Gromoll, J., & Nieschlag, E. (2004). X-chromosome inactivation patterns and androgen receptor functionality influence phenotype and social characteristics as well as pharmacogenetics of testosterone therapy in Klinefelter patients. *Journal of Clinical Endocrinology and Metabolism, 89*(12), 6208–6217.

Neuroscience of Developmental Disabilities

Curt A. Sandman
Aaron S. Kemp

DEVELOPMENTAL DISABILITY AND NEUROSCIENCE

Defining "neuroscience" and "developmental disability" is, on the face of it, simple and straightforward. Neuroscience is the science of the nervous system (Zigmond et al., 1999). Although the scientific study of the nervous system dates at least to the 16th century, with the remarkable neuroanatomical studies of Thomas Willis, the formal field of neuroscience is a much more recent development. The term "neuroscience" was coined in the 1960s, and shortly thereafter, in 1970, the Society for Neuroscience was formed with 500 charter members. In 1971, the Society for Neuroscience convened its first meeting. Today it has more than 34,000 members. The scope of this relatively new field is exceptionally broad, encompassing research of every nuance on the relation between layers of the nervous system and multiple forms of "behavior." This research provides the basis for understanding the medical fields that are concerned with treating nervous system disorders, including developmental disabilities.

Willis's goal was the same as the goals of contemporary neuroscientists: to understand the mysteries of the nervous system—the organ of time, place, and orientation, the basis of personality, the structure of intellect, the seat of curiosity and perceiver of good and evil. Construed in this framework, modern-day neuroscience has the same obstacles (Is the human mind capable of examining the human mind?) and even the same foes ("intelligent design"), encountered by Willis (the church) in his attempts to understand the human mind with physical rather than spiritual explanations.

"Developmental disability" (DD) encompasses an equally broad definition. Technically, it refers to any condition that delays or impairs an individual's physical, cognitive, physiological, and/or psychological development. The condition must be present before the age of 18 years, but the influence can extend throughout the lifespan. The conditions are unlimited and include genetic, traumatic, metabolic, environmental, prenatal, and psychological factors, among others. The most common *known* causes of DD are genetic, but the etiology that comprises over 60% of the cases of DD is "*unknown perinatal complications*" (Barron & Sandman, 1984). This vague etiological explanation implies that "something" has happened between conception and the early neonatal period with the majority of individuals who exhibit developmental delay and that this event or condition has lifelong and deleterious consequences for the individual.

It is a sobering reminder that nearly every condition entertained by contemporary neuroscience as a factor in DD was discussed either as a "genetic" or "physical" factor in the classic textbook, *The Mentally Retarded Child* (Robinson & Robinson, 1965). Prenatal effects, including psychosocial stress, nutrition, infection, allergic reactions, cervical anomalies, maternal age, parity, drugs, radiation, and anoxia, among others, all are discussed as possible factors influencing fetal brain development. The risk of adverse birth outcomes and the distinction between pre- and postnatal conditions are delineated in this classic work. The relation is considered between brain development and intelligence and between physical limitations such as microencephaly or hydrocephaly and adaptive function.

It would be a mistake to conclude from this observation that there has not been any progress in the study of the nervous system of developmentally delayed individuals. Quite the contrary, there has been enormous progress, especially in methods for examining the nervous system in conscious, living individuals. Thus the primary focus of this chapter is to highlight these new methods with special relevance for the study of developmental delays. The facts will change with time. Thus the findings presented in this chapter should be considered only examples from the contemporary methods that are, or could be, applied to the study of the nervous system in individuals with developmental problems. Two basic questions should be addressed before we describe the methods available for the neuroscientific study of the human brain.

What Does the Brain Have to Do with Developmental Disabilities?

The implicit question is, What does the brain have to do with intelligence? The simple answer is "everything." But what does that mean? Is a big brain more intelligent than a small brain? Do some areas of the brain relate to intelligence more strongly than others? Are neural connections more important than brain mass? Then, of course, what is intelligence? This last question has enormous significance for the future of neuroscience because psychometric measurement of intelligence can be unreliable due to factors unrelated to intellectual potential (e.g. compliance; Walsh et al., 2007), especially in individuals who are severely and profoundly retarded. Without a reliable and stable phenotype, the search for biological correlates is futile. An objective index of intelligence, that is, a measure (or a phenotype) based on structural and/or functional measures of the nervous system, may improve the separation of levels of ability, especially at the low end of the intelligence scale, and offers the promise of precision regarding etiology, diagnosis, and prognosis for the majority of individuals with intellectual impairments of unknown causes.

The provocative report of Ertl and Schafer (1969) indicated that intellectual ability was coded in the electrical activity of the brain. The electroencephalogram (EEG) is a noninvasive measure of the electrical activity of the brain taken from the scalp. As illustrated in Figure 7.1, there are many frequencies in the EEG, and different frequencies are associated with unique states of consciousness. Ertl and Schafer (1969) showed that "stretching" the EEG to create a string (a more complex EEG would stretch further) was associated with IQ. They reported that longer strings were related to higher IQ. Recent research has suggested that alpha power (Klimesch, Vogt, & Doppelmayr, 2000; Doppelmayr, Klimesch, Stadler, Pollhuber, & Heine, 2002), alpha frequency (Anokhin & Vogel, 1996; Clark et al., 2004), and increases in the upper alpha band of about 10–12 Hz (termed alpha event-related desynchronization; ERD) were related to higher measured intelligence. It is assumed that increased ERD reflects cortical activation (Anokhin & Vogel, 1996; Klimesch et al., 2000; Dopplemayr et al., 2002, 2005; Clark et al., 2004) so these findings are not substantially different from the conclusions of Ertl and Schafer (1969).

Event-related potentials (ERPs) of the brain provide another way to assess the relation between the nervous system and intelligence. ERPs are stimulus-linked responses of the EEG that are averaged over many trials (Figure 7.2). The ERP is an evoked neural response that emerges from random background EEG activity. As illustrated in Figure 7.2, characteristic components of the ERP reflect positive (P) and negative (N) current.

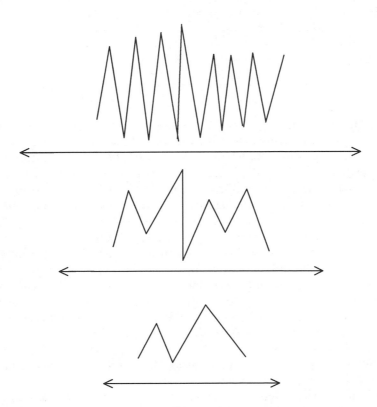

FIGURE 7.1. Graphic representation of EEG "stretching." More complex EEGs (faster activity) result in a longer string (lines with arrows) than slower, higher amplitude activity. Longer strings are associated with higher intelligence.

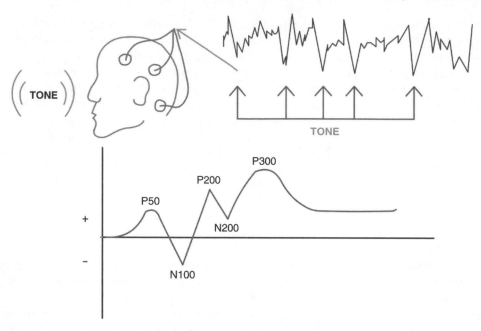

FIGURE 7.2. Representation of event-related potential (ERP) methodology. When the EEG is averaged across multiple presentations of a stimulus (tone), a characteristic event-related waveform develops. The peaks and valleys labeled as N (negative) and P (positive) refer to the direction of the electrical current, and the numbers (50, 100, etc.) refer to the approximate time after the event that the peaks develop (sometimes referred to as 1, 2 and 3, reflecting order and not time).

Distinctive components arising at different latencies after stimulation reflect the type and depth of information processing. In general, higher intelligence has been associated with (1) shorter component latencies of the ERP, (2) increased component amplitude, (3) faster habituation of the brain responses to repeated stimulation, (4) greater waveform complexity, (5) decreased trial-to-trial variability, and (6) greater hemispheric asymmetry. The wide variations in measures of ability, however, make comparisons tenuous among tests, studies, and individuals (Sandman & Barron, 1986).

Subsequent studies have yielded mixed results, partly because many parameters of the EEG have been compared with different measures or features of intelligence. For instance, adaptive ability (Sandman & Barron, 1986) or the acquisition of a skill (Shucard & Horn, 1973) had higher relations with EEG measures than did scores on an intelligence test. Moreover, some studies of the EEG coupled with complex tasks have suggested that intelligence is related to the efficiency of the frontal lobes to orchestrate posterior and temporal neural resources (Thatcher, Northa, & Bivera, 2005), and others suggest that intelligence reflects the function of a specific neural system (Duncan et al., 2000). Some suggest that the relationship between intelligence and the EEG is apparent only when there is no specific task to solve.

Does size make a difference? Evidence indicates that larger brains are related to higher levels of function. Genes (*ASPM* and *MCPH1*) that regulate brain size have emerged and continue to evolve because of strong positive selection. The pressure for these genes to evolve is believed to be related to (or responsible for) the remarkable adaptation (intelligence) of *Homo sapiens* (Mekel-Bobrov et al., 2005; Evans et al., 2005). A recent review (Miller, 2006) reported that children who scored high on an intelligence test had *delayed*, but prolonged, "growth spurts" in the cerebral cortex. A postmortem study of 100 men and women indicated that, in general, larger brains were associated with higher intelligence, but sex differences and asymmetries also were discovered. An interesting decline in visuospatial ability with age was correlated with an age-related decline in brain volume, further implicating brain size and ability (Witelson, Beresh, & Kigar, 2006).

A comprehensive analysis (Toga & Thompson, 2005) of the relation between brain structure and intelligence concludes that "~10% of the population variability in IQ can be predicted from brain volume measures alone" (p. 16). They cite a paper presentation (McDaniel & Nguyen, 2002, as cited in Toga & Thompson, 2005) that reported that 27 of 28 MRI studies of intelligence, using 1,375 participants, reported significant correlations between intelligence and brain volume. Improved relations between the brain and intelligence are obtained by examining specific areas (parcellation) of the brain. The general finding is that intelligence is linked with cortical mass (gray matter) in the frontal regions of the brain (Postuma et al., 2002).

Does the Nervous System Change with Experience?: Neurogenesis and Plasticity of the Nervous System

The concept of a static brain no longer is tenable. It is well established that the brain forms new neurons in response to environmental stimulation (Dong & Greenough, 2004). Remarkably, exposure to novel information can rewire the brain. For instance, visual information can be "rewired" to auditory cortex. The novel projection in the rewired brain may be less efficient than genetically determined pathways, but evidence indicates that cortical function "depends on inputs for physiological and behavioral instruction" (Sur & Rubenstein, 2005, p. 805). This effect of experience on the brain appears to be pervasive. Although it has been known for some time that experience can change the structure of the brain and the number of synapses, recently it has been shown that astrocytes, oligodendrocytes, and the vasculature of the brain also can be altered by environmental stimulation (Dong & Greenough, 2004). Dong and Greenough (2004) argue that developmental conditions such as epilepsy or autism may involve abnormal plasticity of both nonneuronal tissue and neurons. There is another proposal that autism and Rett syndrome can be traced to exaggerated experience-dependent synaptic plasticity that occurs months after periods of normal growth (Zoghbi, 2003). Most developmental problems, however, occur during developmental periods when the rate of growth is extremely high. The fastest periods of growth, and thus the most vulnerable periods, are the embryonic/fetal and neonatal periods.

The human fetus expresses an estimated eightfold more cell divisions before term than during the remainder of life (Barker, 1998). The fetal human brain particularly is undergoing dramatic growth. Between gestational age (GA) 8–16 weeks, migrating neurons form the subplate zone, awaiting connections from afferent neurons originating in the thalamus, basal forebrain, and brainstem. Concurrently, cells accumulating in the outer cerebral wall form the cortical plate, which eventually will become the cerebral cortex. By week 20 GA, axons form synapses with the cortical plate. This process continues so that by 24 weeks GA cortical circuits are organized (Kostovic, Judas, Rados, & Hrabac, 2002; Bourgeois, Goldman-Rakic, & Rakic, 1994). The enormous growth of the nervous system is characterized by the proliferation of neurons. By week 28 GA, the number of neurons in the human fetal brain is 40% greater than in the adult (Huttenlocker & Dabholkar, 1997; Huttenlocher, de Courten, Garey, & Van der Loos, 1982; Becker, Armstrong, Chan, & Wood, 1984; Bourgeois et al., 1994). The rate of synaptogenesis reaches an astonishing peak at week 34 GA through 24 months postpartum of 40,000 synapses per second (Levitt et al., 2003). Because of this, the human fetus and neonate are particularly vulnerable to both organizing and disorganizing influences. These influences have been described as "programming" (Nathanielsz, 1999).

Programming is a process by which a stimulus or insult during a critical developmental period has a long-lasting or permanent influence on health and well-being. Exposure to adversity early in life imprints a pattern of neural activity that results in a "program" of disorders. These programs alter the set point for release of critical neurochemical messengers and influence health and the subsequent behavioral and physiological repertoire of the individual (Barker, 1998). The effects of toxins and teratogens on development are well documented, but even exposure to maternal stress, as suggested by Robinson and Robinson (1965), is known to influence development (Sandman, Glynn, et al., 2003). Prenatal stress in rodents results in permanent changes in the brain (Weinstock, Poltyrev, Schorer-Apelbaum, Men, & McCarty, 1996). Maternal stress (crowding) is associated with persistent changes in serotonin binding in the cortex and hippocampus of offspring (Peters, 1988). Prenatally stressed rats have reduced concentrations of dopamine and norepinephrine in the cortex and locus coeruleus (Takahashi, Turner & Kalin, 1992), reduced concentrations of brain N-acetyl aspartate in the frontal cortex (Poland, 1999), alterations in forebrain cholinergic systems, higher levels of corticotrophin-releasing hormone (CRH) in the amygdala, fewer hippocampal glucocorticoid receptors, reduced numbers of opioid receptors in the brain (Insel, Kinsley, Mann, & Bridges, 1990), increased opioid levels in the hypothalamus (Sanchez, Milanes, Fuente, & Laorden, 1993), and reduced benzodiazepine inhibitory activity (Fride, Dan, Gavish, & Weinstock, 1985). In an elegant and direct assessment of the effects of maternal stress on offspring, pregnant rhesus monkeys were acutely stressed on a daily basis with acoustical stimulation (Coe et al., 2003). Reduced hippocampal volume and inhibition of neurogenesis in the dentate gyrus were observed in the offspring of the stressed animals at 2–3 years of age. Thus even subtle effects during periods of development can influence the brain and inhibit the critical processes of neurogenesis later in life.

Recent conclusions from definitive research indicate that neurogenesis in the adult brain is restricted to the dentate gyrus (Nowakowski, 2006). This research indicates that no new neurons are produced in the adult cortex and that all neurons in the human neocortex are generated before birth. According to this research, plasticity in the adult cortex is limited to the reorganization of brain circuitry, not the generation of new neurons. The implications of these findings argue not only for the evolutionary stability of human traits reflected in cortical function but also for the essential role the prenatal environment plays in endowing the intellectual potential of the individual.

METHODS OF NEUROSCIENCE

Animal Models

Nonhuman animal models have long been a standard methodological avenue of investigation in neuroscience, because they afford a degree of experimental manipulation and control that is not feasible or ethical to introduce in human participants. Most human behaviors are far more complex than those that may be accurately modeled in nonhuman species; thus considerable methodological constraints require that animal models be thoroughly evaluated to establish consensus on construct and predictive validity, as well as replicability and reliability, before any findings may be deemed generalizable to humans (van der Staay, 2006). The question, then, with regard to animal studies of mental retardation is, what should be modeled? One of the most thorough and focused animal studies of "mental retardation" was reported by Thompson, Huestis, Crinella, and Yu (1986, 1987). These investigators argued that mental retardation is a "generalized learning impairment" and that assessment of a general learning system in the white rat would be the most fruitful model for approximating the human condition. They studied the learning abilities of 25 groups of rats with various lesions on a large series of learning and problem-solving tasks. They concluded that subcortical lesions produced the largest learning impairment.

A simpler approach, and one that has generated considerable interest, is to use animal models for studying genetic syndromes related to mental retardation. Branchi, Bichler, Berger-Sweeney, and Ricceri (2003) review models for three disorders that have reasonably homogenous genetic etiologies: Down syndrome (DS), Rett syndrome, and X-linked mental retardation. The most abundant animal model investigations of mental retardation appear to have been conducted with full and segmental trisomy-16 mice models for DS. According to Galdzicki and Siarey (2003), the distal segment of mouse chromosome 16 is homologous to nearly the entire long arm of human chromosome 21 (HC21), the full or segmental triplication of which has long been associated with the etiology of DS (Lejeune, Turpin, & Gautier, 1959). The reported phenotypic similarities to DS identified in this model include developmental delay, sterility, skeletal malformation, impaired behavioral functions, abnormal synaptic plasticity, abnormal cerebellum and hippocampus, and abnormal pain responsiveness. A more recent review (Reeves, 2006) highlights the development of the "Tc1" mouse model for DS, which carries a full copy of HC21 (with the exception of two small gaps), giving it approximately 92% of the genes from HC21, whereas the trisomy-16 model contains orthologs of only 50%. In addition to the phenotypic DS features displayed in trisomy-16 models, Tc1 mice also exhibit heart defects similar to those that make trisomy 21 the leading cause of congenital heart disease in humans.

Similar attempts to develop mouse models for specific developmental disorders that present without clear genetic etiologies or identifiable biomarkers also have been the subject of several recent reviews. Andres (2002), Murcia, Gulden, and Herrup (2005), Belzung, Leman, Vourch, and Andres (2005), and Sadamatsu, Kanai, Xu, Liu, and Kato (2006) all provide reviews of recently proposed animal models for autistic spectrum disorders. Though none report that any one model has yet gained acceptance, these reviews provide thorough and intriguing discussions of the significant challenges of identifying animal behaviors that may be comparable to the complex and often heterogeneous clinical manifestations observed. Nonetheless, there remains considerable interest among researchers who are eager to confront such challenges, because the approach bears tremendous potential for both increasing our understanding of the disorders and providing an empirical basis of assessing putative pharmacological treatments (Gerlai & Gerlai, 2004; Kim et al., 2006; Johnston, 2006).

In addition to rodents, nonhuman primates also have been the focus of several proposed animal model investigations of developmental disabilities. Although nonhuman primates present additional limitations regarding cost and availability, they do confer significant advantages in that they are much more closely related to humans in both genetic and behavioral repertoires than rodents are. Machado and Bachevalier (2003) address such issues in proposing the use of macaque monkeys to model the development of complex behavioral constructs such as social cognition and emotional regulation, which are characteristically disturbed in several childhood psychopathologies. Several groups of researchers (e.g., Bayne, Haines, Dexter, Woodman, & Evans, 1995; Novak, Crockett, & Sackett, 2002) have also shown that macaque monkeys sometimes display self-injurious behaviors (SIB), which also are characteristic of many individuals with various developmental disabilities. The occurrence of SIB in this population is very poorly understood, so the identification of an animal model for this behavior has the potential to elucidate mechanisms (Kraemer & Clarke, 1990; Kraemer, Schmidt, & Ebert, 1997; Tiefenbacher, Novak, Jorgensen, & Meyer, 2000; Tiefenbacher et al., 2004; Tiefenbacher, Novak, Lutz, & Meyer, 2005; Novak, 2003) and remediation (Weld et al., 1998; Eaton et al., 1999; Tiefenbacher, Fahey, et al., 2005; Taylor, Bass, Flory, & Hankenson, 2005; Fontenot et al., 2005).

Neuropathology

The neuroscientific discipline of neuropathology encompasses a variety of empirical techniques for the identification of morphological, cellular, and molecular abnormalities in living and postmortem tissue specimens. The primary line of neuropathological research, histopathology, relates to the microscopic study of tissue obtained from individuals with specific disorders (or from animal models) using the tools and methods of histology, such as the fixation, embedding, serial sectioning, and staining of the samples. Recent advances in immunohistochemistry and fluorescent reagents, combined with technological innovations in light-transmission microscopy (e.g., scanning electron and laser scanning), have led to a wealth of research on the cellular processes that characterize normal and abnormal brain development (Haydar, 2005).

A broad review of how various neuropathological research methods have been central to the characterization of various disorders of cerebral development has been provided by Francis et al. (2006). A more specific example of how these methods have been applied to the study of developmental disorders, however, is the postmortem investigations of Bauman and Kemper (2005) in their attempts to identify neuropathological abnormalities in individuals with autism. The most robust findings to date appear to be reduced cell size and increased packing density in the limbic system (hippocampus, amygdala, and entorhinal cortex), significantly reduced numbers of Purkinje cells in the cerebellum, age-related changes in cerebellar nuclei and inferior olives, and increased brain size, particularly in childhood (see also Bailey et al., 1998; Pickett & London, 2005; Courchesne, Redcay, Morgan, & Kennedy, 2005; Courchesne & Pierce, 2005). These findings indicate that complications may arise during prenatal brain development but that the neuropathology of autism is almost certainly an ongoing process.

Neuropathological research also employs novel *in vitro* methods of investigation using cell cultures from samples related to specific disorders. Saud et al. (2006), for example, have developed techniques for the stable *in vitro* immortalization of cell lines derived from various brain tissues of normal and trisomy-16 mice. By comparing the cell lines from each, they discovered abnormal intracellular responding to several neurotransmitters in the trisomy-16 cell lines from the cerebral cortex, hippocampus, spinal cord, and dorsal root ganglion. Such *in vitro* research into specific neuronal dysfunctions may significantly expand the utility of animal model investigations, particularly when genetic modifications result in unviable offspring. Furthermore, these methods have considerable potential to provide an empirical basis for evaluating candidate pharmacological interventions.

Neurochemistry

Neurochemistry is a branch of neuroscience devoted to the study of organic molecules that participate in neural activity. This involves a very broad spectrum of studies that include neurotransmitters, neuropeptides, hormones, immune and infectious agents, and medications that influence the function of neurons. There are many examples of attempts to implicate neurochemical systems in mental retardation and even more studies that have used various medications to treat (the symptoms of) mental retardation. This section focuses on two examples of neurochemical research: one mature idea in which a biomarker (or mechanism) for a specific behavior (self-injury) associated with mental retardation and autism has been the focus and a second area in which neuroprotective agents are proposed to overcome impairment.

The majority of contemporary studies support a biological basis for some forms of self-injuring behavior. One significant research focus has been on the stress system and specifically proopiomelanocortin (POMC; Sandman & Touchette, 2002; Sandman, Spence & Smith, 1999). In humans, most POMC is produced in the pars distalis of the anterior pituitary. POMC also is produced by other neurons, including many hypothalamic neurons and neurons in the amygdala and pituitary stalk. POMC gives rise to a variety of neuropeptides, including ACTH, MSH, LPH, and endorphin, which are prominent in the hypothalamic–pituitary–adrenal (HPA) axis. Two enzymes for converting POMC into these HPA-active agents are present in the fetus by midgestation, but there are differences in the timing of their regional distribution, resulting in variable levels of susceptibility to stress in the immature brain. As organisms reach adulthood, this uneven distribution disappears, resulting in adaptive coupling of the stress system (Sandman, Touchette, Lenjavi, Marion, & Chicz-DeMet, 2003). However, the finding that the POMC products are not coupled among the majority of individuals exhibiting self-injury could be evidence of disturbance in expression or activity of the enzymes early in fetal life. Significant disregulation of POMC relations is associated with a unique self-injuring phenotype (Sandman, Touchette, Marion, Lenjavi, & Chicz-DeMet, 2002; Sandman, Touchette, et al., 2003). Medication that blocked the POMC system altered the phenotype (reduced self-injury), suggesting that this stress system plays a fundamental role in the maintenance of this dramatic behavior (Sandman & Touchette, 2002).

Activity-dependent neuroprotective protein (ADNP) is a 14–amino-acid peptide that protects neurons against a wide variety of toxic substances (Chen, Charness, Wilkemeyer, & Sulik, 2005) and attenuates damage in animal models of neuronal injury (Zaltzman, Alexandrovich, Trembovler, Shohami, & Gozes, 2005). Evidence indicates that this peptide (and smaller sequences) is essential for neuronal survival and that it protects neurons because it blocks apoptosis (Sari & Gozes, 2006). Its release from astroglia is stimulated by vasoactive intestinal peptide, and it is believed that the protective effects are related to the regulation of calcium and transcription factor activation (Sari & Gozes, 2006). The intriguing feature about this family of peptides is the wide range of protective properties they possess. Protection against fetal/infant exposure to alcohol, hypoxia, brain injury, viral exposure, age-related decline, and fetal waste all have been demonstrated with pre-, co- or posttreatment with the ADNP family (Rotstein et al., 2006; Smith-Swintosky, Gozes, Brenneman, D'Andrea, & Plata-Salaman, 2005;

)06). The possibilities for treatment of, and perhaps inoculation against,
eurological injuries and neurotoxic exposures would dramatically alter
elopmental disability. The progress of this line of research deserves care-

ging

ing" refers to the application of a variety of advanced techniques for creat-
ical representations of brain structures and detailed maps of functional acti-
terns. Although the widely variable etiologies of developmental disorders
mplex, diffuse, and often nonuniform abnormalities of brain development,
vances in neuroimaging technologies are nonetheless critical in defining comes in brain structure and functions that may be central to the further character-
of phenotypic biomarkers of many disorders. By applying neuroimaging tech-
to advance our understanding of the complex neural networks subserving
diverse brain functions, cognitive and behavioral neuroscientists hope to identify key
indicators of abnormal development in the neuroanatomical substrates of several specific disabilities. In addition to this promise of *in vivo* research tools to elucidate
pathophysiological indices in brain development, the recent maturation of several neuroimaging technologies also has begun to have a direct impact on clinical diagnostic
practice by aiding in the identification of congenital malformations, recognizable syndromes, specific disease processes, and prognostic indicators of neurodevelopmental
outcome in developmentally delayed and encephalopathic children (Williams, 2004).

Because of the logistic difficulties in identifying subtle brain abnormalities in heterogeneous samples, many studies have focused on findings within relatively homogenous diagnostic groups. Reiss, Eliez, Schmitt, Patwardhan, and Haberecht (2000) provide a review of neuroimaging findings in five genetic conditions that commonly give
rise to developmental or neuropsychiatric disabilities: fragile X syndrome, velocardiofacial syndrome, Williams syndrome, Turner syndrome, and Klinefelter syndrome. A
more recent review by Gothelf, Furfaro, Penniman, Glover, and Reiss (2005) also highlights studies that focus on developmental disorders with known genetic etiologies as
the preferred alternative to neuroimaging in idiopathic cases in which the tremendous
heterogeneity of pathophysiological characteristics would require the study of enormous samples before any consistency of findings could hope to elucidate commonalities of abnormal brain morphology or function.

Despite these implicit limitations, however, several other reviews have identified
converging evidence within neuroimaging results in disorders typified by uncertain etiology and inherent difficulties in diagnostic specificity, such as autism. Indeed, Frank
and Pavlakis (2001), Boddaert and Zilbovicius (2002), Brambilla et al. (2003), Greicius
(2003), Sokol and Edwards-Brown (2004), Toal, Murphy, and Murphy (2005), and most
recently Lainhart (2006), have all provided detailed reviews of the application of neuroimaging to the study of autistic spectrum disorders. Though plagued by a decade of discrepant findings with poor replicability, some consistent findings have begun to
emerge. Specifically, these reviews appear to agree on the consistency of reports of
accelerated brain growth followed by atypical developmental trajectories of brain volume and functional connectivity, though the specific longitudinal course of such findings is still a subject of debate. Further complicating the desire to find commonalities is
an overall lack of uniformity in not only the demographics of the participants and the
diagnostic criteria employed but also in the use of the specific scanning sequences and

activation paradigms applied. For these reasons, neuroimaging research in autistic spectrum disorders has not yet attained a level of consensus sufficient to recommend clinical application as a diagnostic aid, but it has at least provided a promising avenue of *in vivo* investigation into the neuropathological substrates believed to characterize these disorders.

Clearly, neuroimaging research offers critically important emerging tools in the neuroscience of developmental disorders. The following sections are brief overviews of the various neuroimaging techniques that have been devoted to the study of developmental disorders. The summary of studies discussed for each method is therefore not intended to provide an exhaustive review of extant findings but rather a representative sampling of how each has been applied in the field.

Ultrasonography

Due in large part to its portability, noninvasive ease of use, and relatively inexpensive availability, ultrasonography (US) has become one of the most widely used methods of imaging the developing human brain. US, which has been in medical use since the 1940s, relies on the principles of ultrasonic (frequencies beyond the range of human hearing) sound waves echoing differentially from various tissues. A phased array of piezoelectronic transducers is used to emit pulsed sound waves from a handheld probe that can be manually directed. These transducers then transmit the resulting echo pulses to the ultrasound scanner to be processed and transformed into a digital image of the underlying tissues. Relatively recent advances in US technologies, such as 3-D and 4-D imaging, including color-coded images of the dynamic movement of various tissues (usually blood flow), have relied on improvements in the transducer arrays and on the application of sophisticated analytic techniques such as the calculation of Doppler effects.

Both transabdominal and transvaginal US have been utilized to image the developing fetal brain, and standardization of the planes and sections acquired has enabled researchers to produce images that can be compared with neonatal transfontanelle US (Timor-Tritsch & Monteagudo, 1996, 2001; Pooh, Pooh, Nakagawa, Nishida, & Ohno, 2000). Such capabilities have allowed neuroscientists and neurologists to establish standards of practice that have dramatically facilitated the early (both prenatal and neonatal) diagnosis of a variety of cerebral malformations and abnormalities that may be the first indication of a neurodevelopmental disability (Aubry, Aubry, & Dommergues, 2003; Angtuaco, 2005). Furthermore, the ease of administration of US allows researchers to apply it in longitudinal designs much more readily than other neuroimaging methods, thus enabling serial investigations to establish milestones in fetal cortical development (Cohen-Sacher, Lerman-Sagie, Lev, & Malinger, 2006). The clinical application of such "neurosonographic" landmarks will further enhance the diagnostic and prognostic validity of US and solidify its utility as the first-line indicator of developmental brain abnormalities. At present, however, the clinical application of US warrants mindful consideration of the spatial resolution limitations of the method for identification of subtle malformations (Correa et al., 2006).

In addition to structural imaging with conventional US, functional measures of regional cerebral blood flow (rCBF) dynamics (e.g., velocity, pulsatility, and resistance indices) can also be acquired using transcranial Doppler US (tDUS), suggesting utility in a range of interesting research and clinical applications (Aaslid, Markwalder, & Nornes, 1982). Bruneau, Doumeau, Garreau, Pourcelot, and Lelord (1992), for example, employed tDUS to compare rCBF responses to auditory stimuli in 12 children diagnosed with autism, 10 with nonautistic mental retardation, and 12 considered normal controls. They report that the auditory stimulation evoked asymmetric increases in blood flow and decreases in resistance indices in the left hemisphere for both normal control children and those with mental retardation. Children with autism, however, displayed significantly different patterns of rCBF, responding with symmetric decreases in blood flow and increases in resistance indices in both hemispheres. Examples of how tDUS may be applied clinically to monitor rCBF and cerebral spinal fluid dynamics in the neonate are also reviewed by Kirimi, Tuncer, Atas, Sakarya, and Ceylan (2002), Galarza and Lazareff (2004), and White and Venkatesh (2006), but caution is recommended, as more research is needed to establish the diagnostic and prognostic merits of this approach.

Computed Tomography

Computed axial tomography (CAT or CT) relies on a series of X-rays obtained from a rotating detector array, allowing multiplanar tomographic reconstruction of 2-D slices into high-resolution, digital 3-D images. The advent of magnetic resonance imaging (MRI) has all but replaced the utility of CT scanning in most investigations of structural brain abnormalities due to its increased sensitivity; however, CT still has important uses, particularly when the imaging of calcification is important (Hoon & Melhem, 2000). In a review comparing various neuroimaging methods, Barkovich (1997) states that CT is most limited in the imaging of neonates, particularly preterm neonates, because the high water content of the neonatal brain significantly reduces the contrast between normal and injured tissue. The fact that CT is relatively widely available and provides greater ease of use than MRI, in that it generally does not require sedation and can usually accommodate life-support equipment, makes this method of neuroimaging nonetheless clinically important, especially for emergency assessment of hydrocephaly, hemorrhage, or gross neurological abnormalities when MRI is not a viable alternative.

Single Photon Emission Computed Tomography

Single photon emission computed tomography (SPECT) is similar to CT in that it uses a rotating array of gamma ray detectors and computer algorithms for tomographic reconstruction of 3-D images from 2-D planar slices and is also very similar to positron emission tomography (PET) in that it relies on the injection of radioactive tracer isotopes to image perfusion (such as rCBF). Because uptake of most SPECT radiotracer agents is generally complete in less than a minute, imaging with this method is particularly well suited for patients with severe epilepsy or seizure disorders whose erratic movements might make other imaging modalities untenable. In addition to rCBF studies, further advances in SPECT (as well as PET) include the use of radioligands with specific affinities for selective neurotransmitter receptors or transporters, facilitating the investigation of putative pharmaceutical interventions to target deficiencies that may characterize some developmental or neuropsychiatric disabilities (Santosh, 2000).

Sufficient research is still lacking to warrant routine clinical application of SPECT for developmental disorders; however, several interesting investigations have been conducted with this method that contribute to the growing understanding of candidate mechanisms of the neural dysfunctions involved. Ohnishi et al. (2000) used SPECT to investigate the associations between rCBF and behavioral syndrome profiles (derived from factor analyses) in 23 children with infantile autism and 26 age- and IQ-matched children with nonautistic mental retardation. In comparisons between the groups, they found decreases in rCBF in the children with autism in the bilateral insula, superior temporal gyri, and left prefrontal cortices. They also report significant correlations between *impairments in communication and social interaction* and abnormal perfusion in the medial prefrontal cortex and anterior cingulate gyrus, and between *the obsessive desire for sameness* and altered perfusion in the right medial temporal lobe. In a similar study, Kaya et al. (2002) compared rCBF with scores on the Ritvo–Freeman Real Life Rating Scale in 18 children with autism and 11 controls without autism. They report hypoperfusion in children with autism relative to controls in frontal, frontotemporal, temporal, and temporo-occipital regions but found no significant correlations between rCBF and Ritvo–Freeman ratings. Further research with this method may serve to elucidate the neural circuits believed to subserve some of the characteristic dysfunctions of such disorders; however, the relatively unknown risk of childhood exposure to radioactive isotopes has raised some ethical concerns about the potential for routine clinical application of both SPECT and PET in this population (Bookheimer, 2000).

Positron Emission Tomography

Since its emergence in the 1970s, PET has remained at the forefront of functional neuroimaging technologies. PET scanning involves the injection or inhalation of a relatively short-lived radioisotope that decays by emitting a positron. Such positrons collide with nearby electrons, and the resulting annihilation event produces a pair of photons traveling approximately 180 degrees from one another. When these photons are detected in coincidence by scintillations in a ring of detector crystals, the source of the annihilation event is calculated, and a multicolor 3-D image is generated to reveal the relative spatial concentrations of the radiotracer (Figure 7.3). In addition to basal measures of resting brain activity, activation tasks also may be performed during the uptake of the radiotracers to assess functional aspects of evoked brain patterns. Furthermore, the recent and ongoing development of novel radioligands with specific binding affinities, in addition to the traditional use of radioisotopes bound to glucose, water, or oxygen, enable the use of PET to provide invaluable information about the biochemical, meta-

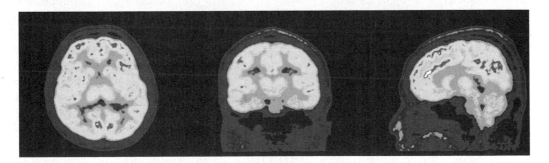

FIGURE 7.3. These images illustrate the use of positron emission tomography (PET) to map regional brain concentrations of radiotracer compounds, such as fluorodeoxyglucose (FDG). The shading of the images (normally represented with color coding) reveals the magnitude of the concentrations of FDG, thereby indicating regional metabolic activity. (Color images available by request from the authors.) Images provided by Steven G. Potkin, Brain Imaging Center, University of California, Irvine.

bolic, and molecular processes of regional brain activation as contrasted across functional task conditions and/or between diagnostic groups. Thus PET constitutes a powerful neuroimaging technology for investigating gene–brain–behavior relations in a variety of neuropathological conditions.

Sundaram, Chugani, and Chugani (2005) provide an excellent review of previous research and future directions in the application of PET to the study of mental retardation and developmental disabilities. The authors state that PET research may be key in identifying the physiological consequences and expression of the genes associated with various forms of mental retardation. Specialty PET scanners designed for rodents, for example, have facilitated the study of transgenic mouse models of human genetic disorders, and greater benefits of higher spatial resolution are anticipated with new developments in "micro" PET technology. Sundaram et al.'s (2005) review of PET studies of human brain development include investigations showing that regional changes in glucose metabolism correlate with the maturation of behavioral, neurophysiological, and neuroanatomical events in infants and that measures of serotonin synthesis capacity and $GABA_A$ receptor distribution decrease dramatically with age in children before reaching adult levels. Several findings of abnormal development on each of these measures include studies of glucose metabolism in Rett syndrome, focal and global abnormalities of serotonin synthesis in autism, and decreased $GABA_A$ receptor binding in Angelman and Prader–Willi syndromes. The authors also provide arguments that the ethical concerns regarding the use of radiopharmaceuticals in children (mentioned earlier) may constitute unnecessary limitations on the tremendous potential of PET investigations, citing several indicators that the radiological risks conveyed by a typical PET scan are negligibly low. As such, they encourage the implementation of PET studies to identify key biomarkers of abnormal development in glucose metabolism, neurotransmitter and gene-regulated protein synthesis, and receptor binding profiles, but suggest rational screening of participants to exclude children with high levels of prior exposure to radiation or a strong family history of cancer.

Magnetic Resonance Imaging

Regarded as perhaps the quintessential neuroimaging modality, magnetic resonance imaging (MRI) affords tremendous latitude to construct high-contrast, multiplanar, 3-D images of a variety of living tissues, including structural, functional, biochemical, and diffusivity measures of the human brain, without the risk of exposure to ionizing radiation. MRI is based on principles of nuclear magnetic resonance (NMR) concerning the directional alignment of hydrogen atoms in a magnetic field, which precess at characteristic resonance frequencies. The energy released when the nuclei of these atoms "relax" to an equilibrium precession state following perturbation by radio frequency pulse waves is the basis of the MRI signal. The application of such principles has spawned an entire field of dauntingly complex mathematical methods for pulse sequencing and signal processing that continues to evolve advanced MRI technologies.

Although the traditional usage of MRI has been to provide detailed structural or morphometric images (Figure 7.4), relatively recent advances have enabled a range of additional applications. Such advanced variants of MRI include the imaging of regional brain activation patterns with functional magnetic resonance imaging (fMRI), neurometabolic biochemistry with magnetic resonance spectroscopy (MRS), mean regional diffusivity measures using diffusion-weighted imaging (DWI), and directional diffusion fiber mapping using diffusion-tensor imaging (DTI). Collectively, these methodologies

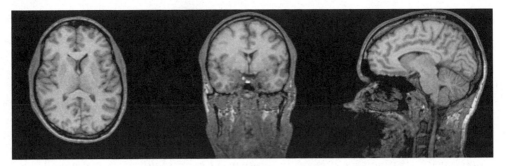

FIGURE 7.4. These anatomical images were obtained using structural magnetic resonance imaging (sMRI). The high spatial resolution of such images yields detailed morphometric data that can be used in a variety of analytic techniques, such as parcellation and mapping of cortical thickness. Images provided by Steven G. Potkin, Brain Imaging Center, University of California, Irvine.

represent an impressive array of neuroimaging tools that make MRI the preferred technology for investigating the pathophysiological substrates of developmental disabilities, with the promise of facilitating diagnostic specificity and predicting outcome.

Due to the detection of subtle changes in signal intensity depending on the amount of oxygen present in hemoglobin, Ogawa, Lee, Kay, and Tank (1990) established that regional variations in blood oxygen levels could be used to image functional brain activation patterns. This blood-oxygenation-level-dependent (BOLD) signal is the basis for fMRI, which has had a dramatic impact on neuroscience investigations through the use of clever contrast designs comparing regional neural activity levels during various task conditions on the cognitive, affective, or behavioral activation paradigms employed (for examples of fMRI activation maps, see Figure 7.5). Additionally, the use of arterial

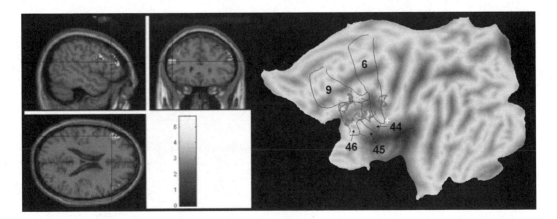

FIGURE 7.5. This combination of images illustrates the types of functional activation maps that are derived from functional magnetic resonance imaging (fMRI). Comparing subtle changes in the blood-oxygenation-level-dependent (BOLD) signal acquired during performance of various activation task conditions yields regions of interest (normally color coded), where contrast differences reach a defined statistical threshold of significance (e.g., $p < .01$). (Color images available by request from the authors.) Images provided by Jessica Turner and David B. Keator, Brain Imaging Center, University of California, Irvine.

spin labeling (ASL) or weighting the MRI signal by rCBF or regional cerebral blood volume (rCBV) by injecting paramagnetic contrast agents has provided alternative methods of fMRI, conferring additional sensitivity or quantitative information to BOLD signal contrasts that could extend the clinical utility of this method beyond research applications (Wang & Licht, 2006).

MRS has been used to assess neurometabolic indicators, such as the ratios of N-acetylaspartate (NAA) or choline (Cho) to creatine (Cr), which are thought to reflect neurodevelomental processes of myelination, dendritic proliferation, and synaptogenesis. For example, Filippi, Ulug, Deck, Zimmerman, and Heier (2002) applied MRS to the characterization of subtle brain abnormalities in children with clinically significant developmental delays who present without notable abnormalities on conventional, structural MRI. They report decreased NAA/Cr ratios and increased Cho/Cr ratios in frontal and parieto-occipital subcortical white matter in developmentally delayed children over the age of 2 years, but not in those less than 2 years old, relative to age-matched controls. Based on these initial findings they suggest further longitudinal studies to evaluate the potential for such measures to be used as diagnostic tools or neuroimaging biomarkers to assess functional outcome in children with developmental delays who are older than 2 years.

Diffusion MRI methods allow researchers to measure regional differences in the diffusion of water molecules throughout connecting fibers in the brain. With DWI, three magnetic gradients are generally used to derive nondirectional, isotropic values of mean diffusivity, whereas DTI may utilize as many as six gradients to calculate directional, anisotropic diffusion values within each image voxel, which may then be used to derive tensor maps of white-matter connections (tractography; for examples of such images, see Figure 7.6). In another excellent example of how these methods may be applied, Filippi et al. (2003) compared children with a clinical presentation of developmental delay, but no abnormal structural MRI findings, with age-matched healthy controls on regional measures of mean diffusivity and anisotropy. Their results indicated

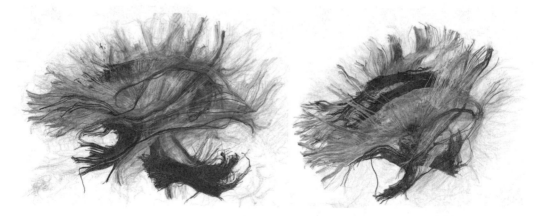

FIGURE 7.6. These images are examples of fiber-mapping tractography derived from the use of diffusion tensor imaging (DTI). The generation of such incredible images relies on as many as six magnetic gradients for precise mapping of the anisotropic diffusion of water molecules along white-matter tracts, where the shading (normally represented with color coding) indicates the direction of diffusion, weighted by the degree of anisotropy in a given image voxel. (Color images available by request from the authors.) Images provided by James A. Fallon, Brain Imaging Center, University of California, Irvine.

that children with developmental delay, relative to controls, show significantly *increased* mean diffusion in all structures measured and significantly *decreased* values of anisotropy in all white-matter fiber tracts studied except the posterior limb of the internal capsule. As the normal developmental progression of myelination with white-matter maturation is associated with *decreases* in mean water diffusion and *increases* in directional anisotropy (see Mascalchi et al., 2005, for a review), the authors interpret their findings as indicative of abnormal myelination or white-matter development. As with the MRS study mentioned earlier, the authors recommend further longitudinal and normative studies to determine the predictive validity and diagnostic specificity of these measures, but the potential value is already quite evident.

The sheer volume of MRI investigations of various developmental disorders conducted within the past 5 years alone prohibits a thorough review in this chapter but nonetheless provides encouraging indications that research in this area will soon begin to coalesce around the most salient findings with the potential to have direct impact on prognostic and diagnostic clinical practices in the field. Though far from exhaustive, Table 7.1 provides a representative summary of recent structural and functional MRI findings in one area of DD research (autistic spectrum disorders). Toga, Thompson, and Sowell (2006) provide a fairly comprehensive review of how various MRI acquisition and analysis techniques have begun to elucidate the longitudinal course of normal brain maturation and how this, in turn, will serve to further the characterization of biomarkers for abnormal development in various disorders. The authors state that multicenter scan databases are only beginning to reach the enormous sample sizes required to stratify key indicators of brain development by symptom profiles, known genotypes, or currently identified risk factors; but such progress may portend the widespread clinical and diagnostic utility of MRI technologies.

Already, structural MRI has gained routine acceptance in the identification of neonatal brain abnormalities, with considerable advantages in resolution and contrast over CT and US, without the risk of radiation. Reviews by Robertson and Wyatt (2004) and Garel (2006) tout the value of structural MRI in the clinical assessment of neonatal and fetal brain development and foretell the additional advantages that advanced MRI methods such as fMRI, MRS, DWI, and DTI may soon confer. Indeed, studies such as those recently conducted by Barkovich et al. (2006) and Boichot et al. (2006) comparing the prognostic value of conventional MRI with MRS, DWI, and DTI in encephalopathic neonates will be vital in determining the safety and practicality of each of these methods for routine clinical use. Thus ongoing investigations with MRI techniques and the other neuroimaging methodologies described earlier are essential for the refinement of the research tools to further the neuroscience of developmental disorders and as guideposts in eventual clinical applications to provide early indicators of abnormal development.

FUTURE RESEARCH DIRECTIONS

There are several areas we believe should be given special attention. In addition to the specific areas discussed in this section, it is clear from this review that the prenatal period has become an increasingly critical period for projecting human potential. A significant proportion of variation in infant and adult health outcomes and disease risk is attributable to developmental processes during fetal life in response to a variety of environmental, social, psychological, physiological, and genetic influences. Fetal exposures

TABLE 7.1. Representative Summary of Structural and Functional MRI Findings for Autism Spectrum Disorders

Publication	Participants	Key findings
Carper & Courchesne (2005)	25 patients (mean age = 5.3) and 18 controls (mean age = 5.1)	The dorsolateral region showed a reduced age effect in patients when compared with control participants, with a predicted 10% increase in volume from 2 years of age to 9 years of age compared with a predicted 48% increase for control participants. In a separate analysis, dorsolateral and medial frontal regions were significantly enlarged in patients ages 2 to 5 years compared with control participants of the same age, but the precentral gyrus and orbital cortex were not.
Hazlett et al. (2005)	51 patients and 25 controls (11 with atypical and 14 with typical development; 18–35 months)	Significant enlargement was detected in cerebral cortical volumes but not cerebellar volumes in the patient group. Enlargement was present in both white and gray matter, and it was generalized throughout the cerebral cortex. Head circumference appears normal at birth, with a significantly increased rate of head circumference growth appearing to begin around 12 months of age.
Hendry et al. (2006)	19 patients (ages 6–16) and 20 controls (ages 6–16)	Patients had an increase in average cerebral white matter, although no group differences were seen in average cerebral gray matter. Patients also had bilateral regional increases in the gray matter and associated white matter of the parietal lobes (primary sensory association areas) and occipital lobes (visual association areas) and in the white matter within the supplementary motor areas in the frontal lobes.
Herbert et al. (2005)	16 patients and 30 controls (15 with DLD and 15 with typical development) (ages 5.7–11.3)	Asymmetries were masked with larger units of analysis but progressively more apparent with smaller units, and within the cerebral cortex the differences were greatest in higher order association cortex. The larger units of analysis, including the cerebral hemispheres, the major grey and white matter structures and the cortical lobes, showed no asymmetries in patients or individuals with DLD and few asymmetries in controls. However, at the level of cortical parcellation units, patients and individuals with DLD showed more asymmetry than controls.
Levitt et al. (2003)	22 patients (mean age = 10.7) and 20 controls (mean age = 11.3)	Found anterior and superior shifting of the superior frontal sulci bilaterally, anterior shifting of the right Sylvian fissure, the superior temporal sulcus and the left inferior frontal sulcus in the patient group relative to the control group.
McAlonan et al. (2005)	17 patients (mean age = 12) and 17 controls (mean age = 11)	Patients had a significant reduction in total gray matter volume and significant increase in CSF volume. They had significant localized gray matter reductions within frontostriatal and parietal networks and decreases in ventral and superior temporal gray matter. White matter was reduced in the cerebellum, left internal capsule, and fornices.

Lotspeich et al. (2004)	3 patient groups: LFA, HFA, ASP and matched controls (age range = 7.8–17.9)	Cerebral gray matter volume was enlarged in both HFA and LFA compared with controls. Cerebral gray matter volume in ASP was intermediate between that of HFA and controls, but nonsignificant. Exploratory analyses revealed a negative correlation between cerebral gray matter volume and performance IQ within HFA but not ASP. A positive correlation between cerebral white matter volume and performance IQ was observed within ASP but not HFA.
Gomot et al. (2006)	12 patients (mean age = 13.5) and 12 controls (mean age = 13.8)	During deviance detection, significant activation common to both groups was located in the superior temporal and inferior frontal gyri. During "novelty detection" both groups showed activity in the superior temporal gyrus, the temporoparietal junction, the superior and inferior frontal gyri, and the cingulate gyrus. Patients showed reduced activation of the left anterior cingulate cortex during both deviance and novelty detection. During novelty detection, patients also showed reduced activation in the bilateral temporoparietal region and in the right inferior and middle frontal areas.
Muller et al. (2004)	8 patients (mean age = 28.4) and 8 controls (mean age = 28.1)	Patients showed overall less prefrontal activation during late visuomotor learning; however, the main finding was a complementary one of enhanced activation in right pericentral and premotor cortex. In the patient group, Brodmann areas 3, 4, and 6 of the right hemisphere became more involved during late learning stages (trials 25–48), compared with early stages (trials 1–24). This effect was not seen in the control group.
Allen & Courchesne (2003)	8 patients (mean age = 26.89) and 8 controls (mean age = 26.77)	Patients showed significantly greater cerebellar motor activation and significantly less cerebellar attention activation.
Allen, Muller, & Courchesne (2004)	8 patients (mean age = 26.89) and 8 controls (mean age = 26.77)	Patients showed significantly increased motor activation in the ipsilateral anterior cerebellar hemisphere relative to normal participants, in addition to atypical activation in contralateral and posterior cerebellar regions. Moreover, increased activation was correlated with the degree of cerebellar structural abnormality.
Baron-Cohen et al. (1999)	6 patients (mean age = 26.3) and 12 controls (mean age = 25.5)	The superior temporal gyrus and amygdala show increased activation when using social intelligence. Some areas of prefrontal cortex also showed activation. In contrast, patients activated the frontotemporal regions, but not the amygdala, when making mentalistic inferences from the eyes.
Critchley et al. (2000)	9 patients (mean age = 37) and 9 controls (mean age = 27)	Patients did not activate a cortical "face area" when explicitly appraising expressions nor the left amygdala region or left cerebellum when implicitly processing emotional facial expressions

(continued)

TABLE 7.1. *(continued)*

Publication	Participants	Key findings
Harris et al. (2006)	14 patients (mean age = 36) and 22 controls (mean age = 31)	Semantic processing in the controls produced robust activation in Broca's area (left inferior frontal gyrus) and in superior medial frontal gyrus and right cerebellum. The patient group had substantially reduced Broca's activation but increased left temporal (Wernicke's) activation. Furthermore, the patients showed diminished activation differences between concrete and abstract words, consistent with behavioral studies.
Kennedy, Redcay, & Courchesne (2006)	15 patients (mean age = 25.49) and 14 controls (mean age = 26.07)	Several regions of the brain are known to have high metabolic activity during rest, which is suppressed during cognitively demanding tasks. However, it was found that the autism group failed to demonstrate this suppression effect. Furthermore, there was a strong correlation between a clinical measure of social impairment and functional activity within the ventral medial prefrontal cortex.
Ring et al. (1999)	6 patients (mean age = 26.3) and 12 controls (mean age = 5.5)	Normal controls demonstrated generally more extensive task-related activation and activated prefrontal cortical areas that were not recruited in the patient group. Conversely, the patients demonstrated greater activation of ventral occipitotemporal regions.
Schmitz et al. (2006)	10 patients of normal intelligence (mean age = 38) and 12 controls (mean age = 39)	Compared with control participants, patients showed significantly increased brain activation in (1) left inferior and orbital frontal gyrus (motor inhibition); (2) left insula (interference-inhibition); and (3) parietal lobes (set shifting). Moreover, increased frontal gray matter density and increased functional activation shared the same anatomical location in the patient group.
Wang, Lee, Sigman, & Dapretto (2006)	18 patients (mean age = 11.9) and 18 controls (mean age = 11.9)	Although the patients performed well above chance, they were less accurate than the controls at interpreting the communicative intent behind a potentially ironic remark, particularly with regard to taking advantage of available contextual information. In contrast to prior research, patients showed significantly greater activity than the controls in the right inferior frontal gyrus as well as in bilateral temporal regions.

Note. DD, developmentally delayed; HFA, high-functioning autism; LFA, low-functioning autism; DLD, developmental language disorder; ASP, Asperger's syndrome.

148

may fix, by birth, stem-cell populations and factors controlling neurogenesis. Elucidation of the nature and magnitude of the relation between these fetal exposures and subsequent health outcomes has become a national priority in the United States with the planning and announcement by the National Institutes of Health of the National Children's Study (NCS). The NCS is a proposed longitudinal study of approximately 100,000 individuals from preconception and conception to age 21, examining environmental and genetic influences on a variety of health outcomes.

Refining the Phenotypes

Can the neuroscientific study of DD proceed without refinement of the phenotype? What neural, biological, or genetic marker can be investigated if the modal diagnosis of DD is "unknown perinatal complications"? (Clearly, this is not a problem for well-defined genetic syndromes.) One suggestion offered earlier in this chapter was to use imaging procedures to redefine DD in terms of brain systems that were impaired. The logistical challenge of imaging the entire population of individuals with DD makes this strategy implausible, and besides there are many cases in which level of function is unrelated to apparent neuropathology. An alternative strategy adopted in our research is to refine the behavioral phenotype. Instead of exploring biological markers among vague categories of DD individuals, we have chosen to examine clusters of individuals with specific behavioral profiles. Moreover, instead of simply reporting rates or frequencies of various behaviors, we have examined the relations among behaviors and the context in which the behaviors occur using time-series procedures (Marion, Touchette, & Sandman, 2003; Kroeker, Touchette, Engleman, & Sandman, 2004). We have discovered that the phenotype derived from this more complex analysis improved the association between biological markers and behavior (Sandman et al., 2002; Sandman & Touchette, 2002; Kemp et al., 2007).

Stem Cells

Will stem cells provide a therapeutic avenue to repairing intellectual function? At the simplest level, a stem cell is a cell without an identity or function. Every cell in the body "stems" or originates from this cell. A stem cell has the ability to divide itself *and* produce a specialized cell throughout the lifetime of the organism. Because the context or medium defines its function, there is the promise that stem cells may be transplanted into host tissue to repair damage. There are several categories of stem cells, each with unique potential as therapeutic interventions. *Embryonic stem cells* are totipotent because they can become any cell in the body. They arise at the first step in development—when the zygote begins to divide, producing an embryo. These cells are the most promising for repair of function, but the current political atmosphere has greatly limited research with these lines. *Blastocyst embryonic stem cells* arise 7 days after fertilization, when the embryo forms the blastocyst that contains cells that will become the fetus and the placenta. These cells are pluripotent and can become *almost* any kind of cell in the body. *Fetal stem cells* arise after the 8th week of gestation. These cells also are pluripotent and have been used with limited effectiveness in models of Parkinson's disease. Many ethical issues have been raised about the use of fetal tissues, and the future of this research is unknown. *Umbilical-cord stem cells* are multipotent (they can differentiate into a limited range of cell types) and are genetically identical to the cells of the newborn. There is interest in "banking" umbilical blood for possible use of this tissue and the stem cells, if needed, for possible repair later in life. This approach obviates the possibility of tissue rejection. *Adult stem cells* are found in developed tissues to direct growth and repair in both children and adults. These multipotent cells are rare, and their origin is unknown. It is believed that they may be "set aside" during development and their expression "restrained" as an investment for future use. Despite recent highly controversial reports, there is no evidence to date that these cells give rise to cells in a host tissue.

Protecting/Repairing the Nervous System

In this chapter we have considered several ways that the damaged nervous system might be protected or repaired. The burgeoning research on activity-dependent neuroprotective proteins may produce compounds that ultimately can be used to inoculate individuals against a wide range of neurological insults. The recent findings presented in this chapter (Nowakowski, 2006) temper enthusiasm for the possibility that new neurons can be stimulated to grow in the brain. However, there is continued support for neurogenesis in the dentate gyrus, and there is compelling evidence for lifelong synaptogenesis. Demonstrations that an impaired function can be revived by rewiring the brain offer another avenue for repair of the nervous system.

Neuroprosthetics

Can an artificial device be used to replace a missing or impaired function in the nervous system? An auditory prosthesis, the cochlear implant, has been used for years to improve the sensation of hearing (Nicolelis, 2001), but what about functions such as memory and attention? In a provocative review, Keiper (2006) proposes a coming age of new devices that will improve the functioning of the nervous system and have obvious implications for developmentally delayed individuals. Among the procedures and devices he described, the proposal to develop computer chips to perform higher functions of the nervous system has special significance for individuals with intellectual impairment. Computer chips would function as artificial neurons. These chips could be loaded with information for the brain to access much as we search the Internet now for information. Not only could these chips serve as a brain-accessed database, but recently learned information could also be stored on these chips to serve as a surrogate memory system for patients with memory impairment. This may seem far-fetched, but serious programs of research are dedicated to these possibilities (Birbaumer, 2006; Berger & Glanzman, 2005; Berger et al., 2005).

ACKNOWLEDGMENTS

Preparation of this chapter was supported in part by award HD-48947 to Curt A. Sandman from the National Institutes of Child Health and Human Development. We are grateful for the expert assistance of Mohammed Lenjavi, Shervin Bazmi, and David B. Keator.

REFERENCES

Aaslid, R., Markwalder, T. M., & Nornes, H. (1982). Noninvasive transcranial Doppler ultrasound recording of flow velocity in basal cerebral arteries. *Journal of Neurosurgery, 57,* 769–774.
Allen, G., & Courchesne, E. (2003). Differential effects of developmental cerebellar abnormality on

cognitive and motor functions in the cerebellum: An fMRI study of autism. *American Journal of Psychiatry, 160*(2), 262–273.

Allen, G., Muller, R. A., & Courchesne E. (2004). Cerebellar function in autism: Functional magnetic resonance image activation during a simple motor task. *Biological Psychiatry, 56*(4), 269–278.

Andres, C. (2002). Molecular genetics and animal models in autistic disorder. *Brain Research Bulletin, 57*(1), 109–119.

Angtuaco, T. L. (2005). Ultrasound imaging of fetal brain abnormalities: Three essential anatomical levels. *Ultrasound Quarterly, 21*, 287–294.

Anokhin, A., & Vogel, F. (1996). EEG alpha rhythm frequency and intelligence in normal adults. *Intelligence, 23*, 1–14.

Aubry, M. C., Aubry, J. C., & Dommergues, M. (2003). Sonographic prenatal diagnosis of central nervous system abnormalities. *Child's Nervous System, 19*, 391–402.

Bailey, A., Luthert, P., Dean, A., Harding, B., Janota, I., Montgomery, M., et al. (1998). A clinicopathological study of autism. *Brain, 121*, 889–905.

Barker, D. J. (1998). *Mothers, babies and health in later life* (2nd ed.). Edinburgh, UK: Churchill Livingstone.

Barkovich, A. J. (1997). The encephalopathic neonate: Choosing the proper imaging technique. *American Journal of Neuroradiology, 18*, 1816–1820.

Barkovich, A. J., Miller, S. P., Bartha, A., Newton, N., Hamrick, S. E. G., Mukherjee, P., et al. (2006). MR imaging, MR spectroscopy, and diffusion tensor imaging of sequential studies in neonates with encephalopathy. *American Journal of Neuroradiology, 27*, 533–547.

Baron-Cohen, S., Ring, H. A., Wheelwright, S., Bullmore, E. T., Brammer, M. J., Simmons, A., et al. (1999). Social intelligence in the normal and autistic brain: An fMRI study. *European Journal of Neuroscience, 11*(6), 1891–1898.

Barron, J. L., & Sandman, C. A. (1984). Self-injurious behavior and stereotypy in institutionalized mentally retarded population. *Applied Research in Mental Retardation, 5*, 499–511.

Bauman, M. L., & Kemper, T. L. (2005). Neuroanatomic observations of the brain in autism: A review and future directions. *International Journal of Developmental Neuroscience, 23*, 183–187.

Bayne, K., Haines, M., Dexter, S., Woodman, D., & Evans, C. (1995). Nonhuman primate wounding prevalence: A retrospective analysis. *Lab Animal, 24*, 40–44.

Becker, L. E., Armstrong, D. L., Chan, F., & Wood, M. M. (1984). Dendritic development in human occipital cortical neurons. *Brain Research, 315*(1), 117–124.

Belzung, C., Leman, S., Vourch, P., & Andres, C. (2005). Rodent models for autism: A critical review. *Drug Discovery Today: Disease Models, 2*(2), 93–101.

Berger, T. W., Ahuja, A., Courelis, S. H., Deadwyler, S. A., Erinjippurath, G., Gerhardt, G. A., et al. (2005). Restoring lost cognitive function: Hippocampal-cortical neural prostheses. *IEEE Engineering in Medicine and Biology, 24*(5), 30–44.

Berger, T. W., & Glanzman, D. L. (2005). *Toward replacement parts for the brain: Implantable biomimetic electronics as neural prostheses.* Cambridge, MA: MIT Press.

Birbaumer, N. (2006). Brain–computer interface research: Coming of age. *Clinical Neurophysiology, 117*, 479–483.

Boddaert, N., & Zilbovicius, M. (2002). Functional neuroimaging and childhood autism. *Pediatric Radiology, 32*, 1–7.

Boichot, C., Walker, P. M., Durand, C., Grimaldi, M., Chapuis, S., Gouyon, J. B., et al. (2006). Term neonate prognoses after perinatal asphyxia: Contributions of MR imaging, MR spectroscopy, relaxation times, and apparent diffusion coefficients. *Radiology, 239*(3), 839–848.

Bookheimer, S. Y. (2000). Methodological issues in pediatric neuroimaging. *Mental Retardation and Developmental Disabilities Research Reviews, 6*, 161–165.

Bourgeois, J. P., Goldman-Rakic, P. S., & Rakic, P. (1994). Synaptogenesis in the prefrontal cortex of rhesus monkeys. *Cerebral Cortex, 4*(1), 78–96.

Brambilla, P., Hardan, A., Ucelli di Nemi, S., Perez, J., Soares, J. C., & Barale, F. (2003). Brain anatomy and development in autism: Review of structural MRI studies. *Brain Research Bulletin, 61*, 557–569.

Branchi, I., Bichler, Z., Berger-Sweeney, J., & Ricceri, L. (2003). Animal models of mental retardation: From gene to cognitive function. *Neuroscience and Biobehavioral Reviews, 27*, 141–153.

Bruneau, N., Doumeau, M. C., Garreau, B., Pourcelot, L., & Lelord, G. (1992). Blood flow response to auditory stimulations in normal, mentally retarded, and autistic children: A preliminary transcranial Doppler ultrasonographic study of the middle cerebral arteries. *Biological Psychiatry, 32,* 691–699.

Carper, R. A., & Courchesne, E. (2005). Localized enlargement of the frontal cortex in early autism. *Biological Psychiatry, 57*(2), 126–133.

Chen, S. Y., Charness, M. E., Wilkemeyer, M. F., & Sulik, K. K. (2005). Peptide-mediated protection from ethanol-induced neural tube defects. *Developmental Neuroscience, 27,* 13–19.

Clark, C. R., Veltmeyer, M. D., Hamilton, R. J., Simms, E., Paul, R., Hermens, D., et al. (2004). Spontaneous alpha peak frequency predicts working memory performance across the age span. *International Journal of Psychophysiology, 53,* 1–9.

Coe, C. L., Kramer, M., Czeh, B., Gould, E., Reeves, A. J., Kirschbaum, C., et al. (2003). Prenatal stress diminishes neurogenesis in the dentate gyrus in juvenile rhesus monkeys. *Biological Psychiatry, 54,* 1025–1034.

Cohen-Sacher, B., Lerman-Sagie, T., Lev, D., & Malinger, G. (2006). Sonographic developmental milestones of the fetal cerebral cortex: A longitudinal study. *Ultrasound in Obstetrics and Gynecology, 27,* 494–502.

Correa, F. F., Lara, C., Bellver, J., Remohi, J., Pellicer, A., & Serra, V. (2006). Potential pitfalls in fetal neurosonography. *Prenatal Diagnosis, 26,* 52–56.

Courchesne, E., & Pierce, K. (2005). Brain overgrowth in autism during a critical time in development: Implications for frontal pyramidal neuron and interneuron development and connectivity. *International Journal of Developmental Neuroscience, 23,* 153–170.

Courchesne, E., Redcay, E., Morgan, J. T., & Kennedy, D. P. (2005). Autism at the beginning: Microstructural and growth abnormalities underlying the cognitive and behavioral phenotype of autism. *Development and Psychopathology, 17,* 577–597.

Critchley, H. D., Daly, E. M., Bullmore, E. T., Williams, S. C., Van Amelsvoort, T., Robertson, D. M., et al. (2000). The functional neuroanatomy of social behaviour: Changes in cerebral blood flow when people with autistic disorder process facial expressions. *Brain, 123*(Pt. 11), 2203–2212.

Dong, W. K., & Greenough, W. T. (2004). Plasticity of noneuronal brain tissue: Roles in developmental disorders. *Mental Retardation and Developmental Disabilities Research Reviews, 10,* 85–90.

Doppelmayr, M., Klimesch, W., Sauseng, P., Hodlmoser, K., Stadler, W., & Hanslmayr, S. (2005). Intelligence related differences in EEG-bandpower. *Neuroscience Letters, 381,* 309–313.

Doppelmayr, M., Klimesch, W., Stadler, W., Pollhuber, D., & Heine, C. (2002). EEG alpha power and intelligence. *Intelligence, 30,* 289–302.

Duncan, J., Seltz, R. J., Kolodny, J., Bor, D., Herzog, H., Ahmed, A., et al. (2000). A neural basis for general intelligence. *American Journal of Ophthalmology, 130*(5), 687.

Eaton, G. G., Worlein, J. M., Kelley, S. T., Vijayaraghavan, S., Hess, D. L., Axthelm, M. K., et al. (1999). Self-injurious behavior is decreased by cyproterone acetate in adult male rhesus (*Macaca mulatta*). *Hormones Behavior, 35,* 195–203.

Ertl, J. P., & Schafer, E. W. (1969). Brain response correlates of psychometric intelligence. *Nature, 223,* 421–422.

Evans, P. D., Gilbert, S. L., Mekel-Bobrov, N., Vallender, E. J., Anderson, J. R., Vaez-Azizi, L. M., et al. (2005). Microcephalin, a gene regulating brain size, continues to evolve adaptively in humans. *Science, 309,* 1717–1720.

Filippi, C. G., Lin, D. M., Tsiouris, A. J., Watts, R., Packard, A. M., Heier, L. A., et al. (2003). Diffusion-tensor MR imaging in children with developmental delay: Preliminary findings. *Radiology, 229,* 44–50.

Filippi, C. G., Ulug, A. M., Deck, M. F., Zimmerman, R. D., & Heier, L. A. (2002). Developmental delay in children: Assessment with proton MR spectroscopy. *American Journal of Neuroradiology, 23,* 882–888.

Fontenot, M. B., Padgett, E. E., Dupuy, A. M., Lynch, C. R., De Petrillo, P. B., & Higley, J. D. (2005). The effects of fluoxetine and buspirone on self-injurious and stereotypic behavior in adult male rhesus macaques. *Comparative Medicine, 55*(1), 67–74.

Francis, F., Meyer, G., Fallet-Bianco, C., Moreno, S., Kappeler, C., Socorro, A. C., et al. (2006). Human disorders of cortical development: From past to present. *European Journal of Neuroscience, 23,* 877–893.

Frank, Y., & Pavlakis, S. G. (2001). Brain imaging in neurobehavioral disorders. *Pediatric Neurology*, *25*, 278–287.

Fride, E., Dan, Y., Gavish, M., & Weinstock, M. (1985). Prenatal stress impairs maternal behavior in a conflict situation and reduces hippocampal benzodiazepine receptors. *Life Sciences*, *36*(22), 2103–2109.

Galarza, M., & Lazareff, J. A. (2004). Transcranial Doppler in infantile cerebrospinal fluid disorders: Clinical validity. *Neurological Research*, *26*, 409–413.

Galdzicki, Z., & Siarey, R. J. (2003). Understanding mental retardation in Down's syndrome using trisomy 16 mouse models. *Genes, Brain and Behavior*, *2*, 167–178.

Garel, C. (2006). New advances in fetal MR neuroimaging. *Pediatric Radiology*, *36*, 621–625.

Gerlai, R., & Gerlai, J. (2004). Autism: A target of pharmacotherapies? *Drug Discovery Today*, *9*(8), 366–374.

Gomot, M., Bernard, F. A., Davis, M. H., Belmonte, M. K., Ashwin, C., Bullmore, E. T., et al. (2006). Change detection in children with autism: An auditory event-related fMRI study. *Neuroimage*, *29*(2), 475–484

Gothelf, D., Furfaro, J. A., Penniman, L. C., Glover, G. H., & Reiss, A. L. (2005). The contribution of novel brain imaging techniques to understanding the neurobiology of mental retardation and developmental disabilities. *Mental Retardation and Developmental Disabilities Research Reviews*, *11*, 331–339.

Greicius, M. D. (2003). Neuroimaging in developmental disorders. *Current Opinion in Neurology*, *16*, 143–146.

Harris, G. J., Chabris, C. F., Clark, J., Urban, T., Aharon, I., Steele, S., et al. (2006). Brain activation during semantic processing in autism spectrum disorders via functional magnetic resonance imaging. *Brain and Cognition*, *61*(1), 54–68.

Haydar, T. (2005). Advanced microscopic imaging methods to investigate cortical development and the etiology of mental retardation. *Mental Retardation and Developmental Disabilities Research Reviews*, *11*, 303–316.

Hazlett, H. C., Poe, M., Gerig, G., Smith, R. G., Provenzale, J., Ross, A., et al. (2005). Magnetic resonance imaging and head circumference study of brain size in autism: Birth through age 2 years. *Archives of General Psychiatry*, *62*(12), 1366–1376.

Hendry, J., DeVito, T., Gelman, N., Densmore, M., Rajakumar, N., Pavlosky, W., et al. (2006). White matter abnormalities in autism detected through transverse relaxation time imaging. *Neuroimage*, *29*(4), 1049–1057.

Herbert, M. R., Ziegler, D. A., Deutsch, C. K., O'Brien, L. M., Kennedy, D. N., Filipek, P. A., et al. (2005). Brain asymmetries in autism and developmental language disorder: A nested whole-brain analysis. *Brain*, *128*(Pt. 1), 213–226.

Hoon, A. H., & Melhem, E. R. (2000). Neuroimaging: Applications in disorders of early brain development. *Journal of Developmental and Behavioral Pediatrics*, *21*(4), 291.

Huttenlocher, P. R., & Dabholkar, A. S. (1997). Regional differences in synaptogenesis in human cerebral cortex. *Journal of Comparative Neurology*, *387*(2), 167–178.

Huttenlocher, P. R., de Courten, C., Garey, L. J., & Van der Loos, H. (1982). Synaptogenesis in human visual cortex; evidence for synapse elimination during normal development. *Neuroscience Letters*, *33*(3), 247–252.

Insel, T., Kinsley, C. H., Mann, P. E., & Bridges, R. S. (1990). Prenatal stress has long-term effects on brain opiate receptors. *Brain Research*, *511*, 93–97.

Johnston, M. V. (2006). Fresh ideas for treating developmental cognitive disorders. *Current Opinion in Neurology*, *19*, 115–118.

Kaya, M., Karasalihoglu, S., Ustun, F., Gultekin, A., Cermik, T. F., Fazlioglu, Y., et al. (2002). The relationship between 99mTc-HMPAO brain SPECT and the scores of real life rating scale in autistic children. *Brain and Development*, *24*, 77–81.

Keiper, A. (2006). The age of neuroelectronics. *New Atlantis*, *11*, 4–41.

Kemp, A. S., Fillmore, P., Lenjavi, M. R., Lyon, M., Chicz-DeMet, A., Touchette, P. E., et al. (2007). Temporal patterns of self-injurious behavior correlate with stress hormone levels in the developmentally disabled. *Psychiatry Research*, doi:10.1016/j.psychres.2007.04.003

Kennedy, D. P., Redcay, E., & Courchesne, E. (2006). Failing to deactivate: Resting functional abnormalities in autism. *Proceedings of the National Academy of Sciences of the USA*, *103*(21), 8275–8280.

Kim, N. D., Yoon, J., Kim, J. H., Lee, J. T., Chon, Y. S., Hwang, M. K., et al. (2006). Putative therapeutic agents for the learning and memory deficits of people with Down syndrome. *Bioorganic and Medicinal Chemistry Letters, 16,* 3772–3776.

Kirimi, E., Tuncer, O., Atas, B., Sakarya, M. E., & Ceylan, A. (2002). Clinical value of color Doppler ultrasonography measurements of full-term newborns with perinatal asphyxia and hypoxic ischemic encephalopathy in the first 12 hours of life and long-term prognosis. *Tohoku Journal of Experimental Medicine, 197,* 27–33.

Klimesch, W., Vogt, F., & Doppelmayr, M. (2000). Interindividual differences in alpha and theta power reflect memory performance. *Intelligence, 27*(4), 347–362.

Kostovic, I., Judas, M., Rados, M., & Hrabac, P. (2002). Laminar organization of the human fetal cerebrum revealed by histochemical markers and magnetic resonance imaging. *Cerebral Cortex, 12*(5), 536–544.

Kraemer, G. W., & Clarke, A. S. (1990). The behavioral neurobiology of self-injurious behavior in rhesus monkeys. *Progress in Neuropsychopharmacology and Biological Psychiatry, 14*(Suppl.), S141–S168.

Kraemer, G. W., Schmidt, D. E., & Ebert, M. H. (1997). The behavioral neurobiology of self-injurious behavior in rhesus monkeys: Current concepts and relations to impulsive behavior in humans. *Annals of the New York Academy of Sciences, 836,* 12–38.

Kroeker, R., Touchette, P. E., Engleman, L., & Sandman, C. A. (2004). Quantifying temporal distributions of self-injurious behavior: Defining bouts versus discrete events. *American Journal of Mental Retardation, 109*(1), 1–8.

Lainhart, J. E. (2006). Advances in autism neuroimaging: Research for the clinician and geneticist. *American Journal of Medical Genetics, 142C,* 33–39.

Lejeune, J., Turpin, R., & Gautier, M. (1959). Le mongolisme premier exemple d'aberration autosomique humaine. *Annales de Génétique, 1*(2), 41–49.

Levitt, J. G., Blanton, R. E., Smalley, S., Thompson, P. M., Guthrie, D., McCracken, J. T., et al. (2003). Cortical sulcal maps in autism. *Cerebral Cortex, 13*(7), 728–735.

Lotspeich, L. J., Kwon, H., Schumann, C. M., Fryer, S. L., Goodlin-Jones, B. L., Buonocore, M. H., et al. (2004). Investigation of neuroanatomical differences between autism and Asperger syndrome. *Archives of General Psychiatry, 61*(3), 291–298.

Machado, C. J., & Bachevalier, J. (2003). Non-human primate models of childhood psychopathology: The promise and the limitations. *Journal of Child Psychology and Psychiatry, 44*(1), 64–87.

Marion, S. D., Touchette, P. E., & Sandman, C. A. (2003). Sequential analysis reveals a unique structure for self-injurious behavior. *American Journal of Mental Retardation, 108*(5), 301–313.

Mascalchi, M., Filippi, M., Floris, R., Fonda, C., Gasparotti, R., & Villari, N. (2005). Diffusion-weighted MR of the brain: Methodology and clinical application. *La Radiologia Medica, 109,* 155–197.

McAlonan, G. M., Cheung, V., Cheung, C., Suckling, J., Lam, G. Y., Tai, K. S., et al. (2005). Mapping the brain in autism: A voxel-based MRI study of volumetric differences and intercorrelations in autism. *Brain, 128*(Pt. 2), 268–276.

Mekel-Bobrov, N., Gilbert, S. L., Evans, P. D., Vallender, E. J., Anderson, J. R., Hudson, R. R., et al. (2005). Ongoing adaptive evolution of ASPM, a brain size determinant in *Homo sapiens. Science, 309*(5741), 1662–1663.

Miller, G. (2006). The thick and thin of brainpower: Developmental timing linked to IQ. *Science, 311,* 1851.

Muller, R. A., Cauich, C., Rubio, M. A., Mizuno, A., & Courchesne, E. (2004). Abnormal activity patterns in premotor cortex during sequence learning in autistic patients. *Biological Psychiatry, 56*(5), 323–332.

Murcia, C. L., Gulden, F., & Herrup, K. (2005). A question of balance: A proposal for new mouse models of autism. *International Journal of Developmental Neuroscience, 23,* 265–275.

Nathanielsz, P. W. (1999). *Life in the womb: The origin of health and disease.* Ithaca, NY: Promethean Press.

Nicolelis, M. A. L. (2001). Actions from thoughts. *Nature, 409,* 403–407.

Novak, M. A. (2003). Self-injurious behavior in rhesus monkeys: new insights into its etiology, physiology, and treatment. *American Journal of Primatology, 59*(1), 3–19.

Novak, M. A., Crockett, C. M., & Sackett, G. P. (2002). Self-injurious behavior in captive macaque monkeys. In S. R. Schroeder, M. L. Oster-Granite, & T. Thompson (Eds.), *Self-injurious behavior: Gene–brain–behavior relationships* (pp. 151–161). Washington, DC: American Psychological Association.

Nowakowski, R. S. (2006). Stable neuron numbers from cradle to grave. *Proceedings of the National Academy of Sciences of the USA, 103*(33), 12219–12220.

Ogawa, S., Lee, T. M., Kay, A. R., & Tank, D. W. (1990). Brain magnetic resonance imaging with contrast dependent on blood oxygenation. *Proceedings of the National Academy of Sciences of the USA, 87*(24), 9868–9872.

Ohnishi, T., Matsuda, H., Hashimoto, T., Kunihiro, T., Nishikawa, M., Uema, T., et al. (2000). Abnormal regional cerebral blood flow in childhood autism. *Brain, 123,* 1838–1844.

Peters, D. A. (1988). Effects of maternal stress during different gestational periods on the serotonergic system in adult rat offspring. *Pharmacology, Biochemistry, and Behavior, 31*(4), 839–843.

Pickett, J., & London, E. (2005). The neuropathology of autism: A review. *Journal of Neuropathology and Experimental Neurology, 64*(11), 925–935.

Poland, R. E. (1999) Brain N-acetyl aspartate concentration measured by H MRS are reduced in adult male rats subjected to perinatal stress: Preliminary observations and hypothetical implications for neurodevelopmental disorders. *Journal of Psychiatric Research, 33,* 41–51.

Pooh, R. K., Pooh, K., Nakagawa, Y., Nishida, S., & Ohno, Y. (2000). Clinical application of three-dimensional ultrasound in fetal brain assessment. *Croatian Medical Journal, 41,* 245–251.

Postuma, D., De Geus, E. J. C., Baare, W. F. C., Pol, H. E. H., Kahn, R. S., & Boomsma, D. I. (2002). The association between brain volume and intelligence is of genetic origin. *Nature Neuroscience, 5,* 83–84.

Reeves, R. H. (2006). Down syndrome mouse models are looking up. *Trends in Molecular Medicine, 12,* 237–240.

Reiss, A. L., Eliez, S., Schmitt, J. E., Patwardhan, A., & Haberecht, M. (2000). Brain imaging in neurogenetic conditions: Realizing the potential of behavioral neurogenetics research. *Mental Retardation and Developmental Disabilities Research Reviews, 6,* 186–197.

Ring, H. A., Baron-Cohen, S., Wheelwright, S., Williams, S. C., Brammer, M., Andrew, C., et al. (1999). Cerebral correlates of preserved cognitive skills in autism: A functional MRI study of embedded figures task performance. *Brain, 122*(Pt. 7), 1305–1315.

Robertson, N. J., & Wyatt, J. S. (2004). The magnetic resonance revolution in brain imaging: Impact on neonatal intensive care. *Archives of Disease in Childhood: Fetal and Neonatal Edition, 89,* 193–197.

Robinson, H. B., & Robinson, N. M. (1965). *The mentally retarded child: A psychological approach.* New York: McGraw-Hill.

Rotstein, M., Bassan, H., Kariv, N., Speiser, Z., Harel, S., & Gozes, I. (2006). NAP enhances neurodevelopment of newborn apolipoprotein E deficient mice subjected to hypoxia. *Journal of Pharmacology and Experimental Therapeutics, 319,* 332–339.

Sadamatsu, M., Kanai, H., Xu, X., Liu, Y., & Kato, N. (2006). Review of animal models for autism: Implication of thyroid hormone. *Congenital Anomalies, 46,* 1–9.

Sanchez, M. D., Milanes, M. V., Fuente, T., & Laorden, M. L. (1993). The B-endorphin response to prenatal stress during postnatal development in the rat. *Developmental Brain Research, 74,* 142–145.

Sandman, C. A., & Barron, J. L. (1986). Parameters of the event-related potential are related to functioning in the mentally retarded. *International Journal of Neuroscience, 29,* 37–44.

Sandman, C. A., Glynn, L., Wadhwa, P. D., Chicz-DeMet, A., Porto, M., & Garite, T. (2003). Maternal hypothalamic–pituitary–adrenal disregulation during the third trimester influences human fetal responses. *Developmental Neuroscience, 25*(1), 41–49.

Sandman, C. A., Spence, M. A., & Smith, M. (1999). Proopiomelanocortin (POMC) disregulation and response to opiate blockers. *Mental Retardation and Developmental Disabilities Research Reviews, 5,* 314–321.

Sandman, C. A., & Touchette, P. (2002). Opioids and the maintenance of self-injurious behavior. In S. R. Schroeder, M. L. Oster-Granite, & T. Thompson (Eds.), *Self-injurious behavior: Gene–brain–behavior relationships* (pp. 191–204). Washington, DC: American Psychological Association.

Sandman, C. A., Touchette, P., Lenjavi, M., Marion, S., & Chicz-DeMet, A. (2003). Beta-endorphin and ACTH are dissociated after self-injury in adults with developmental disabilities. *American Journal of Mental Retardation, 108*(6), 414–424.

Sandman, C. A., Touchette, P., Marion, S., Lenjavi, M., & Chicz-DeMet, A. (2002). Disregulation of proopiomelanocortin and contagious maladaptive behavior. *Regulatory Peptides, 108*(2–3), 179–185.

Santosh, P. J. (2000). Neuroimaging in child and adolescent psychiatric disorders. *Archives of Disease in Childhood, 82,* 412–419.

Sari, Y., & Gozes, I. (2006). Brain deficits associated with fetal alcohol exposure may be protected, in part, by peptides derived from activity-dependent neurotrophic factor and activity-dependent neuroprotective protein. *Brain Research Reviews, 52*(1), 107–118.

Saud, K., Arriagada, C., Cardenas, A. M., Shimahara, T., Allen, D. D., Caviedes, R., et al. (2006). Neuronal dysfunction in Down syndrome: Contribution of neuronal models in cell culture. *Journal of Physiology–Paris, 9,* 201–210.

Schmitz, N., Rubia, K., Daly, E., Smith, A., Williams, S., & Murphy, D. G. (2006). Neural correlates of executive function in autistic spectrum disorders. *Biological Psychiatry, 59*(1), 7–16.

Shucard, E. W., & Horn, J. L. (1973). Evoked potential amplitude change related to intelligence and arousal. *Psychophysiology, 10,* 445–452.

Smith-Swintosky, V. L., Gozes, I., Brenneman, D. E., D'Andrea, M. R., & Plata-Salaman, C. R. (2005). Activity-dependent neurotrophic factor-9 and NAP promote neurite outgrowth in rat hippocampal and cortical cultures. *Journal of Molecular Neuroscience, 25*(3), 225–238.

Sokol, D. K., & Edwards-Brown, M. (2004). Neuroimaging in autistic spectrum disorder. *Journal of Neuroimaging, 14,* 8–15.

Sundaram, S. K., Chugani, H. T., & Chugani, D. C. (2005). Positron emission tomography methods with potential for increased understanding of mental retardation and developmental disabilities. *Mental Retardation and Developmental Disabilities Research Reviews, 11,* 325–330.

Sur, M., & Rubenstein, J. L. (2005). Patterning and plasticity of the cerebral cortex. *Science, 310,* 805–810.

Takahashi, L. K., Turner, J. G., & Kalin, N. H. (1992). Prenatal stress alters brain catecholaminergic activity and potentiates stress-induced behavior in adult rats. *Brain Research, 574*(1–2), 131–137.

Taylor, D. K., Bass, T., Flory, G. S., & Hankenson, F. C. (2005). Use of low-dose chlorpromazine in conjunction with environmental enrichment to eliminate self-injurious behavior in a rhesus macaque (*Macaca mulatta*). *Comparative Medicine, 55*(3), 282–288.

Thatcher, R. W., Northa, D., & Bivera, C. (2005). EEG and intelligence: Relations between EEG coherence, EEG phase delay and power. *Clinical Neurophysiology, 116,* 2129–2141.

Thompson, R., Huestis, P. W., Crinella, F. M., & Yu, J. (1986). The neuroanatomy of mental retardation in the white rat. *Neuroscience and Biobehavioral Reviews, 10,* 317–338.

Thompson, R., Huestis, P. W., Crinella, F. M., & Yu, J. (1987). Further lesion studies on the neuroanatomy of mental retardation in the white rat. *Neuroscience and Biobehavioral Reviews, 11,* 415–440.

Tiefenbacher, S., Fahey, M. A., Rowlett, J. K., Meyer, J. S., Pouliot, A. L., Jones, B. M., et al. (2005). The efficacy of diazepam treatment for the management of acute wounding episodes in captive rhesus macaques. *Comparative Medicine, 55*(4), 387–392.

Tiefenbacher, S., Novak, M. A., Jorgensen, M. J., & Meyer, J. S. (2000). Physiological correlates of self-injurious behavior in captive, socially-reared rhesus monkeys. *Psychoneuroendocrinology, 25,* 799–817.

Tiefenbacher, S., Novak, M. A., Lutz, C. K., & Meyer, J. S. (2005). The physiology and neurochemistry of self-injurious behavior: A nonhuman primate model. *Frontiers in Bioscience, 10,* 1–11.

Tiefenbacher, S., Novak, M. A., Marinus, L. M., Chase, W. K., Miller, J. A., & Meyer, J. S. (2004). Altered hypothalamic–pituitary–adrenocortical function in rhesus monkeys (*Macaca mulatta*) with self-injurious behavior. *Psychoneuroendocrinology, 29*(4), 501–515.

Timor-Trisch, I. E., & Monteagudo, A. (1996). Transvaginal fetal neurosonography: Standardization of the planes and sections by anatomic landmarks. *Ultrasound in Obstetrics and Gynecology, 8,* 42–47.

Timor-Trisch, I. E., & Monteagudo, A. (2001). Normal two-dimensional neurosonography of the prenatal brain. In I. E. Timor-Trisch, A. Monteagudo, H. L. Cohen (Eds.), *Ultrasonography of the prenatal and neonatal brain* (pp. 13–91). New York: McGraw-Hill.

Toal, F. A., Murphy, D. G. M., & Murphy, K. C. (2005). Autistic-spectrum disorders: Lessons from neuroimaging. *British Journal of Psychiatry, 187,* 395–397.

Toga, A. W., & Thompson, P. M. (2005). Genetics of brain structure and intelligence. *Annual Review of Neuroscience, 28,* 1–23.

Toga, A. W., Thompson, P. M., & Sowell, E. R. (2006). Mapping brain maturation. *Trends in Neurosciences, 29*(3), 148–159.

van der Staay, F. J. (2006). Animal models of behavioral dysfunctions: Basic concepts and classifications, and an evaluation strategy. *Brain Research Reviews, 87,* 659–665.

Walsh, D. M., Finwall, J., Touchette, P. E., McGregor, M., Fernandez, G., Lott, I., & Sandman, C. A. (2007). Rapid assessment of severe cognitive impairment in individuals with developmental disabilities. *Journal of Intellectual Disability Research, 51,* 91–100.

Wang, A. T., Lee, S. S., Sigman, M., & Dapretto, M. (2006). Neural basis of irony comprehension in children with autism: The role of prosody and context. *Brain, 129*(Pt. 4), 932–943.

Wang, J., & Licht, D. J. (2006). Pediatric perfusion MR imaging using arterial spin labeling. *Neuroimaging Clinics of North America, 16*(1), 149–167.

Weinstock, M., Poltyrev, T., Schorer-Apelbaum, D., Men, D., & McCarty, R. (1996). Effect of prenatal stress on plasma corticosterone and catecholamines in response to footshock in rats. *Physiology and Behavior, 64,* 439–444.

Weld, K. P., Mench, J. A., Woodward, R. A., Bolesta, M. S., Suomi, S. J., & Higley, J. D. (1998). Effect of tryptophan treatment on self-biting and central nervous system serotonin metabolism in rhesus monkeys (*Macaca mulatta*). *Neuropsychopharmacology, 19*(4), 314–321.

White, H., & Venkatesh, B. (2006). Applications of transcranial Doppler in the ICU: A review. *Intensive Care Medicine, 32,* 981–994.

Williams, H. J. (2004). Imaging the child with developmental delay. *Imaging, 16,* 174–185.

Witelson, S. F., Beresh, H., & Kigar, D. L. (2006). Intelligence and brain size in 100 postmortem brains: Sex, lateralization and age factors. *Brain, 129,* 386–398.

Zaltzman, R., Alexandrovich, A., Trembovler, V., Shohami, E., & Gozes, I. (2005). The influence of the peptide NAP on Mac-1–deficient mice following closed head injury. *Peptides, 26,* 1520–1527.

Zigmond, M. J., Bloom, F. E., Lanois, S. C., Roberts, J. L., Squire, L. R., & Woolley, R. S. (1999). *Fundamental neuroscience.* San Diego, CA: Academic Press.

Zoghbi, H. Y. (2003). Postnatal neurodevelopmental disorders: Meeting at the synapse. *Science, 302,* 826–830.

EARLY INTERVENTION

An African proverb says "as the twig is bent, so grows the tree," the connotation being that providing support for a straight sprout early on will have direct and important implications later. A belief that exists across cultures and nations is that providing nurturing experiences, health care, and nutrition to infants and young children with developmental disabilities and support for their families is fundamentally important for growth and development (Odom & Kaul, 2003). Chapters in this section provide broad coverage of early intervention for infants, toddlers, and preschoolers with developmental disabilities. In addition, two areas of research that are particularly exemplary of "cutting edge" research and likely to have strong impacts on the field are reviewed.

In his examination of research and service options for infants and toddlers with developmental disabilities and their families, Dunst lays out a set of principles that underlie early intervention for infants and toddlers and their families. Basing his analysis on the work of Bronfenbrenner and others, Dunst describes a model for synthesizing the literature that leads to four strongly supported early-intervention practices: (1) response-contingent child learning, (2) parent responsiveness to child behavior, (3) everyday natural learning opportunities, and (4) capacity-building help-giving practices. He then contrasts the current provision of early-intervention services to infants, toddlers, and families with the empirically supported efficacious practices, finding a large discrepancy between the two.

From early intervention in the infant and toddler years, research and policy extends to preschool-age children with developmental disabilities. Carta and Kong, in their chapter, describe the evolution of social policy that underlies support for this older group of young children and highlight the types of models for providing services. Importantly, they describe the initiative in early childhood special education to establish outcome-based intervention approaches. Returning to a theme from an earlier chapter by Klingner et al., Carta and Kong emphasize the importance of culturally compatible intervention approaches for young children and families. As in Dunst's chapter, the authors identify the theme of evidence-based practices as central to the current work in the field and highlight the importance of naturalistic intervention approaches that are grounded in the routines of classrooms and community. Carta and Kong extend this concept for preschool children by describing intervention strategies for individualizing the level of support preschool children may need in order to participate and learn in the naturalistic setting.

One of the largest changes in the developmental disabilities area has been the marked increase in prevalence of children with autism or autism spectrum disorders. The increase has spawned one of the most active research literatures in early intervention. Odom, Rogers, McDougle, Hume, and McGee examine three areas in which the greatest strides in research have been and are being made. As the developmental literature provides more information about children with autism, the potential for identifying children with autism earlier than ever (down to the 12- to 18-month age level) is being realized, and the authors of this chapter examined such early screening and diagnostic approaches. Again, reflecting the themes from the preceding two chapters, Odom et al. identify focused interventions and comprehensive treatment models for preschool children that have evidence of efficacy and the emerging intervention approaches appropriate for infants and toddlers. In addition to behavioral treatment models, the research on psychopharmacology for preschool children is just emerging, with the active scientific literature for older children having the future potential for young children with autism who experience certain specific symptoms and behaviors.

Intervention approaches to promote early communication is a research area that responds to one of the most critical needs for young children with developmental disabilities. Kaiser and Trent propose that naturalistic approaches (mentioned in each of the three previous chapters) have been the most thoroughly examined and hold the greatest promise for young children with developmental disabilities. Their critical examination of different naturalistic approaches reveals a set of strongly supported efficacious practices that would serve as valuable tools for practitioners working with young children and families and for researchers interested in examining the acquisition of communication and language. Importantly, they note the powerful effect of the responsiveness of the caregiver in supporting the success of these interventions for young children.

REFERENCE

Odom, S. L., & Kaul, S. (2003). Early intervention themes and variations from around the world. In S. Odom, M. Hanson, J. Blackman, & S. Kaul (Eds.), *Early intervention practices around the world* (pp. 333–346). Baltimore: Brookes.

8

Early Intervention
for Infants and Toddlers
with Developmental Disabilities

Carl J. Dunst

Although claims that early intervention is a necessary condition to optimize the developmental outcomes of infants and toddlers with disabilities generally go unchallenged today, this was not always the case. For most of the first 50 to 60 years of the 20th century, there was a strongly held belief that human growth and development to a large degree were not alterable by differential environmental experiences and that this especially held true for children with disabilities or other identified conditions (e.g., McNemer, 1940). The classic study by Skeels and Dye (1939) of young children with mental retardation living in an institution was one of the first experimental investigations to demonstrate that supplemental experiences provided to children with disabilities can, in fact, influence their early development.

J. McVicker Hunt's (1961) highly influential book *Intelligence and Experience* proved a tipping point in building a convincing case that human development was malleable and that environmental enrichment and deprivation can, respectively, have positive and negative effects on child behavior and development. The contention that the experiences afforded infants and toddlers can shape the course of growth and development was demonstrated in a series of studies subsequently conducted by Hunt and his colleagues (see Uzgiris & Hunt, 1987, for a review of this research).

The 1980s proved to be an important decade for amassing evidence either supporting or refuting the benefits of early intervention for young children with disabilities. A plethora of research reviews were published that attempted to answer the question, Is early intervention effective? (see, e.g., Dunst, Snyder, & Mankinen, 1988). Notwithstanding claims for or against the effectiveness of early intervention for infants and toddlers with disabilities, the largest majority of these reviews were analyses of early intervention at a macro-, or program, level and not at a micro-, or practice, level. An examination of these previous reviews is beyond the scope of this chapter. Suffice it to say that the equivocal conclusions made by different reviewers were due, in part, to a failure to disentangle the *practice characteristics* associated with differential behavioral and developmental benefits.

The purpose of this chapter is to present an integrated set of research findings about one particular approach to early intervention with infants and toddlers with developmental disabilities and other identified conditions associated with poor developmental outcomes. The chapter includes five major sections: (1) a definition of early intervention that delimits the kind of research that constitutes the focus of review and analysis, (2) a framework for operationalizing the kinds of experiences and opportunities afforded infants and toddlers with disabilities that are intended to alter behavioral and developmental trajectories, (3) a presentation of findings from a series of practice-based research syntheses (Dunst, Trivette, & Cutspec, 2002) and corroborating studies that highlight those practice characteristics that are now known to positively affect child and parent functioning both directly and indirectly, (4) a critical analysis of the Individuals with Disabilities Education Act (IDEA) early-intervention program in light of available research evidence, and (5) a discussion of the implications of state-of-the-art knowledge for improving policy and practice. The chapter concludes with some thoughts about the reasons that evidence-based information is generally not being used to inform practice.

DEFINITION OF EARLY INTERVENTION

For purposes of this chapter, early intervention is defined as the *experiences and opportunities afforded infants and toddlers with disabilities by the children's parents and other primary caregivers that are intended to promote the children's acquisition and use of behavioral competencies to shape and influence their prosocial interactions with people and objects.* This definition excludes research on early intervention that does not include parents and other primary caregivers as primary sources of children's learning opportunities. It also excludes research on practices that do not support and strengthen either *parents' capacity* to provide their children with development-instigating learning experiences and opportunities or *children's capacity* to engage in child-initiated and child-directed interactions with people and the physical environment.

Guiding Principles

The particular approach to early intervention that constitutes the focus of this chapter is consistent with the intent of the IDEA early-intervention program that places primary emphasis on strengthening parents' capacity to promote their children's learning and development. The definition of early intervention used in this chapter is based on three principles that guide the ways in which early intervention is operationalized and practiced.

   • *Principle 1. The experiences and opportunities afforded infants and toddlers with disabilities should strengthen children's self-initiated and self-directed learning and development to promote acquisition of functional behavioral competencies and children's recognition of their abili-*

ties to produce desired and expected effects and consequences. A fundamental distinction is made between experiences and opportunities that are contexts for a child's acquisition and use of behavior that is intended to have desired consequences (e.g., a child who learns to use a pointing gesture to get an adult to retrieve a desired object) and those intended to elicit a child's behavior (e.g., having a child name objects shown to him or her or by an adult). The former and not the latter is the type of early-intervention practice that constitutes the focus of this chapter.

 • *Principle 2. Parent-mediated child learning is effective to the extent that it strengthens parents' confidence and competence in providing their children with development-instigating and development-enhancing learning experiences and opportunities.* This principle makes explicit that the benefits of early intervention should be realized by both children and their parents or other primary caregivers. The likelihood that parents and other primary caregivers will provide children with the kinds of experiences and opportunities that influence their development is maximized when adults recognize and understand the important role they play in influencing their children's growth and development.

 • *Principle 3. The role of early-intervention practitioners in parent-mediated child learning is to support and strengthen parent capacity to provide their children with experiences and opportunities of known qualities and characteristics (i.e., evidence based) that are most likely to support and strengthen both parent and child capacity.* Knowledgeable practitioners are aware of what research "tells us" about the characteristics of practices that are associated with optimal positive benefits. Practitioners intervene directly with children only to the extent that it serves to model for parents the use of evidence-based practices with their children.

The approach to early intervention that constitutes the focus of this chapter is based on the assumption that responsibility for child rearing rests within the family and that professionals working with a family intervene in ways that support and strengthen parent capacity to carry out child-rearing responsibilities effectively and efficiently. This approach in no way is intended to argue against or refute professionally implemented interventions with infants and toddlers with disabilities. Notwithstanding this assertion, there is, as will be shown, a converging body of evidence regarding the practice characteristics that are a foundation for a parent-mediated approach to early-childhood intervention.

FRAMEWORK FOR INVESTIGATING EARLY-INTERVENTION PRACTICES

According to Bronfenbrenner (1992), the aim of a science of human development is the "systematic understanding of the *processes* and *outcomes* of human development" (p. 188), in which "variations in developmental processes and outcomes are [considered] a *joint* function of the environment and of a [developing] person" (p. 197). Bronfenbrenner (1993) also noted:

> Among the personal characteristics likely to be most potent in affecting the course . . . of development . . . are those that set in motion, sustain, and encourage processes of interaction between the [developing] person and two aspects of the proximal environment: first, the people present in the setting; and second, the physical and symbolic features of the setting that invite, permit, or inhibit engagement in sustained, progressively more complex interaction with an activity in the immediate environment. (p. 11)

Given these assertions, the factors that influence child development include, but are not limited to, the characteristics of the developing child (e.g., type and severity of disability, gender, personal preferences), the characteristics of the child's parents (e.g., parenting style, parenting confidence, parenting beliefs about child rearing), and the characteristics of the experiences and opportunities that a child is afforded (e.g., material availability, interestingness, responsiveness). Consequently, the effects of experiences and opportunities afforded infants and toddlers with disabilities would be expected to vary as a function of any number of different factors and combinations of factors. For example, the developmental trajectories of infants and toddlers with disabilities or developmental delays who receive early intervention vary as a function of their etiologies and diagnoses in clearly discernable and expected ways (Dunst, 1998), in which variations in trajectories among children with the same type of disabilities are attributable to both intervention and nonintervention variables (Dunst & Trivette, 1994).

Although similar to other models and frameworks (e.g., Guralnick, 2005) that call for conditional tests of the relationships between intervention and nonintervention factors and their consequences (e.g., Does XYZ practice influence children with different disabilities in the same way?), the Bronfenbrenner framework focuses attention on the specific features of the experiences and opportunities afforded children with a focus on the *proximal characteristics* that account for observed effects. This is what was described earlier as a microlevel approach to examining early-intervention practice research. The goal of a *science of early intervention* is a better understanding of the practice characteristics that influence child learning and development and the identification of those processes that best explain the obtained or observed relationship between the practices and their consequences.

Practice-Based Research Syntheses

Bronfenbrenner's (1992, 1993) characteristics–consequences framework has been used to conduct what have come to be called *practice-based research syntheses* of early-intervention and related practices research studies (Dunst, Trivette, & Cutspec, 2002). A practice-based research synthesis involves the systematic analysis of a narrowly defined body of research that has investigated the same or similar practice with a focus on the extent to which the relationship between the practice characteristics and their consequences replicate across studies. The practice itself, to the extent possible, is *unpacked* and *disentangled* to identify the features, elements, and factors that account for the largest amount of covariation between the use of the practice characteristics and their effects or outcomes. For example, an analysis of the extent to which the clarity of a response-contingent relationship in infant operant-learning studies affects rate of learning is illustrative of this kind of investigative process (Dunst, 2003).

RESEARCH FOUNDATIONS FOR EARLY-INTERVENTION PRACTICES

Four different kinds of intervention practices are used to illustrate what is known about the characteristics of practices that positively affect the learning and development of infants and toddlers with disabilities: (1) response-contingent child learning, (2), parent responsiveness to child behavior, (3) everyday natural learning opportunities, and (4) capacity-building help-giving practices. These are by no means the only practices that constitute the content and scope of early intervention (see, e.g., Guralnick, 2005; Odom & Wolery, 2003). They do, however, make up a conceptually and operationally coherent set of practices that, taken together, provide one way of thinking about parent-mediated, evidence-based early-childhood intervention (Dunst, 2000, 2004).

Response-Contingent Child Learning

The term "response-contingent child learning" refers to environmental arrangements by which a child's production of a behavior produces or elicits a reinforcing or interesting consequence that increases the rate, frequency, or strength of behavior responding (e.g., Hulsebus, 1973). The movement and sound of a mobile that occurs as a result of an infant swiping the apparatus is an example of this type of learning. Infants without disabilities or delays typically learn and remember this kind of relationship by 2 to 3 months of age (e.g., Lipsitt & Werner, 1981). Infants' recognition of the relationship between what they do and what happens in response to their behavior is called "contingency awareness" (Watson, 1966) or "contingency detection" (Rochat, 2001). This awareness or detection is often manifested by concomitant social–emotional behavior. Haith (1972) noted that an infant's ability to understand that he or she is the agent of an environmental consequence produces social–emotional responding because cognitive achievement is pleasurable.

The extent to which infants and young children with disabilities are able to learn the relationship between their behavior and its consequences has been the focus of investigation in more than 50 studies spanning some 40 years (see e.g., Dunst, 2003; Hutto, 2003). Participants in these studies included children with Down syndrome, cerebral palsy, sensory impairments, hydrocephaly, microcephaly, seizure disorders, multiple disabilities, and other syndromes, etiologies, and diagnoses associated with developmental disabilities or delays.

The characteristics of response-contingent learning opportunities associated with variations in rates and patterns of learning in children with disabilities has been examined in three research syntheses of this practice (Dunst, 2003; Dunst, Storck, Hutto, & Snyder, 2006; Hutto, 2003). These syntheses included analyses of how long it takes children with disabilities to learn a response-contingent relationship, the correlates of rapidity of learning, the relative effectiveness of different types of environmental arrangements and reinforcers, and whether children with disabilities manifest social-emotional responding as a result of contingency awareness or detection in a manner similar to their typically developing peers. Taken together, findings from available studies clearly show that children with disabilities are capable of response-contingent learning and that these kinds of learning opportunities constitute a useful early-intervention practice for these children (e.g., Lancioni, 1980). In almost every published and unpublished study of children with disabilities, rates of behavior responding increased, sometimes three- or fourfold, once the children were reinforced for their efforts. There are, however, important differences in patterns of learning among children with disabilities compared with their typically developing peers.

Infants without disabilities typically demonstrate response-contingent learning in as few as 2 to 4 minutes. In contrast, it more often than not takes children with disabilities considerably longer to demonstrate the same kind of learning (Hutto, 2003) in which rapidity of learning is differentially affected by a number of factors. As might be expected, the more profoundly delayed a child is when he or she is first provided with response-contingent learning opportunities, the longer it takes the child to learn the relationship between his or her behavior and its consequences. Furthermore, children with physical disabilities take longer to learn a contingency than do children who have other kinds of disabilities presumably because of their difficulty in executing motor responses.

The characteristics of the response-contingent learning opportunities themselves influence learning, as well. These include the type of behavior used to produce a reinforcing consequence, the type of reinforcement (e.g., social or nonsocial), and the type of contingency relationship (e.g., episodic vs. conjugate). In general, studies in which some type of manual response (e.g., arm or hand movements) was required to produce or elicit a reinforcer showed that a child with a disability took longer to learn a contingency. This is especially the case for children with physical disabilities. In contrast, rapidity of learning is very similar when leg kicks, vocalizations, head turns, or smiling are used to produce or elicit reinforcing consequences.

Social reinforcers are somewhat more effective than are nonsocial reinforcers in influencing learning (Dunst, Storck, et al., 2006; Hutto, 2003), as the social learning opportunities are more likely to evoke social–emotional child responding (Dunst, 2003). Somewhat ironically, in situations in which response-contingent learning opportunities are used as an intervention for children with disabilities, the children are much more likely to be provided with nonsocial learning opportunities (e.g., Dunst, Raab, Wilson, & Parkey, 1997).

The large majority of response-contingent learning studies have been conducted using either episodic or conjugate reinforcement paradigms (Dunst, Storck, et al., 2006). In episodic reinforcement studies, the reinforcement is delivered in a predetermined manner and amount following the child's production of a contingency behavior. In conjugate reinforcement studies, the amount or intensity of the reinforcement is proportional to the strength of the contingency behavior. Research shows that for children both with and without disabilities, patterns of learning are almost identical in episodic reinforcement studies, but that children with disabilities take up to three times longer to demonstrate learning in conjugate reinforcement studies (Dunst, Storck, et al., 2006).

Dunst (2003) examined the manner in which contingency awareness or detection was associated with positive social–emotional child responding in studies of children with and without disabilities. Findings showed that patterns of social–emotional responding among children with disabilities was much like those among children without disabilities but that the sheer amount of social–emotional behavior manifested by children with disabilities was considerably less than that of their typically developing peers. For both groups of children, the clarity of the relationship between a child's behavior and its consequence was an important determinant of social–emotional responding. In those cases in which a child's behavior produced a consequence within a few seconds and the behavior–response relationship did not overlap in real time, the probability was higher that the children would detect the contingency and display positive affect in response to their newly learned capabilities.

Response-contingent learning opportunities either arise naturally as part of children's everyday interactions with people or objects or can be intentionally arranged so that children have opportunities to learn the relationship between their behavior and its consequences. These kinds of learning opportunities are especially important for infants and toddlers with disabilities because they promote children's acquisition of behavior that can be used to initiate and produce desired effects.

Parent Responsiveness

Parents' sensitivity and responsiveness to their infant or toddler's behavior during parent–child interactions is a potent determinant of child development (Shonkoff & Phillips, 2000). Encouraging and supporting parents' use of a responsive interactional style with children with disabilities has been recognized as an important early-intervention practice for more than 25 years (e.g., Affleck, McGrade, McQueeney, & Allen, 1982; Marfo, 1988).

It is generally recognized that parent responsiveness is a complex process that includes different elements and features that both individually and in combination influence child learning and development (De Wolff & van IJzendoorn, 1997). This process includes, but is not limited to, parental response quality, timing, appropriateness, affect, and comforting. In the context of the characteristics–consequences framework described earlier, parents' responsiveness to their children's behavior is considered an environmental (intervention) factor that contributes to variations in behavioral and developmental outcomes.

Findings from three practice-based research syntheses of different aspects of parent sensitivity and responsiveness highlight the features of this practice that matter most in terms of benefits to the child (Kassow & Dunst, 2004, 2005) and the strategies that are most effective for promoting parents' use of a responsive interactional style (Kassow & Dunst, 2005). Parents' contingent responsiveness to their children's behavior is associated with improved child functioning. The effectiveness of the parents' behavior is maximized when the parent is attuned to the child's signals and intent to communicate, when the parent promptly and appropriately responds to the child's behavior, and when parent–child interactions are synchronous and mutually reinforcing (Kassow & Dunst, 2004, 2005). Findings from a companion research synthesis indicated that behaviorally based interventions that specifically target parental awareness, interpretation, and responsiveness to their children's behavior are especially effective, and the effectiveness is enhanced when videotapes are used either to illustrate responsive parent–child interaction styles or to provide feedback to parents regarding their own interactional styles (Dunst & Kassow, 2004).

The extent to which parents' responsiveness to the behavior of children with disabilities influences the children's behavioral and developmental outcomes has been assessed in three practice-based research syntheses (Trivette, 2003; Trivette, 2004; Trivette & O'Herin, 2006). The studies included children with Down syndrome, Williams syndrome, hydrocephaly, physical disabilities, mental retardation, developmental delays, and multiple disabilities and children at risk for poor outcomes due to birth-related complications. The outcomes that constituted the focus of investigation included measures of children's cognitive, language, and social–emotional functioning.

In studies of children with disabilities, parents' responsiveness to the children's behavior shows very much the same kind of relationship with the outcomes that constitute the focus of investigation as is found in studies of children without disabilities. In almost every case, measures of parents' responsiveness during interactions with their children were positively associated with subsequent performance by the children on the outcomes measured in the studies. Notwithstanding differences in the absolute levels of functioning of the children with and without disabilities, the amount of covariation, or effect sizes, between parent responsiveness and child functioning were more alike than different for the two groups of children.

The reasons that parent responsiveness is associated with positive child benefits is perhaps best understood by considering what it "teaches" a child. A parent who is responsive to a child's efforts and success, who is helpful and supportive when necessary, and who is encouraging and facilitative helps a child learn that the parent is nurturing and dependable, which are exactly the kind of environmental conditions that are ripe for optimal learning and development. This would seem especially necessary for infants and toddlers with disabilities, who more often than not need an extra boost to learn about their own capabilities, as well as the behavioral propensities of others.

Natural Learning Opportunities

Children's lives throughout the world are made up of everyday activities that are the contexts for learning culturally meaningful behavior (Göncü, 1999). These everyday activities, or "microsystems" in Bronfenbrenner's (1992) terminology, invite or inhibit child learning depending on the characteristics of the setting and the behavior of the people in the settings. According to Farver (1999), the experiences and opportunities afforded children as part of everyday life are "ordinary settings in which children's social interaction and behavior occurs. They are the who, what, where, when, and why of daily life" (p. 201). Everyday activities, by definition, are natural learning environments in which contextually meaningful and functional behavior is learned, further increasing children's participation in family and community life (Dunst, Hamby, Trivette, Raab, & Bruder, 2000).

The extent to which infants and toddlers with disabilities participate in everyday activities and benefit from these natural learning opportunities has been examined in a number of practice-based research syntheses (Dunst, 2006; Masiello & Gorman, 2006; Raab & Dunst, 2006b; Trivette & Click, 2006) and other investigations (e.g., Dunst et al., 2001; Dunst et al., 2000; Dunst, Hamby, Trivette, Raab, & Bruder, 2002). These studies included children with Down syndrome and other chromosomal aberrations, physical disabilities, sensory impairments, autism, multiple disabilities, and other conditions associated with developmental delays.

Findings from research on naturally occurring learning opportunities indicate that everyday life is made up of some 22 different categories of natural learning opportunities (Dunst et al., 2000) and that preschool children with and without disabilities, on average, participate in about 40 to 50 different kinds of activities on a fairly regular basis (Dunst & Bruder, 1999). During the first 3 years of a child's life, participation in everyday family and community activities increases in a relatively linear fashion, albeit at different rates depending on the everyday activity (Dunst, Hamby, et al., 2002). More specifically, infants with disabilities from birth to 6 months of age are typically involved in about 19 ($SD = 13$) family activities and about 11 ($SD = 11$) community activities, and toddlers with disabilities 30–36 months of age are involved in about 34 ($SD = 9$) family activities and about 21 ($SD = 7$) community activities.

Infants and toddlers with disabilities on average tend to participate in somewhat fewer everyday activities compared with their typically developing counterparts. The differences in the experiences and opportunities afforded children with disabilities, however, are due less to their disabilities and more to their parents' beliefs about the value of everyday learning opportunities (Trivette, Dunst, & Hamby, 2004). In one study, for example, the children with the most profound developmental delays and associated disabilities and complications participated in even more family and community activities than did most of the typically developing children, a fact that was easily traced to the parents' belief systems (Dunst, Bruder, Trivette, Raab, & McLean, 1998).

The extent to which the characteristics of the everyday experiences and opportunities afforded children with and without disabilities influence child behavior and development was examined as part of a research synthesis of interest-based child learning (Raab & Dunst, 2006b). Results showed that learning opportunities that either provided a context for interest expression or had interest-evoking features were associated with increased positive and decreased negative child functioning. Moreover, the benefits were greatest in situations in which interest-based learning occurred in the context of everyday activities, in which the pattern of relationships between the characteristics of the activities and benefits to the child were very much the same for children with and without disabilities.

The extent to which different approaches to conceptualizing and implementing natural-learning-environment practices have similar or different consequences has been the focus of several studies of infants and toddlers participating in Part C early-intervention programs (Dunst, Bruder, Trivette, & Hamby, 2006; Dunst, Trivette, Hamby, & Bruder, 2006). In both investigations, one or two samples of parents were asked to report the number and frequency of times they used different everyday activities as learning opportunities for their children, and one or two samples of parents were asked to report the number and frequency of times early-intervention practitioners implemented their practices in everyday activities. The outcomes constituting the focus of investigation included parent and child well-being, parent self-efficacy appraisals, parenting competence, and parents' judgments of their children's capabilities.

In both studies, parents' use of everyday activities as sources of natural learning opportunities was associated with positive consequences in nearly all the outcome measures, whereas early-intervention practitioners' implementing their practices in everyday activities had little or no positive effects and, in several cases, had negative effects on parent functioning. In the one instance in which both types of natural-environment practices were associated with positive child functioning, the effect size for parents' use of everyday activities as an early intervention was three times larger than that for practitioners' use of early intervention in everyday activities.

The everyday activities that make up the fabric of a child's life include, but are not limited to, the kinds of response-contingent and parent–child interaction learning opportunities described previously. Everyday activities are powerful contexts for child learning, and when used as sources of learning opportunities for children with disabilities, they can, and generally do, have positive child benefits, as well as parent benefits (e.g., improved sense of parent competence).

Capacity-Building Help-Giving Practices

The approach to early-childhood intervention that constitutes the focus of this chapter considers intervention effective when parents' as well as children's competence and confidence are strengthened as a result of the efforts of practitioners. Parents' sense of their own parenting abilities is considered a mediating factor influencing the kinds and characteristics of learning opportunities afforded their children (Dunst, Trivette, & Hamby, 2006b).

The extent to which practitioner help-giving practices influence (1) parents' competence in performing their roles and tasks, (2) parents' confidence in carrying out parenting responsibilities, (3) and parents' enjoyment in interacting with and playing with their children was assessed as part of three research syntheses of family-centered help-giving practices (Dunst, Trivette, & Hamby, 2006a, 2006b; Dunst, Trivette, Hamby, & Snyder, 2006). More than half of the studies in the different syntheses were conducted with parents of children with disabilities who were involved in early-childhood intervention programs. The children's disabilities included Down syndrome, cerebral palsy, sensory impairments, autism, multiple disabilities, developmental delays due to birth-related complications, and other disabilities associated with different etiologies and diagnoses.

Three different kinds of family-centered help-giving practices were examined as potential determinants of parenting abilities: relational help giving, participatory help giving, and parent–practitioner collaboration. Relational help giving involves practices typically associated with good clinical practice (active and reflective listening, empathy and compassion, reassurance, etc.). Participatory help giving involves practices that promote parent decision making and action based on choices necessary to obtain desired resources or attain desired goals. Parent–practitioner collaboration involves practices in which partners work together to plan courses of action and to decide what will be the foci of intervention.

A consistent pattern of findings occurred in those studies that examined the relationship between family-centered help giving and parenting. Collaboration had no discernable direct or mediational effects on parenting competence, confidence, or enjoyment (e.g., Dunst & Dempsey, in press). Relational help giving had small direct effects and somewhat larger mediational effects on the three parenting measures. Participatory help giving had both large direct effects and large mediational effects on parenting competence, confidence, and enjoyment. Moreover, the nature of the relationships between help giving and parenting was much alike for parents of children with or without disabilities.

In those cases in which family-centered help-giving practices had indirect or mediational effects on parenting competence, confidence, and enjoyment, the strongest mediational variable was parents' beliefs about their ability to execute courses of action necessary to achieve desired outcomes or attainments (Bandura, 1997). In almost every analysis that constituted the focus of review, practitioner participatory (and to a lesser degree relational) help-giving practices were positively related to parents' self-efficacy beliefs, which in turn influenced the parents' judgments of their parenting abilities.

The fact that participatory help giving proved the more important determinant of parenting competence, confidence, and enjoyment was not unexpected. Practitioners who use participatory help-giving practices with families encourage and support parents' involvement in experiences that provide contexts for them to successfully provide their children with learning opportunities that benefit parents, as well as children. In other words, when practitioners support parents and parents in turn support their children, both parents and children realize a heightened sense of competence and confidence.

EARLY INTERVENTION AS WE NOW KNOW IT

Early intervention for infants and toddlers with disabilities in the United States has become synonymous with the Individuals with Disabilities Education Act (IDEA), Part C, early-intervention program. Evidence from a number of sources indicate that early-intervention practitioners working in Part C programs generally do not use either evidence-based or recommended practices and that many infants and toddlers participating in Part C early-intervention programs are not provided with the kinds of experiences and opportunities that are likely to have optimally beneficial effects (e.g., Campbell & Halbert, 2002).

Part C early intervention *as we now know it* is, for all intents and purposes, a service-based program (or, as some states claim, a *system*) that more often than not involves practitioners from different disciplines working directly with infants or toddlers generally in an uncoordinated fashion. The latter is especially the case in states that use private-provider models in which practitioners from different programs and organizations separately work with eligible children. In those states that rely heavily on Medicaid reimbursement as a way of funding early intervention, the likelihood that practitioners will intervene directly with children in the absence of meaningful parent involvement is increased considerably. This is often but not always the case because practitioners are not reimbursed for their services if they do not deliver "hands on" therapy or intervention.

Sixteen services are mandated by law as constituting the focus of Part C intervention. Findings from different national surveys, however, indicate that most infants and toddlers participating in Part C early intervention receive primarily service coordination, special instruction, speech therapy, occupational therapy, and physical therapy (e.g., Bruder & Dunst, 2006; U.S. Department of Education, 2002). To the best of my knowledge (based on an extensive literature search), there have been no efficacy or effectiveness studies of service-based Part C early intervention, nor have there been any studies relating variations in Part C service provision to variations to child or parent benefits. As noted, Part C early intervention lacks any substantive evidence of effectiveness, and it is implemented based on the faulty assumption that the services provided by programs and practitioners are *de facto* efficacious. The evidence that is available suggests that service-based early intervention is not effective and in some cases has negative effects (see, e.g., Dunst, Brookfield, & Epstein, 1998; Dunst, Hamby, & Brookfield, 2006; McWilliam et al., 1995; Trivette, Dunst, & Deal, 1997). For example, Dunst, Brookfield, and Epstein (1998) found that more services provided more frequently by more practitioners was negatively related to parent well-being and functioning.

Part C service-based early intervention is based on yet another faulty assumption that has generally gone unchallenged. Proponents of Part C early intervention *as we now know it* often cite the Perry Preschool Study, the Abecedarian Study, and other infant and early-intervention studies as the sources of evidence justifying service-based early intervention. This is clearly not warranted. Early intervention as practiced in Part C programs bears no relationship whatsoever to how early intervention was implemented and evaluated in these studies. The leap of faith that Part C proponents make in terms of "building the case" for service-based early intervention is simply not defensible.

Three sets of findings are briefly examined here to illustrate that early intervention as currently implemented by early-childhood practitioners is not aligned with recommended or generally accepted practices, including those examined earlier in this chapter. The findings are from the Division for Early Childhood (DEC) recommended practices validation studies (McLean, Snyder, Smith, & Sandall, 2002; Odom, McLean, Johnson, & LaMontagne, 1995), an Everyday Children's Learning Opportunities Early Childhood Research Institute study (Dunst, Bruder, et al., 1998), and the National Early Intervention Longitudinal Study (Bailey, Scarborough, Hebbeler, Spiker, & Mallik, 2004; U.S. Department of Education, 2002).

Division for Early Childhood Recommended Practices Surveys

As part of the original development and subsequent revision of the recommended practices for early-childhood intervention by the Division for Early Childhood of the Council for Exceptional Children (DEC Task Force on Recommended Practices, 1993; Odom
& McLean, 1996), social validation surveys of DEC members were conducted to ascertain whether members agreed that the recommended practices were considered valued
and desirable and the extent to which the practices were currently used by early intervention and preschool special education practitioners (McLean et al., 2002; Odom et
al., 1995). Findings from both surveys indicated that the largest number of recommended practices were judged *best or valued practices* but that very few were considered
mainstay early-intervention practices.

Simple recalculations of data presented in McLean et al. (2002) finds that for the
four child and parent intervention practices constituting the focus of analysis (assessment, child-focused interventions, family-based practices, and technology applications),
respondents *strongly agreed* that 69% of the more than 20,000 indicators were recommended practices. However, only 28% of the same practices were deemed *frequently*
used by early-childhood intervention programs and practitioners. Odom et al. (1995)
noted in their analyses of the discrepancy between valued and used practices that very
few indicators were judged as frequently used by survey respondents.

Individualized Family Service Plan
Natural-Environment-Practices Study

As part of the Everyday Children's Learning Opportunities Early Childhood Research
Institute, Dunst, Bruder, et al. (1998) conducted analyses of the extent to which individualized family service plan (IFSP) (as well as individualized education plan [IEP]) outcome statements and activities were implemented in the context of everyday family and
community settings. The focus of analysis was 106 IFSPs from Part C program participants in nine states. The IFSPs included 1,466 outcome statements that specifically
addressed child-level interventions.

Findings showed that less than 1% of the outcome statements were described as
occurring in the context of any family or community activity. So striking was the
noncontextual nature of the outcome statements that only 3% of the outcomes were
judged as having a high probability of increasing the children's interactions with either
people or objects. Furthermore, only 40% of the IFSPs were judged as focusing on the
development of functional behaviors that might promote or encourage child participation in everyday activity.

Dunst, Bruder, et al. (1998) also investigated the kinds of instructional practices
that early-intervention practitioners either used with Part C program participants or
suggested that parents use with their children. The most frequently mentioned practice
was repeated presentation of the same task, or repetitious practice. Yet repeated practice is not generally recognized as an evidence-based teaching strategy (Wolery &
Sainato, 1996).

National Early Intervention Longitudinal Study

The National Early Intervention Longitudinal Study (NEILS), a prospective study of
more than 3,000 infants and toddlers enrolled in Part C early-intervention programs in

20 states, includes a wealth of data useful for discerning the consequences of early intervention (Bailey, Hebbeler, Scarborough, Spiker, & Mallik, 2004; U.S. Department of Education, 2002). A critical examination of findings from NEILS indicates that Part C early intervention may not be having optimal positive benefits for either children or their parents.

Many of the children with identified disabilities in the NEILS study entered early intervention under 1 year of age, and they constitute the focus of discussion here. Child developmental progress, behavior, and functional skills were measured at entry into early intervention and at yearly intervals thereafter. The majority of children made motor, self-help, communication, and cognitive progress between measurement occasions 1 year apart. This is not surprising, because most children with disabilities demonstrate improved functioning even without the benefits of early intervention (see, e.g., Dunst & Rheingrover, 1981; Shonkoff, Hauser-Cram, Wyngarden-Krauss, & Upshur, 1992). What is surprising is the lack of improvements over the course of 1 year in certain areas of functional capabilities. For example, results showed that for the behavior marker "pays attention and stays focused" (a proxy measure of child engagement; McWilliam & Ware, 1994), there were no changes in the percentage of parents of infants ages birth–6 months or 6–12 months who indicated that the statement was "very much like their child." Inasmuch as research indicates that young children with disabilities show improved engagement when they experience high-quality environments (e.g., Ichinose & Clark, 1990) and that parent and teacher behavior contribute to high levels of engagement (e.g., Lussier, Crimmins, & Alberti, 1994), the lack of change in this kind of behavior in the NEILS study participants suggest that there may be less than optimal benefits associated with Part C early intervention.

Parents of infants and toddlers who receive early intervention report, for the most part, overwhelmingly positive appraisals of their experiences (see, e.g., Kontos & Diamond, 2002; McNaughton, 1994). Findings from the NEILS study (Bailey, Scarborough, et al., 2004) indicate that parents do not make these types of positive attributions about their experiences, as are typically found in other studies.

One of the main purposes of Part C early intervention is supporting parents so they can promote child learning and development. It therefore seems reasonable to expect that the largest percentage of parents of children who have participated in Part C early-intervention programs should make positive judgments of their experiences in order to consider early intervention successful. The generally accepted standard for ascertaining success is at least 85% of respondents giving the highest rating on a scale that measures program or practice quality (Reichheld, 2003). Not a single NEILS program quality measure got close to this percentage. In response to the question, "How would you rate the help and information your family received through early intervention?" just over half of the parents (56%) gave the highest rating ("excellent"). Similarly, in response to the question, "How has the help and information received [from early intervention] affected your family?" only 59% of the parents said that their families were "much better off" as a result of early intervention.

Parents' judgments of their ability to help their children learn and develop is perhaps the *sine qua non* for ascertaining the success of Part C early intervention. The results in the NEILS study are not impressive. Only about two-thirds (64%) of the participants "strongly agreed" that they felt capable of helping their children learn as a result of early intervention.

Summary

Taken together, different sources of evidence indicate that Part C early intervention is not aligned with either recommended or evidence-based practices and that the benefits realized by program participants are less than desirable. Available evidence "paints a picture" that early intervention *as we now know it* bears only a faint resemblance to what we know are evidence-based practices.

IMPLICATIONS FOR POLICY AND PRACTICE

Knowledge about the characteristics and consequences of intervention practices that have development-enhancing qualities and benefits, as well as knowledge about early intervention as it is generally practiced in many states, has implications for improving policy and for informing parents and practitioners about the key features of evidence-based practices. The research summarized in this chapter, as well as that reported elsewhere (e.g., Bailey, Aytch, Odom, Symons, & Wolery, 1999; Odom & Wolery, 2003), may be considered the standards against which current policy and practice are judged as either consistent or inconsistent with available research.

Policy

Current knowledge about optimally effective early-intervention practices has implications for policy at both the federal and state levels. There is an urgent need to completely update the federal Part C infant/toddler program legislation and rules and regulations in light of available research evidence. In the 20 years since the passage of the Public Law 99-457 Part H program that established the current early intervention system in the United States, there have been tremendous advances in our understanding of the factors that influence the growth and development of infants and toddlers with disabilities. But even a cursory examination of the various reauthorizations of Part H, and, subsequently, the Part C early-intervention program, indicates that the changes that have been made have not kept pace with the current knowledge base.

Two of the many changes that are needed in the federal legislation are briefly discussed here to highlight what evidence-based policy would look like. The first would be a redefinition of early intervention as a set of practices (rather than services) and a description of the kinds of practices that would be authorized by the Part C legislation. The second would be a reemphasis on the original purpose of the legislation—to support parents' capacity to promote their children's learning and development in *ways that strengthen parenting competence and confidence*. Some simple calculations indicate that twice-a-week hourly intervention or therapy, in the absence of parent involvement, accounts for only 2% of the total waking hours of a 1-year-old child (Roffwarg, Muzio, & Dement, 1966), hardly enough time for any kind of intervention to make a meaningful difference in a child's life (McWilliam, 2000).

The largest majority of state early-intervention programs and systems have been developed in ways that include features and elements that run counter to current knowledge about evidence-based early intervention. Take, for example, the faulty logic in the use of dedicated-service-coordination models in which service coordinators provide only service coordination but not early-intervention services and private-provider early-intervention models in which early intervention is provided by contracting with individuals who often work for different agencies. Research findings from the Research and Training Center on Service Coordination indicate that dedicated-service coordination results in the provision of fewer service-coordinator practices (Dunst & Bruder, 2006) and that there is very little relationship between what service coordinators do and what services infants and toddlers receive (Bruder & Dunst, 2006).

Medicaid-funded early intervention, especially in states with private-provider models or in which services must be delivered by "qualified professionals" to be reimbursed, often excludes parents from the interventions with their children. This, at least in part, may account for the fact that professionally centered early intervention sometimes has negative effects on parent functioning (Dunst, Bruder, et al., 2006; Dunst, Trivette, et al., 2006): Parents' beliefs about their capacities to help their children learn may be compromised when professional practices take over parenting functions.

One use of research evidence for informing policy is in discerning where financial resources ought to be allocated to maximize the benefits of the funding. There has been a recent trend in states toward using federal and state Part C dollars to fund service coordination and nonintervention services (e.g., multidisciplinary evaluations) and to use Medicaid to fund the provision of early intervention (typically through a reimbursement system). There is little or no evidence that service coordination is an evidence-based practice (Bruder et al., 2005) or that multidisciplinary evaluations are useful for their intended purposes (Neisworth & Bagnato, 2004), yet tremendous amounts of public dollars are used to fund these kinds of activities. States would do a much better job of using available resources by funding evidence-based practices that support and strengthen parents' capacity to promote their children's learning and development.

Practice

Knowledge about the characteristics of practices that have desired benefits can be useful as well to both practitioners and parents. Practitioners can use evidence-based information as a standard for discerning the extent to which their work with infants and toddlers and their parents is consistent with the characteristics of practices most likely to have optimal positive benefits (see e.g., Raab & Dunst, 2006a; Wilson & Dunst, 2004).

Parents should find information about evidence-based practices useful for judging whether their children and family are receiving high-quality early intervention. A common theme that has emerged from the conduct of different practice-based research syntheses of early-childhood intervention practices is that intervention practices in which children are producers of their own behavior are ones that strengthen existing skills and promote acquisition of new skills that have capacity-building consequences (e.g., Brandtstädter & Lerner, 1999). In contrast, interventions in which participants are passively involved or in which things are done to them (e.g., noncontingent stimulation) are not associated with positive benefits. If, for example, parents see that their children are being passively manipulated or stimulated or are being asked only to produce or repeat adult-desired behavior, they should question the practice. Similarly, if parents are being asked only to follow professionally prescribed practices and are not acquiring knowledge and skills that can be used more broadly to provide their children with development-enhancing learning opportunities, the practices should be questioned as well.

CONCLUSION

Research on early intervention has increased almost exponentially over the past 40–50 years. The sheer amount of research informing early-childhood intervention is almost overwhelming. Trying to keep abreast of the knowledge base can be a daunting task. It is, however, essential that scholars, practitioners, and policy makers know how and in what manner early experiences are likely to influence infant and toddler learning and development. Yet research evidence that informs practices is often disregarded or treated with indifference (Campbell & Halbert, 2002).

In an informative and thoughtful article about why people "explain away" evidence when it contradicts their (often strongly held) beliefs, Chinn and Brewer (1993) list seven types of responses to anomalous data. "Anomalous data" refers to evidence that contradicts people's personal theories, beliefs, or paradigms. The seven responses include such things as ignoring, rejecting, reinterpreting, and refusing to "hear" or acknowledge the data. Readers may respond in similar ways to at least some of the findings and assertions presented in this chapter. For example, some readers may take issue with the critical assessment of Part C early intervention. Perhaps it will stimulate healthy debate about the ways in which states currently practice early intervention and what can be done to better align state efforts with existing research evidence. Also, the parent-mediated approach to early intervention that constitutes the focus of this chapter may also be challenged based on the contention that professionally implemented interventions are more likely to be effective.

Hewlett and West (1998), in their book *The War Against Parents*, note that the

> unintended consequence of the well-meaning crusade [of help-giving professionals] to save our children was the emergence of a new class of professionals—social workers, therapists, foster care providers, family court lawyers—who have a vested interest in taking over parent functions. Bureaucracies everywhere have a remorseless drive to expand—to widen their client base. If children are the clients, parents can quite easily become the adversaries—the people who threaten to take business away." (p. 109)

Something akin to this seems to be happening in early intervention and is especially the case in states that are privatizing early intervention. The research foundations for supporting parents and families strongly indicate a much better way of conducting early intervention. Can that research continue to be ignored if the consequences are undermining the confidence of parents and their abilities to provide their children with learning experiences and opportunities of known quality?

REFERENCES

Affleck, G., McGrade, B. J., McQueeney, M., & Allen, D. (1982). Promise of relationship-focused early intervention in developmental disabilities. *Journal of Special Education, 16,* 413–430.

Bailey, D., Scarborough, A., Hebbeler, K., Spiker, D., & Mallik, S. (2004, October). *National Early Intervention Longitudinal Study: Family outcomes at the end of early intervention* (NEILS Data Report No. 6; SRI Project No. 11247). Retrieved January 19, 2006, from *www.sri.com/neils/pdfs/FamilyOutcomes-Report_011405.pdf*.

Bailey, D. B., Jr., Aytch, L. S., Odom, S. L., Symons, F., & Wolery, M. (1999). Early intervention as we know it. *Mental Retardation and Developmental Disabilities Research Reviews, 5,* 11–20.

Bailey, D. B., Jr., Hebbeler, K., Scarborough, A., Spiker, D., & Mallik, S. (2004). First experiences with early intervention: A national perspective. *Pediatrics, 113,* 887–896.

Bandura, A. (1997). *Self-efficacy: The exercise of control.* New York: Freeman.

Brandtstädter, J., & Lerner, R. M. (Eds.). (1999). *Action and self-development: Theory and research through the life span.* Thousand Oaks, CA: Sage.

Bronfenbrenner, U. (1992). Ecological systems theory. In R. Vasta (Ed.), *Six theories of child development: Revised formulations and current issues* (pp. 187–248). Philadelphia: Kingsley.

Bronfenbrenner, U. (1993). The ecology of cognitive development: Research models and fugitive findings. In R. H. Wozniak & K. W. Fischer (Eds.), *Development in context: Acting and thinking in specific environments* (pp. 3–44). Hillsdale, NJ: Erlbaum.

Bruder, M. B., & Dunst, C. J. (2006). *Relationship between service coordinator practices and early intervention services.* Manuscript submitted for publication.

Bruder, M. B., Harbin, G. L., Whitbread, K., Conn-Powers, M., Roberts, R., Dunst, C. J., et al. (2005). Establishing outcomes for service coordination: A step toward evidence-based practice. *Topics in Early Childhood Special Education, 25,* 177–188.

Campbell, P. H., & Halbert, J. (2002). Between research and practice: Provider perspectives on early intervention. *Topics in Early Childhood Special Education, 22,* 213–226.

Chinn, C. A., & Brewer, W. F. (1993). The role of anomalous data in knowledge acquisition: A theoretical framework and implications for science instruction. *Review of Educational Research, 63*(1), 1–49.

De Wolff, M. S., & van IJzendoorn, M. H. (1997). Sensitivity and attachment: A meta-analysis on parental antecedents of infant attachment. *Child Development, 68,* 571–591.

DEC Task Force on Recommended Practices. (1993). *DEC recommended practices: Indicators of quality in programs for infants and young children with special needs and their families.* Reston, VA: Council for Exceptional Children.

Dunst, C. J. (1998). Sensorimotor development and developmental disabilities. In B. Hodapp, E. Zigler, & J. Burack (Eds.), *Handbook of mental retardation and development* (pp. 135–182). New York: Cambridge University Press.

Dunst, C. J. (2000). Revisiting "Rethinking early intervention." *Topics in Early Childhood Special Education, 20,* 95–104.

Dunst, C. J. (2003). Social–emotional consequences of response-contingent learning opportunities. *Bridges, 1*(1), 1–17. Retrieved April 3, 2006, from *www.evidencebasedpractices.org/bridges/bridges_vol1_no1.pdf.*

Dunst, C. J. (2004). An integrated framework for practicing early childhood intervention and family support. *Perspectives in Education, 22*(2), 1–16.

Dunst, C. J. (2006). *Daily occupations as the context for child learning and development.* Manuscript in preparation.

Dunst, C. J., Brookfield, J., & Epstein, J. (1998, December). *Family-centered early intervention and child, parent and family benefits: Final report.* Asheville, NC: Orelena Hawks Puckett Institute.

Dunst, C. J., & Bruder, M. B. (1999). Family and community activity settings, natural learning environments, and children's learning opportunities. *Children's Learning Opportunities Report, 1*(2), 1–2. Retrieved April 3, 2006, from *www.everydaylearning.info/reports/lov1–2.pdf.*

Dunst, C. J., & Bruder, M. B. (2006). Early intervention service coordination models and service coordinator practices. *Journal of Early Intervention, 28,* 155–165.

Dunst, C. J., Bruder, M. B., Trivette, C. M., Hamby, D., Raab, M., & McLean, M. (2001). Characteristics and consequences of everyday natural learning opportunities. *Topics in Early Childhood Special Education, 21,* 68–92.

Dunst, C. J., Bruder, M. B., Trivette, C. M., & Hamby, D. W. (2006). Everyday activity settings, natural learning environments, and early intervention practices. *Journal of Policy and Practice in Intellectual Disabilities, 3,* 3–10.

Dunst, C. J., Bruder, M. B., Trivette, C. M., Raab, M., & McLean, M. (1998, May). *Increasing children's learning opportunities through families and communities Early Childhood Research Institute: Year 2 progress report.* Asheville, NC: Orelena Hawks Puckett Institute.

Dunst, C. J., & Dempsey, I. (in press). Family/professional partnerships and parenting competence, confidence, and enjoyment. *International Journal of Development, Disability and Education.*

Dunst, C. J., Hamby, D. W., & Brookfield, J. (2006). *Modeling the effects of early intervention variables on parent and family well-being.* Manuscript submitted for publication.

Dunst, C. J., Hamby, D., Trivette, C. M., Raab, M., & Bruder, M. B. (2000). Everyday family and community life and children's naturally occurring learning opportunities. *Journal of Early Intervention, 23,* 151–164.

Dunst, C. J., Hamby, D., Trivette, C. M., Raab, M., & Bruder, M. B. (2002). Young children's participation in everyday family and community activity. *Psychological Reports, 91,* 875–897.

Dunst, C. J., & Kassow, D. Z. (2004). Characteristics of interventions promoting parental sensitivity to child behavior. *Bridges, 3*(3), 1–17. Retrieved April 3, 2006, from *www.evidencebasedpractices.org/ bridges/bridges_vol3_no3.pdf.*

Dunst, C. J., Raab, M., Wilson, L., & Parkey, C. (1997, November). *The response-contingent learning capabilities of young children with disabilities and their social-emotional concomitants.* Paper presented at the International Division for Early Childhood Conference on Children with Special Needs, New Orleans, LA.

Dunst, C. J., & Rheingrover, R. M. (1981). An analysis of the efficacy of infant intervention programs with organically handicapped children. *Evaluation and Program Planning, 4,* 287–323.

Dunst, C. J., Snyder, S. W., & Mankinen, M. (1988). Efficacy of early intervention. In M. Wang, H. Walberg, & M. Reynolds (Eds.), *Handbook of special education: Research and practice* (pp. 259–294). Oxford, UK: Pergamon Press.

Dunst, C. J., Storck, A. J., Hutto, M. D., & Snyder, D. (2006). Relative effectiveness of episodic and conjugate reinforcement on child operant learning. *Bridges, 4*(3), 1–15. Retrieved April 3, 2006, from *www.evidencebasedpractices.org/bridges/bridges_vol4_no3.pdf.*

Dunst, C. J., & Trivette, C. M. (1994). Methodological considerations and strategies for studying the long-term effects of early intervention. In S. Friedman & H. C. Haywood (Eds.), *Developmental follow-up: Concepts, domains and methods* (pp. 277–313). San Diego, CA: Academic Press.

Dunst, C. J., Trivette, C. M., & Cutspec, P. A. (2002). Toward an operational definition of evidence-based practices. *Centerscope, 1*(1), 1–10. Retrieved April 3, 2006, from *www.evidencebasedpractices. org/centerscope/centerscopevol1no1.pdf.*

Dunst, C. J., Trivette, C. M., & Hamby, D. W. (2006a). *Characteristics and consequences of family-centered help giving on child, parent and family functioning.* Manuscript in preparation.

Dunst, C. J., Trivette, C. M., & Hamby, D. W. (2006b). *Family support program quality and parent, family and child benefits.* Asheville, NC: Winterberry Press.

Dunst, C. J., Trivette, C. M., & Hamby, D. W. (in press). Meta-analysis of family-centered help-giving practices research. *Mental Retardation and Developmental Disabilities Research Review.*

Dunst, C. J., Trivette, C. M., Hamby, D. W., & Bruder, M. B. (2006). Influences of contrasting natural learning environment experiences on child, parent, and family well-being [Electronic version]. *Journal of Developmental and Physical Disabilities, 18*(2).

Farver, J. A. M. (1999). Activity setting analysis: A model for examining the role of culture in development. In A. Göncü (Ed.), *Children's engagement in the world: Sociocultural perspectives* (pp. 99–127). Cambridge, UK: Cambridge University Press.

Göncü, A. (Ed.). (1999). *Children's engagement in the world: Sociocultural perspectives.* Cambridge, UK: Cambridge University Press.

Guralnick, M. J. (Ed.). (2005). *The developmental systems approach to early intervention.* Baltimore: Brookes.

Haith, M. M. (1972). The forgotten message of the infant smile. *Merrill–Palmer Quarterly, 18,* 321–322.

Hewlett, S. A., & West, C. (1998). *The war against parents: What we can do for America's beleaguered moms and dads.* Boston: Houghton Mifflin.

Hulsebus, R. C. (1973). Operant conditioning of infant behavior: A review. *Advances in Child Development and Behavior, 8,* 111–158.

Hunt, J. M. (1961). *Intelligence and experience.* New York: Ronald Press.

Hutto, M. D. (2003). Latency to learn in contingency studies of young children with disabilities or developmental delays. *Bridges, 1*(2), 1–16. Retrieved April 3, 2006, from *www.evidencebasedpractices. org/bridges/bridges_vol1_no2.pdf.*

Ichinose, C. K., & Clark, H. B. (1990). A review of ecological factors that influence the play and activity engagement of handicapped children. *Child and Family Behavior Therapy, 12*(3), 49–76.

Kassow, D. Z., & Dunst, C. J. (2004). Relationship between parent contingent-responsiveness and attachment outcomes. *Bridges, 2*(6), 1–17. Retrieved April 3, 2006, from *www.evidencebasedpractices.org/ bridges/bridges_vol2_no6.pdf.*

Kassow, D. Z., & Dunst, C. J. (2005). Characteristics of parental sensitivity related to secure infant attachment. *Bridges, 3*(2), 1–13. Retrieved April 3, 2006, from *www.researchtopractice.info/bridges/bridges_vol3_no2.pdf*.

Kontos, S., & Diamond, K. (2002). Measuring the quality of early intervention services for infants and toddlers: Problems and prospects. *International Journal of Disability, Development and Education, 49,* 337–351.

Lancioni, G. E. (1980). Infant operant conditioning and its implications for early intervention. *Psychological Bulletin, 88,* 516–534.

Lipsitt, L. P., & Werner, J. S. (1981). The infancy of human learning processes. In E. S. Gollin (Ed.), *Developmental plasticity: Behavioral and biological aspects of variations in development* (pp. 101–133). New York: Academic Press.

Lussier, B. J., Crimmins, D. B., & Alberti, D. (1994). Effect of three adult interaction styles on infant engagement. *Journal of Early Intervention, 18,* 12–24.

Marfo, K. (Ed.). (1988). *Parent–child interaction and developmental disabilities: Theory, research, and intervention.* New York: Praeger.

Masiello, T. L., & Gorman, E. (2006). *Family activity settings and the behavior and development of young children.* Manuscript in preparation.

McLean, M. E., Snyder, P., Smith, B. J., & Sandall, S. R. (2002). The DEC recommended practices in early intervention/early childhood special education: Social validation. *Journal of Early Intervention, 25,* 120–128.

McNaughton, D. (1994). Measuring parent satisfaction with early childhood intervention programs: Current practice, problems, and future perspectives. *Topics in Early Childhood Special Education, 14,* 26–48.

McNemer, Q. (1940). A critical examination of the University of Iowa studies of environmental influences upon the IQ. *Psychological Bulletin, 37,* 63–92.

McWilliam, R. A. (2000). It's only natural . . . to have early intervention in the environments where it's needed. *Young Exceptional Children: Monograph Series No. 2. Natural Environments and Inclusion,* 17–26.

McWilliam, R. A., Lang, L., Vandiviere, P., Angell, R., Collins, L., & Underdown, G. (1995). Satisfaction and struggles: Family perceptions of early intervention services. *Journal of Early Intervention, 19,* 43–60.

McWilliam, R. A., & Ware, W. B. (1994). The reliability of observations of young children's engagement: An application of generalizability theory. *Journal of Early Intervention, 18,* 34–47.

Neisworth, J. T., & Bagnato, S. J. (2004). The mismeasure of young children: The authentic assessment alternative. *Infants and Young Children, 17*(3), 198–212.

Odom, S. L., & McLean, M. E. (Eds.). (1996). *Early intervention/early childhood special education: Recommended practices.* Austin, TX: PRO-ED.

Odom, S. L., McLean, M. E., Johnson, L. J., & LaMontagne, M. J. (1995). Recommended practices in early childhood special education: Validation and current use. *Journal of Early Intervention, 19,* 1–17.

Odom, S. L., & Wolery, M. (2003). A unified theory of practice in early intervention/early childhood special education: Evidence-based practices. *Journal of Special Education, 37,* 164–173.

Raab, M., & Dunst, C. J. (2006a). Checklists for promoting parent-mediated everyday child learning opportunities. *CASEtools, 2*(1), 1–9. Retrieved April 3, 2006, from *www.fippcase.org/casetools/casetools_vol2_no1.pdf*.

Raab, M., & Dunst, C. J. (2006b). Influence of child interests on variations in child behavior and functioning. *Bridges, 4*(2), 1–22. Retrieved April 3, 2006, from *www.researchtopractice.info/bridges/bridges_vol4_no2.pdf*.

Reichheld, F. F. (2003, December). The one number you need to grow. *Harvard Business Review,* 46–54.

Rochat, P. R. (2001). Social contingency detection and infant development. *Bulletin of the Menninger Clinic, 65,* 347–360.

Roffwarg, H. P., Muzio, J. N., & Dement, W. C. (1966). Ontogenetic development of the human sleep–dream cycle. *Science, 152,* 604–618.

Shonkoff, J., Hauser-Cram, P., Wyngarden-Krauss, M. W., & Upshur, C. C. (1992). Development of infants with disabilities and their families: Implications for theory and service delivery. *Monographs of the Society for Research in Child Development, 57*(6, Serial No. 230).

Shonkoff, J. P., & Phillips, D. A. (Eds.). (2000). *From neurons to neighborhoods: The science of early childhood development.* Washington, DC: National Academies Press.

Skeels, H. M., & Dye, H. B. (1939). Psychology: A study of the effects of differential stimulation on mentally retarded children. *Proceedings and Addresses of the American Association on Mental Deficiency, 44*,
114–136.

Trivette, C. M. (2003). Influence of caregiver responsiveness on the development of young children
with or at risk for developmental disabilities. *Bridges, 1*(3), 1–13. Retrieved April 3, 2006, from
www.evidencebasedpractices.org/bridges/bridges_vol1_no3.pdf.

Trivette, C. M. (2004). Influence of home environment on the social–emotional development of young
children. *Bridges, 2*(7), 1–15. Retrieved April 3, 2006, from *www.evidencebasedpractices.org/bridges/
bridges_vol2_no7.pdf.*

Trivette, C. M., & Click, F. (2006). *Behavioral and developmental consequences of routine-based interventions
with young children.* Manuscript in preparation.

Trivette, C. M., Dunst, C. J., & Deal, A. G. (1997). Resource-based approach to early intervention. In S.
K. Thurman, J. R. Cornwell, & S. R. Gottwald (Eds.), *Contexts of early intervention: Systems and settings* (pp. 73–92). Baltimore: Brookes.

Trivette, C. M., Dunst, C. J., & Hamby, D. (2004). Sources of variation in and consequences of everyday
activity settings on child and parenting functioning. *Perspectives in Education, 22*(2), 17–35.

Trivette, C. M., & O'Herin, C. E. (2006). *Characteristics of caregiver responsiveness and child competence.*
Manuscript in preparation.

U.S. Department of Education. (2002). *Twenty-fourth annual report to Congress on the implementation of the
Individuals with Disabilities Education Act: Section IV. Results experienced by children and families 1 year
after beginning early intervention.* Washington DC: Author.

Uzgiris, I. C., & Hunt, J. M. (Eds.). (1987). *Infant performance and experience: New findings with the ordinal
scales.* Urbana: University of Illinois Press.

Watson, J. S. (1966). The development and generalization of "contingency awareness" in early infancy:
Some hypotheses. *Merrill-Palmer Quarterly, 12*, 123–135.

Wilson, L. L., & Dunst, C. J. (2004). Checking out family-centered help giving practices. In E. Horn, M.
M. Ostrosky, & H. Jones (Eds.), *Young Exceptional Children: Monograph Series No. 5. Family-Based
Practices* (pp. 13–26). Longmont, CO: Sopris West.

Wolery, M., & Sainato, D. M. (1996). General curriculum and intervention strategies. In S. L. Odom &
M. E. McLean (Eds.), *Early intervention/early childhood special education: Recommended practices*
(pp. 125–158). Austin, TX: PRO-ED.

9

Trends and Issues in Interventions for Preschoolers with Developmental Disabilities

Judith J. Carta
Na Young Kong

Growing evidence from many fields has substantiated the importance of early intervention for laying the foundation for lifelong learning, behavior, and health outcomes (Shonkoff & Phillips, 2000). Effective early intervention approaches are those that prevent or arrest problems early in a child's life or at early stages in the development of problem situations. The importance of prevention and intervention for our nation's most vulnerable citizens (those with developmental delays or disabilities) was formally recognized in the United States with the passage of the Individuals with Disabilities Education Act (IDEA) and its amended version, Public Law 99-457. With this amendment to IDEA in 1986, the nation mandated that children from 3 to 5 years with developmental delays and disabilities should be granted a free, appropriate public education (FAPE)—mandates that had previously been limited to students in kindergarten through 12th grade. The extension of FAPE to children prior to school entry was a recognition of the large body of evidence that supports the notion that children's participation in intervention prior to kindergarten is associated with positive outcomes (Ramey & Ramey, 1998) and that declines in intellectual development can be substantially reduced by interventions implemented during the first 5 years of life (Guralnick, 1998).

Since the passage of that law, the way early intervention is carried out in programs serving preschool children with disabilities has changed dramatically. This is true for at least two reasons. Research, supported in large part by the federal government and specifically by the Office of Special Education Programs, has shaped the current practice of early intervention. In addition, however, a range of issues, trends, and values has influenced how these practices are actually implemented in the real-world environ-

181

ments of classrooms, homes, and other community settings. The purpose of this chapter is to provide a broad overview of the trends and issues that are shaping the field of early education for preschoolers with disabilities in the current decade. In the course of that examination, we describe how early intervention is currently delivered. We provide a discussion of the trends that influence the settings in which intervention takes place for young children with disabilities, the teaching content that is addressed in preschool interventions, and the approaches or methods of intervention. In short, we discuss the *where, what,* and *how* of early education for preschoolers with disabilities.

TRENDS AFFECTING *WHERE* INSTRUCTION OCCURS

In 1997, the IDEA of 1990 was reauthorized once again and signed into law as Public Law 105-17. The mandates of the original special education law of 1975 were reaffirmed, and federal statutory requirements for full inclusion of children were strengthened. Part B of IDEA (2004) states that community-based settings with typically developing same-age peers should be available for preschool children with disabilities. The intent of this legislation is to maximize opportunities for children with disabilities to be educated with their peers. Many strategies and models have been developed for teaching children with disabilities and other special needs in inclusive settings (Odom, Horn, et al., 1999). Guralnick (2001) has described four inclusion models for preschool children. The first model is full inclusion. In this model, activities are adapted whenever necessary to allow children with disabilities to be full participants with their nondisabled peers. This model is sometimes called the "itinerant-teacher model" or "consultant model" because support is provided by related services specialists and other specialized staff. The second type of program, the cluster model, or coteaching model, involves bringing together two classes (one with disabilities and one without disabilities) and their respective teachers who share all planning and teaching responsibilities. The third model, reverse inclusion, is a specialized program usually staffed by early childhood special educators in which a small group of typically developing children joins a larger group of young children with disabilities. The fourth model, the social inclusion model, provides the fewest opportunities for interaction for children with and without disabilities. This model houses an early childhood program and an early childhood special education program in the same building but in different classrooms with different staffs and different curricula. The two classes may come together for free play, art, or recess.

To apply any of these models, teachers and caregivers need a range of supports, including ongoing professional development. These supports are necessary because the goal is not simply to place children with disabilities in inclusive settings but to support their participation and learning in meaningful ways in those settings. Yet the extent to which young children with disabilities are receiving appropriate services in the most inclusive setting possible is far from ideal. Across the country, a patchwork of systems, programs, and agencies serves preschoolers with disabilities and their families. Families whose young children have special needs face significant obstacles when they try to access child care for their children. These obstacles often include transportation difficulties, coordination of child care with early services, and programs that refuse to accept their children (Kelly & Booth, 1999). A major barrier in this regard is a lack of qualified personnel in inclusive settings with the special education training to provide effective individualized intervention for their children with disabilities (Wolery et al.,

1994). Although child care providers are in a unique position to identify young children who may not be diagnosed with a disability but who experience developmental delays or have special needs, they seldom have the training to allow them to make such early identifications (Gilliam, Meisels, & Mayes, 2005). Many challenges remain as local education programs struggle to find ways to provide the least restrictive early education to young children with disabilities by professionally trained staff who can provide high-quality instruction in those settings.

TRENDS AFFECTING *WHAT* WE TEACH: THE PUSH FOR OUTCOMES-BASED INTERVENTION

Outcomes, or what is taught to young children with special needs, are, according to McWilliam, Wolery, and Odom (2001), "a function of the field's beliefs and values (particularly those of the child's team) and the accumulation of knowledge and experience about what seems possible to teach and, thus, what should be taught" (p. 507). In the current decade, identifying clear outcomes for programs and establishing the means for monitoring progress toward outcomes has taken center stage. Probably no issue has affected special education in general or early childhood special education more specifically than the call for programs to become more outcomes-based and to be able to demonstrate their effectiveness. On July 1, 2002, the President's commission on Excellence in Special Education issued a report in which it argued that IDEA be reauthorized based on reforms outlined in the No Child Left Behind Act and Changing America's Special Education System "from a culture of compliance to a culture of accountability for results" (The President's Commission on Excellence in Special Education, 2002, p. 2). The commission encouraged "identification and assessment methods that prevent disabilities and identify needs early and accurately"(p. 9) and promoted "educational reforms based on scientifically rigorous research" (p. 12). Although the report did not address specific issues regarding early childhood special education, the message to programs serving young children with special needs was clear: Develop more effective intervention practices and focus on results.

Yet a consensus about what the outcomes of early education programs should be has not been forthcoming. Traditionally, most early childhood educators share a philosophy that learning environments, teaching practices, and other instructional approaches aimed at young children should be based on what is expected of typically developing children. Often, this perspective is extended to children with special needs. According to this view, young children with developmental problems acquire skills in sequences that mirror those of children without disabilities, but their rate of acquiring these skills is slower than the typical rate (Bennett-Gates & Zigler, 1998). The implication of this perspective (sometimes referred to as the "similar sequence hypothesis"; cf. McWilliam et al., 2001) is that curricular outcomes for preschoolers with special needs should be centered on the mastery of skills that follow a developmental sequence. These sequences are typically organized into a common set of domains: language and communication skills, social skills, cognitive abilities, fine and gross motor skills, and adaptive or self-care skills.

A somewhat different view of what should be taught to preschoolers with disabilities is the functional perspective. This approach selects early childhood outcomes based on a set of skills that allow the child to participate more fully in a variety of community settings. This perspective reinforces the idea that curriculum should be adapted to meet the child's needs and that there should be a clear reason for teaching each skill. These skills, identified through criterion-referenced assessment instruments and ecological inventories or environmental assessments, are those that help the child meet the demands of his or her current and future environments. In early childhood settings, functional targeted skills might be those that would assist the child in interacting more independently and positively within the physical and social environment. Several researchers have recommended outcome areas that might tap functional skills. Bricker, Pretti-Frontczak, and McComas (1998) suggested that important skills to target should be functional, usable across settings and with different people and materials, observable and measurable, and part of the child's natural daily environment. Bailey and Wolery (1992) proposed focus areas such as those that promote children's engagement and mastery of their environment and their abilities to apply and generalize newly acquired skills to a variety of real-world settings.

A third perspective on outcomes focuses on skills needed in future settings. A strong influence in this regard has been the federal initiative Good Start, Grow Smart (GSGS). The goal of GSGS is ensuring that young children enter kindergarten with the skills they need to succeed—especially preacademic outcomes in early literacy, early mathematics, and early language (Good Start, Grow Smart Interagency Workgroup, 2006). Whereas child development experts once theorized that young children were incapable of learning early academic and preliteracy skills and that exposure to academic concepts could even be harmful, more recent research has demonstrated that young children are capable of learning far more complex skills and concepts than previously believed (Bowman, Donovan, & Burns, 2000). The GSGS national initiative has influenced many states to adopt prekindergarten standards that include preacademic and early literacy outcomes (Bodrova, Leong, & Shore, 2004).

This federal push for outcomes in early education has extended to all programs that serve young children, including those aimed at young children with developmental delays and disabilities. One demonstration of this influence is the recent federal reporting requirement that states report child and family outcomes on a yearly basis for children being served by IDEA Part C and Part B-619 programs (National Early Childhood Technical Assistance Center [NECTAC], 2006). Acknowledging that the overarching goal of early childhood special education services is to enable young children to be active participants in their homes and communities during the early childhood years, as well as in the future, the Office of Special Education Programs (OSEP) has selected a set of functional outcomes that are not domain-based but instead refer to an integrated set of behaviors and actions that are meaningful to the child in the context of everyday living. Starting in 2006, OSEP has begun a process of yearly measurement of children in Part C and Part B-619 programs on the following functional outcomes: (1) positive social–emotional skills (including social relationships), (2) acquisition and use of knowledge and skills (including language/communication and literacy), and (3) use of appropriate behaviors to meet their needs. Reports on this common set of functional outcomes for all children in Part C and Part B programs will provide an index of the proportion of children who are improving in their performance each year. (Information about this process is available on the Early Childhood Outcomes Center website at *www.fpg.unc.edu/~eco/index.cfm.*)

In summary, whereas the three functional outcomes are being measured by every program in the United States, most programs today are focusing on a broad set of outcomes that incorporate all three approaches to outcomes. Ultimately, instructional teams composed of the teaching professionals and the child's parents decide on specific outcomes for each child based on an analysis of current needs in present and future environments.

TRENDS AFFECTING *HOW* WE TEACH

For many years, special education and early childhood special education practices have been influenced by the behavioral tradition (cf. Strain et al., 1992). In this approach, teachers or interventionists frequently have taken a direct role in instruction and in that regard have structured the classroom environment in various ways to promote learning and support children's development. Although these and other strategies based on behavioral principles are commonly used in today's early education programs, some concern has been voiced by practitioners, parents, and researchers when behavioral approaches have been employed in early childhood settings in the form of highly structured, teacher-driven direct-instruction approaches. One criticism of strict behavioral practices has been that skills learned in highly structured approaches often fail to generalize to everyday settings. As a result, the trend in instruction in education for young children with disabilities is toward more "naturalistic" intervention approaches that teach skills in sequence with other skills as they would typically occur (Sailor & Guess, 1983), using natural stimuli and consequences (Falvey, Brown, Lyon, Baumgart, & Schroeder, 1980), and at times when they are most needed (Hart & Risley, 1968). Some of the trends driving these changes in how instruction occurs are discussed next.

Using Developmentally and Individually Appropriate Practices

A major influence on interventions for preschoolers with disabilities is the principle of developmentally appropriate practice. "Developmentally appropriate practices" (DAP) describes an approach to education that recognizes the child as an active participant in the learning process who constructs meaning and knowledge through interaction with people and materials in the environment (Bredekamp & Copple, 1997). The teacher's role is to facilitate the child's acquisition of meaning from the various activities and interactions he or she encounters throughout the day. This approach to educating young children was articulated in a position statement on developmentally appropriate practices first published by the National Association for the Education of Young Children (NAEYC) in 1987 (Bredekamp, 1987). NAEYC developed the position statement to give early childhood educators a clear sense of appropriate early childhood practices. DAP emerged out of a concern that early childhood programs were becoming too academically focused and were adopting instructional styles that were too formal and structured. The original 1987 NAEYC document argued for an educational approach that was primarily child-directed on the basis that children learn best when they have real materials they can manipulate and explore and when they have opportunities to learn about topics that are personally meaningful and interesting.

Some individuals from the early childhood special education community expressed concerns that the original NAEYC DAP guidelines published in 1987 were not sufficient for promoting optimal development for young children with disabilities and did not adequately address the issue of individual appropriateness, that is, the importance of instructional practices that address child-specific goals and objectives (Carta, Schwartz, Atwater, & McConnell, 1991). A more recent NAEYC document (Bredekamp & Copple, 1997) outlining the principles of DAP now recommends a balance between child-directed and teacher-directed activities and highlights both developmental appropriateness and individual appropriateness of instruction that takes into consideration the unique features of each child.

Discovering what works best for all children requires knowledge of each child, knowledge of how children learn, and clear learning outcomes. The discussion about DAP and its relevance and sufficiency for young children with disabilities continues and has helped define the dimensions of quality instruction for young children with disabilities (Wolery, Strain, & Bailey, 1992). Carta and Greenwood (1997) identified the following dimensions for defining quality instruction of young children with developmental delays: (1) the curriculum should consider children's future environments; (2) goals and objectives should be identified for individual children, with some means of monitoring progress on those objectives; and (3) effectiveness and efficiency in assisting children in achieving socially valued outcomes should be emphasized.

Making Instruction Contextually Relevant

Another trend in early childhood special education practice is a focus on naturalistic curriculum models (e.g., Noonan & McCormick, 2006). This type of model is based on the idea that because learning occurs in many contexts, teaching should occur in the many environments in which a young child's learning typically takes place. This principle is articulated in the notion of "natural environments" in Part C of IDEA (1997), which requires that, to the maximum extent possible, young children with special needs receive intervention in the home and community settings in which children without disabilities typically participate. Although this feature of programs is mandated in IDEA for infants and toddlers receiving Part C services (see Dunst, Chapter 8, this volume), the same feature applies in principle to preschool-age children. To promote generalization of learning to all the contexts of life, program developers are beginning to extend learning opportunities beyond the classroom. Opportunities for learning must occur in the home, neighborhood, and community so children can learn to be active participants in those settings (Dunst et al., 2001).

As previously noted, another aspect of contextually relevant instruction is the use of more naturalistic teaching strategies in classroom settings. Naturalistic intervention is "specialized instruction provided in the context of naturally occurring routines and events. Instructors facilitate learning and ensure the mastery of functional skills that have immediate application across settings" (McCormick, 2006, p. 16). An important value of naturalistic teaching strategies is taking advantage of those "teachable moments" when children need to perform the goal behavior to meet some intention they have and when instruction can be provided with specific and relevant stimuli to prompt or encourage the goal behavior. This allows the instruction to be relevant to the context in which the child is engaged, which is thought to take advantage of children's existing motivation. More detail about research on naturalistic intervention strategies appears later in the chapter.

Promoting Culturally Compatible Instruction

Another trend that relates directly to contextually relevant instruction is culturally compatible education—an instructional approach characterized by modifications of the communication, social, and behavioral expectations of a child's learning environment (Noonan, 2006; Tharp, 2006). The objective of these modifications is designing educational environments that align with children's cultural expectations, promote their engagement in instruction, and improve learning. As the United States becomes increasingly more culturally and linguistically diverse, there is growing acknowledgment that cultural and linguistic variables are an inextricable part of learning and so must be considered in order to promote the effectiveness of instruction (see Klingner, Blanchett, & Harry, Chapter 4, this volume) Whereas instructional accommodations need to be individualized to address each child's language and culture, some specific cultural modifications have been demonstrated to improve children's engagement in learning. Noonan (2006) provides a detailed list of strategies for supporting language learning in early education settings for children from diverse language and cultural backgrounds. Some examples of these include responding to children's nonverbal communication attempts, using visual cues and other concrete cues when teaching in English, and using cooperative learning methods such as peer helpers and peer tutors.

Focus on Evidence-Based Practice

With the introduction of No Child Left Behind, the U.S. Department of Education began a new emphasis on scientifically based, or evidence-based, education. Evidence-based practice (EBP) involves using scientifically based research to guide educational decisions regarding teaching and learning approaches, strategies, and interventions. Whereas medicine (e.g., Sackett, Richardson, Rosenberg, & Haynes, 1997) and other fields, such as mental health (Geddes, Reynolds, Streiner, & Szatmari, 1997), have embraced EBP for a number of years, it is only recently that the EBP movement has begun to influence early childhood special education (Dunst, Trivette, & Cutspec, 2002).

The intent behind the EBP movement in general and more specifically in education has been to provide information that educators could use to distinguish practices that are supported by rigorous evidence from those that are not. In determinations about what is evidence-based, "rigorous evidence" has been defined not only as the quantity of evidence supporting a practice but also as the quality of research studies that support its merit. This emphasis on EBP reflects the belief that teachers should know what research evidence exists for methods they employ in classrooms and should use those practices that research indicates will be most likely to produce positive outcomes.

To promote the use of evidence-based practice, professional organizations (such as the National Association of School Psychologists) have reviewed the research literature and identified evidence-based practices. Research synthesis groups (e.g., Center for Evidence-Based Practice: Young Children with Challenging Behavior; National Dissemination Center for Children with Disabilities; Research and Training Center on Early Childhood Development; What Works Clearinghouse) also systematically review the research literature to provide usable information on EBP. The Division of Early Childhood (DEC) of the Council for Exceptional Children recently completed a synthesis of the early intervention/early childhood special education (EI/ECSE) research (Smith et al., 2003). This synthesis has been used by DEC to develop a set of recommended-practice guidelines (Sandall, Hemmeter, Smith, & McLean, 2005).

One example of an early childhood EBP is dialogic reading. This technique, a specialized set of procedures for shared book reading with young children, was conceptualized by Whitehurst and colleagues (Whitehurst et al., 1994) and validated through a series of studies (see Justice & Pullen, 2003, for a review). A growing body of evidence indicates that when adults use specific dialogic reading procedures, children make improvements in receptive and expressive vocabulary, narrative skills, and specific early-literacy skills (e.g., Whitehurst et al., 1994). Dialogic reading was recently listed by the What Works Clearinghouse as a practice that produced positive outcomes in oral language (Institute for Education Sciences, 2006).

Promoting Readiness for School

A growing awareness and urgency exists about the importance of the earliest years in a child's life for laying the foundation for later learning, academic success, and positive life outcomes. Studies show that at least half of the educational achievement gaps already exist at kindergarten entry (Lee & Burkham, 2002). Children from low-income families are more likely to start school with limited language skills, health problems, and social and emotional problems that interfere with learning. People who develop programs for young children are realizing that the larger the performance gap is at school entry, the harder it is to close (Shonkoff & Phillips, 2000). As a result, more emphasis than ever is being placed on equipping children with a solid foundation of skills they will need to prepare them for kindergarten and on preparing schools for the greater diversity of children who enter elementary grades (Shore, 1998). Currently, most elementary schools and preschools do not collaborate regularly and have few incentives to do so. The schools relate to different delivery systems, have few resources for collaboration, and have different "cultures." As a result, children entering kindergarten often encounter a classroom and expectations that are qualitatively different from those of their preschool experience, which can disrupt their learning and development (Shore, 1998).

To address this issue, a number of states are advancing the readiness initiative and have identified a set of readiness indicators that encompass children's readiness for school, school readiness for children, and the capacity of communities and families to provide developmental opportunities for their young children (National Schools Readiness Initiative, 2006). The 17 states cooperating in this initiative are using a set of common indicators to track school readiness over time to stimulate policy and program actions to improve all children's ability to read at grade level by third grade. School readiness for children is being measured as related to children's social and emotional development, language development, cognition and general knowledge, approaches to learning, and physical well-being and motor development. Initiatives such as these are pushing early education programs to improve children's readiness to meet kindergarten expectations. As a result, more preschool programs are seeking out and implementing evidence-based practices to help young children learn the skills they need to become more able, confident learners. In addition, community-wide initiatives are supporting more transition planning between elementary school and early education programs.

One critical area for enhancing school readiness that has developed quite rapidly over the past decade is interventions for promoting emergent literacy, that is, the knowledge of and skills in reading and writing that young children obtain prior to achieving conventional literacy. Much has been written about the fact that literacy development starts early in life and is highly correlated with school achievement. Children with disabilities or developmental delays are particularly at risk for experiencing later reading difficulties (Bishop & Adams, 1990; Burns, Griffin, & Snow, 1999). Thus there is growing awareness that interventions for early literacy skills should be part of the set of a preschool curriculum for young children with disabilities or for those who may be at risk for later learning problems (Dickinson, McCabe & Essex, 2006).

A large body of literature points to specific skills of children in the prekindergarten years that predict later reading outcomes (for a review, see Scarborough, 1998). This research has helped define and focus intervention on those skills that are most likely to lead to later success in reading. Phonological awareness and written language awareness, two domains of emergent literacy knowledge, are particularly important to inform models of early identification and early intervention (Justice & Ezell, 2001). Although these areas of knowledge are acquired incidentally by many children through frequent natural interactions with parents and other caregivers (Kaderavek & Justice, 2002), they are much less easily acquired by certain groups (e.g., children with developmental disabilities, children learning English as a second language, children growing up in poverty; Lonigan, Burgess, Anthony, & Barker, 1998). Although a thorough examination of interventions that focus on early literacy is beyond the scope of this chapter, a recent review of these strategies by Justice and Pullen (2003) pointed to three promising evidence-based interventions that have demonstrated their probable efficacy or effectiveness for encouraging emergent literacy outcomes in young children. These were adult–child shared storybook reading (e.g., Crain-Thoreson & Dale, 1999); the use of literacy props and materials in children's dramatic play (e.g., Neuman & Roskos, 1993); and teacher-led games promoting phonological awareness through activities focusing on rhyming, blending, segmenting, and phoneme identity (e.g., van Kleek, Gillam & McFadden, 1998). Each of these practices is increasingly available and appropriate for supporting the early literacy development of many young children with special needs.

Another area in which readiness can be promoted is children's social–emotional learning. Considerable research has been conducted to indicate specific curriculum features that promote social–emotional outcomes in preschoolers (Collaborative for Academic, Social, and Emotional Learning, 2002). Critical elements of effective programs include family involvement, partnerships between professionals and families, implementation across natural environments, assessment-based positive behavior support, and functional and communication-based approaches (Fox, Dunlap, & Cushing, 2002; Walker et al., 1998). In a recent review, Joseph and Strain (2003) used nine criteria to review eight comprehensive social–emotional curricula for preschoolers and to estimate the degree of confidence that the various programs could be positively replicated within an early childhood program. The two programs that received a high confidence rating (i.e., seven or more of the selected criteria) were First Step to Success (Walker et al., 1998), and the Incredible Years Child Training Program (Webster-Stratton, 1990). The Incredible Years: Child Training (CT) program is designed to address the interpersonal difficulties of young children with conduct disorders through direct teaching, videotape modeling, role plays, and ongoing practice. First Step to Success is an early intervention program for at-risk kindergartners who exhibit early signs of antisocial behavior. The program employs universal screening of all kindergartners, classroom intervention, and parent training to promote children's school adjustment.

The ability to interact with peers is an important contributor to children's social–emotional development (Rubin, Bukowski & Parker, 1998). Skills such as gaining the attention of a peer, asking for assistance, or communicating feelings are often a struggle for preschoolers with developmental delays (Guralnick, 1999). Peer-mediated teaching is a validated approach to the direct instruction of social skills (Odom, McConnell, et al., 1999). In this approach, peers are taught to initiate and reciprocate interactions with children with disabilities. Some key examples are social strategies such as making eye contact, inviting a peer to share toys, suggesting play ideas or organizing play, and being responsive or sharing in the play of peers with disabilities (e.g., Goldstein, English, Shafer, & Kaczmarek, 1997; Goldstein, Kaczmarek, Pennington, & Shafer, 1992; Werts, Caldwell, & Wolery, 1996).

Individualizing Level of Support to Child's Level of Need

Although individualizing instruction to young children to match their cultural or language backgrounds is a principle embraced by early education in general, those who teach young children with special needs realize that an additional level of individualization is critical for young children who have disabilities or who are at risk for developmental delays. Individualizing the level of instructional support to match children's level of need has long been a staple in special education practice, and there has been a renewed interest in defining how intervention practices might vary for individual children within inclusive early education settings (Sandall & Schwartz, 2002).

The field of early childhood special education continues to struggle to identify the level of structure appropriate for young children with disabilities. Although naturalistic approaches are used with greater frequency in current practice, they are a contrast to more structured and teacher-driven instructional procedures that were previously recommended for young children with disabilities. Based on behavioral paradigms, intervention programs for preschoolers in earlier decades emphasized addressing children's learning objectives through one-to-one instruction and presenting stimuli in a massed-trial format using errorless learning procedures and relying on high rates of reinforcement. Recent thinking about how to deliver instruction on a specific outcome to a young child with special needs recognizes that each learning objective for each child requires an individualized determination of the level of support or intensity required to give the child the opportunity to acquire, generalize, and maintain the behavior or skill of interest. The least intensive are those based on environmental arrangement (Davis & Fox, 1999), and the most intense or structured often use specific stimulus modification and response prompting techniques in a one-to-one format (Bailey & Wolery, 1992). Although Bailey and McWilliam argued in 1990 that each type of instruction was potentially legitimate and effective for use with young children with disabilities, they also suggested that teachers select the level of intensity and structure that is most "normalized," as well as effective, for each child. What follows is a short description of the continuum of instructional supports that form the array of options for individualizing instruction: arranging the environment, specialized procedures, and integrated approaches.

Arranging the Environment

At the least intrusive level of intervention, changing various aspects of the environment may set the occasion or provide opportunities for children to learn or practice learning goals or objectives. These are deliberate manipulations in specific aspects of the environment, such as: (1) the amount and types of materials made available; (2) the types, sequence, or schedule of activities; (3) the amount or arrangement of space; and (4) the number and characteristics of peers and adults present. In a recent review of environmental supports for promoting social interaction and preventing challenging behaviors, Hemmeter and Ostrosky (2003) reported that children demonstrated higher levels of social interactions in a smaller space than in a larger space, when engaged with social toys versus isolate toys, when involved in socially designed learning centers versus more isolated areas, and in integrated rather than segregated settings. In addition, researchers were able to demonstrate that specific classroom reorganization resulted in higher levels of engagement, play behaviors, compliance, and vocalizations. Much more detail about environmental arrangements is available from other sources (Lawry, Danko, & Strain, 1999; Noonan & McCormick, 2006; Sainato & Carta, 1992).

Several researchers have underscored the point that even when aspects of the environment are carefully arranged to promote acquisition of specific behaviors, the expected changes in target behaviors do not necessarily occur without more direct intervention (Goldstein & Kaczmarek, 1992). For example, putting children in a carefully defined play area with adequate toys does not necessarily result in increases in their social interactions (Kohler & Strain, 1999). Instead, adult prompting of conversations using specialized procedures, described in the next section, might be necessary to increase child–child talk (e.g., Filla, Wolery, & Anthony, 1999).

Specialized Procedures

A second level of intervention strategies to teach children goals and objectives includes a set of more specific and direct intervention strategies. These can be grouped into the following categories: (1) responsive-interaction strategies; (2) naturalistic or milieu teaching strategies; and (3) reinforcement-based procedures. Although the research on these procedures is not new, the procedures are the foundation for some of the more complex and comprehensive interventions that have been developed more recently.

Responsive-interaction procedures are a set of strategies aimed at fostering communication between a child and adults in a conversational context within the child's natural environment. These procedures are especially useful when the goal is to promote children's attempts at communicating their wants and needs, to teach them how to explore their environment, and to learn cause-and-effect relationships (Dunst et al., 1987). Responsive-interaction strategies include following the child's lead about the focus and pace of interactions, responding contingently to the child's behavior with animated and exaggerated expressions, providing models of more elaborate behavior, and taking turns in interactions with the child. An extensive literature documents not only that responsive-interaction strategies are effective for promoting communication (e.g., Yoder et al., 1995) but also that parents and other caregivers can learn to implement these strategies and embed them into natural routines in homes and classrooms (see Dunst & Kassow, 2004, for a review).

Naturalistic or milieu teaching strategies are a set of procedures that were developed based on the way parents and other caregivers typically interact with their young children. Derived from research by Hart and Risley (1968, 1975), the procedures are based on the notion that parents typically talk about objects and events that attract their children's attention, imitate and expand on their children's attempts at communication, and repeat and clarify words that their children do not seem to understand. Their research spawned a set of strategies for promoting communication that form the basis of naturalistic or enhanced milieu teaching procedures. Three specific procedures are typically included in milieu teaching: (1) the mand-model procedure, (2) naturalistic time delay, and (3) incidental teaching (Kaiser & Trent, Chapter 11, this volume). Although these procedures were developed and initially implemented for use in promoting communication skills, they have been shown to be effective in teaching social and other skills (e.g., Brown, McEvoy, & Bishop, 1991) and for teaching children in settings that range from classrooms to homes to child-care settings (Noonan & McCormick, 2006).

Several reinforcement-based procedures exist, including differential reinforcement; response shaping; behavioral momentum, or high-probability, procedures (e.g., Davis & Brady, 1993); and correspondence training (Wolery & Sainato, 1996). These procedures are often useful for increasing the complexity, frequency, and duration of children's behavior, for promoting more engagement and play, and for encouraging appropriate behavior. One example of these, behavior momentum, relies on delivering a set of simple requests (usually three–five) to which there is a high probability that the child will respond (a "high-p" request), followed immediately by a request to which the child is *not* likely to respond (a "low-p" request) . This procedure appears to work because the initial sequence of high-p requests generates an increased rate of positive responses and a corresponding high rate of reinforcement. Together these create a behavioral momentum that increases the probability that the child will respond to a low-p request. These procedures were initially used to reduce noncompliance in classrooms and other settings (Davis & Brady, 1993), but over time they have been extended to a broad range of behavioral outcomes, including teaching social skills, responding to indirect questions and comments, and increased use of augmentative communication devices (e.g., Davis & Reichle, 1996; Santos & Lignugaris/Kraft, 1999).

Integrated Approaches

Most recent trends in instructional approaches for preschoolers with disabilities focus on methods that integrate multiple types of intervention procedures and attempt to individualize instruction within the context of classroom teaching. One approach, called activity-based instruction (ABI; Pretti-Frontczak & Bricker, 2004), is characterized by its method of individualizing instruction by integrating intervention approaches and embedding them in the course of natural interactions across the classroom day. ABI is considered a naturalistic child-directed approach to intervention because of the emphasis on following the child's interests and actions. Key features of ABI include the use of routine, planned, or child-initiated activities; embedding a child's individual goals or objectives in routine, planned, or child-initiated activities; using logically occurring antecedents and consequences; and selecting target skills that are functional and generative. Although the empirical literature documenting the effectiveness of these approaches is in its infancy, some studies suggest that they are more effective than didactic procedures in promoting skill generalization (e.g., Losardo & Bricker, 1994).

A second integrated approach to intervention is the use of three-tiered models. This cutting-edge trend employs more systematic approaches to identifying children who are at risk for problems in learning and behavior and responds with appropriate levels of evidence-based intervention. This approach, sometimes referred to as a "three-tiered model of intervention" or response to intervention (RTI) model, is being widely used with school-age children as a means of preventing and intervening in learning disabilities or serious behavior problems. This model is based on three components: (1) high-quality instruction/intervention, matched to student need, that has been demonstrated through research and practice to produce high rates of learning; (2) decision making about the intensity of intervention a student needs based on measurement of student's growth and level of learning and behavior; (3) multiple tiers of intervention that vary in intensity and determining students' needed level of intensity based on data about their responses to intervention (National Association of State Directors of Special Education and Council of Administrators of Special Education, 2006).

Although some of the components of three-tiered models have been applied to programs for children younger than school age, no early childhood model has yet emerged that contains all three of the components listed. Fox and her colleagues (Fox, Dunlap, Hemmeter, Joseph, & Strain, 2003) have developed a model of prevention and intervention called the "teaching pyramid," which is probably the model that comes closest to a three-tiered model. The teaching pyramid describes early education practices needed to promote social–emotional development and behavior of all children. Their model borrows some of the same features of the three-tiered models but lays them out into a four-level hierarchy that includes: (1) promoting positive relationships with children, families, and colleagues; (2) implementing classroom preventive practices; (3) utilizing of social–emotional teaching strategies; and (4) using positive behavior support. Although research on the use of the entire model has not yet been conducted, each level of the hierarchy is based on a set of evidence-based and effective practices and is available to practitioners in early intervention, early education, and community-based child-care settings (Center for the Social–Emotional Foundation for Early Learning, 2006).

SUMMARY AND CONCLUSION

Although several trends affect where, what, and how young children with disabilities receive instruction, probably nothing affects the quality of the intervention they receive more than the level of training that adults who care for them receive. As research continues to expand the options of the strategies and practices that are evidence based and developmentally appropriate, one of the biggest challenges is the high-fidelity implementation of these practices on a frequent basis in the variety of environments (classrooms, child-care settings, homes, and other community settings) in which young children spend their days. Young children with disabilities typically receive instruction from a number of different "teachers." In past decades, early intervention to preschoolers with disabilities was delivered by an early childhood special educator and occasionally by a range of therapists. These persons are still instrumental in educating these young children, but their roles are changing as more young children with disabilities receive instruction and care in inclusive community-based settings. The role of the interventionist becomes one of instructing adults in these settings in how to help the children with disabilities in their charge.

Thus research is needed in how to translate evidence-based practices to individuals with a range of (and oftentimes limited) background knowledge and training. Promoting faster rates of translation of research about effective interventions into actual practice is a major focus of other fields, such as medicine, and is part of a major initiative in the National Institutes of Health (Zerhouni, 2005). There is a growing acknowledgment that, to close the gap between available research-based strategies and their actual implementation, new and creative approaches to dissemination are needed. We need a clearer identification and articulation of practices that are evidence based, and we need professional development, training, and technical assistance in their use. Practitioners in early intervention and early childhood educators who serve young children with special needs and their families need an "on demand" training and technical assistance system that: (1) focuses on the best available information, including easy-to-access and highly reliable summaries of effective intervention procedures and programs; (2) develops multiple methods for distributing this information in forms well suited to particular audiences; (3) pairs information distribution with focused, effective professional development interventions in ways that make it easier, and much more likely, that procedures will be adopted in various settings. Our focus in the coming decade must be on ways to ensure the high fidelity and intensive implementation of known effective interventions in ways that contribute directly to improved outcomes for children with disabilities throughout the country.

REFERENCES

Bailey, D. B., & McWilliam, R. A. (1990). Normalizing early intervention. *Topics in Early Childhood Special Education, 10*(2), 33–47.

Bailey, D. B., & Wolery, M. (1992). *Teaching infants and preschoolers with disabilities* (2nd ed.). New York: Macmillan.

Bennett-Gates, D., & Zigler, E. (1998). Resolving the developmental-difference debate: An evaluation of the triarchic and systems theory models. In J. A. Burack, R. M., Hodapp, & E. Zigler (Eds.), *Handbook of mental retardation and development* (pp. 115–131). New York: Cambridge University Press.

Bishop, D. V. M., & Adams, C. (1990). A prospective study of the relationship between specific language impairment, phonological disorders and reading retardation. *Journal of Child Psychology and Psychiatry, 31,* 1027–1050.

Bodrova, E., Leong, D., & Shore, R. (2004). *Child outcome standards in pre-k programs: What are standards; what is needed to make them work?* Retrieved October 2, 2006, from *http://nieer.org/resources/policybriefs/5.pdf.*

Bowman, B. T., Donovan, M. S., & Burns, M. S. (Eds.). (2000). *Eager to learn: Educating our preschoolers.* Washington, DC: National Academy Press.

Bredekamp, S. (1987). *Developmentally appropriate practice in early childhood programs serving children from birth through age 8* (expanded ed.). Washington, DC: National Association for the Education of Young Children.

Bredekamp, S., & Copple, C. (1997). *Developmentally appropriate practice in early childhood programs* (rev. ed.). Washington, DC: National Association for the Education of Young Children.

Bricker, D., Pretti-Frontczak, K., & McComas, N. (1998). *An activity-based approach to early intervention* (2nd ed.). Baltimore: Brookes.

Brown, W. H., McEvoy, M.A., & Bishop, N. (1991). Incidental teaching of social behavior. *Teaching Exceptional Children, 24*(1), 35–38.

Burns, M. S., Griffin, P., & Snow, C. E. (Eds.). (1999). *Starting out right: A guide to promoting children's reading success.* Washington, DC: National Academy Press.

Carta, J. J., & Greenwood, C. R. (1997). Barriers to implementation of effective educational practices for young children with disabilities. In J. W. Lloyd, E. J. Kame'enui, & D. Chard (Eds.), *Issues in educating students with disabilities* (pp. 261–274). Mahwah, NJ: Erlbaum.

Carta, J. J., Schwartz, I. S., Atwater, J. B., & McConnell, S. R. (1991). Developmentally appropriate practice: Appraising its usefulness for young children with disabilities. *Topics in Early Childhood Special Education, 11*(1), 1–20.

Center for the Social–Emotional Foundation for Early Learning (CSEFEL). (2006). Retrieved October 31, 2006, from *csefel.uiuc.edu.*

Collaborative for Academic, Social, and Emotional Learning. (2002). *Safe and sound: Educational leader's guide to evidence-based social and emotional learning programs.* Retrieved July 18, 2002, from *www.casel.org.*

Crain-Thoreson, C., & Dale, P. S. (1999). Enhancing linguistic performance: Parents and teachers as book reading partners for children with language delays. *Topics in Early Childhood Special Education, 19,* 28–39.

Davis, C. A., & Brady, M. P. (1993). Expanding the utility of behavioral momentum with young children: Where we've been, where we need to go. *Journal of Early Intervention, 17,* 211–223.

Davis, C. A., & Fox, J. (1999). Evaluating environmental arrangement as setting events: Review and implications for measurement. *Journal of Behavioral Education, 9,* 77–96.

Davis, C. A., & Reichle, J. (1996). Variant and invariant high-probability requests: Increasing appropriate behaviors in children with emotional–behavioral disorders. *Journal of Applied Behavior Analysis, 19,* 471–482.

Dickinson, D., McCabe, A. A., & Essex, M. J. (2006). A window of opportunity we must open to all: The case for preschool with high-quality support for language and literacy. In S. B. Neuman & D. K. Dickinson (Eds.), *Handbook of early literacy research* (2nd ed., pp. 11–28). New York: Guilford Press.

Dunst, C. J., Bruder, M. B., Trivette, C. M., Hamby, D. W., Raab, M., & McLean, M. (2001). Characteristics and consequences of everyday natural learning opportunities. *Topics in Early Childhood Special Education, 21,* 68–92.

Dunst, C. J., & Kassow, D. Z. (2004). Characteristics of interventions promoting parental sensitivity to child behavior. *Bridges, 3*(3), 1–17. Retrieved February 7, 2006, from *www.researchtopractice.info/ bridges/bridges_vol2_no5.pdf.*

Dunst, C. J., Lesko, J. J., Holbert, K. A.,Wilson, I. I., Sharpe, K. L., & Liles, R. F. (1987). A systematic approach to infant intervention. *Topics in Early Childhood Special Education, 7*(2), 19–37.

Dunst, C. J., Trivette, C. M., & Cutspec, P. A. (2002). An evidence-based approach to documenting the characteristics and consequences of early intervention practices. *Centerscope, 1*(2), 1–6. Retrieved February 7, 2006, from *www.evidencebasedpractices.org/centerscope/centerscopevol1no2.pdf.*

Falvey, M., Brown, L., Lyon, S., Baumgart, D., & Schroeder, J. (1980). Strategies for using cues and correction procedures. In W. Sailor, B. Wilcox, & L. Brown (Eds.), *Method of instruction for severely handicapped students* (pp. 109–133). Baltimore: Brookes.

Filla, A., Wolery, M., & Anthony, L. (1999). Promoting children's conversations during play with adult prompts. *Journal of Early Intervention, 22,* 93–108.

Fox, L. G., Dunlap, G., & Cushing, L. (2002). Early intervention, positive behavior support, and transition to school. *Journal of Emotional and Behavior Disorders, 10,* 149–157.

Fox, L., Dunlap, G., Hemmeter, M. L., Joseph, G., & Strain, P. (2003). The teaching pyramid: A model for supporting social competence and preventing challenging behavior in young children. *Young Children, 58*(4), 48–52.

Geddes, J., Reynolds, S., Streiner, D., & Szatmari, P. (1997). Evidence based practice in mental health. *British Medical Journal, 315,* 1483–1484.

Gilliam, W. S., Meisels, S. J., & Mayes, L. C. (2005). Screening and surveillance in early intervention systems. In M. J. Guralnick (Ed.), *The developmental systems approach to early intervention* (pp. 73–98). Baltimore: Brookes.

Goldstein, H., English, K., Shafer, K., & Kaczmarek, L. (1997). Interaction among preschoolers with and without disabilities: Effects of across-the-day peer intervention. *Journal of Speech, Language, and Hearing Research, 40,* 33–48.

Goldstein, H., & Kaczmarek, L. (1992) Promoting communicative interaction among children in integrated intervention settings. In S. F. Warren & J. Reichle (Series & Vol. Eds.), *Communication and language intervention: Vol. 1. Causes and effects in communication and language intervention* (pp. 81–111). Baltimore: Brookes.

Goldstein, H., Kaczmarek, L., Pennington, R., & Shafer, K. (1992). Peer-mediated intervention: Attending to, commenting on, and acknowledging the behavior of preschoolers with autism. *Journal of Applied Behavior Analysis, 25,* 289–305.

Good Start, Grow Start Interagency Workgroup. (2006). *Good Start, Grow Smart: A guide to Good Start, Grow Smart and other federal early learning initiatives.* Retrieved October 31, 2006, from *www. acf.hhs.gov/programs/ccb/ta/gsgs/fedpubs/GSGSBooklet.pdf.*

Guralnick, M. J. (1998). Effectiveness of early intervention for vulnerable children: A developmental perspective. *American Journal on Mental Retardation, 102,* 319–345.

Guralnick, M. J. (1999). Family and child influences on the peer related social competence of young children with developmental delays. *Mental Retardation and Developmental Disabilities Research Reviews, 5,* 21–29.

Guralnick, M. J. (2001). Framework for change in early childhood inclusion. In M. J. Guralnick (Ed.), *Early childhood inclusion* (pp. 1–35). Baltimore: Brookes.

Hart, B. M., & Risley, T. R. (1968). Establishing the use of descriptive adjectives in the spontaneous speech of disadvantaged preschool children. *Journal of Applied Behavior Analysis, 1,* 109–120.

Hart, B. M., & Risley, T. R. (1975). Incidental teaching of language in the preschool. *Journal of Applied Behavior Analysis, 8,* 411–420.

Hemmeter, M. L., & Ostrosky, M. (2003). Executive summary: Classroom preventive practices. In G. Dunlap, M. Conroy, L. Kern, G. DuPaul, J. VanBrakle, P. Strain, G. E. Joseph, M. L. Hemmeter, & M. Ostrosky (Eds.), *Research synthesis on effective intervention procedures: Executive summary.* Tampa, FL: University of South Florida, Center for Evidence-Based Practice: Young Children with Challenging Behavior.

Institute for Education Sciences. (2006, October 12). *WWC intervention report: Dialogic reading.* Retrieved October 31, 2006, from *www.whatworks.ed.gov/PDF/Intervention/WWC_Dialogic_Reading_101206.pdf.*

Joseph, G. E., & Strain, P. S. (2003). Comprehensive evidence-based social–emotional curricula for young children: An analysis of efficacious adoption potential. *Topics in Early Childhood Special Education, 23,* 65–76.

Justice, L. M., & Ezell, H. K. (2001). Written language awareness in preschool children from low-income households: A descriptive analysis. *Communication Disorders Quarterly, 22,* 123–134.

Justice, L. M., & Pullen, P. C. (2003). Promising intervention for promoting emergent literacy skills: Three evidence-based approaches. *Topics in Early Childhood Special Education, 23,* 99–113.

Kaderavek, J., & Justice, L. M. (2002). Use of storybook reading to increase print awareness in at-risk children. *American Journal of Speech–Language Pathology, 9,* 257–269.

Kelly, J., & Booth, C. (1999). Child care for infants with special needs: Issues and applications. *Infants and Young Children, 12,* 26–33.

Kohler, F. W., & Strain, P. S. (1999). Maximizing peer-mediated resources in integrated preschool classrooms. *Topics in Early Childhood Special Education, 19,* 319–345.

Lawry, J., Danko, C., & Strain, P. (1999). Examining the role of the classroom environment in the prevention of problem behaviors. In S. Sandall & M. Ostrosky (Eds.), *Young exceptional children: Practical ideas for addressing challenging behaviors* (pp. 49–62). Longmont, CO: Sopris West, Denver, CO: Division for Early Childhood.

Lee, V., & Burkham, D. T. (2002). *Inequality at the starting gate: Social background differences in achievement as children begin kindergarten.* Washington, DC: Washington Economic Policy Institute.

Lonigan, C. J., Burgess, S. R., Anthony, J. L., & Barker, T. A. (1998). Development of phonological sensitivity in 2- to 5-year old children. *Journal of Educational Psychology, 90,* 294–311.

Losardo, A., & Bricker, D. (1994). Activity-based intervention and direct instruction: A comparison study. *American Journal on Mental Retardation, 98,* 744–765.

McCormick, L. (2006). Perspectives, policies, and practices. In M. J. Noonan & L. McCormick (Eds.), *Young children with disabilities in natural environments* (pp. 1–25). Baltimore: Brookes.

McWilliam, R., Wolery, M., & Odom, S. L. (2001). *Instructional perspectives in inclusive preschool classrooms.* In M. J. Guralnick (Ed.), *Early childhood inclusion: Focus on change* (pp. 506–530). Baltimore: Brookes.

National Association of State Directors of Special Education and Council of Administrators of Special Education. (2006). *Response to intervention: NASDSE and CASE White Paper on RTI.* Retrieved October 31, 2006, from *www.nasdse.org/documents/RTIAnadministratorsPerspective1-06.pdf.*

National Early Childhood Technical Assistance Center. (2006). *Child and family outcomes.* Retrieved October 17, 2006, from *www.nectac.org/topics/quality/childfam.asp.*

National Schools Readiness Initiative. (2006). *Who we are.* Retrieved July 3, 2006, from *www.gettingready.org.*

Neuman, S. B., & Roskos, K. (1993). Access to print for children of poverty: Differential effects of adult mediation and literacy-enriched play settings on environmental and functional print tasks. *American Educational Research Journal, 30,* 95–122.

No Child Left Behind Act of 2001, Public Law No. 107–110. Retrieved October 31, 2006, from *www.ed.gov/nclb/overview/intro/factsheet.html.*

Noonan, M. J. (2006). Designing culturally relevant instruction. In M. J. Noonan & L. McCormick (Eds.), *Young children with disabilities in natural environments* (pp. 151–169). Baltimore: Brookes.

Noonan, M. J., & McCormick, L. (2006). *Young children with disabilities in natural environments.* Baltimore: Brookes.

Odom, S. L., Horn, E. M., Marquart, J. M., Hanson, M. J., Wolfberg, P., Beckman, P., et al. (1999). On the forms of inclusion: Organizational context and individualized service models. *Journal of Early Intervention, 22*, 185–199.

Odom, S. L., McConnell, S. R., McEvoy, M. A., Peterson, C., Ostrosky, M., Chandler, L. K., et al. (1999). Relative effects of interventions supporting the social competence of young children with disabilities in early childhood special education. *Topics in Early Childhood Special Education, 19*(2), 75–91.

The President's Commission on Excellence in Special Education. (2002). *A new era-revitalizing special education for children and families.* Retrieved February 4, 2007, from *www.ed.gov/inits/commissions-boards/whspecialeducation/reports/images/Pres_Rep.pdf.*

Pretti-Frontczak, K., & Bricker, D. (2004). *An activity-based approach to early intervention* (3rd ed.). Baltimore: Brookes.

Ramey, C. T., & Ramey, S. L. (1998). Early intervention and early experience. *American Psychologist, 53*, 109–120.

Rubin, K. H., Bukowski, W., & Parker, J. G. (1998). Peer interactions, relationships, and groups. In W. Damon (Ed.), *Handbook of child psychology* (5th ed., Vol. 3, pp. 619–700). New York: Wiley.

Sackett, D. L., Richardson, W. S., Rosenberg, W., & Haynes, R. B. (1997). *Evidence-based medicine: How to practice and teach EBM.* New York: Churchill Livingstone.

Sailor, W., & Guess, D. (1983). *Severely handicapped students: An instructional design.* Boston: Houghton Mifflin.

Sainato, D. M., & Carta, J. J. (1992). Classroom influences on the development and social competence in young children with disabilities. In S. L. Odom, S. R. McConnell, & M. A. McEvoy (Eds.), *Social competence of young children with disabilities: Issues and strategies for intervention* (pp. 93–109). Baltimore: Brookes.

Sandall, S. R., Hemmeter, M. L., Smith, B., & McLean, M. (2005). *DEC recommended practices: A comprehensive guide.* Missoula, MT: Division for Early Childhood.

Sandall, S. R., & Schwartz, I. S. (2002). *Building blocks for teaching preschoolers with special needs.* Baltimore: Brookes.

Santos, R. M., & Lignugaris/Kraft, B. (1999). The effects of direct questions on preschool children's responses to indirect requests. *Journal of Behavioral Education, 9*, 193–210.

Scarborough, H. S. (1998). Early identification of children at risk for reading difficulties: Phonological awareness and some other promising predictors. In B. K. Shapiro, P. J. Accardo, & A. J. Capute (Eds.), *Specific reading disability: A view of the spectrum* (pp. 75–99). Timonium, MD: York Press.

Shonkoff, J., & Phillips, D. A (Eds.). (2000). *From neurons to neighborhoods: The science of early childhood development.* Washington, DC: National Academy of Sciences.

Shore, R. (1998). *Ready schools: A report of the Goal 1 Ready Schools Resource Group.* Retrieved July 3, 2006, from *www.ode.state.or.us/superintendent/priorities/ready4school/readysch.pdf.*

Smith, B. J., Strain, P. S., Snyder, P., Sandall, S. R., McLean, M. E., Ramsey, A. B., et al. (2003). DEC recommended practices: A review of 9 years of EI/ECSE research literature. *Journal of Early Intervention, 25*, 108–119.

Strain, P., McConnell, S. R., Carta, J. J., Fowler, S. A., Neisworth, J. T., & Wolery, M. (1992). Behaviorism in early intervention. *Topics in Early Childhood Special Education, 12*, 121–141.

Tharp, R. G. (2006). Psychocultural variables and constants: Effects on teaching and learning in schools. *American Psychologist, 44*, 349–359.

van Kleck, A., Gillam, R. B., & McFadden, T. U. (1998). A study of classroom-based phonological awareness training for preschoolers with speech and/or language disorders. *American Journal of Speech–Language Pathology, 7*, 65–76.

Walker, H., Kavanaugh, K., Stiller, B., Golly, A., Severson, H., & Feil, E. (1998). First step to success: An early intervention approach for preventing school antisocial behavior. *Journal of Emotional and Behavioral Disorders, 6*, 66–81.

Webster-Stratton, C. (1990). *Dinosaur social skills and problem-solving training manual.* Seattle, WA: Incredible Years.

Werts, M. G., Caldwell, N. K., & Wolery, M. (1996). Peer modeling of response chains: Observational learning by students with disabilities. *Journal of Applied Behavior Analysis, 29*, 53–66.

Whitehurst, G. J., Arnold, D. S., Epstein, J. N., Angell, A. L., Smith, M., & Fischel, J. E. (1994). A picture book reading intervention in day care and home for children from low-income families. *Developmental Psychology, 30,* 679–689.

Wolery, M., Huffman, A., Holcombe, C. B., Martin, J., Brookfield, J., Schroeder, C., et al. (1994). Preschool mainstreaming: Perceptions of barriers and benefits by faculty in general early childhood education. *Teacher Education and Special Education, 17*(1), 1–9.

Wolery, M., & Sainato, D. M. (1996). General curriculum and intervention strategies. In S. L. Odom & M. McLean (Eds.), *Recommended practices in early intervention* (pp. 125–158). Austin, TX: PRO-ED.

Wolery, M., Strain, P. S., & Bailey, D. B. (1992). Reaching potential of children with special needs. In S. Bredekamp & T. Rosengrant (Eds.), *Reaching potentials: Appropriate curriculum and assessment for young children* (Vol. 1, pp. 92–111). Washington, DC: NAEYC.

Yoder, P., Kaiser, A., Goldstein, H., Alpert, C., Mousetis, L., Kaczmarek, L., et al. (1995). An exploratory comparison of milieu teaching and responsive interaction in classroom applications. *Journal of Early Intervention, 19,* 218–242.

Zerhouni, E. A. (2005). Translational and clinical science: Time for a new vision. *New England Journal of Medicine, 353,* 1621–1623.

Early Intervention for Children with Autism Spectrum Disorder

Samuel L. Odom
Sally Rogers
Christopher J. McDougle
Kara Hume
Gail McGee

From its first discovery within a clinical sample of 11 children seen at a psychiatric clinic at Johns Hopkins University (Kanner, 1943), autism has emerged as a highly prevalent developmental disability and has captured the attention of a world audience. A belief that is supported by mounting evidence is that provision of organized, effective intervention services when children with autism are very young will have significant positive effects on their current and subsequent development in later years. Researchers have conducted detailed and exhaustive reviews of early-intervention techniques and programs (National Research Council, 2001; Harris, Handleman, & Jennett, 2005). Rather than repeating their efforts, the purpose of this chapter is to examine the most critical new knowledge associated with early intervention for children with autism and the implications of this research for social policy and practice. After a brief discussion of diagnostic and definitional terminology and prevalence, we examine the most current research on early diagnosis, comprehensive and focused intervention approaches for preschool children, emerging interventions for infants and toddlers, and psycho-pharmacological treatment for young children. In the conclusion, we offer implications for future research, social policy, and treatment practice.

DIAGNOSIS, CLASSIFICATION, CHARACTERISTICS, AND PREVALENCE

As with the definition of developmental disabilities (see Odom, Horner, Snell, & Blacher, Chapter 1, this volume), multiple definitions of autism exist and are associated with their use or function. Clinical definitions are important for precise medical diagnoses and specification of participant samples in biomedical and behavior research. The most widely cited clinical definition in the United States is from the American Psychiatric Association's (1994) *Diagnostic and Statistical Manual of Mental Disorders* (DSM-IV), which defines "autistic disorder" as evidence for qualitative impairments in social interaction and communication; restrictive, repetitive, and/or stereotyped behavior, interests, or activities; onset before 3 years of age; and presenting characteristics not attributable to Rett's syndrome or childhood disintegrative disorder. The *International Classification of Diseases* (ICD-10) issued by the World Health Organization (1992) has a nearly identical set of criteria for "autism disorder," although the specific diagnostic features differ slightly. Sophisticated, detailed, and psychometrically sound diagnostic instruments, such as the Autism Diagnostic Observation Schedule (ADOS; Lord, Rutter, DiLavore, & Risi, 1999) and the Childhood Autism Rating Scale (CARS; Schopler, Reichler, & Renner, 1988), have been developed and used for preschool- and school-age children (see Lord & Corsello, 2005, for a comprehensive review).

Definitions of autism also qualify children for educational services. In the United States, the Individuals with Disabilities Education Improvement Act (IDEIA; U.S. Department of Education, 2004), establishes an eligibility definition of "autism" as "a developmental disability significantly affecting verbal and nonverbal communication and social interaction, generally evident before age 3, that adversely affects a child's educational performance" (Part A, Section 300.7).

U.S. and international discussions often use the term "autism spectrum disorder" (ASD). ASD extend the conceptualization of autism to a set of related characteristics that may exist across a spectrum or continuum. Although not an official clinical diagnosis, ASD now commonly includes specific disabilities that appear in DSM-IV under a broader heading of "pervasive developmental disorders" (Strock, 2004). The disabilities include autistic disorder (as noted), pervasive development disorder—not otherwise specified (PDD-NOS), Asperger syndrome, Rett syndrome, and childhood disintegrative disorder. In describing research in this chapter, we use the term "autism" to refer to the DSM-IV and ICH-10 definitions noted previously and "ASD" to refer to the common definition just noted. Our usage of the term, when citing specific research, reflects the researchers' terminology in their published articles.

For children with ASD, several demographic characteristics of the population have been identified. Children with ASD are predominantly male (75%), and the disability is not related to ethnicity or social class. Etiology is now commonly assumed to be genetic, neurological, and/or physiological, although specific etiology or sets of etiologies have yet to be determined (see Tartaglia, Hansen, & Hagerman, Chapter 6, this volume). Although early studies estimated that 70–80% of individuals with autism had mental retardation (MR), the broadening of the disability to ASD and improved assessment techniques have resulted in a much lower MR comorbidity estimate (25–52%; Shea & Mesibov, 2005).

Prevalence (i.e., the proportion of the population with ASD) and incidence (i.e., the number of new cases of ASD during a given year) have been an issue of much public debate. The prevalence of autism and ASD has increased tremendously over the past two decades. Studies from the 1960s through the mid-1980s (i.e., before ASD became prominent) found prevalence rates of 0.7/10,000 to around 2/10,000 (Zahner & Pauls, 1987). In 2005, Fombonne estimated the current prevalence rates for ASD as between 35/10,000 and 60/10,000. Although popular discussions of ASD address the "epidemic" of autism, Fombonne (2003) proposed that at least four variables are related to the increase in prevalence: (1) expansion of the definition from autism to ASD; (2) improved methods of surveillance, resulting in more cases being found; (3) diagnostic "substitution" (i.e., some children previously diagnosed with mental retardation now being diagnosed with ASD); and (4) increased secular interest in ASD. As is noted in a subsequent section, the increasingly sophisticated and accurate methods for early identification and diagnosis may well add to the increased incidence and prevalence in the future.

EARLY IDENTIFICATION AND DIAGNOSIS

In their "road map" for research in ASD, the Interagency Autism Coordinating Committee (IACC; 2003), organized through the National Institute of Mental Health (NIMH), predicted that feasible, sensitive screening methods for young infants with ASD would be developed in the next 7–10 years. During the past 5 years, researchers have examined the validity and reliability of diagnosing autism spectrum disorders in 2-year-olds. Longitudinal studies carried out by several groups in both the United States and the United Kingdom have confirmed the validity and reliability of ASD diagnoses at age 2 when carried out by clinicians experienced in ASD diagnosis in general and specifically for 2-year-olds with autism.

Studies by Lord (1995) and Stone et al. (1999) report consistent differences in many developmental areas in 2-year-olds with ASD compared with 2-year-olds with general delays. Deficits in language development and in use of preverbal communicative gestures are a primary symptom of ASD at this age. Lord (1997) reported that 97% of a large group of 2-year-olds with autism scored one or more standard deviations below the mean in expressive language and that they had much greater language developmental deficits relative to their nonverbal abilities than did children with other delays. Receptive language was as delayed as expressive language in this sample. Imitative behavior is also affected in autism, with more immature productions and less frequent imitation of actions on objects, gestural, facial, oral, and vocal imitation (Rogers, Hepburn, Stackhouse, & Wehner, 2003). Decreased variety and frequency of functional and symbolic play (Wetherby, Prizant, & Hutchinson, 1998; Lord, 1995) has been consistently reported, although sensorimotor play has not consistently shown differences (Mundy, Sigman, Ungerer, & Sherman, 1987). Abnormal sensory behaviors have been found to distinguish 2-year-olds with autism from groups of children with other delays in some studies (Lord, 1995; Rogers, Hepburn, & Wehner, 2003) but not others (Cox et al., 1999; Stone & Hogan, 1993).

Thus a specific phenotype of ASD exists at age 2, and it appears to be stable across the early childhood years. Lord (1995) examined 30 children, half diagnosed with autism and half with other delays, at age 2 and again 1 year later. Only 3 out of these 30 changed diagnostic groups over this time period. Similarly, Cox et al. (1999) followed nine 20-month-olds diagnosed with autism to age 42 months, when all continued to meet ASD criteria. Stone et al. (1999) reported that 96% of 2-year-olds diagnosed with an ASD continued to have ASD when seen again at age 3. However, finer discrimination among early diagnoses of autistic disorder and PDD-NOS are not reliable, either in terms of interrater agreement or stability over time (Stone et al., 1999; Cox et al., 1999).

Use of typical autism diagnostic tools with 2-year-olds is a concern, as most were validated on older samples. Well-validated tools such as the Autism Diagnostic Interview—Revised (ADI-R; Lord, Rutter, & Le Couteur, 1994) and the Childhood

Autism Rating Scale (CARS; Schopler et al., 1988) were developed for a somewhat older sample and have been found to be overinclusive when used with 2-year-olds and with nonverbal children with mental ages under 18 months (Lord & Corsello, 2005). Even the DSM-IV criteria for diagnosing autistic disorder may underdiagnose 2-year-olds, as several of the symptoms listed are not expected in children so young (Rogers, 2001; Stone et al., 1999). Current tools for which some published supportive data exist regarding use with 2-year-olds include the Autism Diagnostic Observation Schedule (ADOS), which involves a 25-minute interactive play-based interview (Lord, Rutter, & DiLavore, 1997), the Screening Tool for Autism in Two-Year-Olds (STAT; Stone, Coonrod, Turner, & Pozdol, 2004), described subsequently, and the Parent Interview for Autism (Stone & Hogan, 1993).

Before diagnosis, young children with delays typically undergo a screening process, and screening tools with strong sensitivity and specificity for autism are the focus of significant research at this time. General screening tools such as the Ages and Stages Questionnaire (Bricker & Squires, 1999) or the Parents' Evaluation of Developmental Status (PEDS; Glascoe, 1998) will identify toddlers at risk for developmental delays—including those with autism—due to immature milestones in one or another developmental area. But these tools will not differentiate toddlers at risk for autism from those with other developmental risks.

The first tool developed to detect autism risk in a general population, the Checklist for Autism in Toddlers (CHAT; Baron-Cohen, Allen, & Gillberg, 1992), designed for 18-month-olds, has been found to have strong specificity but only moderate sensitivity when used in population screening. The CHAT is a very brief tool that involves several questions to the mother and several behavioral probes with the child. Slight alterations in scoring procedures may increase the sensitivity of this tool in clinical populations (Scambler, Rogers, & Wehner, 2001). A parent questionnaire version with additional questions, the M-CHAT (Robins, Fein, Barton, & Green, 2001), has also been developed. Initial research has demonstrated high levels of specificity and sensitivity when used with a clinically referred large sample of children, but there have not yet been population-based studies of this instrument (Coonrod & Stone, 2005).

The STAT is a recently published screening tool that is administered individually (Stone, Coonrod, & Ousley, 2000). Unlike the above level-1 screening tools, which are developed for the purpose of detecting autism risk in a population sample, the STAT is a level-2 screener, constructed to differentiate autism from other developmental disorders. The STAT is individually administered in about 20 minutes, but training is required to use the measure. Psychometric studies of this tool in an autism clinic setting demonstrated acceptable levels of sensitivity, specificity, and positive and negative predictive value and very high agreement with ADOS scores (Stone et al., 2004).

The extent to which we can reliably and validly identify or diagnose children with autism younger than 24 months old is still an empirical question. Infants with autism often demonstrate symptoms in the first year of life. Studies involving parental reports and video analysis consistently report differences between behaviors of children who will be diagnosed with autism from those of children who have other kinds of delays. Parents report differences in imitation, social responsivity, sensory and repetitive behaviors, and communicative behaviors (Rogers, 2001). Studies of home videos taken on or before the first birthday reveal differences in the amount of time spent looking at others and in responses to their names being called. Interestingly, neither the presence of repetitive behaviors nor the lack of joint attention behavior appears to discriminate children who will later be diagnosed with autism from those who will later be diagnosed with other kinds of delays (Osterling, Dawson, & Munson, 2002; Baranek, 1999).

A new strategy for studying early signs of autism risk involves prospective study of the development of autism in infant siblings of children with autism, for whom a recurrence rate of 9% is expected (Szatmari, Jones, Zwaigenbaum, & MacLean, 1998). Two different groups have published papers on infant symptoms of these siblings who later develop autism, compared with those who do not. Landa and Garrett-Mayer (2006) examined 60 infant siblings and 27 comparison low-risk infants from 6 to 24 months. Of this group, 24 developed an ASD, 11 had language delays, and the remaining 52 showed typical development at 24 months. There were no significant differences on developmental measures for the autism group at 6 months compared with the typical outcome group.

Similarly, Zwaigenbaum and colleagues (2005) followed 65 infant siblings and 23 low-risk infants from ages 6 to 24 months, assessing them each 6 months on a new instrument, the Autism Observation Scale for Infants (AOSI; Bryson, McDermott, Rombough, Brina, & Zwaigenbaum, 2006). Measures of general development, temperament, and attentional flexibility were also used. When behaviors measured at 6 months were compared with ADOS autism classification categories at 24 months, no group differences in symptoms at 6 months were found between those infants who met ADOS criteria for an ASD at 24 months and those who did not. There were no differences on developmental measures or visual orienting measures, either, though there were some temperamental differences involving lower activity level. The authors state "our current behavioral data do not support predictions after diagnosis based on observations at 6 months" (Zwaigenbaum et al., 2005, p. 147).

However, by 12 months, a significant relationship appeared between AOSI scores and ADOS classifications at 24 months. Six of 7 children who tested positive for autism at 24 months had scores of 7 or more on the AOSI at 12 months. None of the control children had scores this high. Infants who were positive for autism at 24 months had demonstrated a variety of related symptoms at 12 months: expressive language delays, greater temperamental distress and longer periods of orienting to objects, atypical eye contact, imitation deficits, visual tracking and visual disengagement differences, sensory-oriented behaviors, and a variety of social behaviors (Zwaigenbaum et al., 2005). Similarly, at 14 months, the group who would later develop an ASD in the Landa and Garrett-Mayer's (2006) sample had statistically significant delays on all subtests of the Mullen Scales of Early Learning (Mullen, 1995) except Visual Reception. However, the only scores in the ASD group that did not fall in the normal range were their receptive and expressive language scores.

Currently, there is an active search for infant symptoms of autism that are detectable in a screening or well-child visit before 12 months. Several infant sibling studies are currently under way, examining both behavioral and biological variables. Thus far, no symptoms have been identified as early as 6 months of age, though differences on developmental measures are becoming apparent at 12 months. One study has documented stable diagnosis of autism in 1-year-olds (Cox et al., 1999), and clinical tools designed to screen and assess autism in 1-year-olds are currently being developed and tested, including the AOSI (Bryson et al., 2006), the STAT (Stone et al., 2004), a version of the ADOS for toddlers (Richler, Niehus, & Lord, 2006), and a screen for symptoms identified during communication assessment (Wetherby et al., 2004). With the number of studies currently ongoing and with the patterns of findings being reported, the next few years hold great promise for sensitive assessment tools and procedures to identify autism in 1-year-olds. Identification of infants in early infancy appears to be farther off in the future.

COMPREHENSIVE EARLY-INTERVENTION MODELS

One of the most active research literatures related to ASD is on intervention, instructional, and/or treatment approaches for preschool-age children with autism. Researchers have developed and examined comprehensive intervention models, which are broad and usually have multiple components, and focused intervention approaches, which address more specific intervention techniques.

Comprehensive Treatment Models for Preschool Children with ASD

Comprehensive treatment models typically consist of multiple components (e.g., child-focused instruction, family-focused support), a broad scope (i.e., addressing several developmental domain or skill areas), intensity (i.e., often occurring over an entire instructional day or in multiple settings, such as a school or clinic and home), and longevity (i.e., occurring over a month or even years). In 2001, the Committee on Educational Interventions for Children with Autism of the National Research Council (NRC) followed a systematic process for identifying comprehensive intervention models. In this section, we have followed up on the models identified nearly 7 years ago, documenting the current version of each. Also, we have used the NRC committee criteria (see Table 10.1) for identifying comprehensive treatment models that have been developed and evaluated since the initial review. For each model, we have directly contacted program

TABLE 10.1. Criteria from National Research Council

A. Internal validity	B. External validity	C. Generalization
I. Prospective study comparing the intervention or placebo in which evaluators of outcome are blind to treatment status	I. Random assignment of well-defined cohorts and adequate sample size for comparisons	I. Documented changes in at least one natural setting outside of treatment setting
II. Multiple baseline, ABAB design, or reversal/withdrawal with measurement of outcome blind to treatment conditions or pre–post deign with independent evaluation	II. Nonrandom assignment, but well-defined cohorts with inclusion/exclusion criteria and documentation of attrition/failures; adequate sample size for group designs or replication across 3 participants for single-subject design	II. Generalization to one other setting or maintenance beyond experimental intervention in natural setting in which intervention took place
III. Pre–post or historical designs or multiple baselines, ABAB, withdrawal/reversal not blind to treatment conditions	III. Well-defined population of 3 or more subjects participants in single-subject designs or sample of adequate size in group designs	III. Intervention occurred in natural setting to use of outcome measures with documented relationship to functional outcome
IV. Other	IV. Other	IV. Other or not addressed

developers and reviewed published information to obtain details about current program features. Space prohibits a detailed narrative summary of each model, but brief descriptions of the features of such models appear in Table 10.2. Harris and Handleman (2006) contains extended descriptions of most of these models. Themes that occur across models are summarized in the subsequent sections.

Theoretical Orientation

The majority of the comprehensive treatment models utilize behavioral approaches grounded in the theory of applied behavior analysis. The UCLA Young Autism Project, the Princeton Child Development Institute (PCDI), the Douglass Developmental Center, and the Institute for Child Development provide traditional behavioral interventions (i.e., discrete-trial training, small-group instruction). The Learning Experiences and Alternative Program for Preschoolers and Their Parents (LEAP) model, Walden Early Childhood Program, Project DATA (Developmentally Appropriate Treatment for Autism), and the Children's Toddler School utilize behavioral interventions in naturalistic and inclusive instructional settings to emphasize generalization and social interaction. The Denver model and the DIR (Developmental, Individual-Difference, Relationship-Based) program have a developmental orientation, whereas Division TEACCH incorporates both behavioral and developmental approaches.

Developmental Domain or Skill Focus

The behaviorally based models follow a developmentally sequenced curriculum initially focused on teaching compliance, cognitive and communication skills, basic social skills, toilet training, and the reduction of challenging behaviors. Inclusive behavioral models place more emphasis on social development, sustained engagement, language development, and peer interaction. The developmental models emphasize play as a means of targeting social, emotional, communicative, and cognitive skills. Division TEACCH (Treatment and Education of Autistic and Related Communication-Handicapped Children), focuses on engagement, communication, social skills, and cognitive development as its priorities.

Context

The great majority of comprehensive models provide services in center-based settings, often affiliated with universities or hospitals (with the exception of the LEAP program and the DIR model). Several of the center-based programs provide services in home settings (Young Autism Project, PCDI, Douglass, TEACCH, Denver model, and Project DATA) and/or public school and home settings (LEAP, TEACCH, Denver model).

Family Involvement

All of the comprehensive treatment models emphasize family involvement in a variety of ways, including parent education and training home programming and/or home visits, site visitations, and collaboration in goal selection. In several models, family members may be primarily responsible for the implementation of strategies (DIR, TEACCH) or may be encouraged to follow through with naturalistic techniques in the home (Walden Program), whereas in others parent training and support is the focus (Project

TABLE 10.2. Treatment Models for Preschool Children with ASD

Model	Primary teaching method	Hours/week	Setting	Efficacy evidence
Young Autism Project at University of California Los Angeles (Lovaas, 1987)	Discrete-trial training	20–40	Center, school, & home based	• 6 studies with students with PDD/autism • 2 studies used blind evaluators (AII), 1 study used random assignment (BII), and 3 report generalization to other settings (educational placement; CI) • Additional studies were evaluated at AII and AIII (pre–post designs OR evaluators not blind to treatment conditions), BII and BIII (small sample sizes–6–19 students), and CII and CIII (generalization to other settings or use of functional measures)
LEAP (Learning Experiences and Alternative Program for Preschoolers and Their Parents; Strain & Hoyson, 2000)	Naturalistic teaching methods; peer-mediated intervention	15 hours school based; 10 hours home based	School & home based	• 3 studies • AIII (pre–post and historical designs), BIII (small sample sizes), CI (documented changes in a variety of settings)
Walden Early Childhood Program (McGee, Morrier, & Daley, 1999)	Incidental teaching	35	Center based	• 1 study • AIII (pre–post design), BII (well-defined cohort of 28 students), CIII (intervention in natural and inclusive setting)
PCDI (Princeton Child Development Institute (McClannahan & Krantz, 2001)	Discrete-trial training	15 hours school based; 20 hours home based	Center & home based	• 1 study • AIII (pre–post with control group, evaluator not blind to treatment conditions), BII (18 participants), CII (generalization to other settings)
Douglass Developmental Center (Handleman & Harris, 2006)	Discrete-trial training; incidental teaching; pivotal-response training	25 hours school based; 15 hours home based	Center & home based	• 3 studies • AIII (pre–post design with evaluator not blind to treatment), BII (20 participants), CII (generalization to other settings)

Program/Model	Method	Hours	Setting	Studies/Evidence
TEACCH (Treatment and Education of Autistic and Related Communication-Handicapped Children; Mesibov, Shea, & Schopler, 2005)	Visual information, structure, and organizational strategies	20–25	Center, school, & home based	• 3 studies • AII and AIII (experimental and control groups with evaluators both blind and not blind to treatment conditions), BII and BIII (small sample sizes—9–11 participants), CIII (intervention in natural settings using functional measures)
Denver Model at University of Colorado Health Sciences Center (Rogers, Hall, Osaki, Reaven, & Herbison, 2001)	Naturalistic teaching methods—emphasizing interpersonal exchange	25 hours	School, center, or home based	• 4 studies • AIII (pre–post with one comparison group), BII (sample sizes up to 49 participants), CIII (intervention in natural settings)
Institute for Child Development (Children's Unit) at State University of New York (Romanczyk, Lockshin, & Matey, 2001)	Behavioral methodology (principles from applied behavior analysis and behavior therapy)	27.5	Center based	• No peer-reviewed studies in journals on overall efficacy of model
Children's Toddler School (Stahmer & Ingersoll, 2004)	Incidental teaching, discrete-trial training, pivotal-response training	15	Center based	• 1 study • AIII (pre/post with evaluator not blind to treatment), BII (20 subjects), CIII (intervention in natural setting with functional measures)
Project DATA (Developmentally Appropriate Treatment for Autism; Schwartz, Sandall, McBride, & Boulware, 2004)	Naturalistic, discrete-trial training	23 hours school based; 5 hours home based	Center & home based	• 1 study • AIII (pre/post with evaluator not blind to treatment), BII (48 subjects), CIII (intervention in natural setting with functional measures)
Developmental, Individual-Difference, Relationship-Based model (DIR; Greenspan & Wieder, 2006)	Floor time	Varies	School & home based	• 2 studies (1 in press) • 1 study AIV (retrospective record review) & 1 study AIII (pre/post), BIV (no information about subjects) and BIII (74 subjects), CIII (intervention in natural setting)

DATA, Children's Toddler School, Young Autism Project). School-based programs, such as the Denver model and the LEAP program, emphasize family involvement centered around individualized education plan (IEP) development. Several models (PCDI, Institute for Child Development, TEACCH, Project DATA) collect and report parent satisfaction and parent involvement data as an outcome measure.

Evidence Supporting Effectiveness

The NRC (2001) established guidelines when evaluating studies in an effort to identify the strengths, limitations, and quality of evidence related to autism-specific interventions. The NRC guidelines were used in our review of comprehensive treatment models. The need for well-controlled clinical studies that examine the efficacy of comprehensive treatment models remains, as most studies of comprehensive treatment models have included very small samples of children and provided only before- and after-intervention measures to demonstrate progress, without the benefit of comparison or control groups. Table 10.2 summarizes the internal and external validity, as well as the generalization of results, of peer-reviewed studies related to the comprehensive treatment models.

Comprehensive Programs for Infants and Toddlers

As early screening and diagnosis has improved, children with ASD have been identified at a younger age, which has created a need to establish intervention approaches for toddlers. Several comprehensive intervention model programs have responded to this need by modifying their procedures to make them appropriate for toddler-age children, whereas other models specifically designed for toddlers have also emerged. Further, the developmental literature is beginning to inform researchers about association between early communication and social abilities of infants and the development of language and social abilities at a later age. Such information may serve as a basis in the future for the development of intervention programs for infants and caregivers even before the infants reach toddler age.

Current Comprehensive Toddler Intervention Programs

The Walden Early Childhood Program (McGee, Morrier, & Daly, 1999) is a prime example of a preschool early-intervention model that was adjusted down to become appropriate for toddler-age children (15 months of age). While continuing the emphasis on incidental teaching, verbal communication, and social interactions, the focus adjusted to the less mature skill level of the younger children. For example, instead of focused peer-mediated intervention that involved reciprocal social interaction, the focus on social awareness and appropriate exploration of social exchanges was increased. For "older" toddlers, a full-day program was employed, but for young toddlers (below 2 years), attention and engagement faded during the latter parts of the full day, so currently a half-day program is scheduled. The toddler program continues the heavy emphasis on parent involvement, in that parents agree to follow a structured home-based program that blends work on children's goals into family routines.

Beginning with a replication of the Walden toddler model, Stahmer and Ingersoll (2004) developed a toddler program (the Children's Toddler School) that employs additional behavioral and nonverbal communication intervention techniques and that, like Walden, takes place in inclusive settings. Similarly, the Project DATA program (Schwartz, Sandall, McBride, & Boulware, 2004) adapted its procedures and classroom routines to accommodate toddler-age children with ASD and their families in the BABY DATA program (Boulware, Schwartz, Sandall, & McBride, 2006). This program consists of five components: an inclusive early-childhood program, extended instructional time, technical and social support for families, coordination of family negotiated services, and transition. Developers of these three programs report remarkable progress for toddlers enrolled (Boulware et al., 2006; Stahmer & Ingersoll, 2004), which is promising and consistent with assumptions about the value of intervening earlier than the preschool years. Systematic examinations of age of entry into intervention, however, have not yet been conducted.

Infant Interventions to Promote Early Social and Communicative Development

The comprehensive intervention models for toddlers just described all operate in classroom and home settings. As the field becomes more accurate in identifying autism at an earlier age, the focus of earlier intervention may shift from classroom-based models to ones that can occur primarily in the home and with parents. In their road map for autism research, the Interagency Autism Coordinating Committee (2003) proposed that efficacious intervention models for infants and young toddlers (12- to 18-month-olds) could be developed in the near future. The developmental literature on early social and communicative development of infants has begun to uncover the developmental foundations of communication and social abilities, both of which are seen as general core deficits of young children with ASD. This literature may well inform the development of comprehensive intervention programs for infants and their families (Schertz & Odom, 2004).

Joint attention between infants and adults is a social–communicative behavior that appears during the first year of life (Striano & Bertin, 2005) and is associated with later language development (Charman et al., 2003). Joint attention is noticeably absent or delayed in young children with autism in comparison with children having other developmental disabilities or with typically developing children (Dawson et al., 2004). Analyses of videotapes of children during their first year of life who were later diagnosed with autism have found that (the absence of) social attention to adults may reliably differentiate children who were later diagnosed as having autism (Maestro et al., 2005). In a prospective study, Wetherby and colleagues (2004) have identified the *absence* of a set of behaviors that reflect joint attention in infants as a reliable predictor of a diagnosis of autism at a later age.

Early communication and social participation of infants and young children with autism and their caregivers is a logical focus for a comprehensive intervention model. Specifically designed features that promote responding to and, particularly, initiating joint attention may be productive to use in future intervention efforts with young children (Yoder & McDuffie, 2006), and several researchers have taken steps in that direction with preschool-age children. Kasari, Freeman, and Paparella (2006) found positive effects on joint attention and symbolic play, respectively, for two slightly different intervention approaches that combined discrete-trial training and a naturalistic intervention (i.e., each was compared with a nontreatment control). When using a responsive teaching approach in which mothers were taught to observe and respond to their toddler and preschool-age children's social and language behavior, Mahoney and Perales (2003) found positive effects for young children with autism. Although not yet put to the experimental test, the DIR comprehensive model (Greenspan & Wieder, 2006) contains elements (i.e., floor time) that could potentially affect joint attention.

The transactional approaches (e.g., Prizant, Weatherby, Rubin, & Laurant, 2003), that combine the use of prompts in a natural, game-like context contain features that could positively affect joint attention. Yoder and Warren's (2002) responsive education and milieu teaching intervention has produced important prelinguistic gains for very young children with developmental disabilities, and Hancock and Kaiser (2002) taught parents to use an enhanced milieu training approach to promote early social-communication skills in their young children with autism. Some single-subject-design research has also documented interventions that have focused on promotion of joint attention. Whalen and Schreibman (2003) used a combination of pivotal-response and discrete-trial training to promote joint attention in a clinic context. With toddlers, Dawson and Galpert (1990) taught mothers to use imitation (of their children) to increase their children's social responsiveness, which could lead to increased joint attention.

Basing their work on a mediated learning approach originally employed by Klein and Alony (1993), Schertz and Odom (in press) developed a joint-attention-mediated-learning approach that taught mothers ways to promote joint attention by focusing on faces, turn taking, responding to joint attention, and initiating joint attention in toddlers with autism. They found sustained engagement in both forms of joint attention for two of the three children in the study. In summary, an empirical literature appears to be rapidly emerging that could serve as a basis for developing comprehensive model programs for infants with autism and their families, which will be a future direction for research.

FOCUSED-INTERVENTION APPROACHES

Focused-intervention approaches are narrower in scope than the comprehensive treatment models in that they target specific developmental or behavioral outcomes for children and often specify an individual procedure rather than a comprehensive set of procedures. In fact, often focused-intervention procedures (i.e., discrete-trial training) are components of the large comprehensive treatment procedures (e.g., the UCLA Young Autism Project; Lovaas, 1987). In this section, we briefly summarize both focused-intervention approaches that show extensive evidence of effectiveness and approaches that show less evidence of effectiveness but that are emerging as potentially powerful interventions for the future. This distinction is based on evidence-based practice guidelines established by the Council for Exceptional Children (CEC) Division for Research Task Force on Quality Indicators for Special Education Research (Odom, Brantlinger, Gersten, Horner, Thompson, & Harris, 2005), a previous review of single-subject-design research for young children with autism (Odom et al., 2003), a meta-analysis of single-subject-design research for individuals with disabilities (Karasu & Odom, 2006), and a computer search of group-design-research literature on ASD. Space constraints necessitate that descriptions of interventions be limited, with representative articles cited to illustrate empirical support. Well-established (WE) intervention approaches have been documented by at least two high-quality group designs (Gersten et al., 2005) or five high-quality single-subject designs (Horner et al., 2005). Emerging (EM) intervention approaches have accumulating evidence of effectiveness (e.g., one or two medium-quality group-design studies or at least three medium- or high-quality single-subject-design studies). For detailed descriptions of interventions, we refer readers to Odom et al. (2003); and Rogers and Ozonoff (2006). In addition, at this writing, the National Standards Project, organized through the National Center on Autism, is conducting a systematic review and analysis of the research literature on focused interventions for children and youth with autism, which should provide guidance for the field in the future (National Autism Center, 2006).

Differential Reinforcement (WE)

Adults provide rewards for children based on their performance of a targeted skill or behavior. Perhaps one of the most "tried and true" intervention approaches, this approach can be traced back to initial applications of behavior analysis to the modification of children's behavior (Allen, Hart, Buell, Harris, & Wolf, 1964) and usually follows operant principles of reinforcement. In a single-subject-design study, Nuzzolo-Gomez, Leonard, Ortiz, Rivera, and Greer (2002) provided adult reinforcement for the use of toys and books by young children with autism, noting a change in material use and a reduction in stereotypic behavior.

Discrete-Trial Training (WE)

Also described as didactic behavioral teaching (Rogers & Ozonoff, 2006), discrete-trial training (DTT) is a highly focused intervention that usually involves the use of massed teaching trials with an adult and child in individual teaching sessions. The adult provides a cue (e.g., an instruction or model) to begin the teaching episode, provides the necessary prompts, and usually provides reinforcement on a predetermined schedule. DTT is a key feature of several of the comprehensive treatment models described previously, with much evidence of efficacy existing for its use in such a context (Eikeseth, Smith, Jahr, & Eldevik, 2002). In a single-subject-design study, Grindle and Remington (2002) demonstrated the efficacy of DTT using different reinforcement procedures to teach receptive labeling to preschool children with autism.

Naturalistic Behavioral Interventions (WE)

Incidental teaching, naturalistic language paradigm, activity-based intervention, milieu and enhanced milieu language training, and embedded learning opportunities are intervention strategies that share a common set of characteristics. These interventions follow operant behavioral principles but differ from the two previous approaches in that (1) teaching takes place in children's ongoing routines and environments, (2) the environment is arranged to elicit a child's initiation of a skill to be learned, (3) teachers provide models or prompts in the routine setting if the behavior does not occur, and (4) use of natural consequences or reinforcement for the desired behavior is emphasized. In a single-subject-design study, McGee, Almeida, Sulzer-Azaroff, and Feldman (1992) used an incidental teaching technique to promote the reciprocal social interactions of young children with autism and their peers. Kaiser and Trent (Chapter 11, this volume) provide a detailed review of research on naturalistic communication training approaches for children with a range of developmental disabilities.

Pivotal-Response Training (WE)

Like discrete-trial training, pivotal-response training (PRT) is both a focused intervention and a key feature of a comprehensive intervention approach, as described previously. As also noted previously, PRT is based on the theory that the absence of motivation to respond to complex stimuli is a core deficit in autism and is reflected in several pivotal behaviors: (1) responsiveness to multiple cues, (2) self-management, and (3) self-initiation of social interaction. By intervening on the pivotal behaviors, broader changes in children's communicative and social functioning may well occur. Although it shares some characteristics with naturalistic interventions, PRT is distinct in its focus on pivotal behaviors. Single-subject-design studies have documented the efficacy of PRT in promoting children's self-initiation (Koegel, Carter, & Koegel, 2003), social initiations with adults and peers (Pierce & Schreibman, 1997), and appropriate play (Stahmer, Ingersoll, & Carter, 2003).

Peer-Mediated Interventions (WE)

In peer-mediated interventions, peers are taught to initiate or direct specific types of social behaviors to children with autism in order to encourage the children's use of skills or targeted behaviors. Peers receive explicit training, and teachers sometimes provide prompts and reinforcement to peers. Such external supports to peers are systematically reduced across time. Peer-mediated interventions primarily focus on social or communicative behaviors, and their efficacy has been replicated across many studies (Karasu & Odom, 2006). For example, Goldstein, Kaczmarek, Pennington, and Shafer (1992) taught peers to direct attention to and comment on the behavior of preschool-age classmates with autism and found substantial changes in the communicative interactions of the children with autism.

Positive Behavior Support (WE)

Positive behavior support, a set of intervention approaches that include functional assessment, reinforcement of incompatible behavior, and functional communication training, has been widely applied to promoting positive behavior and reducing problem behavior of individuals with developmental disabilities (Horner, Carr, Strain, Todd, & Reed, 2002). Extensive evidence for the efficacy of positive behavior support (PBS) exists for individuals with developmental disabilities (see Dunlap & Carr, Chapter 23, this volume, for an extensive review), and the evidence for use specifically with preschool-age children with disabilities is building (Odom et al., 2003). For example, Dunlap and Fox (1999), using single-subject designs, documented the efficacy of a PBS model for young children with autism who have serious problem behaviors.

Self-Management (WE)

Emanating from a cognitive-behavioral orientation in self-management interventions, adults directly teach children with autism to monitor, record, and/or reinforce their use of a desired behavior or skill. Usually self-management interventions are designed to lead to independent use of a skill by children with ASD. For young children with ASD and other developmental disabilities, Mithaug and Mithaug (2003) compared teacher-directed and self-management interventions for promoting independent work, finding that children were reliably and substantially more independent in the self-management condition.

Social Stories (EM)

Social stories usually are designed to promote appropriate social behavior or decrease problem behavior. They follow a specific format, are written by a professional or parent from the child's perspective, and often describe appropriate behavior in routine or problem situations (Gray & Garand, 1993). Although more studies have been conducted with elementary school-age children with ASD, evidence for their efficacy with some preschool-age children with ASD is accumulating. For three young children with PDD-NOS, Ivey, Heflin, and Alberto (2004) created social stories to prepare children for novel events in their routines and documented children's greater performance of targeted skills when the social stories were used.

Video Modeling and Self-Modeling (EM)

In video modeling (VM), children with ASD watch a video of a child or children demonstrating appropriate use of a targeted skill or behavior. In video self-modeling (VSM), video clips are obtained of the children with ASD as they correctly or competently perform the targeted behavior (this is accomplished through editing), and those demonstrations are used as "self-model" examples for the children with ASD. Again, an accumulating literature on VM and VSM is emerging. In a meta-analysis of single-subject-design studies, Bellini and Akullian (2007) located more than 20 studies documenting the two approaches. Although many of the studies were conducted with elementary-age children, some research with younger children is also occurring. With four young children with autism, Wert and Neisworth (2003) used a VSM approach to promote spontaneous requesting in school settings.

Picture Exchange Communication System (EM)

The Picture Exchange Communication System (PECS) intervention consists of symbols on cards or tokens that children use to initiate communication when they are exchanged with a partner (Bondy & Frost, 1994). A growing literature demonstrates the efficacy of this widely used intervention with elementary-age children with ASD. In two studies involving groups of preschool children with ASD and other developmental disabilities, Schwartz, Garfinkle, and Bauer (1998) documented the children's rapid acquisition of the PECS system and its use in communicating in generalized settings and with "untrained" language forms.

Visual Support (EM)

Visual cues in the environment often assist children with ASD in learning targeted skills or performing independently in the environment. Visual cues may be a sequence of pictures that describe a child's schedule during the day, a pictorial representation of tasks or steps in a task to be completed, or a sign that the teacher shows the child to remind them of the targeted behavior to be performed. The PECS intervention could be considered a visually supported system in that the picture token has a visual symbol, but the literature on PECS is specific to that intervention. Visual supports are used routinely in many classrooms now, and a literature documenting their effectiveness with preschool children is emerging. With three preschool children with autism, Johnston, Nelson, Evans, and Palazolo (2003) used a visual support system to teach young children with ASD to initiate requests to play and noted changes in their social participation and off-task behavior.

ISSUES AND FUTURE DIRECTIONS IN PRESCHOOL INTERVENTIONS

Research on efficacy of comprehensive models and focused interventions for preschool children is one of the most active areas of behavioral research related to ASD. Focused intervention approaches have documented the effectiveness of specific interventions, and much of that literature consists of single-subject-design studies. As agreement emerges about the amount and quality of evidence needed from single-subject designs to document a practice as evidence based (see Horner et al., 2005), this literature will come together more systematically to inform practice. In addition, advances in developing procedures for conducting meta-analyses on single-subject-design studies (Karasu & Odom, 2006) will assist in the synthesis and interpretation of these data. Yet as the nature of the population changes and intervention studies accumulate, several issues have arisen.

Changing Nature of the Population

Many comprehensive and focused approaches were initially designed for children with autism, but over the years the nature of the population has changed. As noted, early diagnostic approaches may lead to earlier interventions, which in turn may lead to children entering preschool intervention programs with a different and more advanced set of skills. Similarly, the models have been established for children with autism; if increased diagnostic specificity for Asperger syndrome occurs, a higher functioning set of children may be entering traditional comprehensive programs. Either of these scenarios will require adjustments to the models and perhaps reevaluations of the efficacy of the model for a "new" generation of children with ASD and their families.

Individual Predictors of Response to Treatment

Although experimental studies of focused interventions and evaluations of comprehensive treatment models illustrate that young children with ASD can make impressive gains, there are always participants who do not respond favorably. Predicting children's responsiveness to treatment is a critical current issue because it may allow service providers to build strong intervention models, plan the provision of services, and identify children who may need more intensive forms of treatment.

Early intervention itself is an outgrowth of a response-to-treatment relationship in that some evidence indicates that intervention beginning at an earlier age produces more positive outcomes than interventions that begin later, as Fenske, Zalenski, Krantz, and McClannahan (1985) found in follow-up assessments of children who participated in their early-intervention program. Child variables associated with response to treatment include pretreatment IQ scores or language performance (Stevens et al., 2000), specific diagnoses within ASD (e.g., autism disorder, PDD-NOS; Smith, Eikeseth,

Klevstrand, & Lovaas, 1997), and behavioral characteristics such as approach, avoidance, and stereotypy (Sherer & Schreibman, 2005). In addition, in a recent retrospective study, Stoelb et al. (2004) found that dysmorphia (which could be related to undiagnosed genetic syndromes) and history of regression (i.e., early normal development followed by loss of developmental skills) were associated with children's immediate and long-term responses to intensive behavior therapy. In addition, family variables, such as maternal stress, may be a significant predictor of success of treatment for children (Robbins, Dunlap, & Plienis, 1991). It is important to note that predicting responsiveness to treatment requires differentiating changes due to the identified treatment from changes due to other factors, such as supplemental educational, medical, or dietary treatments, as well as maturation and history effects (Yoder & Compton, 2004). Specifically building features into experimental studies of treatment to address the responsiveness question will be an important direction for future research.

PSYCHOPHARMACOLOGICAL TREATMENTS FOR CHILDREN WITH ASD

The psychopharmacology of autistic disorder (autism) and other pervasive developmental disorders (PDDs) can be approached from various perspectives. Here, we focus on the use of drugs to improve specific target symptoms, including both core features and associated behavioral disturbances. We discuss drug treatment strategies directed toward motor hyperactivity and inattention, interfering stereotypical and repetitive behaviors, aggression and self-injurious behaviors (SIB), and the core social impairment of autism and other PDDs. An emphasis is placed on results from published double-blind, placebo-controlled studies. Also, because little research involves children with autism below the age of 5 years, studies involving somewhat older children are reviewed, highlighting the implications for treatment. The reader is referred elsewhere for more comprehensive reviews of the pharmacology of autism and developmental disabilities (McDougle, Posey, & Stigler, 2006; Thompson, Moore, & Symons, Chapter 25, this volume).

Motor Hyperactivity and Inattention

Motor hyperactivity and inattention often can cause significant impairment in children with PDDs, particularly younger children within the school setting. Importantly, in DSM-IV, attention-deficit/hyperactivity disorder (ADHD) is not diagnosed if the symptoms of inattention and hyperactivity occur exclusively during the course of a PDD. Not all drug treatments that are effective for these symptoms in typically developing individuals with ADHD are necessarily useful and well tolerated in children with PDDs.

Psychostimulants such as methylphenidate are first-line agents for the treatment of hyperactivity and inattention in patients with ADHD. The largest controlled study of methylphenidate in individuals with PDDs was recently published by the National Institute of Mental Health (NIMH)–sponsored Research Units on Pediatric Psychopharmacology (RUPP) Autism Network (2005). Seventy-two children (ages 5–14 years) with PDDs accompanied by moderate to severe hyperactivity entered the 4-week double-blind, placebo-controlled crossover study (with low, medium, and high doses of methylphenidate), followed by an 8-week, open-label continuation. Methylphenidate was superior to placebo on the primary outcome measure, the teacher-rated hyperactivity subscale of the Aberrant Behavior Checklist (ABC; Aman, Singh, Stewart, & Field, 1985). Thirty-five participants (49%) responded positively to methylphenidate. Adverse effects (agitation, irritability) led to discontinuation of the study drug in 13 (18%) of the participants. This rate of treatment response and subject discontinuation contrasts with results from the NIMH collaborative multisite multimodal treatment study of children with ADHD (the MTA), in which 69% of participants who were randomized to methylphenidate responded and only 1.4% discontinued the drug due to adverse effects (Greenhill et al., 2001). Based on these studies, it appears that methylphenidate is less efficacious and associated with more frequent adverse effects in children with PDDs than in typically developing children with ADHD.

For children and adolescents with PDDs who do not improve with a psychostimulant or who cannot tolerate one, alternative approaches are available, although there is little published controlled data to support their use. Two small controlled studies of the α_2 agonist clonidine indicate that the drug can improve hyperactivity (Fankhauser, Karumanchi, German, Yates, & Karumanchi, 1992; Jaselskis, Cook, Fletcher, & Leventhal, 1992). Side effects can include sedation and hypotension. Recently published open-label data suggest that another α_2 agonist, guanfacine, may benefit nearly a quarter of children and adolescents with PDDs (Posey, Puntney, et al., 2004). Sedation and hypotension can also occur, but possibly less so than with clonidine. With both clonidine and guanfacine, some question exists regarding the maintenance of treatment response over time. Finally, preliminary data is encouraging regarding treatment of hyperactivity and inattention in children and adolescents with PDDs with the selective norepinephrine uptake inhibitor atomoxetine (Posey et al., 2006).

Interfering Stereotypical and Repetitive Behavior

Restricted repetitive and stereotyped patterns of behavior, interests, and activities are a primary feature of autism. At times, these behaviors can be interfering and warrant consideration of drug treatment. A dysregulation of serotonin function has long been hypothesized in autism (McDougle, Erickson, Stigler, & Posey, 2005). In addition, serotonin reuptake inhibitors (SRIs) are the only class of drugs that has been shown to consistently improve the repetitive thoughts and behaviors associated with obsessive–compulsive disorder. A recently published controlled study of the selective SRI (SSRI) fluoxetine (mean dose, 9.9 ± 4.4 mg/day) in children (mean age, 8.2 ± 3 years) with autism and other PDDs indicated that the drug was more effective than placebo for improving repetitive behavior and was well tolerated (Hollander et al., 2005). A number of previously published open-label reports of fluoxetine and other SSRIs in youth with autism and other PDDs suggested that, whereas these agents are effective in some patients, they can be associated with behavioral activation and worsening in others. Additional, larger controlled studies of SSRIs in young children and adolescents with autism are needed.

Aggression and Self-Injurious Behavior

Although aggression toward self, others, and property more typically manifests in older children and adolescents with autism, it can occur in younger children as well. By far, the largest amount of published controlled data on a drug for this target symptom cluster exists for the atypical antipsychotic risperidone. The landmark study, conducted by the NIMH-sponsored RUPP Autism Network (2002), found risperidone (dosage range

0.5–3.5 mg/day) to be effective for these symptoms in 70% of children and adolescents (mean age, 8.8 ± 2.7 years) compared with a 12% rate of placebo response. Common adverse effects included increased appetite, weight gain (5.9 ± 6.4 lbs. over 8 weeks), fatigue, drowsiness, and drooling. A second published placebo-controlled study found similar results with risperidone in youth with autism and other PDDs (Shea et al., 2004). To date, placebo-controlled studies of other available atypical antipsychotics, including clozapine, olanzapine, quetiapine, ziprasidone, and aripiprazole, in youth with autism have not been published.

Core Social Impairment

The preceding discussion of drug treatment primarily focuses on improving behavioral symptoms that often occur in association with autism. There have been a limited number of controlled trials of drugs, such as fenfluramine and naltrexone, that have targeted the core social impairment of autism. These studies, however, found these agents to be no more effective than placebo for this core disturbance.

Recent interest has arisen in the role that glutamate dysfunction may play in the pathophysiology of autism. Posey, Kem, et al. (2004) published a small, prospective, single-blind study of D-cycloserine for the core social impairment of autism. D-cycloserine is an antibiotic used for the treatment of tuberculosis. In adults with schizophrenia, D-cycloserine has been shown to improve the "negative" symptoms, which some have hypothesized are analogous to the social impairment of autism. In a pilot study of 10 participants, McDougle and colleagues (2006) found that D-cycloserine resulted in a statistically significant improvement on the Social Withdrawal subscale of the ABC. Two participants experienced adverse effects (a transient motor tic and increased echolalia) at the highest dose they received. A larger, double-blind, placebo-controlled study is currently under way.

Future Directions

The future of drug treatment for young children with autism will focus on the development of more effective and safer agents for the core and associated behavioral disturbances. Drugs with a better tolerability profile than the psychostimulants are needed for improving inattention and motor hyperactivity. More effective drugs with a lower propensity for behavioral activation are needed for addressing interfering repetitive behavior. Drugs for treating aggression and SIB are needed that do not have the risks of acute extrapyramidal symptoms and tardive dyskinesia. Importantly, research is needed to identify effective pharmacological agents targeted to the core social and language impairments that characterize the disorder. Studying combined pharmacological and behavioral–educational treatment approaches will also be critical in this process. Last, most of the research cited involved older children with ASD. Although the findings may have direct implications for young children, further research is needed to directly extend the findings of these psychopharmacological studies to younger children with ASD.

CONCLUSION

Rapid scientific advances are occurring for young children with autism and their families. Comprehensive treatment models for preschoolers and toddlers that show promise for being efficacious have been developed, and solid evidence exists for efficacious focused interventions. Systematic, carefully controlled psychopharmacological research is identifying treatments that positively affect many of the behavioral characteristics and even the core deficits associated with ASD in children. Their implications and future applications for young children with ASD may well be a major advance in the future. As these advances proceed, the demographic nature of autism is changing. Instruments for reliably and accurately diagnosing autism earlier than currently occurs are being developed that will identify a younger set of toddlers and even infants who need intervention. Developmental science is providing information on the early foundations of social communication, which may serve as the basis for early-intervention programs in the future. In summary, behavioral, developmental, and medical sciences are making major strides in understanding the nature of autism and ASD and treatments that will improve the lives of children with ASD and their families.

REFERENCES

Allen, K. E., Hart, B., Harris, F. R., & Wolf, M. M. (1964). Effects of social reinforcement on isolate behavior of a nursery school child. *Child Development, 35,* 511–518.

Aman, M. G., Singh, N. N., Stewart, A. W., & Field, C. J. (1985). The Aberrant Behavior Checklist: A behavior rating scale for the assessment of treatment effects. *American Journal on Mental Deficiency, 89,* 485–491.

American Psychiatric Association. (1994). *Diagnostic and statistical manual of mental disorders* (4th ed.). Washington, DC: Author.

Baranek, G. (1999). Autism during infancy: A retrospective video analysis of sensory–motor and social behaviors at 9–12 months of age. *Journal of Autism and Developmental Disorders, 29,* 213–224.

Baron-Cohen, S., Allen, J., & Gillberg, C. (1992). Can autism be detected at 18 months? The needle, the haystack, and the CHAT. *British Journal of Psychiatry, 161,* 839–843.

Bellini, S., & Akullian, J. (2007). A meta-analysis of video modeling and video self-modeling intervention for children and adolescents with autism spectrum disorders. *Exceptional Children, 73,* 264–287.

Bondy, A., & Frost, L. (1994). The picture exchange communication system. *Focus on Autistic Behavior, 9,* 1–19.

Boulware, G. Schwartz, I. S., Sandall, S. R., & McBride, B. J. (2006). Project DATA for toddlers: An inclusive approach to very young children with ASD. *Topics in Early Childhood Special Education, 26,* 94–105.

Bricker, D., & Squires, J. (1999). *Ages and Stages Questionnaires* (2nd ed.). Baltimore: Brookes.

Bryson, S. E., McDermott, C., Rombough, V., Brina, J., & Zwaigenbaum, L. (2006). *The Autism Observation Scale for Infants: Scale development and reliability data.* Unpublished manuscript.

Charman, T., Baron-Cohen, S., Swettenham, J., Baird, G., Drew, A., & Cox, A. (2003). Predicting language outcomes in infants with autism and pervasive developmental disorders. *International Journal of Language and Communication Disorders, 38,* 265–285.

Coonrod, E. E., & Stone, W. L. (2005). Screening for autism in young children. In F. R. Volkmar, R. Paul, A. Klin, & D. J. Cohen (Eds.), *Handbook of autism and pervasive developmental disorders* (pp. 707–729). Hoboken, NJ: Wiley.

Cox, A., Klein, K., Charman, T., Baird, G., Baron-Cohen, S., Swettenham, J., et al. (1999). Autism spectrum disorders at 20 and 42 months of age: Stability of clinical and ADI-R diagnosis. *Journal of Child Psychology and Psychiatry, 40,* 719–732.

Dawson, G., & Galpert, L. (1990). Mothers' use of imitative play for facilitating social responsiveness and toy play in young autistic children. *Development and Psychopathology, 2,* 151–162.

Dawson, G., Toth, K., Abbott, R., Osterling, J., Munson, J., Estes, A., et al. (2004). Early social attention impairments in autism: Social orienting, joint attention, and attention to distress. *Developmental Psychology, 20,* 271–283.

Dunlap, G., & Fox, L. (1999). Supporting families of young children with autism. *Infants and Young Children, 12*(2), 48–54.

Eikeseth, S., Smith, T., Jahr, E., & Eldevik, S. (2002). Intensive behavioral treatment at school for 4- to 7-year-old children with autism: A 1-year comparison controlled study. *Behavior Modification, 26,* 49–68.

Fankhauser, M. P., Karumanchi, V. C., German, M. L., Yates, A., & Karumanchi, S. D. (1992). A double-blind, placebo-controlled study of the efficacy of transdermal clonidine in autism. *Journal of Clinical Psychiatry, 53,* 77–82.

Fenske, E., Zalenski, S., Krantz, P., & McClannahan, L. (1985). Age at intervention and treatment outcomes for autistic children in a comprehensive intervention program. *Analysis and Intervention in Developmental Disabilities, 5,* 49–58.

Fombonne, E. (2003). The prevalence of autism. *Journal of the American Medical Association, 289,* 87–89.

Fombonne, E. (2005). Epidemiological studies of pervasive developmental disorders. In F. Volkmar, R. Paul, A. Klin, & D. Cohen (Eds.), *Handbook of autism and pervasive developmental disorders: Vol. 1. Diagnosis, development, neurobiology, and behavior* (3rd ed., pp. 42–69). Hoboken, NJ: Wiley.

Gersten, R., Fuchs, L., Compton, D., Coyne, M., Greenwood, C., & Innocenti, M. (2005). Quality indicators for group experimental and quasi-experimental research in special education. *Exceptional Children, 71,* 149–164.

Glascoe, F. P. (1998). *Collaborating with parents: Using Parents' Evaluation of Developmental Status to detect and address developmental and behavioral problems.* Nashville, TN: Ellsworth & Vandermeer.

Goldstein, H., Kaczmarek, L., Pennington, R., & Shafer, K. (1992). Peer-mediated intervention: Attending to, commenting on, and acknowledging the behavior of preschoolers with autism. *Journal of Applied Behavior Analysis, 25,* 289–307.

Gray, C. A., & Garand, J. D. (1993). Social stories: Improving responses of students with autism with accurate social information. *Focus on Autistic Behavior, 8*(1), 1–10.

Greenhill, L. L., Pliszka, S., Dulcan, M. K., Bernet, W., Arnold, V., Beitchman, J., et al (2001). Summary of the practice parameter for the use of stimulant medications in the treatment of children, adolescents, and adults. *Journal of the American Academy of Child and Adolescent Psychiatry, 40,* 1352–1355.

Greenspan, S., & Wieder, S. (2006). *Engaging autism: Helping children relate, communicate, and think with the DIR Floortime approach.* New York: De Capo Lifelong Books.

Grindle, C., & Remington, B. (2002). Discrete-trial training for autistic children when reward is delayed: A comparison of conditioned cue value and response marking. *Journal of Applied Behavior Analysis, 35,* 187–190.

Hancock, T. B., & Kaiser, A. P. (2002). The effects of trainer implemented enhanced milieu teaching on the social communication of children with autism. *Topics in Early Childhood Special Education, 22,* 29–54.

Handleman, J. S., & Harris, S. L. (Eds.). (2006). *Preschool education programs for children with autism* (3rd ed.). Austin, TX: PRO-ED.

Harris, S. L., Handleman, J. S., & Jennett, H. K. (2005). Models for educational intervention for students with autism: Home, center, and school-based programming. In F. Volkmar, R. Paul, A. Klin, & D. Cohen (Eds.), *Handbook of autism and developmental disorders* (3rd ed., Vol. 2, pp. 1043–1054). New York: Wiley.

Hollander, E., Phillips, A., Chaplin, W., Zagursky, K., Novotny, S., Wasserman, S., et al. (2005). A placebo controlled crossover trial of liquid fluoxetine on repetitive behaviors in childhood and adolescent autism. *Neuropsychopharmacology, 30,* 582–589.

Horner, R., Carr, E., Halle, J., McGee, G., Odom, S., & Wolery, M. (2005). The use of single subject research to identify evidence-based practice in special education. *Exceptional Children, 71,* 165–180.

Horner, R. H., Carr, E. G., Strain, P. S., Todd, A. W., & Reed, H. K. (2002). Problem behavior interventions for young children with autism: A research synthesis. *Journal of Autism and Developmental Disorders, 32,* 423–446.

Interagency Autism Coordinating Committee. (2003). *IACC autism research road map and matrix.* Bethesda, MD: National Institute of Mental Health.

Ivey, M. L., Heflin, L. J., & Alberto, P. (2004). The use of social stories to promote independent behaviors in novel events for children with PDD-NOS. *Focus on Autism and Other Developmental Disorders, 19*(3), 164–176.

Jaselskis, C. A., Cook, E. H., Jr., Fletcher, K. E., & Leventhal, B. L. (1992). Clonidine treatment of hyperactive and impulsive children with autistic disorder. *Journal of Clinical Psychopharmacology, 12*, 322–327.

Johnston, S., Nelson, C., Evans, J., & Palazolo, K. (2003). The use of visual supports in teaching young children with autism spectrum disorder to initiate interactions. *Augmentative and Alternative Communication, 19*, 86–103.

Kanner, L. (1943). Autistic disturbances of affective contact. *Nervous Child, 2*, 217–250.

Karasu, N., & Odom, S. L. (2006). *A meta-analysis of single subject research of communication and social interventions for children and youth with developmental disabilities.* Manuscript in preparation.

Kasari, C., Freeman, S., & Paparella, T. (2006). Joint attention and symbolic play in young children with autism: A randomized controlled intervention study. *Journal of Child Psychology and Psychiatry, 47*, 611–620.

Klein, P. S., & Alony, S. (1993). Immediate and sustained effects of maternal mediating behaviors on young children. *Journal of Early Intervention, 17*, 177–193.

Koegel, L. K., Carter, C. M., & Koegel, R. L. (2003). Teaching children with autism self-initiations as a pivotal response. *Topics in Language Disorders, 23*, 134–145.

Landa, R., & Garrett-Mayer, E. (2006). Development in infants with autism spectrum disorders: A prospective study. *Journal of Child Psychology and Psychiatry, 47*, 629–638.

Lord, C. (1995). Follow-up of two-year-olds referred for possible autism. *Journal of Child Psychology and Psychiatry, 36*, 1365–1382.

Lord, C. (1997). Diagnostic instruments in autism spectrum disorders. In D. Cohen & F. R. Volkmar (Eds.), *Handbook of autism and pervasive developmental disorders* (pp. 460–483). New York: Wiley.

Lord, C., & Corsello, C. (2005). Diagnostic instruments in autism spectrum disorders. In F. R. Volkmar, R. Paul, A. Klin, & D. Cohen (Eds.), *Handbook of autism and pervasive developmental disorders* (pp. 730–771). Hoboken, NJ: Wiley.

Lord, C., Rutter, M., & DiLavore, P. (1997). *Autism Diagnostic Observation Schedule–Generic.* Chicago: University of Chicago Press.

Lord, C., Rutter, M., DiLavore, P. C., & Risi, S. (1999). *Autism Diagnostic Observation Schedule–WPS Edition (ADOS–WPS).* Los Angeles: Western Psychological Services.

Lord, C., Rutter, M., & Le Couteur, A. (1994). Autism Diagnostic Interview—Revised: A revised version of a diagnostic interview for caregivers of individuals with possible pervasive developmental disorders. *Journal of Autism and Developmental Disorders, 24*, 659–685.

Lovaas, O. I. (1987). Behavioral treatment and normal educational and intellectual functioning in young autistic children. *Journal of Consulting and Clinical Psychology, 55*, 3–9.

Maestro, S., Muratori, F., Cavallaro, M. C., Pecini, C., Cesari, A., Paziente, A., et al. (2005). How young children treat objects and people: An empirical study of the first year of life in autism. *Child Psychiatry and Human Development, 35*, 383–396.

Mahoney, G., & Perales, F. (2003). Using relationship-focused intervention to enhance the social–emotional functioning of young children with autism spectrum disorders. *Topics in Early Childhood Special Education, 23*, 77–89.

McClannahan, L. E., & Krantz, P. J. (2001). Behavior analysis and intervention for preschoolers at the Princeton Child Development Institute. In J. S. Handleman & S. L. Harris (Eds.), *Preschool education programs for children with autism* (rev. ed., pp. 191–213). Austin, TX: PRO-ED.

McDougle, C. J., Erickson, C. A., Stigler, K. A., & Posey, D. J (2005). Neurochemistry in the pathophysiology of autism. *Journal of Clinical Psychiatry, 66*, 9–18.

McDougle, C. J., Posey, D. J., & Stigler, K. A. (2006). Pharmacological treatments. In S. O. Moldin & J. L. R. Rubenstein (Eds.), *Understanding autism: From basic neuroscience to treatment* (pp. 417–442). Boca Raton, FL: CRC Press.

McGee, G., Almeida, C., Sulzer-Azaroff, B., & Feldman, R. S. (1992). Promoting reciprocal interactions via peer incidental teaching. *Journal of Applied Behavior Analysis, 25*, 117–126.

McGee, G., Morrier, M., & Daly, T. (1999). An incidental teaching approach to early intervention for toddlers with autism. *Journal of the Association for Persons with Severe Handicaps, 24*, 133–146.

Mesibov, G., Shea, V., & Schopler, E. (2005). *The TEACCH approach to autism spectrum disorders.* New York: Plenum Press.

Mithaug, D. K., & Mithaug, D. E. (2003). Effects of teacher-directed versus student-directed instruction on self-management of young children with disabilities. *Journal of Applied Behavior Analysis, 36*, 133–136.

Mullen, E. M. (1995). *Mullen Scales of Early Learning* (AGS ed.). Circle Pines, MN: American Guidance Service.

Mundy, P., Sigman, M., Ungerer, J., & Sherman, T. (1987). Nonverbal communication and play correlates of language development in autistic children. *Journal of Autism and Developmental Disorders, 17,* 349–364.

National Autism Center. (2006). *National standards project.* Retrieved June 5, 2006, from *www. nationalautismcenter.org/about.html.*

National Research Council. (2001). *Educating children with autism.* Washington, DC: National Academies Press.

Nuzzolo-Gomez, R., Leonard, M. A., Ortiz, E., Rivera, C. M., & Greer, R. D. (2002). Teaching children with autism to prefer books or toys over stereotypy or passivity. *Journal of Positive Behavior Interventions, 4,* 80–87.

Odom, S. L., Brantlinger, E., Gersten, R., Horner, R., Thompson, B., & Harris, K. (2005). Research in special education: Scientific methods and evidence-based practices. *Exceptional Children, 71,* 137–148.

Odom, S. L., Brown, W. H., Frey, T., Karasu, N., Smith-Canter, L., & Strain, P. S. (2003). Evidence-based practices for young children with autism: Evidence from single-subject design research. *Focus on Autism and Other Developmental Disabilities, 18,* 166–175.

Osterling, J., Dawson, G., & Munson, J. (2002). Early recognition of one-year-old infants with autism spectrum disorder versus mental retardation. *Development and Psychopathology, 14,* 239–251.

Pierce, K., & Schreibman, L. (1997). Multiple peer use of pivotal response training to increase social behaviors of classmates with autism: Results from trained and untrained peers. *Journal of Applied Behavior Analysis, 30,* 157–160.

Posey, D. J., Kem, D. L., Swiczy, N. B., Sweeten, T. L., Wiegand, R. E., & McDougle, C. J. (2004). A pilot study of D-cycloserine in autistic disorder. *American Journal of Psychiatry, 161,* 2115–2117.

Posey, D. J., Puntney, J. I., Sasher, T. M., Kem, D. L., & McDougle, C. J. (2004). Guanfacine treatment of hyperactivity and inattention in pervasive developmental disorders: A retrospective analysis of 80 cases. *Journal of Child Adolescent Psychopharmacology, 14,* 233–241.

Posey, D. J., Wiegand, R. E., Wilkerson, J., Maynard, M., Stigler, K. A., & McDougle, C. J. (2006). A prospective, open-label study of atomoxetine for ADHD symptoms associated with higher functioning pervasive developmental disorders. *Journal of Child and Adolescent Psychopharmacology, 16,* 599–610.

Prizant, B. M., Wetherby, A. M., Rubin, E., & Laurant, A. C. (2003). The SCERTS model: A transactional, family-centered approach to enhancing communication and socioemotional abilities of children with autism spectrum disorder. *Infants and Young Children, 16,* 296–316.

Research Units on Pediatric Psychopharmacology Autism Network. (2002). Risperidone in children with autism and serious behavioral problems. *New England Journal of Medicine, 347,* 314–321.

Research Units on Pediatric Psychopharmacology Autism Network. (2005). Randomized, controlled, crossover trial of methylphenidate in pervasive developmental disorders with hyperactivity. *Archives of General Psychiatry, 62,* 1266–1274.

Richler, J., Niehus, R., & Lord, C. (2006, June). *Measuring social and communicative behaviors in toddlers at risk for autism spectrum disorders.* Poster presented at International Meeting for Autism Research, Montreal, Quebec, Canada.

Robbins, F. R., Dunlap, G., & Plienis, A. J. (1991). Family characteristics, family training, and the progress of young children with autism. *Journal of Early Intervention, 15,* 173–183.

Robins, D. L., Fein, D., Barton, M. L., & Green, J. A. (2001). The modified checklist for autism in toddlers: An initial study investigating the early detection of autism and pervasive developmental disorders. *Journal of Autism and Developmental Disorders, 31,* 131–144.

Rogers, S. J. (2001). Differential diagnosis of autism before age 3. *International Review of Research in Mental Retardation, 23,* 1–31.

Rogers, S., Hall, T., Osaki, D., Reaven, J., & Herbison, J. (2001). The Denver model: A comprehensive, integrated educational approach to young children with autism and their families. In J. S. Handleman & S. L. Harris (Eds.), *Preschool education programs for children with autism* (rev. ed., pp. 95–134). Austin, TX: PRO-ED.

Rogers, S. J., Hepburn, S. L., Stackhouse, T., & Wehner, E. (2003). Imitation performance in toddlers with autism and those with other developmental disorders. *Journal of Child Psychology and Psychiatry and Allied Disciplines, 44,* 763–781.

Rogers, S. J., Hepburn, S., & Wehner, E. (2003). Parent reports of sensory symptoms in toddlers with autism and those with other developmental disorders. *Journal of Autism and Developmental Disorders, 33,* 631–642.

Rogers, S. J., & Ozonoff, S. (2006). Behavioral, educational, and developmental treatments for autism. In S. O. Moldin & J. L. R. Rubenstein (Eds.), *Understanding autism: From basic neuroscience to treatment* (pp. 317–348). Boca Raton, FL: CRC Press.

Romanczyk, R. G., Lockshin, S. B., & Matey, L. (2001). The children's unit for treatment and evaluation. In J. Handleman & S. Harris (Eds.), *Preschool education programs for children with autism* (pp. 49–94). Austin, TX: PRO-ED.

Scambler, D., Rogers, S. J., & Wehner, E. A. (2001). Can the checklist for autism in toddlers differentiate autism from those with developmental delays? *Journal of the American Academy of Child and Adolescent Psychiatry, 40,* 1457–1463.

Schertz, H., & Odom, S. L. (2004). Early diagnosis and intervention in autism: The role of joint attention. *Journal of Early Intervention, 27,* 42–53

Schertz, H. H., & Odom, S. L. (in press). Promoting joint attention in toddlers with autism: A parent-mediated developmental model. *Journal of Autism and Developmental Disorders.*

Schopler, E., Reichler, R. J., & Renner, B. R. (1988). *The Childhood Autism Rating Scale.* Los Angeles: Western Psychological Services.

Schwartz, I., Garfinkle, A., & Bauer, J. (1998). The picture exchange communication system: Communicative outcomes for young children with disabilities. *Topics in Early Childhood Special Education, 18,* 144–159.

Schwartz, I., Sandall, S., McBride, B., & Boulware, G. (2004). Project DATA (Developmentally Appropriate Treatment for Autism): An inclusive school-based approach to educating young children with autism. *Topics in Early Childhood Special Education, 23,* 156–168.

Shea, S., Turgay, A., Carroll, A., Schulz, M., Orlik, H., Smith, I., et al. (2004). Risperidone in the treatment of disruptive behavioral symptoms in children with autistic and other pervasive developmental disorders. *Pediatrics, 114,* e634–e641.

Shea, V., & Mesibov, G. B. (2005). Adolescents and adults with autism. In F. Volkmar, R. Paul, A. Klin, & D. Cohen (Eds.), *Handbook of autism and pervasive developmental disorders: Vol. 1. Diagnosis, development, neurobiology, and behavior* (3rd ed., pp. 288–311). Hoboken, NJ: Wiley.

Sherer, M. R., & Schreibman, L. (2005). Individual behavioral profiles and predictors of treatment effectiveness for children with autism. *Journal of Consulting and Clinical Psychology, 73,* 525–538.

Smith, T., Eikeseth, S., Klevstrand, M., & Lovaas, O. I. (1997). Intensive behavioral treatment for preschoolers with severe mental retardation and pervasive developmental disorders. *American Journal on Mental Retardation, 102,* 238–249.

Stahmer, A., & Ingersoll, B. (2004). Inclusive programming for toddlers with autism spectrum disorders: Outcomes from the Children's Toddler School. *Journal of Positive Behavior Interventions, 6,* 67–82.

Stahmer, A. C., Ingersoll, B., & Carter, C. (2003). Behavioral approaches to promoting play. *Autism, 7,* 401–413.

Stevens, M. C., Fein, D. A., Dunn, M., Allen, D., Waterhouse, L. H., Feinstein, C., et al. (2000). Subgroups of children with autism by cluster analysis: A longitudinal analysis. *Journal of the American Academy of Child and Adolescent Psychiatry, 39,* 346–352.

Stoelb, M., Rodney, Y., Miles, J., Takahasi, T. N., Farmer, J. E., & McCathern, R. B. (2004). Predicting responsiveness to treatment of children with autism: A retrospective study of the importance of dysmorphology. *Focus on Autism and Other Developmental Disabilties, 19,* 66–77.

Stone, W., Coonrod, E. E., & Ousley, O. Y. (2000). Screening Tool for Autism in Two-year-olds (STAT): Development and preliminary data. *Journal of Autism and Developmental Disorders, 30,* 607–612.

Stone, W. L., Coonrod, E. E., Turner, L. M., & Pozdol, S. L. (2004). Psychometric properties of the STAT for early autism screening. *Journal of Autism and Developmental Disorders, 34,* 691–701.

Stone, W. L., & Hogan, K. L. (1993). A structured parent interview for identifying young children with autism. *Journal of Autism and Developmental Disorders, 23,* 639–652.

Stone, W. L., Lee, E. B., Ashford, L., Brissie, J., Hepburn, S. L., Coonrod, E. E., et al. (1999). Can autism be diagnosed accurately in children under three years? *Journal of Child Psychology and Psychiatry, 40,* 219–226.

Strain, P., & Hoyson, M. (2000). The need for longitudinal intensive social skill intervention: LEAP follow-up outcomes for children with autism. *Topics in Early Childhood Special Education, 20,* 116–123.

Striano, T., & Bertin, E. (2005). Social–cognitive skills between 5 and 10 months of age. *British Journal of Developmental Psychology, 23,* 559–568.

Strock, M. (2004). *Autism spectrum disorders (pervasive developmental disorders)* (NIH Publication No. NIH-04-5511). Retrieved June 1, 2006, from *www.nimh.nih.gov/publicat/autism.cfm.*

Szatmari, P., Jones, M. B., Zwaigenbaum, L., & MacLean, J. E. (1998). Genetics in autism: Overview and new directions. *Journal of Autism and Developmental Disorders, 28,* 351–368.

U.S. Department of Education. (2004). *Individuals with Disabilities Education Improvement Act of 2004 (Public Law 108-446).* Retrieved August 21, 2006, from *www.ed.gov/about/offices/list/osers/osep/index.html.*

Wert, B. Y., & Neisworth, J. T. (2003). Effects of video self-modeling on spontaneous requesting in children with autism. *Journal of Positive Behavior Interventions, 5,* 30–34.

Wetherby, A. M., Prizant, B. M., & Hutchinson, T. A. (1998). Communicative, social/affective, and symbolic profiles of young children with autism and pervasive developmental disorders. *American Journal of Speech-Language Pathology, 7,* 79–91.

Wetherby, A. M., Woods, J., Allen, L., Cleary, J., Dickinson, H., & Lord, C. (2004). Early indicators of autism spectrum disorders in the second year of life. *Journal of Autism and Developmental Disorders, 34,* 473–493.

Whalen, C., & Schreibman, L. (2003). Joint attention training for children with autism using behavior modification procedures. *Journal of Child Psychology and Psychiatry, 44,* 456–468.

World Health Organization. (1992). *International classification of diseases: Diagnostic criteria for research* (10th ed.). Geneva, Switzerland: Author.

Yoder, P., & Compton, D. (2004). Identify predictors of treatment response. *Mental Retardation and Developmental Disabilities Research Reviews, 10,* 164–168.

Yoder, P., & McDuffie, A. S. (2006). Treatment of responding to and initiating joint attention. In T. Charman & W. Stone (Eds.), *Social and communication development in autism spectrum disorders* (pp. 117–142). New York: Guilford Press.

Yoder, P., & Warren, S. F. (2002). Effects of prelinguistic milieu teaching and parent responsivity education on dyads involving children with intellectual disabilities. *Journal of Speech, Language, and Hearing Research, 45,* 1158–1174.

Zahner, G. E. P., & Pauls, D. L. (1987). Epidemiological surveys of infantile autism. In D. Cohen, A. M. Donnellan, & R. Paul (Eds.), *Handbook of autism and pervasive developmental disorders* (pp. 199–207). New York: Wiley.

Zwaigenbaum, L., Bryson, S., Rogers, T., Roberts, W., Brian, J., & Szatmari, P. (2005). Behavioral manifestations of autism in the first year of life. *International Journal of Developmental Neuroscience, 23,* 143–152.

11

Communication Intervention for Young Children with Disabilities

Naturalistic Approaches to Promoting Development

Ann P. Kaiser
J. Alacia Trent

Learning to communicate is a significant and complex developmental task for young children. Communication has a foundation in primary social interactions, but effective communication requires the coordinated use of cognitive, social, motor, and linguistic skills. The complexity of the social-linguistic communication system and its interdependence with development in other domains makes the language–communication system relatively vulnerable to developmental delay. If a significant delay occurs in any domain of development, it is likely to affect communication development. Thus most children with cognitive, motor, or social delays resulting from genetic or environmental causes are at risk for delays in the development of language and communication skills.

Early intervention for language and communication is the single, most frequently recommended therapy for young children with developmental disabilities and for children at risk due to impoverished environments. Progress in social communication and language skills is an important indicator of general development and provides the foundation for later cognitive, social, and literacy-related skills. Interventions to promote language and communication often begin relatively early, before 36 months, and may continue throughout childhood and adolescence. Although children with significant disabilities may require continuing intervention to support their communication development, early intervention is nonetheless essential for promoting participation in social and learning environments. For children with mild disabilities and children at risk due to impoverished environments, early intervention to support communication and language development may be sufficient to ensure a normal developmental trajectory for cognitive, social, and academic skills. For children with autism spectrum disorders, early intervention to establish functional social communication may be essential to minimizing the lifelong effects of the disorders.

Nearly four decades of research on interventions to promote early language and social communication has provided a substantive empirical foundation. Beginning in the late 1960s, a series of studies demonstrated that children with significant cognitive disabilities could acquire spoken language when taught with direct-instruction strategies (Guess, Sailor, Rutherford, & Baer, 1968; Waryas & Stremel, 1974). The procedures developed for teaching language via direct instruction have continued to be the hallmark of some early-language-intervention approaches (e.g., McEachin, Smith, & Lovaas, 1993) and are frequently used to teach communication skills to children with more severe disabilities (Bambara & Warren, 1993). In more recent comparisons of treatment studies (Cole & Dale, 1986; Losardo & Bricker, 1994; Yoder, Kaiser, et al., 1995), variations of direct instruction have been shown to be effective in teaching the targeted skills to young children. When acquisition and use in the training setting are the primary criteria for effectiveness, substantial evidence indicates that direct instruction is effective for teaching language skills.

Beginning in the late 1970s, a number of studies examining and promoting generalization and maintenance of newly learned language skills, from the direct-instruction setting to everyday social interactions, identified limited generalization and maintenance of skills taught via direct instruction as a concern (see Warren & Kaiser, 1986, for a comprehensive review). This evidence of limited generalization from direct teaching to functional use in natural environments, together with data from studies using incidental teaching strategies to promote language in low-income preschoolers (Hart & Risley, 1968), led to the emergence of naturalistic interventions in everyday environments (Kaiser, Yoder, & Keetz, 1992). In naturalistic interventions, many of the basic teaching strategies from direct instruction (prompting, reinforcement, fading, shaping) were applied during everyday adult–child interactions to teach communication forms that were immediately functional in the conversational setting. Thus, although the content and context for teaching changed to address the emphasis on the generalized use of functional communication skills in natural environments, behavioral instructional strategies continued to be used in naturalistic intervention models that included prompting procedures.

Just after naturalistic interventions began to appear in the empirical literature in the early to mid-1980s, the federal mandate for early intervention for young children with disabilities was passed (Public Law 99-457; U.S. Congress, 1986). This mandate for services in the least restrictive and most typical environments for children with disabilities was a further impetus to develop effective strategies to teach functional communication skills to children during interactions in home, child care, and preschool settings. Since 1986, research in early communication intervention has expanded to include children at the prelinguistic stage of development, as well as children with a range of developmental disabilities who are learning spoken language. Teacher- and parent-implemented naturalistic strategies have been examined to extend communication intervention further into children's typical environments. Finally, strategies for promoting social communication with peers have been developed to extend the naturalistic teaching approach to a wider range of communication partners and contexts in which young children participate and develop.

The emphasis on teaching in natural environments using strategies derived from basic behavioral teaching procedures has been broadened to include strategies for modeling language and responding to children's communication, derived from a social-linguistic interactionist perspective rooted in studies of mother–child interaction (Moerk, 1992). Blending behavioral and social-interactionist techniques for teaching language forms with a strong emphasis on arranging the environment to promote communication has resulted in hybrid naturalistic strategies designed to promote language development in natural environments with caregivers, teachers, and peers.

The purpose of this chapter is to discuss contemporary research on teaching language and communication skills to young children with significant disabilities. We focus on naturalistic language interventions because this general approach remains at the center of both contemporary research and best practices in early intervention. We begin by reviewing the empirical evidence on naturalistic approaches to teaching communication skills: milieu teaching/enhanced milieu teaching, prelinguistic milieu teaching, responsive interaction, pivotal response training, and specific interventions to teach peer-directed communication skills. For each type of intervention, we define the teaching approach, review the procedures used for instruction, describe the populations and settings that have been used in research, summarize the overall findings of empirical studies, and cite examples of studies that illustrate each approach. We then address four key questions about naturalistic teaching approaches: (1) Is naturalistic teaching an effective method of early-language intervention for young children with developmental disabilities? (2) What are the methodological and evidentiary limitations of the research on naturalistic teaching—specifically, across interventions, what is known and not yet known about the effects? (3) What are the critical topics for future research in early-language intervention? (4) What recommendations for practice can be made on the basis of current evidence?

NATURALISTIC LANGUAGE INTERVENTIONS

Naturalistic interventions in the context of everyday play and routines, as a counter to direct instruction, was very much the zeitgeist in language intervention in the 1980s. Naturalistic instruction continues to be the standard for early-language intervention today. Defining the parameters of naturalistic teaching is challenging (Rule, Losardo, Dinnebeil, Kaiser, & Rowland, 1998). In general, naturalistic teaching occurs in children's typical environments and during activities that are focused primarily on things other than language teaching (e.g., play, meals, caregiving, transitions). The instruction occurs when the child is interested and, often, when the child makes an attempt to communicate. An adult's responsiveness to a child's topic and activity are central. Instructional trials are distributed rather than massed, and instructional strategies are conceptually and procedurally wide ranging. The core instructional strategies are often identical to those used in direct teaching (e.g., prompting, reinforcement, time delay, shaping, fading), but they also may include strategies that come from a social-interactionist perspective (e.g., modeling without prompting imitation, expansions, recasts, responsive communication). Naturalistic language interventions may be used as the primary intervention, as an adjunct to direct teaching, or as a generalization promotion strategy.

Four variations of adult-implemented naturalistic teaching have been researched extensively: milieu language teaching (MT), prelinguistic milieu teaching (PMT), responsive interaction (RI), and pivotal response training (PRT). MT, RI, and PRT have also been implemented with siblings or peers as communication partners. In addition, research has investigated other naturalistic interventions as supports for peer-directed social communication, because peer communication is an important developmental goal for young children with language delays. In the following section, we review the four naturalistic teaching approaches and provide an overview of additional strategies for supporting peer-directed social communication by young children with disabilities.

Milieu Language Teaching

Milieu language teaching (MT) is a naturalistic language intervention designed to facilitate language development through the use of systematic prompts for language production embedded in everyday activities. MT was first defined by Hart and Rogers-Warren (1978) as procedures built on the model of incidental teaching. Subsequently, incidental teaching was elaborated into four specific procedures developed specifically to teach functional language to children with significant communication delays (modeling, mand-modeling, time delay, and incidental teaching). Over two decades, MT strategies have been elaborated to include environmental arrangement and responsive interaction strategies, as well as modeling, mand modeling, time delay, and incidental teaching. Since 1990, the expanded model of MT has been referred to as enhanced milieu teaching (EMT; Kaiser, 1993). Variations in MT are not always described sufficiently in the literature to distinguish the degree to which environmental arrangement and responsiveness strategies have been included with the milieu prompting procedures (Rule et al., 1998). Thus, in this chapter, MT and EMT studies are reviewed together. When EMT procedures were clearly specified in an individual study, we use the EMT designation.

Research on the effects of MT/EMT has demonstrated positive gains for young children with developmental delays and disabilities (Kaiser et al., 1992). Children who participate in MT/EMT interventions typically show increased use of targeted language skills, increases in length and complexity of their utterances, and greater diversity in vocabulary (i.e., Kaiser & Hester, 1994; Woods, Kashinath, & Goldstein, 2004). Variations of MT, such as EMT (Kaiser, 1993) have added a responsiveness and modeling component consistent with a social-interactional perspective on language support. The components of MT/EMT are shown in Table 11.1.

Participants and Procedures

The majority of the literature on the generalized effects of MT/EMT includes children between 11 and 60 months of age. Approximately 60 children with language delays or disabilities have been included in 13 studies on the effects of MT. The participants in these studies have had a variety of developmental disabilities and communication disorders, such as severe mental retardation, Down syndrome, cerebral palsy, Williams syndrome, autism, pervasive developmental disorders, developmental apraxia, specific language delay, general language/speech delay or disorder, and significant physical disabilities. Across studies, participants' IQs were reported to be between 43 and 86. General language delays were between 6 and 36 months, expressive language delays between 7 and 52 months, and receptive language delays between 6 and 40 months. Fourteen studies conducted by five different groups of investigators have contributed to this literature. (See Appendix 11.1.)

The majority of the MT/EMT studies have used single-subject research designs to investigate the effects of MT/EMT on targeted language skills. Targeted language skills included two- to four-word utterances, conjunctions, single-word requests, common nouns, common verbs, functional one-word signs, and two- to three-word phrases, with

TABLE 11.1. Components of Milieu Teaching and Enhanced Milieu Teaching

Intervention component	Procedure
Environmental arrangement	• Selecting materials of interest • Arranging materials to promote requests • Mediating the environment • Engaging in activities with the child
Responsive interaction strategies[a]	• Following the child's lead • Balancing turns • Maintaining the child's topic • Modeling linguistically and topically related language • Matching the child's complexity level • Expanding and repeating the child's utterances • Responding communicatively to the child's verbal and nonverbal communication
Milieu teaching techniques	• Modeling • Mand modeling • Time delay • Incidental teaching

[a]These components are included in EMT and may occur in some studies of MT.

the use of signs or communication boards. Intervention settings have included playrooms at university-based clinics or schools, classrooms, and homes; interventionists have included trainers, parents, teachers, and siblings. Intervention sessions were typically conducted twice each week for 30 to 60 minutes for a total of 10 to 73 sessions. Across studies, time actually spent intervening with the child participants (rather than training parent, siblings, or teachers) ranged between 10 and 20 minutes per session.

Results

In studies in which parents, teachers, or siblings were taught to implement MT/EMT strategies, the trained implementers demonstrated improvements in the use of environmental arrangement, responsive-interaction strategies, and/or milieu prompting strategies. Child participants demonstrated language improvements following intervention. They increased their total turns and spontaneous turns taken during interactions and their use of targets, both prompted and unprompted, and demonstrated increases in complexity and mean length of utterance (MLU), as well as diversity of vocabulary. When standardized tests were used to assess outcomes, participants demonstrated improvements on the Sequenced Inventory of Communication Development (SICD; Hedrick, Prather, & Tobin, 1975), Peabody Picture Vocabulary Test (PPVT; Dunn & Dunn, 1997), Expressive One-Word Picture Vocabulary Test (EOWPVT; Brownell, 2001), Assessment, Evaluation, and Programming System (AEPS; Bricker, 1993), Preschool Language Scale (PLS; Zimmerman, Steiner, & Pond, 2002), and the Expressive Vocabulary Test (EVT; Williams, 1997).

In a study on the effects of embedding caregiver-implemented teaching strategies in daily routines, Woods et al. (2004) taught mothers to implement EMT strategies with their young children with developmental delays and disabilities. Parents were taught to use the strategies through written material, oral descriptions, coaching, feedback, and video modeling; intervention sessions took place in the preferred play routines. Following intervention, parents demonstrated improved performances on EMT techniques, and child participants demonstrated increases in frequencies of total targeted language used per session, as well as improved scores on each scale of the AEPS. Assessments of generalization indicated that both parent and child participants were able to generalize their newly acquired behaviors to additional routines.

Generalization assessments were reported in 11 studies on the effects of MT/EMT. Generalization has been assessed: (1) in homes, clinics, and classrooms; (2) across situations such as snack time, caregiving routines, outdoor play, and small-group activities; and (3) across people, including trained and untrained parents, trained and untrained teachers, peers, and research assistants. Generalized improvements have been reported for more than 50% of all participants on measures that include total utterances, spontaneous utterances, target use, spontaneous target use, MLU, and diversity. Generalization of targeted language skills has been reported consistently across studies. Findings suggest that participants have been able to generalize their training to use early syntactic relationships, two- to four-word utterances, conjunctions, single-word requests, common nouns, common verbs, functional sounds, and signs. Both spontaneous and total target use have increased for most participants across generalization contexts.

In a study on the generalized effects of EMT, Kaiser and Hester (1994) investigated the generalized effects of trainer-implemented EMT. Following the EMT intervention with the trainer, participants were assessed in three generalization settings: at home with a parent, in the classroom with a teacher, and in the classroom with a peer. With teachers, most participants performed above baseline levels in total utterances, target use, and diversity of vocabulary with teachers. None of the participants, however, demonstrated increases in MLU in teacher generalization sessions. With parents, they demonstrated generalized use of total utterances, targets, and diversity of vocabulary from training to generalization sessions. Changes in MLU, however, were small and variable in the parent generalization sessions. Finally, few participants generalized newly learned behaviors to peers. Although 5 of the 6 participants performed higher than baseline levels in peer generalization sessions, fewer than half of the participants performed above baseline levels on total utterances, total target use, or MLU.

Prelinguistic Milieu Teaching

Prelinguistic milieu teaching (PMT) is a modified version of milieu teaching that is designed specifically to facilitate the emergence of intentional communication in children with mental retardation. Components of PMT are quite similar to those of EMT: praise, models, prompts, responsiveness, expansions, turn taking, and environmental arrangement (Yoder & Warren, 2001). PMT was developed to help children transition from prelinguistic forms of communication to spoken language and has been applied primarily with children who demonstrate early forms of intentional communication, such as nonverbal requesting (reaching, giving, gesturing) with or without vocalizations. PMT is implemented to increase initiated joint attention, to make requesting more consistent and clear, and to build nonverbal and vocal commenting. Increasing these forms of prelinguistic communication and mapping communication attempts with language is presumed to promote the transition into the use of verbal communication. PMT is also used with children who have very limited spoken language in order to increase the range of forms and functions they express. PMT specifically promotes commenting as a basis for social-language development. Typically, behavioral targets are selected for children based on their existing performance in their communication samples, an experimenter–child sample, a mother–child sample, or an assessment using the Communication and Symbolic Play Scales (CSBS; Wetherby & Prizant, 1993). PMT has been used to facilitate total requests and comments, spontaneous requests and comments, turn taking, one-word to multiword utterances, and lexical density.

Participants and Procedures

Research on the effects of PMT has studied children between 17 and 36 months of age. More than 110 children with language delays or disabilities have been included in studies on the effects of PMT. The range of disabilities included in the research is diverse. Typical participants in PMT research have had fewer than 10 productive words, expressive-language levels of about 7–11 months, receptive-language levels of about 8–14 months, and cognitive skills in the range of 8–16 months. Participants' diagnoses have included autism, Down syndrome, cerebral palsy, Williams syndrome, encephaly, microcephaly, agenesis of the corpus collosum, and developmental disabilities. Five studies, all conducted by the same research group, constitute this literature. (See Appendix 11.1.)

Both single-subject design and group design research has been used to investigate the effects of PMT. Intervention settings have included playrooms located next to participants' classrooms at university-based clinics or schools. PMT has not been used within classrooms or at home. PMT interventionists have been trained research assistants, graduate students, and speech/language professionals. Intervention sessions have typically been conducted three to four times each week for 20 minutes per session. Intervention usually lasts up to 6 months.

Results

Results of research on PMT suggest that participants demonstrate an accelerated use of child-initiated comments and requests, as well as increases in imitations and lexical density, following intervention. Not all children benefit equally, however, and Yoder and colleagues have examined the predictors of treatment outcomes in several studies. Yoder, Warren, and Hull (1995) found that pretreatment measures of play predicted participants' responses to the intervention. Researchers observed pretreatment play of participants and coded play into four categories: uncodable, person-only engagement, undifferentiated object exploration, and transitional/symbolic play. Results suggested that high rates of play categorized as person-only engagement at pretreatment were predictive of slow increases in intentional communication during and following intervention. Results also suggested that high rates of play categorized as transitive/symbolic at pretreatment were predictive of faster increases in intentional communication during and following intervention. In general, children with higher mental ages showed greater gains during the intervention.

In a study on the relative treatment effects of two prelinguistic communication interventions on language development in toddlers with developmental delays and disabilities, Yoder and Warren (2001) compared the effects of PMT and responsive small groups in which children participated in group play sessions with highly responsive interaction partners. Surprisingly small differences in outcomes between the two groups were found, and both interventions appeared to be effective. Results of the study suggest that high maternal responsiveness and education were related to faster growth in lexical density for children in the PMT group. Lower maternal responsiveness and education were related to faster growth in lexical density for children in the responsive small groups. Further improvements were found at the 6- to 12-month follow-up assessments. These findings led to revisions of the PMT model to include training for parents in basic responsiveness strategies that facilitate children's development following intervention.

Responsive Interaction

Responsive interaction (RI) is a naturalistic, play-based intervention strategy used to promote communication and interaction in young children with developmental delays and disabilities. There are two primary features of responsive interaction: nonverbal mirroring and verbal responding (Kaiser & Delaney, 1998). These two features derive from observations of typical parent–child interaction and appear to be foundational for promoting reciprocal social interactions between children and adults. *Mirroring*, defined as the contingent imitation of nonverbal behavior, requires the more capable interaction partner to attend to the nonverbal behaviors of the child with a disability. Mirroring supports turn taking and may help the interaction partner in making activity-relevant comments and contingent responses during interactions with the child with a disability. Through *verbal responding* the interaction partner is contingently responsive to the child, models language responses appropriate to the child's interest and the context, and offers the child opportunities to initiate and respond as part of verbal turn taking. In addition, RI may include modeling language at the child's target level as part of the verbal responding. Although RI has been integrated into MT (e.g., EMT; Kaiser, 1993) and into PMT (rePMT; Fey et al., 2006), the effects of RI without the accompanying use of prompting techniques have been studied in a small number of investigations. Research on RI has included children with developmental delays and disabilities between the ages of 2 and 7 years in classrooms, clinics, and homes. Four studies, conducted by the same research group and including 53 children, make up the research on RI. (See Appendix 11.1.) Although the number of studies is small, RI has been implemented by a range of communication partners, including teachers, parents, and siblings. Because of the small number of diverse studies, we discuss three examples.

Yoder, Kaiser, et al. (1995) compared the effects of MT and RI on child communication behaviors. In this study, 36 children between the ages of 2 and 7 years were assigned to one of the two treatments. Teachers were trained to be the primary interventionists and conducted approximately three intervention activities per day for a total of 64 school days; each intervention activity lasted about 15 to 30 minutes. No main effects for treatment were found. Participants in both groups showed similar improvements on MLU, diversity of vocabulary, scores on the EOWPVT, PPVT, and SICD, total utterances, and spontaneous utterances. MT, however, was more effective in promoting receptive language and expressive vocabulary if the children began intervention with relatively low receptive- or expressive-language levels. RI was more effective than MT in facilitating receptive language and expressive vocabulary when the children began intervention with relatively high receptive- or expressive-language levels.

Kaiser and Hester (1994) examined the effects of RI implemented by 12 parents trained to use it with their language-delayed preschoolers in a multiple baseline design across groups of parent–child dyads. All children showed some positive effects, although there was variability in the specific outcomes. Children with low rates of talking typically showed increases in rate of communication and target use. Children with higher levels of language at baseline typically demonstrated moderate increases in their spontaneous use of targets, MLU, and standardized test scores. Nine of the 12 children generalized and maintained their improvements in language in observations at home. Children whose parents demonstrated mastery of the RI strategies appeared to do better in training and home sessions than those whose parents did not.

Trent, Kaiser, and Wolery (2005) examined the effects of an RI intervention designed to facilitate interactions between two older, typically developing children and their younger siblings with Down syndrome using a multiple-baseline design across behaviors and participants. Typically developing siblings were taught to use two RI strategies with written materials, modeling, role play, and oral feedback during twice weekly intervention sessions of approximately 30 to 60 minutes each. Following intervention, the typically developing siblings demonstrated the ability to use the RI strategies, and modest changes were observed in the communicative behaviors of their siblings with Down syndrome. The siblings maintained their newly learned behaviors at a 1-month follow-up assessment. This study expands the literature on the effects of teaching siblings to implement naturalistic communication strategies with children who have language delays.

The results of RI studies are similar to results reported by Cole, Mills, Dale, and Jenkins (1996) for developmentally appropriate modeling of new language forms. In the Cole et al. study, the responsiveness components (contingent responding, following the child's lead in play and topic maintenance) were not the primary features of the intervention. Thus contemporary RI interventions differ from earlier modeling interventions by emphasizing the social communicative aspects of the interaction, in addition to language modeling. Presumably, it is the combination of responsiveness and language modeling that contributes to the results of the RI studies.

Pivotal Response Training

Pivotal response training (PRT) is a play-based intervention program developed to increase pivotal behaviors in children with autism. Pivotal behaviors are central to a wide area of functioning, such as responding to multiple cues and motivation (Weiss & Harris, 2001). Increases in these pivotal behaviors often lead to improvements across behavioral domains. For example, PRT has been used to facilitate language skills, symbolic play, and sociodramatic play in children with autism. PRT has been proven effective with children of varying developmental levels and when implemented by therapists, parents, and peers in classrooms, group settings, homes, and clinics. Pivotal behaviors promoted through PRT include motivation, response to multiple cues, child self-initiations, and self-management, as shown in Table 11.2. Although PRT is not limited to teaching specific language targets, it can be used to teach a range of social communicative, play, and functional responses that include language as a key component.

Participants and Procedures

The majority of the research on PRT has been done with children with autism. Within this body of research, participants have ranged from approximately 18 to 58 months of age. Research on PRT has included trainer-, parent-, and peer-implemented interven-

TABLE 11.2. Pivotal Behaviors and Intervention Strategies

Pivotal response	Intervention procedure
Motivation	• Provide the child choice • Vary tasks and intersperse maintenance activities • Reinforce attempts • Use natural reinforcers
Multiple cues	• Encourage multiple-cue learning and responses
Self-initiated responses	• Teach question asking
Self-management	• Teach children to discriminate their own behaviors and to record the occurrence or absence of the behavior

Note. Data from Koegel, Koegel, and Carter (1999).

tion sessions. The intervention itself typically consists of 1 to 3 PRT sessions per week for a range of about 12 to 36 sessions per participant; approximately 10 minutes of each session is spent intervening directly with the target child. Nine studies from three different research groups have been published.

Results

Intervention effects have been positive across studies of PRT. When trainers have been the primary interventionists, participants have demonstrated increases in total one- to three-word utterances, total one- to three-word spontaneous utterances, utterance attempts, pragmatic skills, adaptive behavior, symbolic play, and play complexity, as well as decreases in disruptive behaviors. In a study of generalization and maintenance of PRT effects (Stahmer, 1995), participants demonstrated maintenance of symbolic play and play complexity, as well as generalization to mothers, fathers, and new toys. Assessments of generalization to peers, however, indicated that children were unable to generalize newly acquired play behaviors to peers.

Results of parent- and peer-implemented PRT have also been positive. In a study by Koegel, Symon, and Koegel (2002), distal families (families who did not live near the training center) were taught to use PRT strategies through a brief but intensive parent education program. Parents were trained with written material, oral description, coaching, feedback, and modeling. Parents in this study learned to use the PRT techniques correctly during 80–100% of interactions with their children and demonstrated generalization to and maintenance in the home. Subsequently, child utterances at home increased following intervention.

When peers have been taught PRT strategies through written material, oral descriptions, role play, coaching, and feedback, target children have increased play and conversation initiations, maintenance of interactions, engagement in supported and coordinated joint attention, and word use. In a study assessing generalization of peer-implemented PRT effects, participants engaged in the newly learned social behaviors in generalization settings with untrained peers, novel settings, and novel training stimuli (Pierce & Schreibman, 1997).

Peer-Directed Interventions

Peers have been the primary interventionists in a number of interventions aimed at promoting social communication in children with developmental disabilities in natural environments. In these studies, typically developing peers are taught a series of strategies to promote social communicative interaction and then paired with targeted children during a play activity. Peer-directed interventions can be classified into two types: (1) interventions in which the peer uses strategies similar to MT or PRT to teach the target child specific responses (e.g., waiting for a request, asking for a label, providing the target child with the labeled object, and praising appropriate responses; McGee, Aimeda, Sulzer-Azaroff, & Feldman, 1992) and (2) interventions that teach the peer confederate strategies and content for communicating with the target child. Peer-directed communication intervention strategies have included script training (Goldstein & Cisar, 1992), sensitivity training (Goldstein, English, Shafer, & Kaczmarek, 1997), and training in more specific strategies such as maintaining proximity, establishing mutual attention, commenting about ongoing activities, and general acknowledgement of the target partner's communication acts. Commonly used procedures for increasing peer-directed communication are summarized in Table 11.3.

Participants and Procedures

Most of the research on peer-directed interventions has been done with children with mild to moderate autism, but children with Down syndrome and developmental delays have also been included. Within this body of research, participants have ranged from approximately 35 to 81 months of age. Typical peers have ranged in age from 47 to 64 months of age. Most peer training consisted of 4 to 10 training sessions between the peer and an adult trainer. Peer training was often followed by observations of the peers and target children one to three times per day for a total of 7 to 42 sessions. Because peers have been involved in a large number of studies that

TABLE 11.3. Peer-Directed Communication Interventions

Intervention	Procedure
Script training	• Peer use of sociodramatic scripts (i.e., pet shop, carnival, and magic show) to scaffold communicative interactions in play
Peer-prompting sequences	• Wait for request • Ask target child for label • Give object to target child when labeled • Praise for correct responses
Responsive communication strategies	• Turn taking (verbal and nonverbal) • Maintaining proximity during play • Contingent imitation of actions during play (mirroring) • Mutual attention to play activity • Commenting about ongoing activity • Responsiveness to and acknowledgement of target partner's communicative acts

address primarily social behavior, and because peers have been included in studies of EMT and PRT, as discussed earlier, a precise count of studies and research groups is difficult. More than 10 studies with specific measures of peer-directed communication from at least five research groups can be identified. (See Appendix 11.1.) Not included in this summary are studies of video modeling that included some form of peer-directed social or communicative behavior or those studies that targeted increasing social initiations and responses without the goal of increasing specific language in the target children.

Results

Results of the peer-directed intervention literature are encouraging. Target children have demonstrated increases in initiations and responses during interactions, with some indication of improved performance of target utterances or specific language forms. Peers have demonstrated the ability to implement intervention strategies and have shown increases in initiations to target children. Both target children and peers have become more responsive to communication attempts by their partners. Teachers have rated the social competence of both peers and target children as higher following intervention.

Goldstein and Cisar (1992) investigated the effects of teaching scripts to typically developing preschool peers and classmates with disabilities. They were taught three sociodramatic play scripts (pet shop, carnival, and magic show). Peers were trained through role play with an adult trainer and practice with the target child while receiving coaching and feedback from the trainer. Script training was conducted for 5 to 10 days for approximately 15 minutes per day; then the dyads participated in approximately 29 intervention sessions. Following intervention, target children and peers increased theme-related behavior, with specific verbalizations related to the play themes increasing, whereas unrelated behavior decreased. The effects of the intervention were replicated across all three scripts and were maintained when dyads were regrouped to assess generalization.

Goldstein et al. (1997) investigated the effects of an across-the-day intervention on interactions between preschoolers with and without disabilities. Participants in the study included 8 typically developing children and 8 children with disabilities (e.g., Down syndrome and developmental delay) between the ages of 42 and 61 months; participants were divided into two cohorts. Peers received sensitivity training and training in communication strategy use. Sensitivity training consisted of two 20-minute training sessions aimed at sensitizing peers to types of attention-getting and requesting behaviors that target children might use as attempts to communicate. Strategy-use training consisted of three direct-instruction sessions focusing on a sequential behavior chain, including behavior such as maintaining proximity, establishing mutual attention, maintaining talking, and playing with the target child (i.e., stay, talk, play). Following peer training, data were collected from 7 to 26 intervention sessions between the target children and their peers. In cohort 1, both sensitivity training and strategy-use training took place prior to the beginning of intervention sessions. In cohort 2, the sequence was (1) sensitivity training for peers, (2) intervention sessions with target children, (3) strategy-use training for peers, and (4) a second phase of intervention sessions with the target children. Results from cohort 1 (combined sensitivity and strategy-use training) suggested that peers increased their frequencies of social communicative behavior directed toward the target children. Similarly, target children increased the frequency of their social communication directed toward peers. Target children and peers demonstrated generalization of these behaviors when dyads were regrouped. The overall frequency of interactions between target children and untrained peers, however, remained low. For cohort 2, improvements in the social behaviors of both peers and target children were not demonstrated until both sensitivity training and strategy-use training had been completed.

IMPLICATIONS AND LIMITATIONS OF NATURALISTIC INTERVENTION RESEARCH

Is Naturalistic Teaching Effective?

Using contemporary standards, there is relatively strong evidence of the effectiveness of naturalistic interventions to teach generalized communication skills. MT/EMT, RI, PMT, and PRT are all effective in teaching a range of children to use specific language targets, in increasing total and spontaneous communication, in increasing complexity and length of utterances, and in increasing diversity of vocabulary and multiword utterances. Research on PMT suggests that a modified MT approach may facilitate prelinguistic communication in young children with developmental delays and disabilities. The effects of naturalistic teaching have been replicated across participants, in studies conducted by different research groups, in single-subject and group designs, and using both adult and peer agents to implement the intervention. Given the magnitude of gains reported in communication skills, naturalistic teaching is efficient. The amount of time that children spent in intervention across studies of PRT, MT/EMT, RI, and PMT was relatively short, typically about 15 minutes, two times per week for an average of about 12–16 weeks. Naturalistic teaching strategies have been used by a range of intervention agents (speech therapists, graduate students, trained staff, teachers, parents, and peers), with dependable effects on children's targeted communication. Teaching parents, teachers, siblings, and peers to implement naturalistic intervention strategies may be an efficient strategy for promoting learning and/or use of new communication skills in everyday social contexts.

There is also evidence of the effectiveness of naturalistic interventions involving peers, including peer-implemented PRT, sibling-implemented MT/EMT, and RI, as well as interventions based on scripting, peer prompting, and increasing peer communicative responsiveness. Peer- or sibling-implemented naturalistic interventions consistently result in increased social communicative interactions between children with disabilities and their peers. In some instances, peer-based interventions also result in changes in the content or complexity of communication by the children with disabilities. The range of peer-implemented naturalistic procedures for promoting child–child communication allows for selection of a strategy that fits the needs of the target child with disabilities, the interaction context, and the skills of the peer interventionist. The research base for naturalistic peer-implemented communication interventions is relatively modest compared with the larger set of studies that examine the effects of adult-implemented naturalistic teaching. There are some concerns about the degree of prompt dependence evidenced by some children in these studies. Additional replications across child populations, contexts, and research groups are needed, with attention to independent use of peer communication skills. To date, there have been no investigations integrating peer- and adult-implemented interventions for the same child participants.

Although the findings related to effectiveness of naturalistic teaching characterized here apply to all forms of naturalistic teaching, research on PRT is still somewhat unique. The research on PRT has focused on teaching children with autism to initiate social communication using target forms (see also Odom, Rogers, McDougle, Hume, & McGee, Chapter 10, this volume). The act of initiating, rather than the linguistic form of the initiation, has been a primary emphasis, because PRT proposes that initiation is the pivotal behavior for increasing functions of language and the appearance of normalcy in social interaction. A range of communication forms have been taught along with social play and play complexity, and these skills appear to generalize to other contexts. The effects of the PRT approach may be cumulative. For example, increased motivation, responses to multiple cues, and increased play skills may facilitate a child's participation in classroom interactions, thus promoting further social and communicative interactions. The unique focus of PRT that results from its specific application to children with autism makes comparison of its outcomes to those of other naturalistic interventions somewhat difficult, and there have been no studies investigating the differential effects of PRT versus other naturalistic procedures or studies of PRT with children who did not have autism.

What Are the Limitations of Research on Naturalistic Teaching?

Variability in Outcomes for Children

Although the results of naturalistic language interventions were positive for most participants, some children improved more than others. There is a need to better understand the child and treatment protocol predictors of responses to treatment, as has been done in studies of PMT and in one study of MT in classrooms. For example, children in the early stages of language learning (MLU below 2.0) appear to benefit more when taught by MT than by RI methods, whereas children at later stages of development (MLU above 2.5) benefit more when taught using RI (Yoder et al., 1995). The effects of language on development are more variable than are direct measures of use of specific target behaviors. Typically, vocabulary and simple multiword targets have proven to be easier targets for intervention than increasing generative use of syntax or complex language, suggesting that additional strategies for promoting generative use and development at higher levels of language may be needed. There are modest indications that children's vocabulary development, measured on standardized language measures, can be facilitated by naturalistic teaching; evidence of syntactic development is minimal. Child characteristics may interact with treatment assessment methods to increase the apparent variability in developmental outcomes. For example, children with autism may have particular difficulty performing in standardized testing situations, making assessment of developmental effects using these methods potentially unreliable.

Need for Specification of Naturalistic Teaching Models

Variations in quality of interactive teaching and in the range of examples of each target class may also contribute to differences in child outcomes. Advancing the naturalistic paradigm requires conceptualization and better measurement of interventionist behaviors: (1) specifying all interactional components of naturalistic teaching, (2) precisely implementing the specified model, and (3) providing sufficient opportunities to learn specific targets via multiple exemplars that are the foundation of generative language use. Naturalistic teaching is child centered. It occurs in response to child interests and takes into account the child's changing abilities to respond independent of direct prompting. Scaffolding interactions, entering into play, arranging the environment to promote engagement and requesting, teaching specific forms in their functional context, and responding to the child rather than directing the interaction are the hallmarks of naturalistic teaching.

Measurement of core instructional strategies (e.g., modeling, prompting) and some aspects of responsiveness (e.g., mirroring, turn taking) are relatively straightforward, and these measures are typically reported in studies of naturalistic teaching. Measurement of the fidelity of the complex set of behaviors required of the naturalistic interventionist is more difficult. The set of behaviors may include determining when to change or add to materials, scaffolding and expanding limited play, preventing problem behavior, maintaining child engagement, choosing specific instructional strategies based on the child's independent responding, determining when to prompt a single response repeatedly to promote acquisition versus prompting varied responses to prevent preservative or rote behavior, and providing systematic and sufficient examples of a response class.

Few studies have been designed with a specified criterion number of teaching episodes, the number of different examples of target classes, or the level of spontaneous use (vs. imitated or supported by visual or verbal choices) by the child that would ensure sufficient opportunities for learning. There are no empirical data to guide interventionists in determining these levels. Thus variability in child outcomes may be the result of unmeasured variability in the instruction. Insufficient exemplars may limit the acquisition and generalization of targets. Teaching until the child is able to use multiple examples of the target structure spontaneously may be a necessary condition for both mastery and generalization. In sum, the standard of measuring acquisition, mastery, and fluency that has been used in studies of direct instruction has not yet been applied in measuring the effects of naturalistic teaching. Although the responsive quality of the teaching procedures and natural environment settings make this type of measurement more difficult, such a continuum of measurement may be essential to understanding and reducing variability in child outcomes.

Some researchers using naturalistic language interventions have not reported direct measures of procedural fidelity. This is especially true for studies of PRT and those in which parents or peers were trained to implement interventions. General descriptions of the training method have not included direct measures of the training procedures applied to the implementation agent or criterion performance levels for the adult or peer trainers and for the child participants—making it difficult to determine the relationship between implementation of the training, use of intervention strategies, and child outcomes.

A surprising portion of studies of naturalistic teaching have been conducted in clinical or relatively controlled play settings rather than in classrooms. Although several studies involving parents have included observations of their use of MT/EMT at home, implementation across the day in preschool activities has been reported in only a few studies. Although studies of PMT are based in a naturalistic approach that embeds the language teaching procedures in play activities, no applications of PMT in homes or child care settings have been reported. A well-developed technology for naturalistic teaching requires conducting studies in natural environments and addressing the full range of skills and strategies needed to integrate this teaching approach into classrooms, child care settings, and homes.

Promoting and Assessing Generalization

Although most studies have been designed to measure the diversity of vocabulary, and although two studies have measured the diversity of specific targets (Warren, Gazdag, Bambara, & Jones, 1994; Warren, 1992), no researcher has reported a systematic method for promoting generalization across word classes or syntactic classes. The use of a language matrix proposed by Goldstein (1983) to select exemplars to be presented in intervention sessions could ensure that multiple exemplars of a word class or syntactic class, social, or play behavior are presented to the learner and could assist the interventionist in programming for generalization. Similarly, although there has been systematic assessment of generalization across settings and partners, relatively little research has included steps to promote generalization across social contexts.

The conditions under which generalization has been assessed have varied widely, and the results reported may reflect the varying conditions of assessment as much as differences in child outcomes across studies. Both opportunities to communicate and the responsiveness of the generalization partner affect a child's performance. Generalization in studies in which parents were trained to be responsive is, not surprisingly, stronger than in studies that assessed child communication with untrained peers. Measuring the degree of support provided in the generalization context is an important next step in understanding the generalized effects of naturalistic teaching. Similarly, beginning to program across-setting and across-partner generalization by teaching the skills children need to bootstrap their use of new communication skills in less supportive environments is important. To ensure generalization of targeted language skills across settings and persons, children need experiences interacting with individuals who provide varying levels of support and responsiveness. Kaczmarek, Hepting, and Dzubak (1996) provided an example of programming across-partner generalization that could be included in naturalistic teaching. They used a 4×6 matrix with setting/communication partner on one dimension and situations requiring gradually decreasing demands for listener preparatory behaviors on the other dimension. Children were trained and observed across four levels of gradually decreasing listener support using four combinations of setting and communication partner (i.e., trainer in a training environment, nontrainer in a training environment, trainer in a nontraining environment, and nontrainer in a nontraining environment).

What Research Is Needed on Naturalistic Teaching?

We have already highlighted several areas in which further research is needed. More investigations of the child characteristics and variations in treatment fidelity and protocol that affect generalized developmental outcomes are needed to specify treatment dosage for children with a range of developmental skills. Few studies were conducted entirely in preschool classrooms and child care settings during ongoing activities and at home across daily living activities, and such studies are needed to test the power of naturalistic interventions. Research is needed to investigate the parameters of communication support that contribute to generalization, such as opportunities to talk, the match between target skills and natural opportunities, and the availability of responsive peers. Although the improved generalization of newly learned skills was an initial incentive for naturalistic teaching, additional research is needed to further develop strategies to promote generalization across target classes and settings in which support is limited.

At the end of more than two decades of study in this area, developing comprehensive naturalistic teaching interventions should be foremost on the research agenda. By "comprehensive interventions," we mean interventions that specify a full sequence of target skills (prelinguistic communication, vocabulary, semantics, syntax, and social pragmatic skills ranging from simple to complex) and procedures for teaching generalized skills so that children make significant progress in language development and in remediation of significant delays in communication skills. Most studies of naturalistic teaching have taught a small set or range of skills to children in relatively brief interventions. It is not clear whether naturalistic methods are sufficient for teaching the range of skills that many children with disabilities need for functional communication in social and learning contexts. New research should: (1) determine the intensity and duration of intervention needed to ensure children's mastery of skills; (2) specify the range of target communicative and linguistic skills; (3) embed procedures to promote generalization; and (4) teach ancillary skills that may be essential to children's use of new language (e.g., pragmatics, play skills, peer-directed social interaction skills). Although randomized group designs may be needed to test the effectiveness of comprehensive naturalistic interventions in comparison with other approaches to intervention, developmental work using single-subject designs will also be informative. As part of developing and testing comprehensive communication interventions, we must conceptualize and measure accurately the range of effects of intervention on development in children with disabilities

A second approach to developing comprehensive interventions is to interweave the communication skills perspective with the engagement, behavior, play, and social skills that provide a platform for communicative interactions. Research on PRT provides one framework for doing this for children with autism, but additional research is needed using other naturalistic approaches with children who have social-initiation skills. It is possible to expand current models of naturalistic teaching in three ways: (1) add instructional techniques from behavioral research (e.g., instructive feedback, constant time delay) to the naturalistic language teaching paradigm; (2) use peer-directed communication prompts in addition to adult-directed prompts to teach a wider range of target language, especially vocabulary and advanced syntax; and (3) integrate naturalistic teaching with techniques that promote self-management, activity engagement, and social participation (e.g., visual schedules, social stories, and plan–play–report sequences). Finally, there is a critical need to develop efficient technologies for training naturalistic teachers, as well as for monitoring implementation fidelity and child progress in everyday settings.

What Recommendations Can Be Made for Practice?

Use of naturalistic intervention strategies to teach communication skills to young children with disabilities can be recommended based on the existing empirical evidence. The individual instructional components of naturalistic teaching are well defined. Yet practitioners may find translation from research to practice challenging without detailed information on how to choose target behaviors, how to arrange classroom schedules, activities, and home routines to deliver naturalistic teaching episodes, and how to fully embed teaching in play, routines, and social interactions with peers. Effectively arranging the environment supports the naturalistic teacher as much as it supports the learner. Thus planning when to teach, selecting materials to teach specific targets, concurrent use of strategies to prevent and manage problem behavior, and strategies for including classroom peers in instructional interactions are an essential part of practitioner-implemented naturalistic teaching.

Both the direct evidence from studies of RI and the indirect evidence of differential effects of PMT with responsive caregivers suggest that the responsive behavior of adults and peers will affect the overall impact of naturalistic teaching on children's communication. Thus, optimizing the generalized effects of naturalistic teaching may require increasing responsiveness of other communication partners and arranging opportunities for using newly learned communication skills across the day outside of teaching episodes. Similarly, the effects of naturalistic teaching interventions may be enhanced when the environment provides models of language at the child's target level from adults and peers. Increasing child engagement after the child has learned to attend to modeling during naturalistic intervention may accelerate learning new forms; however, this idea is untested in the empirical literature. In sum, the practitioner has the challenging task of integrating naturalistic teaching fully in the child's environments, selecting the content and contexts for teaching, and providing the ancillary environmental supports to scaffold generalization and extend learning in everyday interactions.

CONCLUSIONS

Nearly three decades of research in naturalistic teaching has yielded four systematic teaching strategies (MT/EMT, PMT, RI, and PRT) and a set of strategies for promoting peer-directed communication. Studies using these strategies indicate that they are moderately to highly effective with a range of young children who face communication challenges in development. Research is needed to maximize the generalization of new vocabulary, syntax, and social use of these skills across contexts and to assemble target content and teaching procedures into a comprehensive model of early-communication intervention.

The next generation of studies on naturalistic language teaching must be informed by applications in everyday settings, as well as by the overarching goal of developing an intervention approach that can teach the range of skills needed to facilitate language development in children with disabilities. Practitioners and applied researchers can play an important role in testing, validating, defining, and ultimately shaping the naturalistic teaching paradigm toward an effective and comprehensive communication intervention delivered in everyday environments.

ACKNOWLEDGMENTS

Preparation of this chapter was supported in part by National Institutes of Health Grant No. R01 HD045745-02 to Ann P. Kaiser.

REFERENCES

Bambara, L. M., & Warren, S. F. (1993). Massed trials revisited: Appropriate applications in functional skill training. In R. A. Gable & S. F. Warren (Eds.), *Advances in metal retardation and developmental disabilities* (pp. 165–190). Philadelphia: Kingsley.

Bricker, D. (1993). *Assessment, Evaluation, and Programming System (AEPS) for infants and children: Measurement from birth to three years* (Vol. 1.). Baltimore: Brookes.

Brownell, R. (2001). *Expressive One-Word Picture Vocabulary Test*. Novato, CA: Academic Therapy Association.

Cole, K. N., & Dale, P. S. (1986). Direct language instruction and interactive language instruction with language delayed preschool children: A comparison study. *Journal of Speech and Hearing Research, 29*, 206–217.

Cole, K. N., Mills, P. E., Dale, P. S., & Jenkins, J. R. (1996). Preschool language facilitation methods and child characteristics. *Journal of Early Intervention, 20*, 113–131.

Dunn, L. M, & Dunn, L. M. (1997). *Peabody Picture Vocabulary Test–III* (3rd ed.). Circle Pines, MN: American Guidance Services.

Fey, M., Warren, S., Brady, N., Finestack, L., Bredin-Oja, S., Fairchild, M., et al. (2006). Early effects of responsivity education/prelinguistic milieu teaching for children with developmental delays and their parents. *Journal of Speech, Language and Hearing Research, 49*(3), 526–548.

Goldstein, H. (1983). Recombinative generalization: Relationships between environmental conditions and the linguistic repertoires of language learners. *Analysis and Intervention in Developmental Disabilities, 3*, 279–293.

Goldstein, H., & Cisar, C. (1992). Promoting interaction during sociodramatic play: Teaching scripts to typical preschoolers and classmates with disabilities. *Journal of Applied Behavioral Analysis, 25*, 265–280.

Goldstein, H., English, K., Shafer, K., & Kaczmarek, L. (1997). Interaction among preschoolers with and without disabilities: Effects of across-the-day peer intervention. *Journal of Speech, Language, and Hearing Research, 40*, 33–48.

Guess, D., Sailor, W., Rutherford, D., & Baer, D. M. (1968). An experimental analysis of linguistic development: The productive use of the plural morpheme. *Journal of Applied Behavioral Analysis, 1*, 297–306.

Hart, B. M., & Risley, T. R. (1968). Establishing use of descriptive adjectives in the spontaneous speech of disadvantaged preschool children. *Journal of Applied Behavior Analysis, 1*, 109–120.

Hart, B. M., & Rogers-Warren, A. K. (1978). A milieu approach to teaching language. In R. L. Schiefelbusch (Ed.), *Language intervention strategies* (Vol. 2, pp. 192–235). Baltimore: University Park Press.

Hedrick, D. L., Prather, E. M., & Tobin, A. R. (1975). *Sequenced Inventory of Communication Development*. Seattle: University of Washington Press.

Kaczmarek, L. A., Hepting, N. H., & Dzubak, M. (1996). Examining the generalization of milieu language objectives in situations requiring listener preparatory behaviors. *Topics in Early Childhood Special Education, 16*, 139–167.

Kaiser, A. P. (1993). Parent-implemented language intervention: An environmental system perspective. In A. P. Kaiser & D. B. Gray (Eds.), *Enhancing children's communication: Research foundations for intervention* (Vol. 2, pp. 63–84). Baltimore: Brookes.

Kaiser, A. P., & Delaney, E. M. (1998). Responsive conversation: Creating opportunities for naturalistic language teaching. *Young Exceptional Children Monograph Series, 3*, 13–23.

Kaiser, A. P., & Hester, P. P. (1994). Generalized effects of enhanced MT. *Journal of Speech and Hearing Research, 37*, 1320–1340.

Kaiser, A. P., Yoder, P. J., & Keetz, A. (1992). Evaluating milieu teaching. In S. F. Warren & J. Reichle (Eds.), *Causes and effects in communication and language intervention* (Vol. 1, pp. 9–47). Baltimore: Brookes.

Koegel, R. L., Symon, J. B., & Koegel, L. K. (2002). Parent education for families of children with autism living in distant areas. *Journal of Positive Behavior Interventions, 4*, 88–103.

Koegel, R. L., Koegel, L. K., & Carter, C. M. (1999). Pivotal teaching interactions for children with autism. *School Psychology Review, 28*, 576–594.

Losardo, A., & Bricker, D. (1994). Activity-based intervention and direct instruction: A comparison study. *American Journal on Mental Retardation, 98*, 744–765.

McEachin, J. J., Smith, T., & Lovaas, O. I. (1993). Long-term outcome for children with autism who received early intensive behavioral treatment. *American Journal on Mental Retardation, 97*, 359–372.

McGee, G. G, Aimeda, M. C., Sulzer-Azaroff, B., & Feldman, R. S. (1992). Promoting reciprocal interactions via peer incidental teaching. *Journal of Applied Behavioral Analysis, 25*, 117–126.

Moerk, E. L. (1992). *First language taught and learned*. Baltimore: Brookes.

Pierce, K., & Schreibman, L. (1997). Multiple peer use of pivotal response training to increase social behaviors of classmates with autism: Results from trained and untrained peers. *Journal of Applied Behavior Analysis, 30,* 157–160.

Rule, S., Losardo, A., Dinnebeil, L., Kaiser, A., & Rowland, C. (1998). Translating research on naturalistic instruction into practice. *Journal of Early Intervention, 21,* 283–293.

Stahmer, A. C. (1995). Teaching symbolic play to children with autism using pivotal response training. *Journal of Autism and Developmental Disorders, 25,* 123–141.

Trent, J. A., Kaiser, A. P., & Wolery, M. (2005). Sibling use of responsive interaction strategies. *Topics in Early Childhood Special Education, 25,* 107–118.

U.S. Congress, House of Representatives. (1986). *House Report 99–457: Education of the Handicapped Act Amendments of 1986.* Washington, DC: U.S. Government Printing Office.

Warren, S. F. (1992). Facilitating basic vocabulary acquisition with MT procedures. *Journal of Early Intervention, 16,* 235–251.

Warren, S. F., Gazdag, G. E., Bambara, L. M., & Jones, H. A. (1994). Changes in the generativity and use of syntactic relationships concurrent with milieu language intervention. *Journal of Speech and Hearing Research, 37,* 924–934.

Warren, S. F., & Kaiser, A. P. (1986). Generalization of treatment effects by young language-delayed children: A longitudinal analysis. *Journal of Speech and Hearing Disorders, 51,* 239–251.

Waryas, C., & Stremel, K. (1974). On the preferred form of the double object construction. *Journal of Psycholinguistic Research, 3,* 271–280.

Weiss, M. J., & Harris, S. L. (2001). Teaching social skills to people with autism. *Behavior Modification, 25,* 785–802.

Wetherby, A. M., & Prizant, B. M. (1993). *Communication and Symbolic Behavior Scales.* Chicago: Applied Symbolix.

Williams, K. T. (1997). *Expressive Vocabulary Test.* Circle Pines, MN: American Guidance Service.

Woods, J., Kashinath, S., & Goldstein, H. (2004). Effects of embedding caregiver-implemented teaching strategies in daily routines on children's communication outcomes. *Journal of Early Intervention, 26,* 175–193.

Yoder, P. J., Kaiser, A. P., Goldstein, H., Alpert, C., Mousetis, L., Kaczmarek, L., et al. (1995). An exploratory comparison of milieu teaching and responsive interaction in classroom applications. *Journal of Early Intervention, 19,* 218–242.

Yoder, P. J., & Warren, S. F. (2001). Relative treatment effects of two prelinguistic communication interventions on language development in toddlers with developmental delays vary by maternal characteristics. *Journal of Speech, Language, and Hearing Research, 44,* 224–257.

Yoder, P. J., Warren, S. F., & Hull, L. (1995). Predicting children's response to prelinguistic communication intervention. *Journal of Early Intervention, 19,* 74–84.

Zimmerman, I. L., Steiner, V. G., & Pond, R. E. (2002). *Preschool Language Scale, Fourth Edition (PLS-4).* San Antonio, TX: Psychological Corporation.

APPENDIX 11.1. RESEARCH STUDIES REVIEWED

EMT

Hancock, T. B., & Kaiser, A. P. (1996). Siblings' use of MT at home. *Topics in Early Childhood Special Education, 16*(2), 168–190.

Hancock, T. B., & Kaiser, A. P. (2002). The effects of trainer-implemented enhanced MT on the social communication of children with autism. *Topics in Early Childhood Special Education, 22*(1), 39–54.

Hancock, T. B., Kaiser, A. P., & Delaney, E. M. (2002). Teaching parents of preschoolers at high risk strategies to support language and positive behavior. *Topics in Early Childhood Special Education, 22*(4), 191–222.

Hemmeter, M. L., & Kaiser, A. P. (1994). Enhanced MT: Effects of parent-implemented language intervention. *Journal of Early Intervention, 18*(3), 269–289.

Hester, P. P., Kaiser, A. P., Alpert, C. L., & Whiteman, B. (1995). The generalized effects of training trainers to teach parents to implement MT. *Journal of Early Intervention, 20*(1), 30–51.

Kaczmarek, L. A., Hepting, N. H., & Dzubak, M. (1996). Examining the generalization of milieu language objectives in situations requiring listener preparatory behaviors. *Topics in Early Childhood Special Education, 16*(2), 139–176.

Kaiser, A. P., Hancock, T. B., & Nietfield, J. P. (2000). The effects of parent-implemented enhanced MT on the social communication of children who have autism. *Early Education and Development, 11*(4), 423–446.

Kaiser, A. P., Hemmeter, M. L., Ostrosky, M. M., Alpert, C. L., & Hancock, T. B. (1995). The effects of group training and individual feedback on parent use of MT. *Journal of Childhood Communication Disorders, 16*(2), 39–48.

Kaiser, A. P., & Hester, P. P. (1994). Generalized effects of enhanced MT. *Journal of Speech and Hearing Research, 37*, 1320–1340.

Kaiser, A. P., Ostrosky, M. M., & Alpert, C. L. (1993). Training teachers to use environmental arrangement and MT with nonvocal preschool children. *Journal of the Association for Persons with Severe Handicaps, 18*(3), 188–199.

Kaiser, A. P., Yoder, P. J., & Keetz, A. (2002). Evaluating milieu teaching. In J. E. Reichle & S. F. Warren (Eds.), *Causes and effects in communication and language intervention* (pp. 9–47). Baltimore: Brookes.

Warren, S. F. (1992). Facilitating basic vocabulary acquisition with MT procedures. *Journal of Early Intervention, 16*(3), 235–251.

Warren, S. F., Gazdag, G. E., Bambara, L. M., & Jones, H. A. (1994). Changes in the generativity and use of syntactic relationships concurrent with milieu language intervention. *Journal of Speech and Hearing Research, 37*, 924–934.

Warren, S. F., Yoder, P. J., Gazdag, G. E., Kyoungran, K., & Jones, H. A. (1993). Facilitating prelinguistic communication skills in young children with developmental delay. *Journal of Speech and Hearing Research, 36*, 83–97.

Woods, J., Kashinath, S., & Goldstein, H. (2004). Effects of embedding caregiver-implemented teaching strategies in daily routines on children's communication outcomes. *Journal of Early Intervention, 26*(3), 175–193.

Yoder, P. J., & Warren, S. F. (1998). Maternal responsivity predicts prelinguistic communication intervention that facilitates generalized intentional communication. *Journal of Speech, Language, and Hearing Research, 41*(5), 1107–1119.

Yoder, P. J., & Warren, S. F. (2001). Relative treatment effects of two prelinguistic communication interventions on language development in toddlers with developmental delays vary by maternal characteristics. *Journal of Speech, Language, and Hearing Research, 44*(1), 224–237.

PRT

Koegel, L. K., Koegel, R. L., Shoshan, Y., & McNerny, E. (1999). Pivotal response intervention II: Preliminary long-term outcome data. *Journal of the Association for Persons with Severe Handicaps, 24*(3), 186–198.

Koegel, R. L., Bimbela, A., & Schriebman, L. (1996). Collateral effects of parent training on family interactions. *Journal of Autism and Developmental Disorders, 26*(3), 347–359.

Koegel, R. L., Koegel, L. K., & Surratt, A. (1992). Language intervention and disruptive behavior in preschool children with autism. *Journal of Autism and Developmental Disorders, 22*(2), 141–153.

Koegel, R. L., Symon, K. B., & Koegel, L. K. (2002). Parent education for families of children with autism living in geographically distant areas. *Journal of Positive Behavior Interventions, 4*(2), 88–103.

Pierce, K., & Schriebman, L. (1995). Increasing complex social behaviors in children with autism: Effects of peer-implemented pivotal response training. *Journal of Applied Behavior Analysis, 28*, 285–295.

Pierce, K., & Schriebman, L. (1997a). Using peer trainers to promote social behavior in autism: Are they effective at enhancing multiple social modalities? *Focus on Autism and Other Developmental Disabilities, 12*(4), 207–218.

Pierce, K., & Schriebman, L. (1997b). Multiple peer use of pivotal response training to increase social behaviors of classmates with autism: Results from trained and untrained peers. *Journal of Applied Behavior Analysis, 30*, 157–160.

Stahmer, A. C. (1995). Teaching symbolic play skills to children with autism using pivotal response training. *Journal of Autism and Developmental Disorders, 23*(2), 123–141.

Stahmer, A. C. (1999). Using pivotal response training to facilitate appropriate play in children with autistic spectrum disorders. *Child Language, Teaching, and Therapy, 15,* 29–40.

RI

Trent, J. A., Kaiser, A. P., & Frey, J. (in press). Sibling use of responsive interaction strategies. *Journal of Early Intervention.*

Trent, J. A., Kaiser, A. P., & Wolery, M. (2005). Sibling use of responsive interaction strategies. *Topics in Early Childhood Special Education, 25*(2), 107–118.

Yoder, P. J., Kaiser, A. P., Goldstein, H., Alpert, C., Mousetis, L., Kaczmarek, L., et al. (1995). An exploratory comparison of milieu teaching and responsive interaction in classroom applications. *Journal of Early Intervention, 19*(3), 218–242.

Peer-Directed

Hepting, N. H., & Goldstein, H. (1996). Requesting by preschoolers with developmental disabilities: Video-taped self-monitoring and learning of new linguistic structures. *Topics in Early Childhood Special Education, 16*(3), 407–427.

Thiemann, K. S., & Goldstein, H. (2001). Social stories, written text cues, and video feedback: Effects on social communication of children with autism. *Journal of Applied Behavior Analysis, 34*(4), 425–446.

PMT

Warren, S. F., Yoder, P .J., Gazdag, G. E., Kim, K., & Jones, H. A. (1993). Facilitating prelinguistic communication skills in young children with developmental delay. *Journal of Speech and Hearing Research, 36,* 83–97.

Yoder, P. J., Davies, B., Bishop, K., & Munson, L. (1994). Effect of adult continuing wh- questions on conversational participation in children with developmental disabilities. *Journal of Speech and Hearing Research, 37,* 193–203.

Yoder, P. J., Kaiser, A. P., Alpert, C., & Fischer, R. (1993). Following the child's lead when teaching nouns to preschoolers with mental retardation. *Journal of Speech and Hearing Research, 36,* 158–167.

Yoder, P. J., & Warren, S. F. (1998). Maternal responsivity predicts the prelinguistic communication intervention that facilitates generalized intentional communication. *Journal of Speech, Language, and Hearing Research, 41,* 1207–1219.

Yoder, P. J., & Warren, S. F. (2001). Relative treatment effects of two prelinguistic communication interventions on language development in toddlers with developmental delays vary by maternal characteristics. *Journal of Speech, Language, and Hearing Research, 44*(1), 224–238.

Yoder, P. J., & Warren, S. F. (2002). Effects of prelinguistic milieu teaching and parent responsivity education on dyads involving children with intellectual disabilities. *Journal of Speech, Language, and Hearing Research, 45*(6), 1158–1175.

Yoder, P. J., Warren, S. F., & Hull, L. (1995). Predicting children's response to prelinguistic communication intervention. *Journal of Early Intervention, 19*(1), 74–84.

IV

SCHOOL-AGE EDUCATION AND INTERVENTION

This section describes our current understanding of effective procedures for teaching individuals with developmental disabilities (DD). Although hundreds of research findings are summarized in the upcoming six chapters, several themes are evident in the instructional interventions that these authors describe. First, all intervention methods involve a series of actions taken by a teacher to direct learning in the student. These actions are either antecedent to the student's target response (giving a request, waiting for a response, giving a prompt), consequent to the target response (reinforcing independent and prompted correct responses), or both. Although most intervention methods described involve the combination of antecedent and consequent strategies, the emphasis has been on antecedent strategies over consequent strategies. Second, as the recommended learning setting for students with DD has shifted from separate to inclusive, the context for research on instruction more frequently has involved school settings, general education classrooms, and communities and the presence or the direct involvement of typical peers. Third, much attention has been devoted to making students more independent. Examples of this research include approaches for teaching students to request using augmentative and alternative communication and the broad area of student-directed learning. Student-directed learning has included teaching students to problem solve, plan their study, set goals, and monitor their behavior; dependent measures assess students' participation in general education classes and their needed level of assistance for success. Interventions that build student-directed learning skills tend to be complex combination interventions. Finally, most intervention research reviewed in this section has been evaluated through single-subject-design methodology involving a small number of individuals, measuring the target behaviors repeatedly and describing students and intervention procedures in detail.

Several of these themes pose challenges for future research. Research that is conducted in special education schools and classrooms will produce outcomes that are less relevant to the field. Instructional procedures must be demonstrated as socially valid by teachers and paraprofessionals; besides being effective, research must establish that teaching methods are feasible for use in the busy classroom by adults with varying levels of entry skills. Researchers need to involve general education teachers and paraprofessionals more often as skills instructors, while also demonstrating acceptable procedural fidelity and social validation of procedures. Research on instruction should track performance on two levels (student learning outcomes and instructor performance), as well as show a functional relationship between the two.

The six chapters here cover the broad front of skill development in individuals with DD during the school years. Snell begins this section with Chapter 12, which traces recent advances in instructional procedures. In Chapter 13, Hunt and McDonnell write about inclusive education, its characteristics, and its history within the context of school reform, and they describe a sample of research on inclusive education practices. Chapter 14, by Browder, Trela, Gibbs, Wakeman, and Harris, explains the impact of the school reform movement on the education of students with DD and reviews research relevant to educators who teach their state's academic content to these students and assess student learning. In Chapter 15, Carter and Hughes examine intervention strategies that have been demonstrated to increase social interactions between students with and without developmental disabilities. In Chapter 16, Fossett and Mirenda set forth evidence-based practices in augmentative and alternative communication to support persons with DD whose speech is insufficient to meet their ongoing daily communication needs. In Chapter 17, Frey reviews the literature on physical activity and school-age youth with DD. This final area was selected because of the lifelong impact that participation in regular physical activity has on physical health and on people's contributions and enjoyment as adults.

12

Advances in Instruction

Martha E. Snell

PAST RESEARCH TRENDS

Records indicate the presence of children and adults with developmental disabilities (DD) throughout history but tell us little about their instruction. In the Western world, Jean-Marc Itard (1774–1838) is regarded as the earliest special educator who reported both the success and failure of his teaching methods. When his student Victor, the *enfant sauvage*, failed to show progress under his tutelage, many became convinced that Victor was untreatable. De Gerando, a colleague of Itard's, disagreed with this view and in 1803 addressed the scholars of the field in Paris: "Certain people having tried their methods out on him [Victor] without success, concluded that he could not be instructed, rather than suspecting inadequacies in the methods themselves . . . " (Lane, 1976, p. 53). Almost two centuries later, in 1981, when similar doubts were raised in the educability debate, Donald Baer spoke with measured optimism of the potential of all learners: "To the extent that we sometimes finally succeed in teaching a child whom we have consistently failed to teach in many previous efforts, we may learn something about teaching technique and about the nature of behavioral prerequisites to behavior changes" (1981, p. 94). Most behavioral researchers today agree that *all* people, including those with DD, can learn; they accept Baer's principle that there is *always* a better way to teach a person who is not making progress. This chapter will highlight some of the recent advances in instructional methodology and provide suggestions for future research and development.

Reviews of behavioral, single-subject-design research on teaching individuals with DD reveal trends that have great value for practitioners, policy makers, and researchers.

Nietupski, Hamre-Nietupski, Curtin, and Shrikanth (1997), in their appraisal of curricular research on students with severe disabilities over a 20-year period, found that the amount of research on functional skill instruction had decreased, whereas research addressing interactions with nondisabled peers in inclusive classrooms had increased. Their review also revealed that non-data-based publications had decreased by half, a significant shift in the field from expert opinion on how to teach toward the use of systematic evaluation of instructional practices. Snell's (1997) review of skill instruction research involving school-age students with mental retardation found that, although research since the 1990s addressed a variety of functional and age-appropriate skills, it did so in segregated settings, with frequent omissions of social validity and procedural fidelity. In a review of time-delay research, Schuster et al. (1998) also reported overuse of separate settings.

A series of reviews and meta-analyses have identified the effectiveness of systematic instruction, with increasing focus on (1) use of natural materials, (2) teaching in typical social and physical contexts, and (3) organizing instruction to promote generalization. Browder and her colleagues examined reading instruction research and discovered an increased emphasis on the importance of real materials and instructive feedback over prompting, but they also found consistently strong support for systematic prompting using constant time delay (Browder, Wakeman, Spooner, Ahlgrim-Delzell, & Algozzine, 2006; Browder & Xin, 1998). Wolery and Schuster's (1997) review also provided strong support for (1) teaching with real materials, with or without simulation, (2) using multiple exemplars to promote skill generalization, (3) using materials to facilitate play or communication, (4) adapting materials to reduce the complexity of academic skills, and (5) using materials such as picture schedules to support skill performance. Their review revealed that increased performance, motivation, and learning in these students seems to be improved (1) when instruction matches current skills, (2) by keeping intertrial intervals short and varying tasks, and (3) by using prompting and contingent reinforcement. Learning appears to be promoted when reinforcement is varied across learning opportunities and with specific reinforcement (i.e., reinforcer has a definite relationship to the desired behavior, such as fulfilling a request of a child learning to request), whereas reinforcement delay can improve skill maintenance. Finally, the researchers found strong research support for self-management, peer-mediated instruction, and response-prompting procedures.

Odom, Brown, Frey, Karasu, Smith-Canter, and Strain's (2003) review of effective interventions for young children with autism identified the practices of (1) adult-directed teaching and differential reinforcement as having a well-established evidence base, (2) peer-mediated interventions, visual supports, self-monitoring, and family member involvement as having emerging evidence, and (3) videotaped models and child choices and preferences embedded into teaching activities as probably being efficacious.

In a more recent review of intervention methods to teach augmentative and alternative skills to students with severe disabilities, Snell, Chen, and Hoover (2006) found a predominance of "naturalistic" strategies meant to influence students' motivation and engagement with the environment, such as teachers being close to students, following their lead, using preferred materials, arranging environments to tempt responding, and embedding teaching into activities. They reported that, rather than single strategies, combinations of these instructional strategies, both antecedent and consequent, often constituted the independent variable.

This chapter will set forth some of the important advances in single-subject behavioral research on instruction for school-age individuals with DD and describe current practices with promising or well-established evidence. Implications for researchers are integrated throughout, and the implications for practitioners, families, and policy makers conclude the chapter.

CURRENT INSTRUCTIONAL ADVANCES

Instructional strategies can focus on the antecedents to instruction, on the student's behavior, or on the consequences for responding. The first part of this chapter addresses recent work in these three areas, and the second part is devoted to interventions that combine a variety of strategies.

Antecedent Instructional Strategies

Providing Opportunities for Making Choices

There is widespread support for giving choice-making opportunities to individuals with DD as a means to improve motivation, performance, behavior, and day-to-day experiences (Kern et al., 1998). In comparison with direct imperatives, Dibley and Lim (1999) found that student protests decreased and task initiations increased for an adolescent with severe DD when she was given opportunities to choose the task materials and the time at which to perform tasks (now or later). Similarly, with women with profound multiple disabilities, Green, Reid, Rollyson, and Passante (2005) found a reduction in physical resistance to the teacher and negative affect when preferred activities were given before, during, and right after teaching sessions.

There is empirical evidence of the differential effects of making a choice over being given preferred items (Dunlap et al., 1994; Hughes, Pitkin, & Lorden, 1998; Vaughn & Horner, 1997). For example, two adolescents with autism completed work tasks more quickly when they selected their reinforcers (from a choice of computer-displayed videos) than when teachers selected tangible reinforcers for them from a pool of known reinforcers (Mechling, Gast, & Cronin, 2006). Understanding the reason that the act of choosing leads to more active involvement in task performance will yield useful guidance for promoting motivation.

Students with severe intellectual disabilities can be taught to make choices (Stafford, Alberto, Fredrick, Helfin, & Heller, 2002), and the power of giving choices to students is well documented, yet surprisingly little is known about natural opportunities for individuals with and without DD to make choices in school settings. Jolivette, Stichter, Sibilsky, Scott, and Ridgley (2002), who observed 14 preschoolers, half with and half without disabilities, found that those with disabilities were offered choice options more often than those without disabilities (0.17 per minute vs. 0.12), whereas both groups initiated choice making at the same rate (0.03 per minute). Teacher trainers will benefit from knowing more about how to improve and maintain teachers' offers of choices to students.

Instructional Requests and Opportunity to Respond

Learning appears to be directly related to the rate of opportunities given to students to respond (i.e., having regular opportunities to use target skills). Current research suggests that students with DD respond better when instructional requests or directions (1) are not complex, (2) seek developmentally realistic performances, and (3) are given when the student is attending. Kim and Hupp (2005) found that teachers of students with DD varied widely in the frequency of their directions and responses to students during one-on-one language arts instruction, averaging 15 directions and 6 responses (acknowledgments, elaborations) per minute. To direct students, teachers used gestural prompts most often, followed by questions. Gestural prompts (as well as commands, directions, and suggestions) were highly correlated with student engagement, but questions were not. Chavez-Brown, Scott, and Ross (2005) did not find clear learning benefits when children with autism were taught by simple verbal antecedents ("Give me car") compared with conversational antecedents ("One of these is a car. Which one is it?").

Prompting

Prompts are artificial antecedent events that momentarily increase the likelihood of correct responding. Teachers use prompts (e.g., pointing) with natural stimuli to help students identify what, where, or how to succeed. Prompting is a fundamental strategy for building new responses. Several response-prompting methods that incorporate a fading strategy have been demonstrated as effective in producing low-error acquisition of new behaviors in students with DD. The most recent method is simultaneous prompting (SP), which involves ongoing antecedent prompts that are eliminated, rather than gradually faded, when probe trials indicate that the student is correctly responding without the prompt. Comparison studies lend support to some prompt procedures over others under certain conditions.

Riesen, McDonnell, Johnson, Polychronis, and Jameson (2003) found constant time delay (CTD) to have comparable success for teaching academic tasks in general education classrooms, with two students learning more effectively with CTD and two with SP. Heckaman, Alber, Hooper, and Heward (1998) compared least-to-most prompts (LMP) with progressive time delay (PTD) in teaching difficult (30% accuracy when unassisted) word-reading and match-to-sample tasks to four students with autism and problem behavior. PTD produced learning with fewer errors for all students and lower rates of problem behavior with two students. Tekin and Kircaali-Ifar (2002) taught three children to tutor their siblings with DD on receptive identification of animal figures. Tutors alternated between using SP and CTD to teach their siblings. Differences in learning were minimal (CTD required fewer trials to criterion and SP resulted in fewer errors); whereas both methods yielded good skill maintenance, CTD yielded better generalization across materials. Both time delay and SP have a strong record of success for teaching new skills to individuals with DD, but understanding how student and task characteristics interact with prompt procedures and learning will provide valuable guidelines for teachers planning instruction.

The principle of parsimony still is an excellent guide to judge the quality of teaching methods: Select the simplest but still effective approach (Etsel & LeBlanc, 1979). Much of the research on prompting methods reports information on efficiency (e.g., number of sessions and minutes to achieve criterion, total and mean errors, and materials cost). Some suggest that SI may be the easiest procedure for teachers to use (i.e., unchanging procedure over trials in terms of reinforcement, timing, and prompt), but CTD has a longer, broader history of success than does SI. Both CTD and SI, however, have been demonstrated as being easy to use, low cost, and efficient, producing low-error learning on many skills, chained and discrete, in both individual and small-group formats, and in a variety of natural settings. PTD, more challenging to use, seems to produce the lowest error rate and thus may be selected when difficult tasks are necessary for students who also exhibit problem behavior under such conditions. Selection of a prompting method should be influenced by: (1) student history—whether one method works better or should be avoided with a given student; (2) teacher's skill level and experience with prompting; and (3) the intrusiveness of the method and its fit with classroom and community settings (Riesen et al., 2003). For example, Batu, Ergenekon, Erbas, and Akmanoglu (2004) used an intrusive most-to-least prompting system (graduated guidance) and simulation to teach street-crossing skills and to prevent accidents in early learning; all five students learned the skills and generalized them to the community.

Some teaching strategies, such as adding preferred materials, giving choices, or changing the number or type of individuals present, operate by influencing control over a student's engagement with the environment, whereas other strategies (e.g., prompting, peer mediation) operate to change specific student behaviors (Wolery & Schuster, 1997). We need to understand simple ways to assess students' success with and preference for these two broad types of teaching strategies. This knowledge is helpful with critical behaviors that are not easily adapted and with students who have a history of poor learning or problem behavior. The principle of parsimony also should influence strategy selection; for example, it may be easier and yield wider effects if teachers improve students' task engagement rather than prompt their behavior.

Stimulus modification procedures (stimulus prompts) involve stimulus shaping or fading and require that teachers gradually manipulate the materials over instructional opportunities to produce low-error learning. Past research supports the effectiveness of these approaches, but they require extensive material preparation, as some learning stimuli cannot be easily manipulated. Computer programs with digital pictures and videos should reduce these difficulties.

Visual and Auditory Instruction

As predicted by Wolery and Schuster in 1997, numerous studies in the past decade have supplemented instruction with various forms of technology (e.g., self-operated auditory prompting, videotape prompting, video prompting by laptop or handheld computers). Researchers have involved students with DD of all ages and taught a variety of skills, including social communication skills, play, academics (spelling words, grocery–word association), and functional tasks (brushing teeth, ordering fast food, cooking). More studies have used models (video modeling [VM]) than have used tapes of the actual learner (video self-modeling [VSM]). Because VSM makes use of edited video images that show the target student appearing to be independent, the cost of this approach is greater. Some VM research involved videos or stills made as if the viewer were performing the task and thus not showing the model. Future research will need to isolate the advantages of one approach over another (VSM, VM) while reporting cost and preparation time.

Graves, Collins, Schuster, and Kleinert (2005) used a simple VM method to teach high school students with moderate mental retardation to prepare food items on a stove, in a microwave, and on a countertop. Videotapes of tasks were made by school staff and students in a video class. Tapes were shot from a subjective viewpoint (as if the viewer were performing the task) and included males and females. Videotapes (for 0- and 5-second CTD levels of instruction) were edited to include, in order: (1) task request, (2) model of whole task, (3) delay interval of 0 seconds, (4) repeat of task request, (5) delay of 0 seconds, (6) verbal prompt with first task step, (7) 20-second blank frame for student to perform first step, and (8) repetition of steps 4–7 for each successive task step. Students were taught in one-to-one sessions using total task instruction and CTD with video prompting; thus teachers began with the 0-second videos and switched to the 5-second-delay videos when students reached 100% performance for 2 days. All students learned the cooking tasks in an average of 10 sessions, each averaging 14 minutes. The shortcomings of this approach included tape preparation, the need for teachers to fast-forward tapes during instruction, and the need for teachers at all.

Mechling, Pridgen, and Cronin (2005) used computer-based video instruction (CBVI) to teach three secondary students with DD to answer cashiers' questions (e.g., "How can I help you?") and to complete the other steps for using fast-food restaurants (picking up a tray, going to the drink machine, etc.). Video simulations of three different restaurants were made, using video captions, still images, and voice recordings, and were shown to students on a laptop computer. Individual instruction took place in the classroom, and generalization probes were carried out in the three restaurants. Teachers used CTD and advanced the computer images manually to teach answers to cashiers' questions, and the computer automatically advanced the images to teach the motor responses. The computer program was less effective in teaching motor skills (e.g., getting the napkin), for which the video required only a screen touch response on the correct picture rather than a performance of the response (e.g., stating an order, taking money from a wallet). If computers made use of speech recognition, students could self-instruct, eliminating the teacher.

Two studies compared video modeling with other approaches. In the first, Branham, Collins, Schuster, and Kleinert (1999) examined different combinations of simulation, VM, and community-based instruction (CBI) to teach community skills (mailing a letter, crossing a street, and cashing a check) to three students with mild to moderate cognitive disabilities. Using one-to-one instruction and CTD, teachers applied one of three combinations: (1) classroom simulation plus CBI, (2) VM plus CBI, and (3) VM plus simulation plus CBI. Videotapes of peers performing the task were made using school equipment and edited so that a complete task performance was followed by still frames of each task step, separated by 10-second response intervals. As in some other VM examples, students' responses did not involve performing the step but verbally stating the step either by repeating the modeled task-step description ("hand check to teller") or by stating the task step before the delayed picture and verbal explanation were played. Although time delay was effective for teaching the skills regardless of the instructional combination used, results showed that simulation plus CBI required the least instructional time. Because VM required more time than simulation, the overall time was higher whenever VM was combined with another technique. However, results also showed that the combination of all three techniques required fewer teaching sessions, although this combination was always used following the other two combinations. Simulation was viewed as an efficient supplement to CBI, particularly when daily CBI was not available.

Charlop-Christy, Le, and Freeman (2000) compared the effectiveness of VM with *in vivo* teacher modeling in teaching children with autism verbal (greeting, answering questions), play (simple card games, coloring), and self-help skills. Both the video and the *in vivo* modeling involved different, but familiar, teachers performing the skills at an intentionally slowed pace. Under both conditions, children were prompted and praised only for attending to the model, not for target responses. VM not only resulted in faster acquisition of skills over *in vivo* modeling but also led to skill generalization, whereas *in vivo* modeling did not. The authors set forth several explanations for the findings: (1)

VM emphasizes relevant cues by zooming in on them and reducing overselectivity to nonrelevant cues; (2) VM improves motivation for watching and learning and may be automatically reinforcing; (3) the social deficit characteristics of children with autism makes VM easier to use, as social interaction is not required; and (4) *in vivo* models are associated with a history of inconsistent reinforcement and prompt dependence. These promising findings warrant careful follow-up and additional study.

As these examples illustrate, the amount and type of accompanying teacher instruction varied across this pool of research, as did student participation (teacher advancing pictures or video versus student responding through touch screen). For example, Mechling et al. (2005) found that observation alone was less effective than having students also perform the response. "Cost" ranged widely in terms of the effort needed to video and edit the tapes and to show the tapes. Several researchers mentioned that the videos were made with school equipment (Branham et al., 1999) and/or staff (Graves et al., 2005), but only Charlop-Christy et al. (2000) figured in the cost and time required, a factor schools must consider when selecting these interventions. It is appropriate to question the added preparation cost of using VM plus a teacher for instructional tasks that are easily modeled, such as making popcorn (Sigafoos et al., 2005), rather than for tasks that are community based. It will be important to assess whether certain media characteristics (e.g., static picture or video; peer, self-, or teacher models; active or passive student responding) are more beneficial to some learners than to others (Cihak, Alberto, Taber-Doughty, & Gama, 2006).

With the rapidly expanding growth of portable auditory (iPods, cell phones) and visual display devices (cell phones and digital cameras with still and video display), technology-assisted instruction expands the alternatives to teaching in the presence of realistic task stimuli. Using readily available technology both to cut costs and to boost student motivation for learning will be important, while also selecting simpler technology or making adaptations so that students can master use of the device. For example, Taber, Alberto, Seltzer, and Hughes (2003) varied their approach to teaching students to deal with being lost in the community, depending on their understanding of being lost and their ability to dial a cell phone. Those who could do neither during baseline were taught to answer the cell phone, to describe where they were, and to stay put. Researchers noted students' high motivation to learn to use cell phones, so they programmed the phones for one-touch speed dialing and selected models that were easier to use (with raised buttons and color-coded send buttons). Technology-assisted instruction has great potential for motivating students and teaching them a variety of skills, but researchers need to report the costs of preparing and using these technologies and to test ways to make their application more efficient, such as involving small groups or making CVM self-instructional.

New Responses

Learning Strategies

There is an abundance of research on students with learning disabilities and learning strategies that promote successful performance (e.g., mnemonics), but less research with students who have DD. Test and Ellis (2005) demonstrated that adolescent students with mild mental retardation could add and subtract fractions using a peer-assisted learning strategy to identify the fraction type and carry out the function. Students learned the eight-step mnemonic strategy through modeling and guided practice and by playing a baseball card game with a peer. Then they learned to apply the strategy using the same instructional steps, with the card game adapted to fraction football and basketball. For a picture memory task, Stromer, Mackay, McVay, and Fowler (1998) found that three students with mental retardation who had the prior ability to write words and to connect words and pictures were able to recall sets of two to six pictures when they used their handwritten word lists to mediate the lapse in time when pictures disappeared. Although some learned quickly and needed the strategy only with larger groups of pictures, others self-instructed using the "write"/"don't write" task directions given for short and long picture groupings. Both studies illustrate the need for more research addressing the advancement of students' use of these strategies to an automatic level, such as solving problems more quickly "in their heads" and knowing when to use a strategy and when not to.

Self-Monitoring

Teaching students with DD self-directed strategies allows them to achieve less dependence on others while also increasing their engagement and motivation and improving the likelihood for learning in school. Several researchers have demonstrated that individuals with a wide range of DD can learn specific strategies to monitor their own target behaviors. For example, high school students with mild to moderate intellectual disabilities learned to use a stimulus, such as money being placed in their hands or a picture prompt card, to direct themselves to perform a relevant behavior (e.g., thank the cashier, keep the head upright, complete assignments, and initiate a conversation) in a variety of school settings (Hughes et al., 2002). These students learned the strategy in two to three sessions when researchers first gave students a rationale for the approach and then used modeling, direct instruction, guided practice, and corrective feedback to teach self-monitoring.

In a second study, peer tutors, using some of the same approaches Hughes et al. (2002) applied, taught five middle school students with severe disabilities to self-monitor their performance of teacher-selected classroom survival skills (e.g., being in class and seat when bell rings, bringing appropriate materials, greeting teachers and peers, asking and answering questions; Gilberts, Agran, Hughes, & Wehmeyer, 2001). Peers taught their fellow students to place checkmarks next to survival-skill words and pictures on a simple recording form whenever they performed the classroom skills. Following training, students' self-recording was close to accurate, and they had all increased their survival skills in general education classrooms. Finally, middle school students with moderate to severe disabilities learned to self-monitor their following of teachers' directions in general education classrooms. Researchers taught them to discriminate directions from nondirections, to self-record their direction following through modeling and guided practice, and to apply self-monitoring through role play (Agran et al., 2005). Following intervention, all students made rapid improvements in following teachers' directions in class. General and special education teachers socially validated the behavior changes in all three studies, and classmates also did so in the study by Gilberts et al. (2001).

This current research adds to the existing database of support for teaching self-directed strategies to students with DD. Researchers will want to compare the benefits of peer-versus-teacher-instructed self-monitoring for teaching relevant skills and to further assess changes in student dependence on others, task engagement, and effects on classroom achievement.

Consequent Strategies

Self-Recruited Reinforcement

We know a lot about how to identify reinforcers for people with mild to significant DD (Hughes et al., 1998; Lohrmann-O'Rourke & Browder, 1998). The behavioral approach emphasizes teachers' contingent use of reinforcement and lends support to more frequent schedules early in learning that are thinned as students master skills, while teachers shift from artificial reinforcers to natural reinforcers. In the busy general education classroom setting, teachers often fail to offer choices and show low rates of praise. Self-recruitment of praise is a strategy researchers have explored with students with DD in special education settings. Craft, Alber, and Heward (1998) demonstrated that fourth graders with DD could be taught by their special education teachers to recruit teacher praise and to generalize the skill to their general education classroom teachers. Instruction involved explaining the rationale, role playing, prompting, and checking at the end of the day, with rewards given when students reported recruiting praise two to three times in a day. Students were taught to use socially valid methods to recruit teacher praise that were consistent with the teacher's practices and then to self-monitor how often they recruited praise (by checking up to three small boxes) so that they did not overrecruit. Along with clear changes in their recruitment of praise, all students made improvements (some modest, others notable) in their work completion and accuracy.

Specific Reinforcement

Specific, or natural contingent, reinforcement refers to reinforcement with consequences that have a specific relationship to the desired behavior, such as providing assistance when a child whose target behavior is to ask for help does so. Often recommended for teaching early language, specific reinforcement was used in all but 1 of the 33 studies reviewed by Snell et al. (2006), in which augmentative and alternative communication (AAC) skills were taught to students with moderate and severe disabilities. Both specific reinforcement and an alternate practice of having students select the reinforcer seem to be used more often within current interventions than the past practice of giving teacher-selected "reinforcers" (food or activities) to students following correct responses. Snell et al. (2006) also found no evidence of research in which punishing consequences for errors made during AAC instruction were applied (time-out, reprimands, repeating the request with mandates).

Combination Methods

As in the past with general case instruction and interrupted chain, "package" interventions that combine a number of effective teaching strategies have been developed and tested. The four multiple-element interventions reviewed next focus either on instruction in general education settings or on naturalistic approaches for teaching students with significant disabilities.

Support Package for Students in General Education

Specific strategies shown to facilitate the inclusion of students with DD in general education classrooms have been applied together, such as the modification of teacher-assigned work sheets, improved team communication and skill monitoring, instruction in assignment completion and self-monitoring, and peer tutoring. Researchers have applied various combinations with elementary and secondary students with DD.

The support package that Copeland, Hughes, Agran, Wehmeyer, and Fowler (2002) devised was directed toward making high school students with mild to moderate DD independent in completing assigned work sheets and in self-monitoring their classroom performance skills while involving them cooperatively in setting and evaluating personal performance goals. Researchers taught students these skills on an individual basis over an average of nine sessions lasting a mean of 14 minutes. In addition, with input from the general education teacher, teacher-assigned work sheets in a cosmetology class were modified in one of several ways: (1) the number of questions was reduced; (2) written prompts were embedded on the work sheet to guide them in answering specific questions and in completing the work (i.e., "get work sheet from folder," "write name," "answer questions," "put work sheets back in folder"), and (3) boxes were provided for students to check after performing each prompted task. In comparison with baseline, all students showed major improvements in their performance of work sheet completion steps, and 3 of the 4 students improved their grades. Students and teachers judged the intervention as being positive and effective.

Another support package for students in general education classes involved peer tutoring, multielement curricula, and accommodations (McDonnell, Mathot-Buckner, Thorson, & Fister, 2001). The 3 participating middle school students with moderate and severe disabilities had poor class participation and varying levels of competing behavior. Three general education teachers learned to implement classwide peer tutoring in which class members, organized into heterogeneous triads, served both as tutors and tutees and learned to tutor using systematic teaching methods. In addition, teachers learned to cooperatively develop, with special educators, (1) instructional objectives linked to the general curriculum but geared to students' ability to learn and (2) accommodations that would increase students' participation in class activities and tutoring sessions (e.g., reducing number of problems; using calculators; shooting baskets in simpler ways; using verbal, not written, directions). All 3 students improved in their academic responding and showed decreased levels of interfering behavior following implementation of the support package, whereas 2 of 3 randomly selected typical classmates also improved.

Extending their earlier research on unified plans of support (UPS), Hunt, Soto, Maier, and Doering (2003) implemented an intervention that emphasized team collaboration and led to increased academic achievement and social participation in six fourth-graders with mild to severe DD enrolled in general education classrooms. The UPS set forth individualized instructional goals and procedures for reading, writing, and math and for participation and interaction (e.g., "adults will prompt Francisco to ask a peer for assistance by signing 'ask a friend' "; p. 319). The UPS teaming elements included (1) regularly scheduled meetings of the student's team, (2) planning and development of supports to increase the student's academic and social participation in the classroom, (3) a system of accountability for team monitoring of student progress, and (4) flexibility in changing and improving supports that a team found ineffective. When this process and UPS plans were consistently used by teams with each student, students made gains in academic skills, classroom engagement, interactions with peers, and self-initiated interactions.

As these studies show, supporting students with DD in general education so that they can participate, interact, and learn is a complex task requiring a combination of proven methods. Some methods focus directly on instructional strategies, whereas other approaches must concern teacher collaboration in identifying reasonable goals and adaptations and in monitoring progress. Researchers have identified many instructional strategies that are effective with students who have DD and who are taught in general education settings. Yet without more understanding of the complex collaborative teacher tasks (e.g., identifying reasonable goals and adaptations, monitoring student progress) that are essential to a support package for these students in general education, little lasting impact will result from just the instructional elements.

Embedding Instruction within Activities

Based on the rationale of promoting stimulus generalization and motivation, young children with disabilities are often taught communication and social skills during scheduled activities and play. The terms "activity-based" or "naturalistic instruction" are used as synonyms for "embedded instruction," which refers to the insertion of teaching trials within regularly occurring routines during the day "without breaking the flow of the routine or ongoing activity" (Schepis, Reid, Ownbey, & Parsons, 2001, p. 314). Embedding instruction means that teaching trials are distributed rather than massed, a condition that is more conducive to learning in individuals with DD. For younger children, instruction is embedded into free play, mealtimes, recess, and self-care activities, whereas school transitions and breaks have been used for older students. Embedding is combined with systematic prompting, reinforcement, and corrective feedback to teach specific skills, frequently communication skills (e.g., incidental teaching, milieu approach). Several recent studies have examined embedding as a strategy for teaching academic skills within inclusive settings.

Riesen et al. (2003) compared CTD and SI within embedded instruction to teach middle school students with DD to read and define academic concepts in science, U.S. history, and German. They trained special education paraprofessionals to carry out the procedures in the general education classroom and to embed teaching trials during natural breaks in ongoing classroom routines (roll call, transition to science lab, transition from lecture to an independent seat activity). Paraprofessionals learned to reliably implement interventions, and all students mastered the skills through embedded instruction and generalized the skills to naturalistic probes. The effectiveness of prompt methods varied by student, with two learning more quickly under one prompting approach than the other.

McDonnell and colleagues (2006) also recruited paraprofessionals in secondary schools to use embedded instruction to teach definitions of vocabulary words drawn from the general education curriculum, but they compared embedded one-to-one instruction in general education classrooms with small-group, spaced-trial instruction in special education classes. Paraprofessionals learned to teach word definitions in two ways. First, they embedded instructional trials on word definitions within general education class breaks and transitions while using CTD, differential reinforcement, and systematic error correction to teach each trial. Second, they applied the same systematic teaching methods to teach comparable definitions using the same number of trials but in a small-group format. Paraprofessionals accurately used the intervention, and their students learned the definitions regardless of the approach and also generalized the skills to work sheets. It will be valuable to compare these instructional formats in the general education setting and to assess social validity.

In a related study, Johnson and McDonnell (2004) demonstrated successful learning by two of three elementary students with DD when their general education teachers embedded systematic instructional trials on matching sight words, on signing "help" to request assistance, and on identifying the larger of two numbers. General education teachers reliably used embedding and judged the procedures as being an acceptable and effective strategy for teaching students with DD.

Finally, Schepis et al. (2001) demonstrated that paraprofessionals could learn to embed systematic instructional trials to teach preschoolers with severe disabilities such tasks as following directions, completing routines, cutting with scissors, playing, and identifying colors in an inclusive preschool. Paraprofessionals learned to identify five types of situations in which to embed instruction (e.g., child-initiated activities, naturally occurring staff-initiated routines, curriculum-based activities) and were successful in implementing the procedures, and all five students demonstrated that they had learned the target skills.

Embedding systematic instruction into routines, play, downtime, and transitions appears to be successful for teaching students with DD of all ages in general education settings. The method can be successfully applied by paraprofessionals and general education teachers with instruction. It will be useful to know more about the embedding situation and its relation to the skill being taught and whether some contexts (e.g., that are related to the skill or preferred by the student) are better for teaching some students and skills.

Embedding Nontarget Information into Instruction

Because of overlapping terminology, embedding nontarget information (ENI) can be confused with embedding instruction into activities. ENI involves the presentation of extra visual or spoken information during systematic instruction of other skills but *without* requiring an active response from the learner and *without* providing immediate feedback on his or her response. By contrast, embedded instruction simply shifts complete instructional trials to noninstructional times. The intent of ENI is to promote incidental learning *without direct instruction* while systematically teaching another target skill. Researchers studying ENI typically have used CTD or simultaneous instruction as the prompt procedure for the target skill. ENI has many variations: (1) task type: discrete or chained; (2) teaching format: one-to-one and group; (3) stimuli presented: verbal statement, visual stimuli (word, picture, model), or both; (4) information that is related or unrelated to the task; and (5) placement of the information within the teaching trial: in the task directions, during the delivery of prompts, or as instructional feedback after the student's response. Number of exposures to the nontarget information seems to be important, as students who quickly learn a target task get fewer trials on nontarget information and show less learning of nontarget information (Ficus, Schuster, Morse, & Collins, 2002). A primary focus of ENI research has been on instructional feedback (embedding nontarget information following the student response), which has proven successful with preschoolers to adolescents across a range of disabilities, settings, and tasks (Werts, Wolery, Holcombe, & Gast, 1995).

Ficus et al. (2002) used one-to-one instruction and CTD to teach four elementary students with moderate and severe disabilities to prepare three foods (e.g., frozen waffles with syrup) in a chained task, while embedding instructive feedback stimuli within the prompt and consequences. The nontarget information was either relevant (pointing to and reading the words in the recipe book) or irrelevant to the target task (pointing to and labeling kitchen utensils). Students learned the cooking tasks and also some to all of the nontarget information; they showed greater success on the unrelated information, perhaps due to its comparatively simpler nature or to its novelty. Teachers demonstrated 100% accuracy in ENI while teaching chained tasks. In a second study, Collins, Hall, Branson, and Holder (1999) studied the acquisition of related factual information ("Every sentence should end with a period," p. 227) and unrelated factual information ("Paul Patton is the governor . . .," p. 227) delivered twice per class by a general education teacher to high school students with moderate DD in English classes. Unlike other applications of ENI, teachers did not specifically teach another skill but embedded the systematic presentation of information to individual students within the class period as students worked on their daily assignments. Students, probed daily in their special education class, acquired three to four of the six facts after an average of 10 exposures (range: 2–24 presentations). Although teachers faithfully presented the nontarget information, it would be worthwhile to study more natural ways for teachers to systematically present irrelevant nontarget information in general education.

Accurate use of ENI by teachers is not trivial. Thus future research should assess whether it is better to teach some skills directly rather than through ENI. In contrast with direct instruction, ENI has some novel characteristics (no response required; applied during downtimes) that may be more conducive to learning with some students. Researchers need to determine when and with what students ENI is more efficient and effective than direct instruction.

Naturalistic Instruction of Early Skills

In the past decade, increased attention was given to the importance of early social-communicative skills (joint attention, prelinguistic communication, motor and language imitation, and eye contact) in children with autism and to the resultant development of their communication and social abilities. Reviews of research on social-interactive interventions (Hwang & Hughes, 2000a; Snell et al., 2006) point to shortcomings with traditional behavioral interventions while suggesting the value of more naturalistic social interactive strategies (child-preferred stimuli; child-initiated responses as the target for intervention; environmental arrangement; natural cues such as expectant delay, questioning looks, and approach; time delay and minimal use of physical prompts; specific reinforcement; contingent imitation). Research lends support to these approaches (e.g., Halle, 1987; Schepis, Reid, Behrmann & Sutton, 1998).

Hwang and Hughes (2000b) applied a social-interactive intervention (SII) to three preschoolers with autism with limited eye contact, joint attention, and imitation skills. Graduate students, trained to implement the procedures as interactive partners, used short one-to-one instructional sessions 3 days a week in naturally occurring activities but apart from other children in the special education classroom. Two of the three classroom teachers were trained to serve as partners during generalization. SII was implemented on a one-to-one basis by several graduate students who interacted with children and their preferred play materials while applying four strategies: (1) providing contingent and immediate imitation of children's actions within their range of vision, (2) using naturally occurring or specific reinforcement, (3) presenting children with an expectant look for 5 seconds before responding to their actions or requests to give the children time to respond first, and (4) arranging the environment in ways that provoked joint attention and interest (e.g., offering choices, using preferred materials, removing materials not of interest) and that required the children to use gestures or vocalizations to elicit their partner's attention. The interventionist immediately imitated children's actions and vocalizations to provoke attention, waited for children to look at them before giving familiar imitative models, and prompted them only if they did not respond in 30 seconds. Interventionists learned to implement SII reliably, and children made increases over baseline performance in their eye contact, joint attention, and motor imitation and generalized treatment effects. Outcomes were socially validated by 30 respondents experienced with children having autism. Although this research supports SII, the outcomes were variable across children, and maintenance was not assessed.

Ingersoll and Schreibman (2006) applied reciprocal imitation training (RIT) to teach imitation to five preschoolers with autism. RIT, a social-interaction approach, involves naturalistic techniques such as contingent imitation, linguistic mapping (i.e., giving the child a running commentary of the interaction), following the child's lead, and using four teaching phases that reflect the developmental progression of imitation acquisition. Familiar actions were modeled about every minute, and children's imitations were reinforced with praise and continued access to the play materials; physical prompting with contingent praise was used only when children did not imitate after the third model. After 6 weeks of eight 20-minute sessions a week with multiple therapists, children made substantial gains in spontaneous object imitation that were maintained after a month and that generalized to different play materials, locations, and therapists. Children showed increases in language, pretend play, and joint attention. Social-validation tests indicated that observers judged children to look more typical after intervention.

Naturalistic methods were applied in both of these studies, but children still were taught in separate settings apart from typical peers by therapists who were not their regular teachers. In order to understand how to promote the generalized use of social-communicative skills across home and school, future research should test these naturalistic approaches in routine, inclusive settings and involve teachers, peers, and parents as the trainers. Researchers should tease out the elements critical for building robust skills in children with autism and should address intensity of training, specific approaches for motivating students, and the most successful instructional elements (e.g., prompts, reinforcement, corrective feedback).

Research Implications for Combination Methods

As predicted by past reviews of instructional methods, there has been more emphasis in the recent decade on how to teach individuals with DD in general education settings, on efficient and effective strategies, and on teaching strategies that yield independent performance in students. With any of these multielement interventions, however, it is not clear what role each element plays in the students' skill improvements. Future research should evaluate the components separately so that unneeded or less important elements can be eliminated, making the approach more efficient and perhaps simpler to use. Research should compare combination approaches with other proven approaches to teaching the same skill (e.g., embedded one-to-one instruction compared with small-group instruction). As in the studies cited, it is important with combination interventions that there be both rigorous measurement of procedural fidelity and social validation of the methods by users.

IMPLICATIONS FOR RESEARCHERS

There are a myriad of factors in any teaching plan that can be modified to improve student motivation (e.g., adding peers; varying task novelty; interspersing easy and hard tasks), as well as the likelihood that a student will learn (e.g., low error prompts, adequate opportunities). Observation to assess a student's response to instruction and the circumstances under which learning problems occur, coupled with close monitoring of learning, can produce the best ways to advance learning (Farlow & Snell, 1994, 2005). For example, if there is resistance to participating or to responding, a number of instructional elements could be responsible (e.g., difficulty or ease of responding; presence of background noise or crowding; being touched or physically prompted) and these can be modified. Other students, although they do not resist instruction, do not learn a skill even after repeated teaching. Other aspects of instruction need to be examined for these students (e.g., response difficulty; visual or auditory demands; inconsistent instruction). Thus the selection of teaching strategies and their interaction with student characteristics (stage of learning, interfering behavior, strategy preference or dislike) merits more study. When is it best, for example, to influence control over a student's engagement with the environment (e.g., giving choices) rather than applying strategies that change specific student behaviors (e.g., prompting)? Should the student's stage of learning for the target skill be given primary attention in strategy selection (e.g., prompting method)? How important is student preference for a teaching strategy to his/her resultant learning? Ultimately, research must go beyond the discovery and refinement of effective teaching methods and study the complex process of how teachers orchestrate learning in individual students (e.g., teacher communication, decision making, monitoring of progress, method–student match).

We know that many single and combined strategies work to promote learning in students who have DD. Why, then, is much of what we know about effective instruction not put into ordinary practice? Two likely reasons concern (1) the effort involved in using these teaching approaches and (2) a lack of knowledge about them. Both possibilities have implications for future research. First, researchers can focus on identifying the critical instructional elements so that combination procedures such as self-monitoring, support packages for included students, and ENI can be stripped to their essential components and possibly simplified for users. Although we know much about systematic prompting, researchers could test guidelines for effective matching of methods to learners and tasks. This type of study must include analyzing efficiency data, conducting rigorous measurement of procedural fidelity, and having users socially validate the methods. Second, more researchers should direct their study toward the science of teaching teachers to use these approaches, to generalize them across tasks, students, and settings, and to maintain their use on a long-term basis. The work of Schepis et al. (2001) on teaching paraprofessionals to embed instruction with preschoolers provides a good example. Traditional in-service training could be vastly improved if it reflected these research outcomes.

IMPLICATIONS FOR PRACTITIONERS AND FAMILIES

University teacher-training programs in special education must reflect evidence-based practices so that students with DD have the best opportunity to learn needed skills. Given the importance and legal emphasis on placement in the least restrictive environment, general education teachers, related services personnel, and school administrators also will influence the success of students with DD, and they need to be equipped with an understanding of the disability, positive attitudes toward students with DD, and training in collaborative teaming. Ongoing in-service training is the primary way that schools have to keep veteran teachers current with proven instructional methods.

Families should be able to assume that their children are being taught in ways that are consistent with current research findings. To check this assumption, parents can ask their child's educational teams several key questions. What useful skills, academic and applied, is my child being taught? Are these skills taught every day and with fairly consistent methods? Is my child taught so that errors are minimized in early learning, prompts eventually are faded, and motivation for learning is good? Do teams regularly gather and monitor performance data on my child so that ineffective teaching programs can be improved? Is my child learning meaningful skills? Does my child enjoy school? Trained teachers should be able to answer these basic questions.

IMPLICATIONS FOR POLICY MAKERS

Probably the greatest political impact on instruction has been federal and state policy requiring all students, including those with DD, to meet regular or adapted standards or alternate assessment criteria on year-end academic tests. It is not clear how much instructional time is devoted to teaching the content on these tests or how these assessments change the balance of what is taught to students, but test performance may determine whether students will graduate and may affect school status. A recent analysis of alternate assessment performance indicators found that some of the better alternate assessments retained a focus on functional skills but also accessed the general curriculum (Browder et al., 2004). Both are important for students with DD, but the balance in the composition of their curricula between functional and general curriculum skills should reflect individual student needs. Policy makers should (1) monitor whether and how such evaluations affect the appropriateness of the curriculum taught and (2) enforce criteria for awarding personnel preparation grants in special education to universities whose curricula reflect evidence-based instructional practices for students with DD.

Consistent with the strong presumption of IDEA that favors educating students with disabilities in general education, a second policy issue that influences instruction is national and local educational placement practice (Williamson, McLeaskey, Hoppey, & Rentz, 2006). Freeman and Alkin's (2000) review of separate class placement for individuals with DD concluded that placement in general education leads to better achievement and social competence for those with mild disabilities and better social outcomes for those with severe disabilities. A recent study of national and state practices on placing students diagnosed with mental retardation indicates that the identification rates remained stable during the 1990s, but placement rates changed consistent with Freeman and Alkin's (2000) recommendation. That is, (1) rates of placement in general education during the 1990s increased from 27.3 to 44.7%, and (2) rates of separate-setting placement decreased from 72.7 to 55.3% (Williamson et al., 2006). However, because of the great variability found in this survey from state to state and the fact that national placement trends also seem to have reached a plateau, Williamson et al. recommended first that states with the lowest rates of placement in general education be monitored and second that the policies of the highest placement state and local education agencies be examined to identify policies that reinforce the development and maintenance of inclusive programs. Special and general education settings feature many differences that affect instruction. Thus it is important that research findings from general education settings be applied in general education settings and vice versa to reduce threats to external validity. Although more than half of the research reviewed in this chapter took place in general education settings, it will be crucial for federal research funds to prioritize research in general education settings, consistent with the legal language that urges placement of individuals with disabilities in the least restrictive environment.

REFERENCES

Agran, M., Sinclair, T., Alper, S., Cavin, M., Wehmeyer, M., & Hughes, C. (2005). Using self-monitoring to increase following-direction skills of students with moderate to severe disabilities in general education. *Education and Training in Developmental Disabilities, 40,* 3–13.

Baer, D. M. (1981). A hung jury and a Scottish verdict: "Not proven. " *Analysis and Intervention in Developmental Disabilities, 1,* 91–97

Batu, S., Ergenekon, Y., Erbas, E., & Akmanoglu, N. (2004). Teaching pedestrian skills to individuals with developmental disabilities. *Journal of Behavioral Education, 13,* 147–164.

Branham, R. S., Collins, B. C., Schuster, J. W., & Kleinert, H. (1999). Teaching community skills to students with moderate disabilities: Comparing combined techniques of classroom simulation, videotape modeling, and community-based instruction. *Education and Training in Mental Retardation and Developmental Disabilities, 34,* 170–181.

Browder, D., Flowers, C., Alhgrim-Delzell, L., Karvonen, M., Spooner, F., & Algozzine, R. (2004). The alignment of alternate assessment content with academic and functional curricula. *Journal of Special Education, 37,* 211–223.

Browder, D., Wakeman, S. Y., Spooner, F., Ahlgrim-Delzell, L., & Algozzine, B. (2006). Research on reading instruction for individuals with significant cognitive disabilities. *Exceptional Children, 72,* 392–408.

Browder, D. M., & Xin, Y. P. (1998). A meta-analysis and review of sight-word research and its implications for teaching functional reading to individuals with moderate and severe disabilities. *Journal of Special Education, 32,* 130–153.

Charlop-Christy, M. H., Le, L., & Freeman, K. (2000). A comparison of video modeling with in vivo modeling for teaching children with autism. *Journal of Autism and Developmental Disorders, 30,* 537–552.

Chavez-Brown, M., Scott, J., & Ross, D. E. (2005). Antecedent selection: Comparing simplified and typical verbal antecedents for children with autism. *Journal of Behavioral Education, 14,* 153–165.

Cihak, D., Alberto, P., Taber-Doughty, T., & Gama, R. (2006). A comparison of static picture prompting and video prompting simulation strategies using group instructional procedures. *Focus on Autism and Other Developmental Disabilities, 21,* 89–99.

Collins, B. C., Hall, M., Branson, T. A., & Holder, M. (1999). Acquisition of related and unrelated factual information delivered by a teacher within an inclusive setting. *Journal of Behavioral Education, 9,* 223–237.

Copeland, S. R., Hughes, C., Agran, G., Wehmeyer, M. L., & Fowler, S. E. (2002). An intervention package to support high school students with mental retardation in general education classrooms. *American Journal on Mental Retardation, 107,* 32–45.

Craft, M. A., Alber, S. R., & Heward, W. L. (1998). Teaching elementary students with developmental disabilities to recruit teacher attention in a general education classroom: Effects on teacher praise and academic productivity. *Journal of Applied Behavior Analysis, 31,* 399–415.

Dibley, S., & Lim, L. L. (1999). Providing choice making opportunities within and between daily school routines. *Journal of Behavioral Education, 9,* 117–132.

Dunlap, G., dePerczel, M., Clarke, S., Wilson, D., Wright, S., White, R., et al. (1994). Choice making to promote adaptive behavior for students with emotional and behavioral challenges. *Journal of Applied Behavior Analysis, 27,* 505–518.

Etsel, B. C., & LeBlanc, J. M. (1979). The simplest treatment alternative: The law of parsimony applied to choosing appropriate instructional control and errorless learning procedures for the difficult-to-teach child. *Journal of Autism and Developmental Disorders, 9,* 361–382.

Farlow, L. J., & Snell, M. E. (1994). *Making the most of student performance data.* Washington, DC: American Association on Mental Retardation.

Farlow, L. J., & Snell, M. E. (2005). Making the most of student performance data. In M. L. Wehmeyer & M. Agran (Eds.), *Mental retardation and intellectual disabilities: Teaching students using innovative and research-based practices* (pp. 27–77). Upper Saddle River, NJ: Merrill/Prentice Hall.

Ficus, R. S., Schuster, J. W., Morse, R. E., & Collins, B. C. (2002). Teaching elementary students with cognitive disabilities food preparation skills while embedding instructive feedback in the prompt and consequent event. *Education and Training in Mental Retardation and Developmental Disabilities, 37,* 55–69.

Freeman, S. F. N., & Alkin, M. C. (2000). Academic and social attainments of children with mental retardation in general and special education settings. *Remedial and Special Education, 21,* 2–18.

Gilberts, G. H., Agran, M., Hughes, C., & Wehmeyer, M. (2001). The effects of peer delivered self-monitoring strategies on the participation of students with severe disabilities in general education classrooms. *Journal of the Association for Persons with Severe Handicaps, 26,* 25–36.

Graves, T. B., Collins, B. C., Schuster, J. W., & Kleinert, H. (2005). Using video prompting to teach cooking skills to secondary students with moderate disabilities. *Education and Training in Developmental Disabilities, 40,* 34–46.

Green, C. W., Reid, D. H., Rollyson, J. H., & Passante, S. C. (2005). An enriched teaching program for reducing resistance and indices of unhappiness among individuals with profound multiple disabilities. *Journal of Applied Behavior Analysis, 38,* 221–233.

Halle, J. (1987). Teaching language in the natural environment: An analysis of spontaneity. *Journal of the Association for Persons with Severe Handicaps, 12,* 28–37.

Heckaman, K. A., Alber, S., Hooper, S., & Heward, W. L. (1998). A comparison of least-to-most prompts and progressive time delay on the disruptive behavior of students with autism. *Journal of Behavioral Education, 8,* 171–201.

Hughes, C., Copeland, S. R., Agran, M., Wehmeyer, M., Rodi, M. S., & Presley, J. A. (2002). Using self-monitoring to improve performance in general education high school classes. *Education and Training in Mental Retardation and Developmental Disabilities, 37,* 262–272.

Hughes, C., Pitkin, S. E., & Lorden, S. W. (1998). Assessing preferences and choices of persons with severe and profound mental retardation. *Education and Training in Developmental Disabilities, 33,* 299–316.

Hunt, P., Soto, G., Maier, J., & Doering, K. (2003). Collaborative teaming to support students at risk and students with severe disabilities in general education classrooms. *Exceptional Children, 69,* 315–332.

Hwang, B., & Hughes, C. (2000a). The effects of social interactive training on early social communicative skills of children with autism. *Journal of Autism and Developmental Disabilities, 30,* 331–343.

Hwang, B., & Hughes, C. (2000b). Increasing early social-communicative skills of preverbal preschool children with autism through social interactive training. *Journal of the Association for Persons with Severe Handicaps, 25,* 18–28.

Ingersoll, B., & Schreibman, L. (2006). Teaching reciprocal imitation skills to young children with autism using a naturalistic behavioral approach: Effects on language, pretend play, and joint attention. *Journal of Autism and Developmental Disorders, 36,* 487–505.

Johnson, J. W., & McDonnell, J. (2004). An exploratory study of the implementation of embedded instruction by general educators with students with developmental disabilities. *Education and Treatment of Children, 27,* 46–63.

Jolivette, K., Stichter, J. P., Sibilsky, S., Scott, T. M., & Ridgley, R. (2002). Naturally occurring opportunities for preschool children with and without disabilities to make choices. *Education and Treatment of Children, 25,* 396–414.

Kern, L., Vorndran, C. M., Hilt, A., Ringdahl, J. E., Adelman, R. E., & Dunlap, G. (1998). Choice as an intervention to improve behavior: A review of the literature. *Journal of Behavioral Education, 8,* 151–169.

Kim, O., & Hupp, S. C. (2005). Teacher interaction styles and task engagement of elementary students with cognitive disabilities. *Education and Training in Developmental Disabilities, 40,* 293–308.

Lane, H. (1976). *The wild boy of Aveyron*. Cambridge, MA: Harvard University Press. Lohrmann-O'Rourke, S., & Browder, D. M. (1998). Empirically based methods to assess the preferences of individuals with severe disabilities. *American Journal on Mental Retardation, 103*, 146–161.

McDonnell, J., Johnson, J., Polycronis, S., Riesen, T. Jameson, M., & Kercher, K. (2006). Comparison of one-to-one embedded instruction in general education classes with small group instruction in special education classes. *Education and Training in Developmental Disabilities, 41*, 125–138.

McDonnell, J., Mathot-Buckner, C., Thorson, N., & Fister, S. (2001). Supporting the inclusion of students with moderate and severe disabilities in junior high school general education classes: The effects of classwide peer tutoring, multielement curriculum, and accommodations. *Education and Treatment of Children, 24*, 141–160.

Mechling, L. C., Gast, D. L., & Cronin, B. A. (2006). The effects of presenting high-preference items, paired with choice, via computer-based video programming on task completion of students with autism. *Focus on Autism and Other Developmental Disabilities, 21*, 7–13.

Mechling, L. C., Pridgen, L. S., & Cronin, B. A. (2005). Computer-based video instruction to teach students with intellectual disabilities to verbally respond to questions and make purchases in fast food restaurants. *Education and Training in Developmental Disabilities, 40*, 47–59.

Odom, S. L., Brown, W. H., Frey, T., Karasu, N., Smith-Canter, L. L., & Strain, P. S. (2003). Evidence-based practices for young children with autism: Contributions for single-subject design research. *Focus on Autism and Other Developmental Disabilities, 18*, 166–175.

Nietupski, J., Hamre-Nietupski, S., Curtin, S., & Shrikanth, K. (1997). A review of curricular research in severe disabilities from 1976 to 1995 in six selected journals. *Journal of Special Education, 31*, 36–55.

Riesen, T., McDonnell, J., Johnson, J. W., Polychronis, S., & Jameson, M. (2003). A comparison of constant time delay and simultaneous prompting within embedded instruction in general education classes with students with moderate to severe disabilities. *Journal of Behavioral Education, 12*, 241–259.

Schepis, M. M., Reid, D. H., Behrmann, M. M., & Sutton, K. A. (1998). Increasing communicative interactions of young children with autism using a voice output communication aid and naturalistic teaching. *Journal of Applied Behavior Analysis, 31*, 561–578.

Schepis, M. M., Reid, D. H., Ownbey, J., & Parsons, M. (2001). Training support staff to embed teaching within natural routines of young children with disabilities in an inclusive preschool. *Journal of Applied Behavior Analysis, 34*, 313–327.

Schuster, J. W., Morse, T. E., Ault, M. J., Doyle, P. M., Crawford, M. R., & Wolery, M. (1998). Constant time delay with chained tasks: A review of the literature. *Education and Treatment of Children, 21*, 74–106.

Sigafoos, J., O'Reilly, M., Cannella, H., Upadhyaya, M., Edrisinha, C., Lancioni, G. E., et al. (2005). Computer-presented video prompting for teaching microwave oven use to three adults with developmental disabilities. *Journal of Behavioral Education, 14*, 189–201.

Snell, M. E. (1997). Teaching children and young adults with mental retardation in school programs: Current research. *Behaviour Change, 14*, 73–105.

Snell, M. E., Chen, L. Y., & Hoover, K. (2006). Teaching augmentative and alternative communication to students with severe disabilities: A review of intervention research, 1997–2003. *Research and Practice for Persons with Severe Disabilities, 31*, 203–214.

Stafford, A. M., Alberto, P. A., Fredrick, L. D., Heflin, L. J., & Heller, K. W. (2002). Preference variability and the instruction of choice making with students with severe intellectual disabilities. *Education and Training in Mental Retardation and Developmental Disabilities, 37*, 70–88.

Stromer, R., Mackay, H. A., McVay, A., & Fowler, T. (1998). Written lists as mediating stimuli in the matching-to-sample performances of individuals with mental retardation. *Journal of Applied Behavior Analysis, 31*, 1–19.

Taber, T. A., Alberto, P. A., Seltzer, A., & Hughes, M. (2003). Obtaining assistance when lost in the community using cell phones. *Research and Practice for Persons with Severe Disabilities, 28*, 105–116.

Tekin, E., & Kircaali-Iftar, K. (2002). Comparison of the effectiveness and efficiency of two response prompting procedures delivered by sibling tutors. *Education and Training in Mental Retardation and Developmental Disabilities, 37*, 283–299.

Test, D. W., & Ellis, M. F. (2005). The effects of LAP fractions on addition and subtraction of fractions with students with mild disabilities. *Education and Treatment of Children, 28*, 11–14.

Vaughn, B. J., & Horner, R. H. (1997). Identifying instructional tasks that occasion problem behaviors and assessing the effects of student versus teacher choice among these tasks. *Journal of Applied Behavior Analysis, 30,* 299–312.

Williamson, P., McLeaskey, J., Hoppey, D., & Rentz, T. (2006). Educating students with mental retardation in general education classrooms. *Exceptional Children, 72,* 347–361.

Werts, M. G., Wolery, M., Holcombe, A., & Gast, D. L. (1995). Instructive feedback: Review of parameters and effects. *Journal of Behavioral Education, 5,* 55–75.

Wolery, M., & Schuster, J. W. (1997). Instructional methods with students who have significant disabilities. *Journal of Special Education, 31,* 61–79.

13

Inclusive Education

Pam Hunt
John McDonnell

When inclusive education is fully embraced, we abandon the idea that children
have to become typical in order to contribute to the world. Instead, we search
for and nourish the gifts that are inherent in all people. We begin to look
beyond typical ways of becoming valued members of the community and, in
doing so, begin to realize the achievable goal of providing all children with the
authentic sense of belonging.

—KUNC (2000, pp. 91–92)

Writing a chapter on inclusive education is a daunting task: What aspects of the educational inclusion of students with disabilities should we address? Taking into account the number of individuals who have made significant contributions to the development of inclusive services, whose advocacy, research, program design, and systems-change efforts should we include? From the rapidly expanding body of research on inclusive education, how do we draw a representative sample? Given these considerations, we offer the reader (1) an overview of the definition of inclusive education and a description of the characteristics of inclusive schools; (2) a synopsis of the "history" of inclusive education within the context of school reform; (3) a sample of research on inclusive education models and practices, with a particular focus on students with developmental disabilities; and (4) a summary discussion of the implications of the current state of special education reform for educational policy makers and for future research.

We dedicate this chapter to inclusive education advocates, researchers, and leaders in systems change and to the students, teachers, parents, and administrators who are creating and continually contributing to inclusive schools in which all students are valued members.

WHAT IS INCLUSIVE EDUCATION?

The term "inclusion" began to appear in the literature with some frequency around 1990 (e.g., Gartner & Lipsky, 1987; Sailor, 1991; Stainback & Stainback, 1990). When inclusive educational practices are implemented, students with disabilities attend their home schools and receive educational services through full-time placement in chronologically age-appropriate general education classes within the context of the core curriculum and general class activities and in integrated community settings. In addition there are (1) a natural proportion of students with disabilities at the school site, (2) a zero-rejection district policy so that no student is excluded on the basis of type or extent of disability, and (3) a staff-to-student ratio for inclusion support teachers (certificated special education teachers) and a level of instructional assistant support that is equivalent to the special class ratio in the district (Halvorsen & Neary, 2001; Sailor, 1991).

Inclusive education is differentiated from "integration," which was identified with the late 1970s and 1980s advocacy movement to educate students with developmental disabilities in regular schools—albeit in self-contained classrooms—rather than in special education schools with little or no contact with general education students, settings, or curricula (Sailor et al., 1989) and from "mainstreaming," in which students with disabilities are members of special education classes but "visit" general education classes to engage in educational and social activities with same-age general education peers (Halvorsen & Neary, 2001; Sailor, 1991). Unlike integrated or mainstreamed students, students who receive inclusive educational services are *members* of the general education classroom community. According to Halvorsen and Neary (2001), "the single most identifiable characteristic of inclusive education is membership. Students who happen to have disabilities are seen first as kids who are a natural part of the school and the age-appropriate general education classroom they attend" (p. 3).

Although inclusive education was initially viewed as a *special education service delivery model*, the current focus is on the creation of *inclusive schools* that unify school resources and integrate programs in ways that benefit all students in general education classrooms (Ferguson, Kozleski, & Smith, 2003; Halvorsen & Neary, 2001; Lipsky & Gartner, 1997; Miles & Darling-Hammond, 1998, Parrish, 2002; Sailor, 1991; Villa & Thousand, 2000). Emphasis is placed on building a sense of community in inclusive schools in which all students are valued members and on educational programs that address the needs of students across cultural, language, and ability differences (Ferguson et al., 2003; Hunt, Hirose-Hatae, Goetz, Doering, & Karasoff, 2000). Some major characteristics of inclusive schools are (1) the reallocation of fiscal and personnel resources to more effectively meet the needs of all students; (2) site-based management, teacher empowerment in the decision-making process, and a culture of change for improvement; (3) general and special education collaborative teaming; (4) instructional practices and assistive technologies that make curricula assessable to all students in heterogeneous classrooms and promote active student participation in the learning process; (5) creation of classroom communities in which all students are valued members and diversity is celebrated; and (6) implementation of social supports to facilitate positive social relationships and promote membership in the school community. These characteristics are discussed in the following sections.

Reallocation of Resources

The reallocation of fiscal and personnel resources from general and special education categorical programs to increase the academic achievement of all students in inclusive schools is possible through recent changes in federal education policy. These changes increased flexibility in coordinating special education funding through the 1997 Individuals with Disabilities Education Act with funding from Title I Schoolwide Programs and bilingual education (McLaughlin & Verstegen, 1998; Parrish, 2002). In addition, Schoolwide Programs, under the reauthorized Elementary and Secondary Education Act of 1994 (renamed the Improving America's Schools Act), can use, in addition to Title I monies, funds from most other federal education programs, as long as the reform activities increase the academic achievement of all students. The reallocation of resources from disparate categorical programs can provide a seamless set of services to meet the needs of all students in general education classrooms, thus promoting inclusive educational practices and greatly increasing the efficient use of resources (Miles & Darling-Hammond, 1998; Parrish, 2002). Resources reallocation in inclusive schools allows (1) reduction of specialized programs to provide more individualized instruction for students in small, integrated groups; (2) more flexible student grouping; (3) longer blocks of instructional time; (4) increased common planning time for staff; and (5) the redefinition of staff roles and work schedules to more effectively and efficiently meet the needs of students in general education classrooms (Miles & Darling-Hammond, 1998).

Site-Based Management

Many inclusive schools have implemented forms of site-based management to provide a context for shared decision making, a climate of continuous school improvement, and a forum for reallocating resources (Ferguson et al., 2003; Lambert, 1998; Sailor, 1991). Site leadership teams or site management councils—often composed of teachers, administrators, parents, community members, and students—work together to review current practices related to the distribution of resources, curriculum and classroom practices, student achievement, discipline factors, professional development needs, and school climate issues. Guided by the collective vision of the school community, members of the leadership team identify high-priority need areas, engage in a prioritization and objective-setting process, identify needed resources and actions to address high-priority objectives, and identify evaluation procedures to document progress toward meeting their goals (Sailor & Roger, 2005).

Collaborative Teaming

Collaborative teaming provides the vehicle for unifying general and special education services to support the academic progress and social participation of all students in inclusive classrooms (Hunt, Soto, Maier, & Doering, 2003; Salisbury, Evans, & Palombaro, 1997; Snell & Janney, 2005). The collaborative teaming process offers ongoing opportunities for general and special educators and parents to "share knowledge and skills to generate new and novel methods for individualizing learning, without the need for dual systems of general and special education" (Villa & Thousand, 2000, p. 255). Collaborative planning meetings and activities might focus on developing and implementing individualized academic and social supports for any students in inclusive classrooms who need them, creating classroom curriculum and activities, and establishing a variety of general and special education cooperative teaching models (Udvari-Solner & Thousand, 1995).

Universal Design and Differentiated Instruction

Instructional practices and assistive technologies that make curricula accessible to all students in heterogeneous classrooms have been referred to as "universal design" (Curry, 2003) and "differentiated instruction" (Tomlinson, 1999). For students with developmental disabilities, universal design and differentiated instruction include developing and implementing curricular and instructional adaptations and modifications needed to align each student's individualized education plan (IEP) goals with the general education curriculum and to support student progress in achieving those goals; embedding instruction within age-appropriate and meaningful activities in classroom, school, and community settings; supporting the active involvement of students in the learning process; facilitating positive interactions with classmates in the context of educational activities; and promoting self-determined and self-regulated learning (Falvey, Blair, Dingle, & Franklin, 2000; McDonnell, Johnson, Polychronis, & Riesen, 2002; Sands & Wehmeyer, 1996).

Classroom Communities

Inclusive schools strive to create classroom communities in which all students are valued members and diversity is celebrated. Community building is facilitated through the employment of strategies to increase students' sense of identity and self-worth and their capacity for cooperation, interdependence, and respect for cultural, language, and ability differences. Concepts related to cultural and ability diversity, equity and democracy, and cooperation and interdependence are incorporated into the classroom curriculum. Students are provided with opportunities to recognize each other's accomplishments, and regularly scheduled class meetings may be used for problem solving and conflict resolution (Gibbs, 1994).

Social Relationships and Friendships

Finally, a high-priority educational outcome for students with developmental disabilities, as for any child in inclusive classrooms, is positive interactions with peers and the development of friendships (Meyer, 2001; Staub, Peck, Gallucci, & Schwartz, 2000). Although teachers cannot "program" the establishment of positive student-to-student relationships, a number of research-based contextual arrangements and social-support strategies promote the membership of students with mild to significant cognitive disabilities in their school community (Meyer, 2001). Meyer, Park, Grenot-Scheyer, Schwartz, and Harry (1998) provided guidelines for implementing social-support interventions, including ensuring that the interventions are (1) practical and "doable" in average classroom contexts, (2) possible with available long-term resources, (3) sustainable over time, (4) created and implemented by school personnel and peers, and (5) culturally responsive and intuitively appealing to those implementing and those receiving support.

The development of inclusive schools represents one aspect of a systemic approach to school reform that calls for the unification of general and special education for a shared educational agenda and a fully integrated and coordinated system of educational services. The following section puts the "history" of inclusive education in the context of school reform.

PUTTING INCLUSIVE EDUCATION IN THE CONTEXT OF SCHOOL REFORM

In 1975 Public Law 94-142, the Education of All Handicapped Children Act (EHA), mandated a free, appropriate public education in the least restrictive environment for all students with disabilities, including those with the most significant disabilities who had been excluded from public education in the past. Since the passage of that law, a dominant theme in special education policy reform has been the nature of the special education service delivery model and the extent of its proximity to general education practices, students, and settings (Sailor, 1991).

The Regular Education Initiative: Opening the Door to a Shared Educational Agenda

In the 1980s, in response to a growing concern over the rapid increase in and the effectiveness of special education services provided through separate, categorical placements and practices, Madeleine Will, the assistant secretary for the Office of Special Education and Rehabilitation Services (OSERS), issued a policy initiative addressing the challenge of providing the best, most effective education possible for children and youth with learning problems (Will, 1985). Through what has become known as her Wingspread Regular Education Initiative (REI) speech and through two subsequent 1986 publications (Will, 1986a, 1986b), Will identified the need for general and special education partnerships to "cooperatively assess the educational needs of students with learning problems and to cooperatively develop effective educational strategies for meeting those needs" (Will, 1986a, p. 415). She also called for early identification and intervention for students with learning problems using curriculum-based assessments, for the use of research-based instructional practices in general education classrooms, and for increased parental involvement in planning processes. The initiative was largely recommended on the basis of a series of studies conducted by Margaret Wang, Herbert Wahlberg, and Maynard Reynolds, which reported positive educational outcomes for students with mild disabilities when they were supported in general education classrooms rather than in "pull out" settings in which they received remedial education services (e.g., Reynolds & Wang, 1983; Wang & Birch, 1984).

The REI generated tremendous controversy within the field of special education, as evidenced by a special issue of the *Journal of Learning Disabilities* (Wiederholt, 1988), devoted entirely to the REI, in which authors expressed the need for caution and provided critical analyses of the assumptions underlying REI and the research supporting general education class placement for students with high-incidence disabilities (see also Gersten & Woodward, 1990; Kauffman, 1989; Semmel & Gerber, 1990). In addition, although it was presented as general education policy, the REI made little impact in generating general education notice or buy-in because it was, essentially, special education driven; however, it was the first U.S. Department of Education policy to address the rapid increase in special education services provided through separate, categorical placements and practices, and it provided an opening for researchers and practitioners calling for an inclusive educational system (e.g., Gartner & Lipsky, 1987; Stainback & Stainback, 1984).

The REI debate soon broadened to include students with moderate and severe cognitive disabilities. Initial arguments for the general education placement of students with significant disabilities were values based; that is, advocates contended that students with disabilities should not be segregated for their education and should have access to interactions and friendships with peers in general education classes. Armed with this civil rights argument for inclusive educational services, parents and professionals were confronted with the reality of public schools and the general lack of inclusive placement options. In response, they aligned themselves with disability-rights lawyers and exercised the due-process rights specified in the amendments to the EHA. Hearings escalated into litigation, and several landmark decisions were made in appellate courts between 1989 and 1994—for example, *Daniel R. R. v. State Board of Education*, 1989, and *Sacramento City Unified School District v. Rachel Holland*, 1994. These decisions upheld the right of children with significant cognitive disabilities to attend general education classes full time when the academic and/or nonacademic benefits for the individual child called for such placement (see Lipton, 1997, for a review). Litigation-based efforts were supported by the growing body of research documenting, for the most part, positive outcomes for students with disabilities who received educational services in general education settings (see later in this chapter for a review of inclusive education research).

Goals 2000: Including All Students in Educational Goals and Reform

In the 1990s there was growing dissatisfaction with the poor outcomes for students receiving special education services because of their limited access to the general education curriculum (National Association of State Boards of Education [NASBE] Study Group on Special Education, 1992; Sailor & Skrtic, 1995; Skrtic, 1991) and the overrepresentation of culturally and linguistically diverse students in a special education system that allowed their exclusion from general education classes (Ferguson et al., 2003). There was a call for the development of multicultural, inclusive schools whose primary mission was to nurture and educate all children regardless of their differences in culture, language, ethnicity, or ability and to ensure equal access to socially valid educational outcomes for all students (Ferguson et al., 2003; Sailor & Skrtic, 1995).

In 1992 the NASBE Study Group on Special Education issued their report, *Winners All: A Call for Inclusive Schools,* after 2 years of reviewing special education and the general education reform movement. In it they called for "an inclusive system of education that strives to produce better outcomes for all students" (p. 4). Authors of the NASBE report recommended changes in three areas, including (1) the creation of a new belief system and vision for education that includes all students; (2) the development of collaborative partnerships between general and special educators and joint training programs to increase teacher capacity to work with a diverse student population; and (3) changes in funding requirements so that they would no longer drive programming and placement decisions.

Two years later, the Clinton administration's education reform legislation, Goals 2000: Educate America Act of 1994 (Public Law 103-227), took the position that all students must achieve at higher levels; and it provided resources to ensure that the lowest achieving students—students with disabilities, students who are English-language learners, students living in poverty—had access to challenging curricula and instruction (Kleinhammer-Tramill & Gallagher, 2002; Villa & Thousand, 2000). The reauthorized Elementary and Secondary Education Act in 1994 (renamed the Improving America's

Schools Act) was aligned with the broader Goals 2000 framework and, according to Kleinhammer-Tramill and Gallagher (2005), "became a vehicle for promoting school improvement and infusion of resources to promote inclusive education and standards-based accountability for student progress" (p. 27).

Reauthorization of IDEA in 1997 and 2004 and the No Child Left Behind Act of 2001: High Expectations for All Students

The reauthorization of IDEA in 1997 heralded a major policy shift toward the alignment of special education services with broader educational reforms, such as those represented in Goals 2000; that is, IDEA 1997 (1) reaffirmed the assumption that students with disabilities are educated in general education classrooms; (2) mandated access to and progress in the general education curriculum for students receiving special education services and inclusion of the students in state and local district educational assessments; and (3) coordinated the implementation of IDEA with other school improvement acts such as Title I Schoolwide Programs to promote unified educational systems (Villa & Thousand, 2000; McLaughlin & Verstegen, 1998). This shift in special education policy continues with the newly reauthorized IDEA of 2004 (renamed the Individuals with Disabilities Education Improvement Act).

The No Child Left Behind Act of 2001 (NCLB), the Bush administration's education legislation, also clearly identified all children in public schools as first and foremost general education students and encouraged the use of whole-school approaches (e.g., evidence-based reading programs, positive behavioral interventions, and early intervention services) to reduce referrals to special education and the need to label students as disabled to meet their needs. In addition, NCLB mandated high expectations and accountability for every child in the public school system by requiring statewide assessment systems based on challenging state standards in reading and language arts, mathematics, and science. Annual testing was required for all students in grades 3–8. In addition, states were required to develop progress objectives to ensure that all groups of students reach proficiency within 12 years. Students with significant cognitive disabilities (approximately 1% of the student population) were included in state testing systems through alternate assessments based on alternate standards; and, more recently, an additional 2% of students (i.e., students who demonstrate "persistent academic difficulties") may be included through alternate assessments with modified standards (Browder et al., 2003; Kleinert, Haig, Kearns, & Kennedy, 2000).

An increased emphasis on educational accountability and the inclusion of students with significant disabilities in alternate assessments holds the promise for increased consideration of these students in school and state policy decisions, as well as enhanced educational expectations, greater access to the general education curriculum, and improved instructional programs for this population of students (Browder et al., 2003); however, to date these promises have not been realized. The validity and reliability of states' alternate assessments have not yet been demonstrated, and, therefore, the data that they produce are of uncertain value. In addition the promise of alternate assessments will be achieved only when the assessment outcomes are related to classroom instruction, tied to the students' IEPs, and used as the basis for increasing the quality of the students' educational programs by increasing access to the general education curriculum, assistive technology, and integrated educational contexts (Browder et al., 2003).

Inclusive School Reform: Where We Go from Here

Although there is increasing evidence that general and special education are moving in the direction of sharing a common educational agenda, as evidenced by the legislation reviewed previously, there continue to be limited systemic reform efforts to create an integrated and coordinated system of educational services, failure to obtain "buy-in" from the general education community, and continued opposition to inclusive education policy and practices within the special education community (Ferguson et al., 2003; Sailor & Roger, 2005). The limited success of the "inclusion initiative" is reflected in the educational placement statistics from the *Twenty-Fourth Annual Report to Congress on the Implementation of the Individuals with Disabilities Education Act* (U.S. Department of Education, 2002). In the 1999–2000 school year, only 47% of the students receiving special education services in regular schools were placed in general education classes (and were removed for services less than 21% of the school day). Only 14% of the students with cognitive disabilities were placed in general education classes. Twenty-nine percent were served in different educational settings for 21 to 60% of the day, and 51% were placed in special classes. In addition, a significantly disproportionate percentage of students of color were receiving special education services in special classes. Realization of an inclusive educational system in which all students are valued members will require substantial changes in existing educational policy and practices, including the development of district-wide, general education-driven, comprehensive school reform models that unify school resources and administration to more efficiently and effectively support all students (see later in this chapter for a discussion of the implications for educational policy makers and for future research; Ferguson et al., 2003; Lipsky & Gartner, 1997; Miles & Darling-Hammond, 1998; Sailor & Roger, 2005; Villa & Thousand, 2000).

RESEARCH ON INCLUSIVE EDUCATION

One area of research that has received increased attention in the past decade is the impact of inclusive education on student learning and the quality of instruction that students with disabilities receive in these settings (Freeman, 2000; Hunt & Goetz, 1997; McDonnell, 1998; McGregor & Vogelsberg, 1998). In this section, we review selected studies that highlight key findings in three areas, including (1) the relative effectiveness of inclusive and separate educational programs, (2) the impact of inclusive education on the achievement of peers without disabilities, and (3) the characteristics of instruction provided to students in general education classes. An examination of studies investigating stakeholder perspectives on inclusive education follows this review.

Comparisons of Inclusive and Separate Education Programs

Several studies have directly compared the academic and social outcomes of inclusive and separate educational programs for students with developmental disabilities (Cole, Waldron, & Majd, 2004; Fisher & Meyer, 2002; Fryxell & Kennedy, 1995; Peetsma, Vergeer, Roeleveld, & Karsten, 2001). For example, Cole et al. (2004) compared the performance in reading and math of matched groups of students with and without mild disabilities (including students with mild cognitive delay) who were enrolled in inclusive or traditional elementary schools. In inclusive schools, students with disabilities received their reading and math instruction in age-appropriate general education classrooms. In traditional schools, students with disabilities received instruction in these areas from a special education teacher in a separate classroom. The researchers found no differences between the groups in either reading or math performance regardless of disability classification. Post hoc analyses for students with mild cognitive delay found that 50% of the students in inclusive schools made progress comparable to or greater than that of their peers without disabilities in math and that 40% did so in reading. In contrast, only 37.7% of the students with mild cognitive delay in traditional schools made gains comparable to or greater than those of their peers in math, and only 29.5% did so in reading.

Fisher and Meyer (2002) compared the development of adaptive behavior in and the social competence of two matched groups of students with moderate to profound disabilities who were educated either in general education classes for the majority of the school day or in self-contained special education classrooms. The results showed that only students in inclusive programs made significant gains in adaptive behavior and social competence. Comparisons between the groups found that gains in adaptive behavior were significantly higher for students in inclusive classes than for those in self-contained classes and that there were no significant differences in gains in social competence.

Fryxell and Kennedy (1995) compared the social interactions of two matched groups of students enrolled full time either in general education classes or in self-contained special education classrooms. They found that the number of social contacts that students in general education classes had with peers without disabilities was more than seven times higher than those of students in self-contained classes. Students enrolled in general education classes also received significantly more social support from others during the school day and provided more social support to others than students in self-contained classes. Finally, the mean number of peers without disabilities identified by students with disabilities as members of their social networks was 17 times higher for students taught in the general education classes than for those taught in self-contained classes.

Impact of Inclusive Education on Students without Disabilities

Several studies have addressed the common criticism that inclusive education will negatively affect the achievement of peers without disabilities (Cole et al., 2004; Sharpe, York, & Knight, 1994). For example, Cole et al. (2004), as part of the study described previously, found that the students without disabilities in inclusive schools made significantly greater academic progress on the reading and mathematics measures used in the study than did the students without disabilities in traditional schools.

McDonnell et al. (2003) examined the educational achievement of 14 students with developmental disabilities who were served in general education classes and of their peers without disabilities enrolled in five elementary schools. The achievement of students with developmental disabilities was measured using a standardized assessment of adaptive behavior in a pre–post design. The academic performance of students without disabilities was measured using scores from a state-mandated, criterion-referenced test in reading and language arts and mathematics. A posttest-only control-group design was used to compare scores of students who were enrolled in classes with a student with developmental disabilities with scores of students enrolled in classes that did not include students with developmental disabilities. The results revealed that 13 of the 14 students with developmental disabilities made significant gains in adaptive behavior, and there were no differences between the two groups of students without disabilities in either reading or math performance.

Characteristics of Curriculum and Instruction in General Education Classes

Although concerns are often expressed about the quality of education that students receive in inclusive programs, studies consistently show that they are actively engaged in the instructional activities of general education classes and that the instruction they receive in these settings is comparable to that of students enrolled in separate classes (Foreman, Arthur-Kelly, & Pascoe, 2004; Hunt, Farron-Davis, Beckstead, Curtis, & Goetz, 1994; Logan & Keefe, 1997; McDonnell, Thorson, McQuivey, & Kiefer-O'Donnell, 1997). For example, Hunt et al. (1994) evaluated the quality of educational programs of two matched groups of students with severe disabilities placed in either general education or special education classrooms. They found that the quality of IEPs of students enrolled in general education classes was superior to that of students served in special education classes and that the goals and objectives were more closely aligned with the general education curriculum. Students enrolled in general education classes, especially those with more significant disabilities, were more engaged in instructional activities than students in special education classes and had more interactions with peers without disabilities.

Logan and Keefe (1997) conducted an observational study examining the instructional context, teacher behavior, and engaged behavior of 30 elementary students with developmental disabilities enrolled in general education and self-contained special education classrooms. Their analysis showed that students enrolled in general education classes received a greater proportion of their instruction through academic rather than functional daily living activities than did students served in special education classes. In addition, they found that students in general education classes received more one-to-one instruction and more attention from the classroom teacher than did students in self-contained classrooms. Finally, no differences were found between the two groups on their level of task engagement.

Areas for Future Research

This group of studies suggests that inclusive education produces better educational and social outcomes for students with developmental disabilities than separate special education settings do; however, the number of studies is small, and there is a need for additional research studies that systematically compare these programs. Future studies should examine the outcomes achieved for students across the full range of variation in classrooms and school structures (e.g., staffing patterns, student-to-staff ratios, type and quality of instruction). Another critical issue is the need to control for the amount of time that students with disabilities spend in general education classes and their level of participation in the general education curriculum. Currently there is extreme variation in these factors across published research studies. This information is critical to future efforts to develop curriculum and instructional approaches that can effectively meet the needs of all students in inclusive classes. Finally, the range of dependent variables used in the next generation of studies must be expanded to directly measure students' participation and progress in the general education curriculum.

EFFECTIVE PRACTICES RESEARCH

Most of the studies conducted on effective practices have examined student-based interventions that are designed to meet the needs of students within the ongoing activities of general education classes or classroom-based interventions that are directed at changing the way instruction is provided to all of the students in the class. In this section we review selected research studies within in each area that illustrate the key findings.

Student-Based Interventions

The five strategies that have the most empirical support in improving the academic and social outcomes of students in general education classes include student-directed learning, embedded instruction, curricular accommodations and modifications, peer supports, and paraeducator supports.

Student-Directed Learning

Studies on student-directed learning have addressed the impact of teaching skills such as problem solving, study planning, goal setting, and self-monitoring on students' participation in general education classes and the general curriculum (Gilberts, Agran, Hughes, & Wehmeyer, 2001; Koegel, Harrower, & Koegel, 1999; Wehmeyer, Yeager, Bolding, Agran, & Hughes, 2003). The purpose of teaching these skills to students is to increase their capacity to participate in the activities of general education classes and to reduce the level of assistance they need to be successful. For example, Gilberts et al. (2001) taught "classroom survival skills" (e.g., bringing appropriate materials to class, greeting other students, asking questions) to five students in general Spanish, history, and art classes using a self-monitoring system. The results indicated that the students' rates of survival skills increased, and they learned to complete the self-monitoring procedures in the general education class with a high degree of accuracy. In addition, the teachers reported that they had observed positive improvements in the participation of four of the students in the activities of their general education classes.

Embedded Instruction

Embedded instruction is designed to teach skills to students with disabilities in general education classrooms by providing systematic instruction during natural opportunities within or across ongoing activities. Research on embedded instruction has shown that it is effective as a supplemental strategy for teaching content drawn from the general education curriculum or as the primary strategy for teaching skills included in students' IEPs (Johnson, McDonnell, Holzwarth, & Hunter, 2004; McDonnell et al., 2002; Wolery, Anthony, Snyder, Werts, & Katzenmeyer, 1997). Johnson et al. (2004) used an embedded-instruction format to teach three students enrolled in general education classes to define basic science concepts drawn from the general science curriculum, to identify sight words drawn from the general reading curriculum, and to use an electronic communication device to make requests of classroom staff. General educators provided instruction to two of the students, and a paraeducator provided instruction to the third student. Results showed that embedded instruction led to acquisition of the target skills by all students. In addition, general education teachers and the paraeducator were able to reliably implement embedded instruction in the routines of the general education classes. Finally, teachers and the paraeducator reported that embedded instruction was an acceptable and effective strategy for meeting the needs of the students in their general education classes.

Curriculum Accommodations and Modifications

The use of curriculum accommodations and modifications with students in general education classes has received a substantial amount of attention in recent years (Fisher & Frey, 2001; Janney & Snell, 1997; Ryndak, Morrison, & Sommerstein, 1999). For example, Fisher and Frey (2001) examined the ways in which an elementary school, middle school, and high school student accessed the general education curriculum through the design and implementation of accommodations and modifications. Data were gathered through direct observations of students in their general education classes and through interviews with parents, general education teachers, special education teachers, and peers without disabilities. The researchers found that all three students were provided a number of individualized, content-specific accommodations and modifications to help them participate successfully in the instructional activities of their general education classes. They also found that collaboration between special and general education teachers was essential to developing accommodations and modifications for students and that peers without disabilities often had important insights in how to make adaptations or modifications more effective.

Establishing Peer Supports

Research has consistently shown that establishing comprehensive peer supports is critical to ensuring the success of students with developmental disabilities in general education classes (Carter, Cushing, Clark, & Kennedy, 2005; Cushing & Kennedy, 1997; Goetz & O'Farrell, 1999; Hunt, Alwell, Farron-Davis, & Goetz, 1996). For example, Goetz and O'Farrell (1999) conducted a qualitative study examining the impact of a social-support intervention package on three elementary students who were deaf-blind and on their peers without disabilities in general education classes. The package included providing information to peers about the strengths and needs of students in ongoing classroom activities, providing students with interactive, multimedia communication systems that were appropriate for their needs in classroom activities, and creating planned and spontaneous opportunities for ongoing social interactions between students and their peers. The results suggested that carefully designing peer-support strategies and environmental engineering led to increased levels of social interaction between students and peers and higher levels of academic engagement.

Although peer supports are clearly beneficial for students with disabilities, they also appear to have educational benefits for peers without disabilities. Cushing and Kennedy (1997) examined the impact of a peer-support strategy on the academic engagement and course-work performance of three middle school students without disabilities who supported three peers with cognitive disabilities in general education classes. The peers were taught how to communicate with the students, to make curricular adaptations necessary for them to complete in-class and homework assignments, and to provide feedback to them on their performance. The results of the study indicated that students without disabilities had higher levels of academic engagement and participated more actively in instruction when they were providing support to their peers than when they were not.

Paraeducator Supports

Although paraeducators are one of the main sources of educational and social support for students in general education classes, a number of recent studies suggest that there is a complex relationship between the roles that paraeducators play and the benefits that students receive (Giangreco, Edelman, Luiselli, & MacFarland, 1997; Shukla, Kennedy, & Cushing, 1999; Young, Simpson, Smith-Myles, & Kamps, 1997). For example, Young et al. (1997) examined the relationship between paraeducator proximity to three students with autism and the students' performance in general education classes. They observed students' behavior when the paraeducator was less than 2 feet away from the student, more than 2 feet away, and out of the room. They found no differences between the conditions on several student behaviors, including rates of on-task behavior, in-seat behavior, inappropriate vocalizations, and self-stimulatory behavior. However, they found that teacher-initiated interactions occurred most frequently when the paraeducators were more than 2 feet away from the student or out of the room. Furthermore, although students' on-task behavior was good, it was generally higher when they were working with peers rather than with the paraeducator.

Classroom-Based Interventions

The classroom-based strategies that have the most empirical support are peer-mediated instruction, collaborative learning, and professional teaming.

Peer-Mediated Instruction

Peer-mediated instruction includes a wide range of programs and approaches that allow students to serve as instructional agents for one another (Harper, Maheady, & Mallette, 1994). Research has clearly documented the effectiveness of peer-mediated instruction for students in general education classes (Carter et al., 2005; McDonnell, Thorson, Allen, & Mathot-Buckner, 2000; Moortweet et al., 1999; Weiner, 2005). For example, Moortweet et al. (1999) compared the effect of classwide peer tutoring and traditional teacher-led instruction on the spelling performance of four students with developmental disabilities and four peers without disabilities. In the peer-tutoring condition, all students in two different general education classes were paired for tutoring sessions. Each student alternated as a tutor and tutee for a 10-minute period. The researchers found that classwide peer tutoring resulted in superior spelling performance and higher levels of academic engagement than traditional teacher-led instruction for students with and without disabilities.

Cooperative Learning

Cooperative learning has been defined as "the instructional use of small groups so that students work together to maximize their own and each other's learning" (Johnson, Johnson, & Holubec, 1993, p. 6). Cooperative learning has been examined extensively as a way to improve the quality of instruction provided to students with developmental disabilities in general education classes (Dugan et al., 1995; Hunt, Staub, Alwell, &

Goetz, 1994; Jacques, Wilton, & Townsend, 1998). Dugan et al. (1995) compared the relative effectiveness of teacher-led lecture activities and cooperative learning with two fourth-grade students with autism and their typical peers. Cooperative learning was implemented four times per week. The students participated in a cooperative learning group that included three peers without disabilities. Group activities included peer tutoring on specific content targets and a team activity drawn from the social studies curriculum. This condition was contrasted with the instructional activities typically provided by the classroom teacher. The results showed that students with and without disabilities performed better on weekly tests, improved academic engagement, and increased social interactions with peers during cooperative learning than during teacher-led activities.

Professional Teaming

The complex educational needs of students with developmental disabilities require that professionals work together as a team to support these students' participation in general education classes. The importance of professional teaming to successful inclusive education has prompted a number of researchers to examine ways to formally support these activities within schools (Hunt, Soto, Maier, & Doering, 2003; Giangreco, Edelman, & Nelson, 1998). For example, Hunt et al. (2003) examined the effectiveness of the unified plan of support (UPS) in promoting collaboration between parents, special and general teachers, and instructional assistants to improve the participation of three students with significant disabilities and three students who were at risk in general education classes. The components of the UPS were (1) regularly scheduled team meetings, (2) collaborative development of student social and academic supports, (3) a specific accountability system, and (4) problem-solving procedures designed to directly address ineffective supports. The results showed that the teams were able to implement the UPS procedures with a high degree of fidelity with each of the students. Observational data indicated that all students demonstrated lower levels of nonengagement, higher rates of initiation of social interactions, and higher rates of reciprocal interactions with peers following the implementation of the UPS. Finally, team members reported that the UPS led to improved outcomes for all students and that it allowed effective and efficient use of the team members' knowledge and expertise.

Areas for Future Research

In spite of the progress made toward developing more effective classroom-based strategies, there a clear need for additional research on ways to improve the efficacy of instruction provided to students. One of the challenges that future research must address is how to "blend" the well-established technology of instruction for students with disabilities into the typical routines and structure of general education classes. Efforts to date in this area have focused on ways that paraeducators and peers can use this technology in general education classes. Additional research is needed to examine ways to promote general educators' adoption of these strategies and integration into their teaching practice for all students. There is also a need to examine additional strategies for increasing the access of students with developmental disabilities to the general education curriculum. Critical areas of need include approaches that allow general educators to differentiate instruction for all students in the class; the application of universal design principles to curriculum, instruction, and classroom organization; and the development of empirically and socially validated strategies for assessing students' progress in the general education curriculum.

Stakeholder Perspectives on Inclusive Education

Teachers, parents, students, and administrators are the critical stakeholders in the movement to create inclusive schools. Indeed, educators and parents led the advocacy efforts to provide inclusive services and have been a major force in shaping the research agenda. Ongoing consideration of their perspectives is essential to the success of systemic school reform efforts. Fortunately, a large body of descriptive research explores stakeholder perspectives through the use of small-sample, in-depth interviews, as well as large-sample interview and survey methods; however, this research presents a challenge to those who attempt to review it because of variability across studies in reports of teachers' and administrators' perceptions of inclusive education. This variability appears to be a function, for the most part, of the respondents' levels of experience in providing services to students with disabilities in general education settings, of perceptions of self-efficacy, and of the availability of resources to support heterogeneous classrooms. There is consensus across these studies, however, on the need for specific resources to support inclusive schooling, including (1) training and technical assistance, (2) administrative leadership and support, (3) collaborative partnerships, and (4) help in the classroom from members of multidisciplinary educational teams.

Training and Technical Assistance

General and special education teachers and administrators have identified comprehensive, district-organized in-service training, as well as site-specific training and technical assistance, as essential in influencing attitudes and enhancing the capacity of teachers to work effectively with a diverse population of students (e.g., Bennett, Deluca, & Bruns, 1997; Minke, Bear, Deemer, & Griffin, 1996; Villa, Thousand, Meyers, & Nevin, 1996; Werts, Wolery, Snyder, & Caldwell, 1996; York & Tundidor, 1995). Staff development and technical assistance that is undertaken as an "interdisciplinary team effort" (Sailor & Skrtic, 1995, p. 424) allows general and special educators to share their expertise and focus on common goals for all students in increasingly heterogeneous classrooms in which "disability" is just one factor.

Administrator Leadership and Support

Stakeholders identified administrator knowledge, leadership, and support of inclusive schooling practices as essential in developing each school's vision for inclusive education and in affecting teacher attitudes (e.g., Bennett et al., 1997; Villa et al., 1996). In addition, they recognized the importance of administrator commitment to funding and release time to support training and technical assistance activities and planning time to promote collaborative partnerships among general and special educators and parents. Finally, they emphasized the need for administrator leadership in the process of reallocating resources to consolidate general and special education services to more efficiently and effectively meet the needs of students in inclusive classrooms.

Collaborative Partnerships and Help in the Classroom

Teachers, administrators, and parents viewed general and special education collaborative teaming, increased parent communication and involvement, and the availability of time for collaboration as critical components of inclusive schooling (e.g., Bennett et al., 1997; Giangreco, Dennis, Cloninger, Edelman, & Schattman, 1993; Minke et al., 1996; Villa et al., 1996; Werts et al., 1996; York & Tundidor, 1995). They considered collaborative partnerships and the presence of other members of multidisciplinary educational teams in the classroom as essential in increasing the capacity of general education classrooms to accommodate a wide range of student skills and abilities.

IMPLICATIONS FOR EDUCATIONAL POLICY MAKERS AND FOR FUTURE RESEARCH

The growing body of research on inclusive education informs our understanding of best practices for supporting students with disabilities in inclusive settings, and several legislative landmarks have offered historic opportunities for the development of inclusive education; however, reform and research are needed in a number of areas before the ideals of inclusive education can be fully realized. These areas include (1) changing special education fiscal policies to implement coordinated services; (2) restructuring districts for an integrated and coordinated system of educational services; (3) establishing and evaluating schoolwide models of inclusive education; (4) building capacity through multidisciplinary professional development activities and teacher preparation programs, and (5) further developing and evaluating universal design and differentiated instructional methods to support all students.

Changing Fiscal Policies to Promote Inclusive Education

There are substantial challenges to the development of coordinated services between Title I, bilingual education, and IDEA. Some barriers were identified by McLaughlin and Verstegen (1998) and include (1) regulations governing fiscal accountability, (2) lack of understanding of what is, and what is not, required by the law, and (3) lack of a cohesive state and federal policy framework. In addition, state accounting systems often do not allow comingling of funds. Finally, and most important, there is no unified vision of a plan for services consolidation nor leadership in this area at the federal or state levels. Miles and Darling-Hammond (1998) suggested that "resources reallocation and the design of an instructional vision and strategy are intertwined" (p. 27). We would add that a commitment to consolidating services to more efficiently and effectively meet the needs of diverse populations of students must exist at all levels of education, from federal and state education policy and regulations to school district accounting systems to school site buy-in.

Restructuring Districts for an Integrated and Coordinated System of Educational Services

Although research on inclusive education has dramatically expanded in the past decade, there is a glaring need to develop and validate approaches to assist districts in restructuring their policies, procedures, and practices to support the expansion of inclusive education for all students (Ferguson et al., 2003; Furney, Hasazi, Clark/Keefe, & Hartnett, 2003; Sailor & Roger, 2005). It is unlikely that individual teachers or schools will be able to make and sustain the changes necessary to support inclusive education without district leadership and support (Hargreaves & Fullan, 1998). A number of areas require immediate attention, including the development of (1) strategies to help districts to identify the potential resources available to support reform and address the barriers to change; (2) approaches to comprehensive planning that promote the development of partnerships with parents, community leaders, institutions of higher education, and other social service agencies; (3) systems of professional development that reflect the realities faced by teachers and administrators; (4) structures for providing ongoing technical assistance to teachers and schools; and (5) comprehensive evaluation systems that ensure accountability and continuous improvement in student outcomes.

Establishing and Evaluating Schoolwide Models of Inclusive Education

Schoolwide models of inclusive school reform represent promising efforts to fully integrate special education and other categorical programs into a universal design that can enable all students to derive academic and social benefits from all available resources at the school site (Ferguson et al., 2003; Miles & Darling-Hammond, 1998; Sailor & Roger, 2005). Creative reallocation of resources, for example, from special education, Title I, and bilingual education—including innovative reorganizations of teachers into a variety of collaborative partnerships—offers the flexibility and additional resources needed to support all students in general education settings. Research is needed to evaluate the extent to which models of inclusive school reform contribute to increased academic progress and positive social participation of all students and increased satisfaction on the part of stakeholders with the overall educational process.

Building Capacity through Multidisciplinary Professional Development Activities and Teacher Preparation Programs

Sailor and Skrtic (1995) recommended a multidisciplinary approach to staff development that focuses on common goals for all students and provides the opportunity for general and special educators to share expertise, thus enabling "more fluid information and resource exchanges to occur across all disciplines, to the benefit of all children at the school site" (p. 424). General educators engaged in an effort to differentiate instruction to meet the needs of heterogeneous groups of students and to implement social supports for learners who present behavioral challenges can benefit from special educators' expertise in curricular adaptations and modifications, research-based literacy intervention, and the development and implementation of positive behavioral supports; and, in turn, general educators, with their knowledge of curricular frameworks, state and national learning standards, and research-based instructional methods have much to offer special educators as they support students in inclusive classrooms and facilitate their access to the general education curriculum.

Similarly, a multidisciplinary approach is needed in teacher preparation programs to "transform teacher education from university-based, categorical training to school-based, team-driven growth and development" (Sailor & Skrtic, 1995, p. 425). If we accept the premise that all teachers share responsibility for meeting the educational needs of all students in their schools, then the overlap between general and special education teacher preparation is clear (Sindelar, Pugach, Griffin, & Seidl, 1995), and the need for shared teacher preparation of course work and extensive fieldwork experiences in the context of inclusive schools is evident (Paul, Epanchin, Rosselli, Duchnowski, & Cranston-Gingras, 2002; Sindelar et al., 1995).

Further Development and Evaluation of a Universal Design for Learning

The continued expansion of inclusive educational services for students with developmental disabilities and the movement to create inclusive schools that unify general and special education resources to support all students will require further development and evaluation of a universal design for learning and differentiated instruction to accommodate the needs of all students in general education classrooms (Hunt & Goetz, 1997; McDonnell, 1998; Orkwis & McLane, 1998). These new approaches must not only be effective for all students, but they must also be acceptable to general and special educators and be practical within the resources typically available in schools. Future efficacy research on universal design and differentiated instruction must be structured so that they address each of these critical issues. Finally, this research must be translated into materials that are accessible and that support the efficient adoption and implementation of these strategies by professionals.

CONCLUDING REFLECTIONS

The empirical evidence that has accumulated over the past decade consistently shows that inclusive education has a number of educational and social benefits for students with developmental disabilities and their peers without disabilities. Further, our understanding of the practices that allow students with developmental disabilities to succeed in general education classes and the general education curriculum has increased dramatically. In spite of this progress, there is a clear need for additional research on improving the quality and effectiveness of the education they receive in these settings. However, it is equally clear that a significant expansion of inclusive education will require a much broader view of the challenges faced by teachers and administrators. Inclusive education represents a significant shift in the ways in which schools and school districts are structured. It requires changes not only in the way that curriculum and instruction are designed but also in the way that resources are allocated at multiple levels within the school system. The changes that are needed in policy and practice are so large and so complex that they defy a "special education" or "general education" solution. Indeed, we believe that the long-term success of inclusive education will require a sustained research and policy agenda that is focused on the eventual elimination of separate systems of education for students with and without disabilities and the development of a unified system that is designed to maximize outcomes for all students.

REFERENCES

Bennett, T., Deluca, D., & Bruns, D. (1997). Putting inclusion into practice: Perspectives of teachers and parents. *Exceptional Children, 64*(1), 115–131.

Browder, D. M., Spooner, F. Algozzine, R., Ahlgrim-Delzell, L., Flowers, C., & Karvonen, M. (2003). What we know and need to know about alternate assessment. *Exceptional Children, 70*(1), 45–61.

Carter, E. W., Cushing, L. S., Clark, N. M., & Kennedy, C. H. (2005). Effects of peer support interventions on students' access to the general curriculum and social interactions. *Research and Practice for Persons with Severe Disabilities, 30,* 15–25.

Cole, C. M., Waldron, N., & Majd, M. (2004). Academic progress of students across inclusive and traditional settings. *Mental Retardation, 42,* 136–144.

Curry, C. (2003). Universal design: Accessibility for all learners. *Educational Leadership, 61*(2), 55–60.

Cushing, L. S., & Kennedy, C. H. (1997). Academic effects of providing peer support in general education classrooms on students without disabilities. *Journal of Applied Behavior Analysis, 30,* 139–152.

Daniel, R. R. v. State Board of Education (874 F.2d 1036 [5th Cir. 1989]).

Dugan, E., Kamps, D., Leonard, B., Watkins, N., Rheinberger, A., & Stackhaus, J. (1995). Effects of cooperative learning groups during social studies for students with autism and fourth-grade peers. *Journal of Applied Behavior Analysis, 28,* 175–188.

Falvey, M. A., Blair, M., Dingle, M. P., & Franklin, N. (2000). Creating a community of learners with varying needs. In R. A. Villa & J. S. Thousand (Eds.), *Restructuring for caring and effective education* (2nd ed., pp. 186–207). Baltimore: Brookes.

Ferguson, D., Kozleski, E., & Smith, A. (2003). Transforming general and special education in urban schools. *Effective Education for Learners with Exceptionalities, 15,* 43–74.

Fisher, D., & Frey, N. (2001). Access to the core curriculum: Critical ingredients for student success. *Remedial and Special Education, 22,* 148–157.

Fisher, M., & Meyer, L. H. (2002). Development and social competence after two years for students enrolled in inclusive and self-contained educational programs. *Research and Practice for Persons with Severe Disabilities, 27,* 165–174.

Foreman, P., Arthur-Kelly, M., & Pascoe, S. (2004). Evaluating the educational experiences of students with profound and multiple disabilities in inclusion and segregated classroom settings: An Australian perspective. *Research and Practice for Persons with Severe Disabilities, 29,* 183–193.

Freeman, S. F. N. (2000). Academic and social attainments of children with mental retardation in general education and special education settings. *Remedial and Special Education, 21,* 3–17.

Fryxell, D., & Kennedy, C. H. (1995). Placement along the continuum of services and its impact on students' social relationships. *Journal of the Association for Persons with Severe Handicaps, 20,* 259–269.

Furney, K. S., Hasazi, S. B., Clark/Keefe, K., & Hartnett, J. (2003). A longitudinal analysis of shifting policy landscapes in special and general education reform. *Exceptional Children, 70,* 81–94.

Gartner, A., & Lipsky, D. K. (1987). Beyond special education: Toward a quality education system for all students. *Harvard Educational Review, 57,* 367–395.

Gersten, R., & Woodward, J. (1990). Rethinking the regular education initiative: Focus on the classroom teacher. *Remedial and Special Education, 11*(3), 7–16.

Giangreco, M. F., Dennis, R., Cloninger, C., Edelman, S., & Schattman, R. (1993). "I've counted Jon": Transformational experiences of teachers educating students with disabilities. *Exceptional Children, 59,* 359–372.

Giangreco, M. F., Edelman, S. W., Luiselli, T. E., & MacFarland, S. Z. C. (1997). Helping or hovering?: Effects of instructional assistance proximity on students with disabilities. *Exceptional Children, 64,* 7–18.

Giangreco, M. F., Edelman, S. W., & Nelson, C. (1998). Impact of planning for support services on students who are deaf–blind. *Journal of Visual Impairment and Blindness, 92,* 18–30.

Gibbs, J. (1994). *Tribes: A new way of learning together.* Santa Rosa, CA: Center Source.

Gilberts, G. H., Agran, M., Hughes, C., & Wehmeyer, M. (2001). The effects of peer-delivered self-monitoring strategies on the participation of students with severe disabilities in general education classrooms. *Journal of the Association for Persons with Severe Handicaps, 26,* 25–36.

Goetz, L., & O'Farrell, N. (1999). Connections: Facilitating social supports for students with deaf–blindness in general education classrooms. *Journal of Visual Impairment and Blindness, 11,* 704–716.

Halvorsen, A. T., & Neary, T. (2001). *Building inclusive schools: Tools and strategies for success.* Boston: Allyn & Bacon.

Hargreaves, A., & Fullan, M. (1998). *What's worth fighting for out there?* New York: Teachers College Press.

Harper, G. F., Maheady, L., & Mallette, B. (1994). The power of peer-mediated instruction: How and why it promotes academic success for all students. In J. S. Thousand, R. A. Villa, & A. I. Nevin (Eds.), *Creativity and collaborative learning: A practical guide to empowering students and teachers* (pp. 229–242). Baltimore: Brookes.

Hunt, P., Alwell, M., Farron-Davis, F., & Goetz, L. (1996). Creating socially supportive environments for fully included students who experience multiple disabilities. *Journal of the Association for Persons with Severe Handicaps, 21,* 53–71.

Hunt, P., Farron-Davis, F., Beckstead, S., Curtis, D., & Goetz, L. (1994). Evaluating the effects of placement of students with severe disabilities in regular education versus special classes. *Journal of the Association for Persons with Severe Handicaps, 19,* 200–214.

Hunt, P., & Goetz, L. (1997). Research on inclusive educational programs, practices, and outcomes for students with severe disabilities. *Journal of Special Education, 31,* 3–29.

Hunt, P., Hirose-Hatae, A., Goetz, L., Doering, K., & Karasoff, P. (2000). " 'Community' is what I think everyone is talking about." *Remedial and Special Education, 21*(5), 305–317.

Hunt, P., Soto, G., Maier, J., & Doering, K. (2003). Collaborative teaming to support students at risk and students with severe disabilities in general education classrooms. *Exceptional Children, 69*(3), 315–332.

Hunt, P., Staub, D., Alwell, M., & Goetz, L. (1994). Achievement by all students within the context of cooperative learning groups. *Journal of the Association for Persons with Severe Handicaps, 19,* 290–301.

Jacques, N., Wilton, K., & Townsend, M. (1998). Cooperative learning and social acceptance of children with mild intellectual disabilities. *Journal of Intellectual Disability Research, 42,* 29–36.

Janney, R. E., & Snell, M. E. (1997). How teachers include students with moderate and severe disabilities in elementary classes: The means and meaning of inclusion. *Journal of the Association for Persons with Severe Handicaps, 22,* 159–169.

Johnson, D. W., Johnson, R. T., & Holubec, E. J. (1993). *Circles of learning: Cooperation in the classroom* (4th ed.). Edina, MI: Interaction Book Company.

Johnson, J. W., McDonnell, J., Holzwarth, V., & Hunter, K. (2004). The efficacy of embedded instruction for students with developmental disabilities enrolled in general education classes. *Journal of Positive Behavior Interventions, 6,* 214–227.

Kauffman, J. M. (1989). The regular education initiative as Reagan–Bush education policy: A trickle-down theory of the hard-to-teach. *Journal of Special Education, 23,* 256–278.

Kleinert, H., Haig, J., Kearns, J. F., & Kennedy, S. (2000). Alternate assessments: Lessons learned and roads to be taken. *Exceptional Children, 67*(1), 51–66.

Kleinhammer-Tramill, P. J., & Gallagher, K. S. (2002). The implications of Goals 2000 for inclusive education. In W. Sailor (Ed.), *Whole-school success and inclusive education: Building partnerships for learning, achievement, and accountability* (pp. 26–41). New York: Columbia University, Teachers College Press.

Koegel, L. K., Harrower, J. K., & Koegel, R. L. (1999). Support for children with developmental disabilities in full inclusion classrooms through self-management. *Journal of Positive Behavioral Interventions, 1,* 26–34.

Kunc, N. (2000). Rediscovering the right to belong. In R. A. Villa & J. S. Thousand (Eds.), *Restructuring for caring and effective education* (2nd ed., pp. 77–92). Baltimore: Brookes.

Lambert, L. (1998). *Building leadership capacity in schools.* Alexandria, VA: Association for Supervision and Curriculum Development.

Lipsky, D. K., & Gartner, A. (1997). *Inclusion and school reform: Transforming America's classrooms.* Baltimore: Brookes.

Lipton, D. (1997). The "full inclusion" court cases: 1989–1994. In D. K. Lipsky & A. Gartner (Eds.), *Inclusion and school reform: Transforming America's classrooms* (pp. 299–314). Baltimore: Brookes.

Logan, K. R., & Keefe, E. B. (1997). A comparison of instructional context, teacher behavior, and engaged behavior for students with severe disabilities in general education and self-contained elementary classrooms. *Journal of the Association for Persons with Severe Handicaps, 22,* 16–27.

McDonnell, J. (1998). Instruction for students with severe disabilities in general education settings. *Education and Training in Mental Retardation and Developmental Disabilities, 33,* 199–215.

McDonnell, J., Johnson, J. W., Polychronis, S., & Riesen, T. (2002). The effects of embedded instruction on students with moderate disabilities enrolled in general education classes. *Education and Training in Mental Retardation and Developmental Disabilities, 37,* 363–377.

McDonnell, J., Thorson, N., Allen, C., & Mathot-Buckner, C. (2000). The effects of partner learning during spelling for students with severe disabilities and their peers. *Journal of Behavioral Education, 10,* 107–122.

McDonnell, J., Thorson, N., Disher, S., Mathot-Buckner, C., Mendel, J., & Ray, L. (2003). The achievement of students with developmental disabilities and their peers without disabilities in inclusive settings: An exploratory study. *Education and Treatment of Children, 26,* 224–236.

McDonnell, J., Thorson, N., McQuivey, C., & Kiefer-O'Donnell, R. (1997). The academic engaged time of students with low incidence disabilities in general education classes. *Mental Retardation, 35,* 18–26.

McGregor, G., & Vogelsberg, R. T. (1998). *Inclusive school practices: Pedagogical and research foundations.* Baltimore: Brookes.

McLaughlin, M. J., & Verstegen, D. (1998). Increasing regulatory flexibility of special education programs: Problems and promising strategies. *Exceptional Children, 64,* 371–384.

Meyer, L. H. (2001). The impact of inclusion on children's lives: Multiple outcomes, and friendships in particular. *International Journal of Disability, Development and Education, 48*(1), 9–31.

Meyer, L. H., Park, H. S., Grenot-Scheyer, M., Schwartz, I. S., & Harry, B. (1998). Participatory research approaches for the study of the social relationships of children and youth. In L. H. Meyer, H. S. Park, M. Grenot-Scheyer, I. S. Schwartz, & B. Harry (Eds.), *Making friends: The influences of culture and development* (pp. 3–30). Baltimore: Brookes.

Miles, K. H., & Darling-Hammond, L. (1998). Rethinking the allocation of teaching resources: Some lessons from high-performing schools. *Educational Evaluation and Policy Analysis, 20*(1), 9–29.

Minke, K. M., Bear, G. G., Deemer, S. A., & Griffin, S. M. (1996). Teachers' experiences with inclusive classrooms: Implications for special education reform. *Journal of Special Education, 30*(2), 152–186.

Moortweet, S. L., Utley, C. A., Walker, D., Dawson, H. L., Delquadri, J. C., Reddy, S. S., et al. (1999). Classwide peer tutoring: Teaching students with mild mental retardation in inclusive classrooms. *Exceptional Children, 65,* 524–536.

National Association of State Boards of Education Study Group on Special Education. (1992). *Winners all: A call for inclusive schools.* Alexandria, VA: Author.

Orkwis, R., & McLane, K. (1998). *A curriculum every student can use: Design principles for student access.* Reston, VA: Council for Exceptional Children.

Parrish, T. B. (2002). Fiscal policies in support of inclusive education. In W. Sailor (Ed.), *Whole-school success and inclusive education: Building partnerships for learning, achievement, and accountability* (pp. 213–227). New York: Columbia University, Teachers College Press.

Paul, J., Epanchin, B., Rosselli, H., Duchnowski, A., & Cranston-Gingras, A. (2002. Developing and nurturing a collaborative culture for change: Implications for higher education. In W. Sailor (Ed.), *Whole-school success and inclusive education: Building partnerships for learning, achievement, and accountability* (pp. 228–245). New York: Columbia University, Teachers College Press.

Peetsma, T., Vergeer, M., Roeleveld, J., & Karsten, S. (2001). Inclusion in education: Comparing pupils' development in special and regular education. *Educational Review, 53,* 125–135.

Reynolds, M. C., & Wang, M. C. (1983). Restructuring "special" school programs: A position paper. *Policy Studies Review, 2*(1), 189–202.

Ryndak, D. L., Morrison, A. P., & Sommerstein, L. (1999). Literacy before and after inclusion in general education settings: A case study. *Journal of the Association for Persons with Severe Handicaps, 24,* 5–22.

Sacramento City Unified School District v. Rachel Holland (14 F.3d 1398 [9th Cir. 1994]).

Sailor, W. (1991). Special education in the restructured school. *Remedial and Special Education, 12*(6), 8–22.

Sailor, W., Anderson, J., Halvorsen, A. T., Doering, K., Filler, J., & Goetz, L. (1989). *The comprehensive local school: Regular education for all students with disabilities.* Baltimore: Brookes.

Sailor, W., & Roger, B. (2005). Rethinking inclusion: Schoolwide applications. *Phi Delta Kappan, 86*(7), 503–509.

Sailor, W., & Skrtic, T. (1995). Modern and postmodern agendas in special education: Implications for teacher education, research, and policy development. In J. Paul, H. Roselli, & D. Evans (Eds.), *Integrating school restructuring and special education reform* (pp. 418–433). New York: Harcourt Brace.

Salisbury, C. L., Evans, I. M., Palombaro, M. M. (1997). Collaborative problem-solving to promote the inclusion of young children with significant disabilities in primary grades. *Exceptional Children, 63,* 195–209.

Sands, D., & Wehmeyer, M. (1996). *Self-determination across the life span: Independence and choice for people with disabilities.* Baltimore: Brookes.

Semmel, M. Y., & Gerber, M. M. (1990). If at first you don't succeed, bye, bye again: A response to general educators' views on the REI. *Remedial and Special Education, 11*(4), 53–59.

Sharpe, M., York, J. L., & Knight, J. (1994). Effects of inclusion on the academic performance of classmates without disabilities: A preliminary study. *Remedial and Special Education, 15,* 281–287.

Shukla, S., Kennedy, C. H., & Cushing, L. S. (1999). Intermediate school students with severe disabilities: Supporting their social participation in general education classrooms. *Journal of Positive Behavior Interventions, 1,* 130–140.

Sindelar, P., Pugach, M., Griffin, C., & Seidl, B. (1995). Reforming teacher education: Challenging the philosophy and practices of educating regular and special educators. In J. Paul, H. Roselli, & D. Evans (Eds.), *Integrating school restructuring and special education reform* (pp. 140–166). New York: Harcourt Brace.

Skrtic, T. (1991). The special education paradox: Equity as a way to excellence. *Harvard Educational Review, 61*(2), 148–206.

Snell, M. E., & Janney, R. E. (2005). *Practices for inclusive schools: Collaborative teaming* (2nd ed.). Baltimore: Brookes.

Stainback, W., & Stainback, S. (1984). A rationale for the merger of regular and special education. *Exceptional Children, 51,* 102–112.

Stainback, W., & Stainback, S. (Eds.). (1990). *Support networks for inclusive schooling: Interdependent integrated education.* Baltimore: Brookes.

Staub, D., Peck, C. A., Gallucci, C., & Schwartz, I. (2000). Peer relationships. In M. E. Snell & F. Brown (Eds.), *Instruction of students with severe disabilities* (5th ed., pp. 381–408). Upper Saddle River, NJ: Prentice-Hall.

Tomlinson, C. A. (1999). *The differentiated classroom: Responding to the needs of all learners.* Alexandria, VA: Association for Supervision and Curriculum Development.

Udvari-Solner, A., & Thousand, J. (1995). Promising practices that foster inclusive education. In R. Villa & J. Thousand (Eds.), *Creating an inclusive school* (pp. 87–109). Alexandria, VA: Association for Supervision and Curriculum Development.

U.S. Department of Education. (2002). *To assure the free appropriate education of all children with disabilities: Twenty-fourth Annual Report to Congress on the Implementation of the Individuals with Disabilities Education Act.* Washington, DC: Author.

Villa, R. A., & Thousand, J. S. (2000). *Restructuring for caring and effective education: Piecing the puzzle together.* Baltimore: Brookes.

Villa, R. A., Thousand, J. S., Meyers, H., & Nevin, A. (1996). Teacher and administrator perceptions of heterogeneous education. *Exceptional Children, 63,* 29–45.

Wang, M. C., & Birch, J. W. (1984). Comparison of a full-time mainstreaming program and a resource room approach. *Exceptional Children, 51,* 33–40.

Wehmeyer, M. L., Yeager, D., Bolding, N., Agran, M., & Hughes, C. (2003). The effects of self-regulation strategies on goal attainment for students with developmental disabilities in general education classes. *Journal of Developmental and Physical Disabilities, 15,* 79–91.

Weiner, J. S. (2005). Peer-mediated conversational repair in students with moderate and severe disabilities. *Research and Practice for Persons with Severe Disabilities, 30,* 26–31.

Werts, M. G., Wolery, M., Snyder, R. D., & Caldwell, N. K. (1996). Teachers' perceptions of the supports critical to the success of inclusion programs. *Journal of the Association for Persons with Severe Handicaps, 21*(1), 9–21.

Wiederholt, L. J. (Ed.). (1988, January). The regular education initiative [Special issue]. *Journal of Learning Disabilities, 21*(1).

Will, M. (1985, December). *Educating children with learning problems: A shared responsibility.* Paper presented at the Wingspread Conference on the Education of Special Needs Students: Research Findings and Implications for Practice, Racine, WI.

Will, M. (1986a). Educating children with learning problems: A shared responsibility. *Exceptional Children, 52,* 411–416.

Will, M. (1986b). *Educating students with learning problems: A shared responsibility.* Washington, DC: U.S. Department of Education, Office of Special Education and Rehabilitative Services.

Wolery, M., Anthony, L., Snyder, E. D., Werts, M. G., & Katzenmeyer, J. (1997). Training elementary teachers to embed instruction during classroom activities. *Education and Treatment of Children, 20,* 40–58.

York, J., & Tundidor, M. (1995). Issues raised in the name of inclusion: Perspectives of educators, parents, and students. *Journal of the Association for Persons with Severe Handicaps, 20*(1), 31–44.

Young, B., Simpson, R. L., Smith-Myles, B., & Kamps, D. M. (1997). An examination of paraprofessional involvement in supporting inclusion of students with autism. *Focus on Autism and Other Developmental Disabilities, 12,* 31–40.

14

Academic Skills
Reading and Mathematics

Diane M. Browder
Katherine Trela
Susan L. Gibbs
Shawnee Wakeman
Amber A. Harris

As part of the school reform movement of the past two decades, educators have set ambitious expectations for all learners to make academic gains. Professional organizations such as the National Council of Teachers of Mathematics (*www.nctm.org*) and National Council of Teachers of English (*www.ncte.org*) proposed national standards for student achievement. States also defined standards that were tied to assessments of student achievement. At first the reform movement seemed silent on students with disabilities, who initially had been exempted from state assessments and expectations of achievement. With the passage of the Individuals with Disabilities Education Act (IDEA) amendments of 1997, states were required to include all students in state and district assessments, utilizing alternate assessments as needed for students unable to participate with accommodations. IDEA 1997 also required that students have access to the general curriculum. As states began to develop alternate assessments, there was some confusion about what standards to assess—academic content standards or functional skills. In 2001, the reauthorized Elementary and Secondary Education Act of 1965 and the No Child Left Behind Act (NCLB; 2001) required states to establish challenging standards, to implement assessments that measured students' performance against those standards, and to hold schools accountable for achievement in reading, math, and science. Final NCLB regulations on including students with the most significant cognitive disabilities permitted states to develop alternate achievement standards for reporting adequate yearly progress for students with significant cognitive disabilities (up to 1% of the general population) but further stipulated that these alternate achievement standards must be aligned with a state's academic content standards, must promote access to the general curriculum, and must reflect the highest achievement standards possible (200.1[d], U.S. Department of Education, 2003). Subsequent non-regulatory guidance noted that alternate assessments "should be clearly related to grade-level content, although it may be restricted in scope or complexity or take the form of introductory or prerequisite skills" (U.S. Department of Education, 2005a, p. 26). In subsequent proposed rules (U.S. Department of Education, 2005b), the Department of Education provided additional flexibility for states to use modified achievement standards but still required that all students receive instruction in the grade-level curriculum being assessed. These regulations have clarified that schools are expected to show achievement by students with significant cognitive disabilities in academic content. Table 14.1 summarizes the options that teams implementing individualized education plans (IEPs) have in considering how students will access the general curriculum.

The expectation that educators will find ways to teach all students and assess them on their state's academic content is having a critical impact on thinking about curricula for students with developmental disabilities. As shown in Table 14.1, all students must receive instruction and assessment on academic content that is linked to the grade-level standards. Browder et al. (2004) describe this historical shift to focusing on academics in curriculum planning for students with developmental disabilities who in the past were given primarily functional skills instruction. Sometimes professionals have distinguished between students who might receive some remedial or early academic instruction (e.g., K–2 academics) and those who would focus only on life skills. In fact, students with developmental disabilities were historically classified by their ability or lack of ability to learn academics (e.g., "educable" vs. "trainable"). Such classifications are no longer consistent with the concept of all students having access to the general curriculum.

TABLE 14.1. Options for IEP Teams to Consider in How Students Show Achievement

What is taught	How it is assessed	Achievement expectation	Who might qualify (state sets eligibility)
Grade-level content	• General assessment • May be with accommodations • Alternate assessment at grade level	• Grade level	• Students with DD who can keep pace with grade level • Not all states use alternate assessment on grade level
Grade-level content	• Alternate assessment or general assessment with modifications	• Modified achievement	• Students with DD who need more time to meet grade-level expectations (2% cap) • Not all states use alternate assessment with modified achievement standards
Academic content linked to grade level	• Alternate assessment	• Alternate achievement	• Students with significant cognitive disabilities (1% cap)
No academic content (not an option)			• No students can be exempted from assessments of state academic standards

However, educators do continue to assume that there should be differential expecta-tions for academic outcomes, as shown in Table 14.1 (e.g., grade level, modified, or alternate achievement). The shift in thinking holds that all students should acquire some skills that link to the academic content of their assigned grades (based on age); some will achieve more of the depth and breadth of the grade-level content, whereas others will focus on more prioritized and adapted content. Many students with develop-mental disabilities will also need supplementary instruction in functional skills or reme-dial academics.

The impact of giving all students the opportunity to learn academics is currently unknown because it has not been fully tried. For example, reading instruction for stu-dents with significant cognitive disabilities has been underemphasized. Qualitative research, including content analyses of textbooks (Katims, 2000b) and ethnographic studies of children's school experiences (Kliewer, 1998), reveals a consistent lack of focus on reading. Comprehensive reviews of the literature in reading (Browder, Wakeman, Spooner, Ahlgrim-Delzell, & Algozzine, 2006), mathematics (Browder, Spooner, Ahlgrim-Delzell, Harris, & Wakeman, in press), and science (Courtade-Little, Spooner, & Browder, in press) for students with significant cognitive disabilities shows that researchers have not addressed most components of academic content in these areas. Similarly, research on students with mild developmental disabilities shows a restricted focus in both reading (Joseph & Seery, 2004) and math (Kroesbergen, 2003.) This research has also examined students' instructional levels in the content areas (e.g., a seventh-grade student acquiring beginning reading skills). How to teach students skills that align with grade-level content so that they demonstrate modified achievement on state assessments is not yet well understood.

The purpose of this chapter is to provide summaries of current research in aca-demic instruction of students with developmental disabilities that can inform practice. Rarely do resources combine research on students with mild versus those with moder-ate to severe developmental disabilities. This chapter does so to address the broad needs of this heterogeneous population while trying to be clear about these two distinct literatures. Because most of the existing research literature on academics for this popu-lation is in reading and mathematics, we limit our focus to these two content areas.

TEACHING STUDENTS WITH DEVELOPMENTAL DISABILITIES TO READ

What We Know about Teaching All Students to Read

Since 1988 researchers have continued to replicate findings that students who do not learn to read by the end of first grade are apt to continue to have poor reading skills, creating a gap that increases as they progress through school (e.g., Juel, 1988; Good, Simmons, & Kame'enui, 2001). Reading disabilities in America's public schools are per-vasive, with 20–25% of the students experiencing reading failure (Stein, Johnson, & Gutlohn, 1999). In 1997, Congress asked the National Institute of Child Health and Human Development (NICHD) to convene a national panel to assess the status of research-based knowledge, including the effectiveness of different approaches for teach-ing students to read (National Reading Panel [NRP], 2000).The NRP report established consensus on the following foundational skills as critical components of beginning reading instruction: (1) phonemic awareness, (2) alphabetic understanding, (3) vocabu-lary, (4) comprehension, and (5) accuracy and fluency with connected text (NRP, 2000). Researchers recently recommended a three-tiered instructional model for K–3 students that includes (1) an effective core instructional program, (2) supplemental interventions designed to accommodate the needs of students who are not responsive to core-level instruction, and (3) intensive or tertiary-level interventions reserved for students who are not responding to core and/or supplemental instruction (e.g., Coyne, Kame'enui, & Simmons, 2001; Dion, Morgan, Fuchs, & Fuchs, 2004).

Experimental studies indicate that most students who are poor readers in the early grades become better readers when provided with explicit instruction in phonological awareness and systematic, explicit phonics instruction (e.g., Good, et al., 2001; O'Connor, Jenkins, Leicester, & Slocum, 1993; Snow, Burns, & Griffin, 1998). *Phonological* awareness is the ability to identify and manipulate parts of spoken language. *Phonemic* awareness is a subcategory of phonological awareness focused on the identification and manipulation of phonemes (i.e., sounds) in words. Systematic, explicit phonics instruction teaches students the most common sounds represented by letters and letter combinations, along with a strategy for sounding out words (Carnine, Silbert, Kame'enui, & Tarver, 2004). Characteristics of students who do not respond to effective phonological awareness and decoding instruction in the early grades have become of recent interest to reading researchers. Al Otaiba and Fuchs (2002) reviewed 23 studies and found the following characteristics to be associated with unresponsiveness to treatment: (1) phonological awareness, (2) phonological memory, (3) rapid naming, (4) intelligence, (5) attention, (6) orthographic processing, and (7) demographics. What is especially noteworthy for students with developmental disabilities is that the significance of intelligence was less clear, with 22% of the researchers reporting some correlation, whereas 30% of the researchers reported no correlation. What may be especially important for students with developmental disabilities is explicit instruction in phonological awareness.

Students with developmental disabilities were not included in the studies identified by the NRB for the meta-analysis that resulted in the NCLB legislation. Within the 38 studies in the meta-analysis, 12 included participants who were identified as at risk, 6 included participants who were identified as low achievers, and 10 included participants who were identified as reading disabled. Although students identified as having mild or moderate cognitive disabilities were not participants in the studies used for the meta-analysis, the information gleaned from this research clearly provides information on best practices for teaching reading. When scientifically based reading research identifies best practices for reading instruction, all children should receive such instruction with appropriate modifications when needed.

Enhancing Reading Success for Students with Mild Developmental Disabilities

Little research has been completed with readers who have mild cognitive disabilities (Conners, Atwell, Rosenquist, & Sligh, 2001). A recent comprehensive review of reading research for students with developmental disabilities (i.e., having IQs from 27 to 76) found only seven studies conducted in the past 10 years (Joseph & Seery, 2004), none of which examined the effect of direct, explicit phonics instruction. Most of the work focused on demonstrating a small subset of phonics skills rather than mastery of decoding. Conners et al. (2001) examined cognitive similarities and differences between participants with intellectual disabilities (i.e., IQs < 70, defined as mental retardation) who had either strong or weak decoding skills (*N* = 65). Analyses indicated that participants with strong decoding skills had significantly better skills in phonemic awareness and in language. The study also determined that when students have substantially limited intelligence, their ability to rehearse phonological codes in working memory has a powerful effect on success in learning to read. The Conners et al. (2001) study supports the suggestion of other researchers (e.g., Siegel, 1992; Stanovich & Siegel, 1994) that a parallel exists between students with and without developmental disabilities who are struggling to learn to read. The underlying problem for both groups lies in phonemic awareness. Juel, Griffith, and Gough's (1986) longitudinal study provides solid evidence that phonemic awareness instruction is more effective than alternative forms of instruction. One of the biggest shifts that needs to occur for students with mild developmental disabilities is to provide early and intensive instruction in phonemic awareness and in systematic, explicit phonics.

In addition to decoding, the NRP (2000) notes the need for instruction in fluency, comprehension, and vocabulary. As might be expected, research on comprehension with this population has usually been limited to some application of sight words, such as matching the word to a picture (Gast, Doyle, Wolery, Ault, & Baklarz, 1991) or reading the word in a functional activity (Schloss et al., 1995). In contrast, comprehension strategies found to be effective for students without disabilities or with learning disabilities include teaching students to monitor their understanding of material (Baumann, Jones, & Seifert-Kessell, 1993), cooperative learning in which students learn strategies together (Vaughn & Klingner, 1999), the use of graphic organizers to assist comprehension (Griffin, Malone, & Kame'enui, 1995), and learning to generate and answer questions with feedback (Ezell & Kohler, 1992). Research is called for that utilizes these additional comprehension strategies for students with developmental disabilities.

Enhancing Reading Success for Students with Moderate and Severe Disabilities

Although the mismatch between research on effective reading instruction and the ways educators have taught students with mild developmental disabilities to read is evident, the contrast is stark indeed for students with moderate and severe disabilities. Browder et al. (2006) conducted a meta-analysis to determine the degree to which students with significant cognitive disabilities have been taught the skills within the NRP reading components. Of the 128 studies identified to have a purpose of teaching at least one component of reading, nearly all ($n = 117$) of those studies addressed word or picture vocabulary. Only a few addressed comprehension ($n = 23$) through having a student use a sight word in the context of a functional activity or task (e.g., Browder & Minarovic, 2000; Mechling & Gast, 2003). In others, individuals demonstrated comprehension through word-to-picture matching (e.g., Driscoll & Kemp, 1996; Rehfeldt, Latimore, & Stromer, 2003). Rarely have researchers tried to teach phonics to this population, but the few studies that exist show strong effect sizes (Barbetta, Heward, & Bradley, 1993; Barudin & Hourcade, 1990; Lane & Critchfield, 1998).

Although fluency has traditionally been viewed as reading orally with speed, accuracy, and expression (NRP, 2000), the study of fluency with students with severe disabilities has been limited to accuracy (Singh & Singh, 1984, 1985, 1988). Singh, Winton, and Singh (1985) studied the effects on students with moderate mental disabilities of delayed and immediate response to errors when reading a passage. Both delayed and immediate teacher attention reduced oral reading errors, but researchers noted that delayed response also increased self-corrections. Singh and Singh (1988) studied the effects of three different response conditions on oral reading errors for students with moderate mental disabilities. Overcorrection and phonic analysis training were effective in reducing oral reading errors, with phonic analysis being more effective with extended training. Other studies have computed errors not in passage reading but in sight-word acquisition (e.g., Farmer, Gast, Wolery, & Winterling, 1991; McGee & McCoy, 1981).

Because words have been the major focus of much of the reading research on students with significant disabilities, clear guidelines can be identified for effective instruction in this component of reading. The strongest evidence for this population shows that systematic prompting and fading, with many opportunities for the student to practice the response, has been effective for teaching sight words. In a meta-analysis of sight-word instruction, Browder and Xin (1998) found that sight-word instruction had been highly effective overall. In a review of the single-subject studies to determine the effect of the reading interventions, Browder et al. (2006) found that of the 57 studies that addressed sight-word or picture vocabulary, 56 met the high evidence-based quality criteria of Horner et al. (2005).

Reading Curricula

Both Reading Mastery (Englemann & Bruner, 1995) and the Edmark Reading Program (2002) have been popular programs for teaching reading to students with developmental disabilities. The Edmark Reading Program addresses prereading, word recognition, direction cards, picture–phrase cards, and storybooks and provides intrinsic motivation through small increments. It is a sight-word program that takes about 5 minutes of one-to-one instruction per day. Students with developmental disabilities have made gains with Edmark Reading, which uses a stimulus-shaping approach to sight-word acquisition (Vandever, Maggart, & Nasser, 1976; Vandever & Stubbs, 1977). However, this program does not contain the instruction in phonemic awareness or phonics that is needed to become literate.

Reading Mastery (formerly DISTAR), a direct-instruction reading program for students in grades K–3, teaches phonemic awareness and systematic, explicit phonics and has been successfully implemented with students with developmental disabilities (Bracey, Maggs, & Morath, 1975; Gersten & Maggs, 1982). Direct instruction is a systematic teaching approach that emphasizes carefully sequenced instruction, ongoing assessment for student understanding, and systematic prompts to ensure student engagement and participation. It is supported by a large body of scientific research (e.g., Carnine, Carnine, & Gersten, 1984; Cunningham, 1990; Lie, 1991; Wagner & Torgeson, 1987). Essential skills addressed in Reading Mastery and other direct-instruction reading programs are (1) explicit instruction in phonemic awareness, (2) systematic and explicit introduction of letter–sound correspondences, (3) instruction in blending sounds into words, (4) the use of code-based text to provide sufficient practice in sounding out words, and (5) the provision of immediate feedback on oral reading errors. Additional components of direct-instruction reading programs are the use of scripted text for teachers, signals to generate choral responses from students, and continuous monitoring of student performance.

Consistent with the NRP recommendations, curricula such as Reading Mastery should be supplemented with instruction for developing vocabulary and comprehension using literature. Students with more severe developmental disabilities may also need instruction in emergent literacy. Researchers recommend that curricular materials for emergent literacy programs for prekindergarten and kindergarten have the following components: (1) phonemic awareness, (2) alphabetic or print awareness, (3) oral language, and (4) emergent writing (Whitehurst & Lonigan, 2001). Emergent literacy curricula are available for 4- and 5-year-old children (i.e., Opening the World of Learning; Schickedanz, Dickinson, & Charlotte-Mecklenburg Schools, 2005) but have not yet been developed for older students who need to develop these skills.

As students age, it will also be important to adapt the literature of their grade level for age-appropriate instruction and linkage with state standards. Table 14.2 provides an example of how a middle school literature unit on a novel can be adapted for students who have lower levels of literacy. Some case studies provide evidence that even students with more severe disabilities benefit from instruction in broader literacy skills. For example, Koppenhaver, Erickson, and Skotko (2001) found that storybook reading promoted communication in children with Rett syndrome. Through a series of qualitative studies, Kliewer and Biklen (2001) found that the printed-language skills of students with severe disabilities proceeded from their social engagement with peers to expressing their own ideas to composing a story.

TEACHING WRITING TO STUDENTS WITH DEVELOPMENTAL DISABILITIES

The Writing Study Group of the National Council of Teachers of English (NCTE) Executive Committee have advocated that "everyone has the capacity to write, writing can be taught, and teachers can help students become better writers" (NCTE, 2004, principle 1). Changes in technologies that support student access to written-work production have inspired NCTE's belief that "composing occurs in different modalities and technologies" (NCTE, 2004, principle 10). When writing is viewed as composing printed communication rather than handwritten passages, more options exist for teaching writing to students with developmental disabilities.

Research in teaching writing to students with disabilities has typically focused on students with high-incidence (e.g., learning disabilities or mild mental retardation) disabilities and on the demands of grade-appropriate literacy instruction and mandatory high-stakes writing assessments (Deshler, Schumaker, & Bui, 2003). One approach to meeting these writing demands for students with mild disabilities is the writer's workshop. In this model, students follow writing as a process approach by which they organize their ideas, write a first draft, confer with peers and teacher for any revisions, and publish their work. Researchers using the writer's workshop model have shown that students with mild disabilities can improve their writing of main ideas and their organization and adherence to writing conventions (Adams et al., 1996).

Although the writer's workshop enhances students' ability to organize and edit their writing, research has shown that adding more explicit instruction, such as self-regulated strategy development (SRSD) or use of graphic organizers, lends the support often needed by students with disabilities (Graham & Harris, 1994). Using SRSD, students learn a strategy for planning, organizing, producing, and revising written work, often through the use of a mnemonic (i.e., POW: **P**lan, **O**rganize, **W**rite; Harris, Graham & Mason, 2003). For motivation, students develop self-statements such as "I can do this if I use my strategy and take my time" to further support their progress through the writing process (Harris & Graham, 1996). Extensive research on the effect of SRSD on students' writing performance has shown that students with learning disabilities increased the length of time they spent planning their essays, the overall length and quality of their essays, and their knowledge and motivation for writing (Graham, Har-

TABLE 14.2. An Example of Adapting Grade-Level Literature for Students with Developmental Disabilities (*The Cay* by Theodore Taylor)

	Strategies and skills given for students on grade level	Application for middle school students with mild/moderate DD reading below grade level (e.g., 2nd-grade level)	Application for middle school students with severe DD at emergent-literacy level (nonreaders)
Middle school (grades 6–8) language arts	Students read chapters of book on grade level.	Students hear chapters read and independently read summaries in printed or digital text format supported by pictures and controlled vocabulary.	Students hear chapter summaries read and participate using pictures, repeated story lines, and controlled vocabulary.
Grade-level standard 1: Distinguish cause from effect	Students make diagram (i.e., fishbone) of story events describing cause and effect with evidence.	Students discuss and diagram a familiar event for cause and effect using fishbone diagram (e.g., release string/balloon floats away). Students choose statements from chapter summary to fill in fishbone diagram.	Teacher demonstrates cause and effect using boat with hole and water (e.g., paper-cup boats); each student makes hole and sees boat sink. Students diagram what happened using pictures or objects. Students select pictures for fishbone diagram after hearing story.
Grade-level standard 2: Distinguish fact from opinion or fiction	Students identify facts and opinions related to the characters (e.g., prejudices vs. physical attributes) and track character changes in opinion throughout the book.	Students sort statements made by characters in the book (written in adapted text) into facts and opinions.	Students refer to pictures and indicate "yes" or "no" about themselves ("Anne has brown hair"). Students use pictures to answer simple yes/no questions about characters in the story (e.g., Was Phillip a boy?)
Grade-level standard 3: Make judgments about setting, characters, and events and support them with evidence from the text	Students write a narrative comparing Phillip's quality of life before and after the boat accident using evidence from the text.	Students sort pictures and phrases into sets to describe Phillip's life before and after the accident and then write a sentence about each picture.	Students compare events from their own lives to events in Phillip's life in the story using a yes/no chart and a Venn diagram.

ris, & Mason, 2005). Konrad, Trela, and Test (2006) applied this strategy and found that students using an SRSD instructional unit increased the quality and content of paragraphs written about their IEP goals.

Graphic organizers are another tool used to support students with disabilities in planning their writing (Boyle, 1996). By definition, a graphic organizer is a visual aid that connects ideas or key vocabulary to diagrams. James, Abbot, and Greenwood (2001) reported using a graphic organizer embedded in a writer's workshop approach in a schoolwide writing instructional model. By the end of the school year, postwriting test scores were similar for high- and low-achieving groups, even though prewriting scores were lower for the low-achieving group.

Writing instruction for students with significant disabilities typically has been embedded in either a functional or a traditional curriculum approach (Katims, 2000a). Opportunities for students following this curriculum to develop writing skills often have been limited to direct applications, such as making a shopping list or filling out a personal identification form. In contrast, an emergent literacy orientation can be followed in which the skills typically developed by younger children can continue to be developed in meaningful ways into adolescence and young adulthood (Katims, 2000a). For example case studies have suggested that students with significant disabilities can use assistive technology to participate in a variety of writing activities to access information, produce work, and socialize with peers (Erikson & Koppenhaver, 1997; Weikle & Hadadian, 2003).

In general, assistive technology can be a critical form of support to help students with developmental disabilities to succeed in writing, because it can reduce the demands of spelling and handwriting (e.g., Co:Writer by Don Johnston Co., 2005; Clicker 4 by Crick Software, 2005). In addition, programs can convert written text to auditory text (e.g., WYNN software by Freedom Scientific Technologies, 2006), supplement text with pictures (e.g., Writing with Symbols software by Mayer-Johnson, 2000), allow students to add text to digital graphic organizers (Inspiration by Inspiration Software, Inc., 2005), and be used to adapt literature with considerable text and auditory feedback (e.g., Start-to-Finish Books by Don Johnston Co., 2005).

TEACHING MATH TO STUDENTS WITH DEVELOPMENTAL DISABILITIES

Instructional practices in mathematics for students with developmental disabilities have often focused on teaching math within functional curricula (e.g., Aeschleman & Schladenauffen, 1984; Haring, Kennedy, Adams, & Pitts-Conway, 1987) or through the use of assistive devices (jigs, calculators) that minimize the need for mathematical understanding (e.g., Frederick-Dugan, Test, & Varn, 1991; Lancioni, Singh, O'Reilly, & Oliva, 2003). Instead of addressing challenging standards that can lead to competence in numeracy, educators have typically focused on less rigorous skills, such as embedding mathematics into the practice of daily living skills (Maccini & Gagnon, 2000). In 1989 the National Council of Teachers of Mathematics (NCTM) developed a comprehensive set of standards based on math goals that address the achievement of all students and include five content standards of mathematics instruction. These content standards are (1) number and operations, (2) measurement, (3) data analysis and probability, (4) geometry, and (5) algebra. To gain skills in numeracy, students with developmental disabilities will need competence in each of these areas.

Teaching Math to Students with Mild Developmental Disabilities

A comprehensive review of 58 studies focusing on mathematics interventions for elementary-age students with developmental disabilities found that the majority of studies focused on basic number and operation skills (Kroesbergen, 2003). These studies suggested that direct instruction and self-instruction were found to be more effective than mediated instruction. Direct instruction was considered to be the most effective intervention for increasing basic math skills, whereas self-instruction was more effective in enhancing problem-solving skills. This review of literature also revealed that direct teacher-led instruction was more effective in teaching numeracy and/or computation skills than peer or computer-assisted learning techniques.

To help students make the transition from one-to-one correspondence to basic computational skills such as addition or subtraction, teachers often introduce a number line. Students count forward or backward to compute sums. A commercial program that builds on the idea of counting to compute is Touch Math (Bullock, Pierce, & McClelland, 1989; Innovative Learning Concepts, *www.touchmath.com*), a multisensory curriculum approach that integrates numbers with corresponding "touch points." Some research suggests that the Touch Math curriculum reinforces mathematics skills using three modalities: visual, auditory, and kinesthetic (Scott, 1993; Simon & Hanrahan, 2004). Scott (1993) found that once students were able to gain retention of math facts, they gave quicker and more accurate responses. Simon and Hanrahan (2004) found that children felt that they could use Touch Math discreetly to solve problems without the embarrassment of counting their fingers or manipulatives in front of their peers.

Current research surrounding abstract problem solving (e.g., word problems, algebra, or geometry) has indicated that students with mild developmental disabilities particularly benefit from highly structured teacher-based instruction (Butler, Miller, Lee, & Pierce, 2001; Kroesbergen, 2003). Methods such as these may include direct or explicit instruction (i.e., modeling) or concrete to representational to abstract sequencing (i.e., manipulatives; Witzel, Mercer, & Miller, 2003). Each of these methods not only provides students with explicit instruction but also allows immediate feedback, along with ample opportunities for drill and practice.

Other empirically validated practices found to be effective for teaching higher order math skills include self-regulated instruction (i.e., mnemonics, structured work sheets, or graphic organizers) and computer-assisted instruction (Bottge, 1999; Scruggs & Mastropieri, 1997; Miller, Butler, & Lee, 1998). Interestingly, students with mild mental retardation may be more responsive than students with learning disabilities to abstract problem-solving interventions (Kroesbergen, 2003; Jitendra & Xin, 1997). One potential explanation that Kroesbergen (2003) offers for this difference is that problem-solving instruction may be new to students with developmental disabilities but associated with prior failure for students with learning disabilities.

Teaching Math to Students with Moderate and Severe Disabilities

In their comprehensive review of methods of teaching mathematics to students with moderate and severe disabilities, Browder et al. (2006) found that most of the existing studies focused on teaching money-management skills. Some addressed number recognition and computation. By including the self-monitoring literature, the researchers also identified studies on teaching data analysis and graphing. There were no studies on algebra and only two on geometry. Research is critically needed in this area, as higher order mathematics skills may be included in expectations for achievement on state alternate assessments.

In their review of research on teaching money skills to students with mental retardation, Browder and Grasso (1999) found 43 studies from 1975 through 1997 that examined one or more of the five aspects of money management: computation, banking, budgeting, purchasing, and saving. A number of studies minimized the need for teacher instruction and the required student mathematical competence by using adaptations such as a calculator to budget purchases, an adapted number line to compare prices, and coin-matching cards to select coins for a vending machine (Sandknop, Schuster, Wolery, & Cross, 1992; Browder, Snell, & Wildonger, 1988). Other studies reduced the academic demands of counting mixed money amounts by using a whole dollar or "next dollar" strategy (Denny & Test, 1995; McDonnell, 1987). Applications of these skills to community settings was taught through the use of videotape and slide presentations depicting purchasing simulations (Haring et al., 1987; Van den Pol et al., 1981). In a review of literature on teaching grocery shopping skills to students with moderate to profound intellectual disabilities, Morse and Schuster (1996) noted a number of successful strategies to incorporate into teaching programs, such as the "next dollar" strategy, social skills training, and locating items from a list in the store. Besides shopping, students may also learn money skills in the context of banking. McDonnell and Ferguson (1989) taught students how to use automatic teller machines and to cash checks. Shafer, Inge, and Hill (1986) used simulated bank machines to teach their use and then generalized the skill to community settings.

Although they are not numerous, some studies have been done with students with moderate and severe disabilities that focused on teaching such skills as computation (Matson & Long, 1986), graphing (Ackerman & Shapiro, 1984), and matching shapes (Mackay, Soraci, Carlin, Dennis, & Strawbridge, 2002). Current federal policy requires that alternate assessments be linked to grade-level content (U.S. Department of Education, 2005). The challenge is finding ways to creatively apply math components in geometry and algebra that are both feasible and meaningful for these students. One option is to identify existing functional activities in which these mathematical concepts are relevant (e.g., using the rectangular place mats rather than the round ones). Other options involve creating opportunities to make mathematical content relevant (e.g., data analysis becomes meaningful when students use graphs to self-monitor their behavior).

IMPLICATIONS OF CURRENT RESEARCH ON TEACHING ACADEMICS

Implications for Future Research

Overall, the research on teaching academics to students with developmental disabilities shows that students have acquired specific target skills through direct and systematic instruction. The scope of this research falls short of the breadth of standards that schools must address in meeting expectations of current federal policy for students with mild or severe disabilities. Research that applies what we know about the science of learning to read to students with developmental disabilities is especially needed (NRP, 2000). Another research priority involves effective approaches to engaging students with the literature of their grade level using assistive technology or compensatory strategies for delayed reading development. Until future research emerges, practitioners are encouraged to continue applying the evidence-based strategies of systematic prompting and fading to sight-word instruction (Browder et al., 2006) while also providing explicit instruction in phonemic awareness and phonics and developing students' comprehension and vocabulary through the use of age-appropriate literature (Good et al., 2001).

Although new strategies have emerged for teaching writing to students with disabilities (Harris et al., 2003), their application to students with developmental disabilities has been extremely limited (Konrad et al., 2006). Similarly, new technology is available that may boost students' writing proficiency by providing support in word finding and spelling (e.g., Co:Writer), but research is needed to demonstrate effective interventions that use technology.

In math, substantial research supports strategies for teaching students with developmental disabilities to use money (Browder & Grasso, 1999). Some studies have also considered computational and problem-solving skills for students with milder disabilities, but often the focus has been on using devices or strategies that eliminate the need for mathematical competence (Kroesbergen, 2003). Where interventions have been tried, outcomes have been promising (Jitendra & Xin, 1997). We need to learn more about teaching the multiple strands of mathematics to students with developmental disabilities (e.g., data analysis, geometry, algebra, measurement, computation). In the interim, practitioners are encouraged to apply the systematic prompting and self-regulated instruction methods previously found effective in research addressing these broader skills. In summary, evidence exists showing that students with both mild and severe developmental disabilities can learn academic content. In contrast, what is known best is how to teach skills that link to functional activities (e.g., sight words, money) or that minimize the need for conceptual learning (e.g., calculator use, using precounted money). Future research is called for in which students with developmental disabilities receive instruction targeted to the achievement of higher levels of numeracy and literacy with practical application. Studies of higher academic goals such as phonics instruction (Joseph & Seery, 2004), problem solving (Jitendra & Xin, 1997), and writing (Konrad et al., 2006), have shown that students with developmental disabilities have the potential to learn more academic content than previously assumed possible.

Implications for Planning Teams

The Individuals with Disabilities Education Improvement Act of 2004 (IDEIA) emphasizes the important role that parents have in the identification, assessment, and planning of their child's individualized education program (Vaughn, Bos, & Schumm, 2006). NCLB emphasizes the important role that scientific research has in planning educational programs for all children. How do educators and parents together reconcile the research on teaching academics to this population with expectations set by policy? The research presented in this chapter includes examples of students with mild to severe developmental disabilities who acquire academic skills; there is evidence to support academic planning for this population. In contrast, this evidence extends only to a narrow scope of the general curriculum, so creative planning will be needed in developing ways to teach students skills such as reading poetry or understanding the mathematical concept of slope. States may have developed curricular frameworks or other guidelines for linking to state standards that can help teams with this planning. In this era of expanding academic horizons for this population, teams must remember the importance of ensuring that these skills have meaning and importance in the lives of the learners. Adding more academic content to a student's school program requires making careful decisions about what other content will be condensed or addressed in new ways. For example, can a student work on some occupational therapy goals in the context of an academic lesson? Can academic lessons be combined with functional activities where feasible (e.g., computing slope as part of a leisure activity such as skateboarding)? Creating the balance needed between functional and academic content requires having student and parental input, as well as knowledge of state expectations for adequate yearly progress.

Implications for Policy Makers

Current federal policy, especially NCLB (2004), places strong emphasis on students making adequate yearly progress in priority academic content areas—reading, math, and science. This legislation, along with IDEIA (2004), has been controversial and has created important discussions about what kind of academic achievement to expect from students with disabilities, particularly those with significant cognitive disabilities. Unfortunately, the intensive energy required for developing and implementing assessments for this population has sometimes faced competition from other priorities. In a recent survey, teachers indicated that alternate assessments had increased expectations for students but also were time-consuming and a paperwork burden (Flowers, Ahlgrim-Delzell, Browder, & Spooner, 2005). In the future better models for assessing adequate yearly progress are needed that are technically sound and efficient for teacher use. These models should promote the alignment of instruction, IEPs, and state standards.

SUMMARY

This is an important era of increasing academic expectations for students with developmental disabilities that is being fueled by current federal policies for American educational reform. The research to date provides important guidance about effective strategies for academic learning. More information is available on how to teach reading, math, and writing to students with mild disabilities, but some research also exists for students with moderate and severe developmental disabilities. As researchers address the gaps in what is known about teaching this content, practitioners and families can build on the foundation of strategies identified as effective for functional academics in planning for broader general curriculum access. In developing policy, increased focus is especially needed on teaching versus testing to promote this access. Discussions also are needed to ensure that the new academic skills acquired have a purpose in the lives of graduates with developmental disabilities.

REFERENCES

Ackerman, A. M., & Shapiro, E. S. (1984). Self-monitoring and work productivity with mentally retarded adults. *Journal of Applied Behavior Analysis, 17,* 403–407.

Adams, D., Powers, B., Reed, M., Reiss, P., & Romaniak, J. (1996). *Improving writing skills and related attitudes among elementary school students.* Tinley Park, IL: Saint Xavier University & IRI/Skylight. (ERIC Document Reproduction Service No. ED398595)

Aeschleman, S. R., & Schladenauffen, J. (1984). Acquisition, generalization, and maintenance of grocery shopping skills by severely retarded adolescents. *Applied Research in Mental Retardation, 5,* 245–258.

Al Otaiba, S., & Fuchs, D. (2002). Characteristics of children who are unresponsive to early literacy intervention. *Remedial and Special Education, 23,* 300–316.

Barbetta, P. M., Heward, W. L., & Bradley, D. M. C. (1993). Relative effects of whole-word and phonetic-prompt error correction on the acquisition and maintenance of sight words by students with developmental disabilities. *Journal of Applied Behavior Analysis, 26,* 99–110.

Barudin, S. I., & Hourcade, J. J. (1990). Relative effectiveness of three methods of reading instruction in developing specific recall and transfer skills in learners with moderate and severe mental retardation. *Education and Training in Mental Retardation, 25,* 286–291.

Baumann, J. F., Jones, L. A., & Seifert-Kessell, N. (1993). Using think alouds to enhance children's comprehension monitoring abilities. *Reading Teacher, 47,* 184–193.

Bottge, B. (1999). Effects of contextualized math instruction on problem solving of average and below-average achieving students. *Journal of Special Education, 33,* 81–96.

Boyle, J. R. (1996). The effects of a cognitive mapping strategy on the literal and inferential comprehension of students with mild disabilities. *Learning Disability Quarterly, 19,* 86–98.

Bracey, S., Maggs, A., & Morath. P. (1975). The effects of direct phonics approach in teaching reading to six moderately retarded children: Acquisition and mastery learning stages. *Slow Learning Child, 22*(2), 83–90.

Browder, D., Flowers, C., Ahlgrim-Delzell, L., Karvonen, M., Spooner, F., & Algozzine, R. (2004). The alignment of alternate assessment content with academic and functional curricula. *Journal of Special Education, 37,* 211–233.

Browder, D. M., & Grasso, E. (1999). Teaching money skills to individuals with mental retardation: A research review with practical applications. *Remedial and Special Education, 20,* 297–308.

Browder, D. M., & Minarovic, T. J. (2000). Utilizing sight words in self-instruction training for employees with moderate mental retardation in competitive jobs. *Education and Training in Mental Retardation and Developmental Disabilities, 35,* 78–89.

Browder, D. M., Snell, M. E., & Wildonger, B. (1988). Simulation and community-based instruction of vending machines with time delay. *Education and Training in Mental Retardation, 23,* 175–185.

Browder, D. M., Spooner, F., Ahlgrim-Delzell, L., Harris, A. A., & Wakeman, S. Y. (in press). A comprehensive review of research on teaching math to students with significant cognitive disabilities. *Exceptional Children.*

Browder, D. M., Wakeman, S. Y., Spooner, F., Ahlgrim-Delzell, L., & Algozzine, B. (2006). Research on reading for individuals with significant cognitive disabilities. *Exceptional Children, 72,* 392–408.

Browder, D. M., & Xin, Y. P. (1998). A meta-analysis and review of sight word research and its implications for teaching functional reading to individuals with moderate and severe disabilities. *Journal of Special Education, 32,* 130–153.

Bullock, J., Pierce, S., & McClelland, L. (1989). *Touch math.* Colorado Springs, CO: Innovative Learning Concepts.

Butler, F. M., Miller, S. P., Lee, K., & Pierce, T. (2001). Teaching mathematics to students with mild-to-moderate mental retardation: A review of literature. *Mental Retardation, 39,* 20–31.

Carnine, D., Silbert, J., Kame'enui, E., & Tarver, S. G. (2004). *Direct instruction reading* (4th ed.). Columbus, OH: Pearson-Merrill.

Carnine, L., Carnine, D., & Gersten, R. (1984). Analysis of oral reading errors made by economically disadvantaged students taught with a synthetic phonics approach. *Reading Research Quarterly, 19,* 343–356.

Clicker 4. (2005). [Computer software]. Redmond, WA: Crick Software.

Conners, F. A., Atwell, J. A., Rosenquist, C. J., & Sligh, A. C. (2001). Abilities underlying decoding differences in children with intellectual disability. *Journal of Intellectual Disability Research, 45,* 292–299.

Courtade-Little, G., Spooner, F., & Browder, D. M. (in press). A review of studies with students with significant cognitive disabilities that link to science content. *Research and Practice for Persons with Severe Disabilities.*

Co:Writer 4000. (2005). [Computer software]. Volo, IL: Don Johnston.

Coyne, M. D., Kame'enui, E. J., & Simmons, D. C. (2001). Prevention and intervention in beginning reading: Two complex systems. *Learning Disabilities Research and Practice, 16,* 62–73.

Cunningham, A. E. (1990). Explicit versus implicit instruction in phonemic awareness. *Journal of Experimental Psychology, 30,* 429–444.

Denny, P. J., & Test, D. W. (1995). Using the one-more-than technique to teach money counting to individuals with moderate mental retardation: A systematic replication. *Education and Treatment of Children, 18,* 422–432.

Deshler, D., Schumaker, J., & Bui, Y. (2003). *The demand writing model: Helping students with disabilities pass statewide writing assessments* (ED/OSERS Contract No. H324B010029). Lawrence: University of Kansas Center for Research on Learning. (ERIC Document Reproduction Service No. ED475513)

Dion, E., Morgan, P. L., Fuchs, D., & Fuchs, L. S. (2004). The promise and limitations of reading instruction in the mainstream: The need for a multilevel approach. *Exceptionality, 12,* 163–173.

Driscoll, C., & Kemp, C. (1996). Establishing the equivalence of single word reading and language in children with disabilities. *Journal of Intellectual and Developmental Disability, 21,* 115–139.

Edmark Reading Program. (2002). San Francisco, CA: Riverdeep. Retrieved February 9, 2007, from *www.riverdeep.net.*

Elementary and Secondary Education Act of 1965, 20 U.S.C. 2701 et seq. (1965).

Englemann, S., & Bruner, E. (1995). *Reading mastery.* Columbus, OH: SRA/McGraw-Hill.

Erikson, K. A., & Koppenhaver, D. A. (1997). Integrated communication and literacy instruction for a child with multiple disabilities. *Focus on Autism and Other Developmental Disabilities, 12,* 142–151.

Ezell, H. K., & Kohler, F. W. (1992). Use of peer-assisted procedures to teach QAR reading comprehension strategies to third-grade children. *Education and Treatment of Children, 15,* 205–228.

Farmer, J. A., Gast, D. L., Wolery, M., & Winterling, V. (1991). Small group instruction for students with severe handicaps: A study of observational learning. *Education and Training in Mental Retardation, 26,* 190–201.

Flowers, C., Ahlgrim-Delzell, L., Browder, D., & Spooner, F. (2005). Teachers' perceptions of alternate assessment. *Research and Practice for Persons with Severe Disabilities, 30,* 81–92.

Frederick-Dugan, A., Test, D. W., & Varn, L. (1991). Acquisition and generalization of purchasing skills using a calculator by students who are mentally retarded. *Education and Training in Mental Retardation, 26,* 381–387.

Gast, D. L., Doyle, P. M., Wolery, M, Ault, M. J., & Baklarz, J. L. (1991). Acquisition of incidental information during small group instruction. *Education and Treatment of Children, 23,* 117–128.

Gersten, R. M., & Maggs, A. (1982). Teaching the general case to moderately retarded children. Evaluation of a five-year project. *Analysis and Intervention in Developmental Disabilities, 2,* 329–343.

Good, R. H., Simmons, D. C., & Kame'enui, E. J. (2001). The importance of decision-making utility of a continuum of fluency-based indicators of foundational reading skills for third-grade high-stakes outcomes. *Scientific Studies of Reading, 5,* 257–288.

Graham, S., & Harris, K. R. (1994). Implications of constructivism for teaching writing to students with special needs. *Journal of Special Education, 28,* 275–289.

Graham, S., Harris, K. R., & Mason, L. (2005). Improving writing performance, knowledge, and self-efficacy of struggling young writers: The effects of self-regulated strategy development. *Contemporary Educational Psychology, 30,* 207–241.

Griffin, C. C., Malone, L. D., & Kame'enui, E. J. (1995). Effects of graphic organizer instruction on fifth-grade students. *Journal of Educational Research, 89,* 98–107.

Haring, T. G., Kennedy, C. H., Adams, M. J., & Pitts-Conway, V. (1987). Teaching generalization of purchasing skills across community settings to autistic youth using videodisc modeling. *Journal of Applied Behavior Analysis, 20*(1), 89–96.

Harris, K. R., & Graham, S. (1996). *Making the writing process work: Strategies for composition and self-regulation.* Cambridge, MA: Brookline Books.

Harris, K. R., Graham, S., & Mason, L. H. (2003). Self-regulated strategy development in the classroom: Part of a balanced approach to writing instruction for students with disabilities. *Focus on Exceptional Children, 35,* 2–16.

Horner, R. H., Carr, E. G., Halle, J., McGee, G., Odom, S., & Wolery, M. (2005). The use of single-subject research to identify evidence-based practice in special education. *Exceptional Children, 71,* 165–180.

Individuals With Disabilities Education Improvement Act of 2004, Public Law No. 108–446, 20 U.S.C. 1400 §611–614.

Inspiration. (2005). [Computer software]. Portland, OR: Inspiration Software.

James, L. A., Abbot, M., & Greenwood, C. R. (2001). How Adam became a writer: Winning writing strategies for low-achieving students. *Teaching Exceptional Children, 33*(3), 30–37.

Jitendra, A., & Xin, Y. P. (1997). Mathematical word problem solving for students with mild disabilities and students at risk of math failure: A research synthesis. *Journal of Special Education, 30*, 412–438.

Joseph, L. M., & Seery, M. E. (2004). Where is the phonics? A review of the literature on the use of phonetic analysis with students with mental retardation. *Remedial and Special Education, 25*, 88–94.

Juel, C. (1988). Learning to read and write: A longitudinal study of 54 children from first through fourth grades. *Journal of Educational Psychology, 90*, 437–477.

Juel, C., Griffith, P. L., & Gough, P. B. (1986). Acquisition of literacy: A longitudinal study of children in first and second grade. *Journal of Educational Psychology, 78*, 243–255.

Katims, D. S. (2000a). *The quest for literacy: Curriculum and instructional procedures for teaching reading and writing to students with mental retardation and developmental disabilities.* Reston, VA: Council for Exceptional Children, Division on Mental Retardation and Developmental Disabilities. (ERIC Document Reproduction Service No. ED445454)

Katims, D. S. (2000b). Literacy instruction for people with mental retardation: Historical highlights and contemporary analysis. *Education and Training in Mental Retardation and Developmental Disabilities, 35*, 3–15.

Kliewer, C. (1998). Citizenship in the literate community: An ethnography of children with Down syndrome and the written word. *Exceptional Children, 64*, 167–180.

Kliewer, C., & Biklen, D. (2001). "School's not really a place for reading": A research synthesis of the literate lives of students with severe disabilities. *Journal of the Association for Persons with Severe Handicaps, 26*, 1–12.

Konrad, M., Trela, K., & Test, D. W. (2006). Using IEP goals and objectives to teach paragraph writing skills to high school students with physical and cognitive disabilities. *Education and Training in Developmental Disabilities, 41*, 111–124.

Koppenhaver, D., Erickson, K., & Skotko, B. (2001). Supporting communication of girls with Rett syndrome and their mothers in storybook reading. *International Journal of Disability, Development and Education, 48*, 395–410.

Kroesbergen, E. H. (2003). Mathematics interventions for children with special educational needs. *Remedial and Special Education, 24*, 97–115.

Lancioni, G. E., Singh, N. N., O'Reilly, M. F., & Oliva, D. (2003). Evaluating optic microswitches with students with profound multiple disabilities. *Journal of Visual Impairment and Blindness, 97*, 1–8.

Lane, S. D., & Critchfield, T. S. (1998). Classification of vowels and consonants by individuals with moderate mental retardation: Development of arbitrary relations via match-to-sample training with compound stimuli. *Journal of Applied Behavior Analysis, 31*, 21–41.

Lie, A. (1991). Effects of a training program for stimulating skills in word analysis in first-grade students. *Reading Research Quarterly, 26*, 234–250.

Maccini, P., & Gagnon, J. C. (2000). Best practices for teaching mathematics to secondary students with special needs: Implications from teacher perceptions and a review of the literature. *Focus on Exceptional Children, 32*, 1–22.

Mackay, H. A., Soraci, S. A., Carlin, M. T., Dennis, N. A., & Strawbridge, C. P. (2002). Guiding visual attention during acquisition of matching-to-sample. *American Journal on Mental Retardation, 107*(6), 445–454.

Matson, J. L., & Long, S. (1986). Teaching computation/shopping skills to mildly mentally retarded adults. *American Journal on Mental Deficiency, 91*, 98–101.

McDonnell, J. (1987). The effects of time delay and increasing prompt hierarchy strategies on the acquisition of purchasing skills by students with severe handicaps. *Journal of the Association for Persons with Severe Handicaps, 12*, 227–236.

McDonnell, J., & Ferguson, B. (1989). A comparison of time delay and decreasing prompt hierarchy strategies in teaching banking skills to students with moderate handicaps. *Journal of Applied Behavioral Analysis, 22*, 85–91.

McGee, G. G., & McCoy, J. F. (1981). Training procedures for acquisition and retention of reading in retarded youth. *Applied Research in Mental Retardation, 2*, 263–276.

Mechling, L. C., & Gast, D. L. (2003). Multi-media instruction to teach grocery word associations and store location: A study of generalization. *Education and Training in Developmental Disabilities, 38,* 62–76.

Miller, S. P., Butler, F. M., & Lee, K. (1998). Validated practices for teaching mathematics to students with learning disabilities: A review of the literature. *Focus on Exceptional Children, 34,* 1–24.

Morse, T. E., & Schuster, J. W. (1996). Grocery shopping skills for persons with moderate to profound intellectual disabilities: A review of the literature. *Education and Treatment of Children, 19,* 487–517.

National Council of Teachers of English, Writing Study Group of the NCTE Executive Committee. (2004). *NCTE beliefs about the teaching of writing.* Retrieved November 10, 2005, from *www.ncte.org.*

National Council of Teachers of Mathematics. (1989). *Curriculum and evaluation standards for school mathematics.* Reston, VA: Author.

National Reading Panel. (2000). *Teaching children to read: An evidence-based assessment of the scientific research literature on reading and its implications for reading instruction* (NIH Publication No. 00–4754). Washington, DC: U.S. Department of Health and Human Services.

No Child Left Behind Act of 2001, Public Law No. 107-110, 115 Stat. 1425 (2002).

O'Connor, R. E., Jenkins, J. R., Leicester, N., & Slocum, T. A. (1993). Teaching phonological awareness to young students with learning disabilities. *Exceptional Children, 59,* 532–546.

Rehfeldt, R. A., Latimore, D., & Stromer, R. (2003). Observational learning and the formation of classes of reading skills by individuals with autism and other developmental disabilities. *Research in Developmental Disabilities, 24,* 333–358.

Sandknop, P. A., Schuster, J. W., Wolery, M., & Cross, D. P. (1992). The use of an adaptive device to teach students with moderate mental retardation to select lower priced grocery items. *Education and Training in Mental Retardation, 27,* 219–229.

Schickendanz, J., Dickinson, D., & Charlotte-Mecklenburg Schools. (2005). *Opening the world of learning.* Parsippany, NJ: Pearson.

Schloss, P., Alper, S., Young, H., Arnold-Reid, G., Aylward, M., & Dudenhoeffer, S. (1995). Acquisition of functional sight words in community-based recreational settings. *Journal of Special Education, 29,* 84–96.

Scott, K. S. (1993). Reflection on "multisensory mathematics for children with mild disabilities." *Exceptionality, 42,* 125–129.

Scruggs, T. E., & Mastropieri, M. A. (1997). Can computers teach problem-solving strategies to students with mild mental retardation? *Remedial and Special Education, 18,* 157–165.

Shafer, M. S., Inge, J. K., & Hill, J. (1986). Acquisition, generalization, and maintenance of automated banking skills. *Education and Training in Mental Retardation, 21,* 265–272.

Siegel, L. S. (1992). An evaluation of the discrepancy definition of dyslexia. *Journal of Learning Disabilities, 25,* 618–629.

Simon, R., & Hanrahan, J., (2004). An evaluation of the Touch Math method for teaching addition to students with learning disabilities in mathematics. *European Journal of Special Needs Education, 19,* 191–209.

Singh, J., & Singh, N. N. (1985). Comparison of word-supply and word-analysis error-correction procedures on oral reading by mentally retarded children. *American Journal of Mental Deficiency, 90,* 64–70.

Singh, N. N., & Singh, J. (1984). Antecedent control of oral reading errors and self-corrections by mentally retarded children. *Journal of Applied Behavior Analysis, 17,* 111–119.

Singh, N. N., & Singh, J. (1988). Increasing oral reading proficiency through overcorrection and phonic analysis. *American Journal on Mental Retardation, 93,* 312–319.

Singh, N. N., Winton, A. S., & Singh, J. (1985). Effects of delayed versus immediate attention to oral reading errors on the reading proficiency of mentally retarded children. *Applied Research in Mental Retardation, 6,* 283–293.

Snow, C., Burns, M. S., & Griffin, P. (1998). (Eds.). *Preventing reading difficulties in young children.* Washington, DC: National Academy of Sciences.

Stanovich, K. E., & Siegel, L. S. (1994). Phenotypic performance of children with reading disabilities: A regression-based test of the phonological-core variable-difference model. *Journal of Educational Psychology, 86,* 24–53.

Start-to-Finish Books. (2005). [Multimedia]. Volo, IL: Don Johnston.

Stein, M., Johnson, B., & Gutlohn, L. (1999). Analyzing beginning reading programs and the relationship between decoding instruction and text. *Remedial and Special Education, 21,* 275–288.

U.S. Department of Education. (2003). Title I: Improving the academic achievement of the disadvantaged: Final rule, 68 Fed. Reg. 236.

U.S. Department of Education. (2005a). *Alternate achievement standards for students with the most significant cognitive disabilities: Non-regulatory guidance* Washington, DC: Author.

U.S. Department of Education. (2005b). Title I: Improving the academic achievement of the disadvantaged; Individuals with disabilities education act (IDEA): Assistance to states for the education of children with disabilities; proposed rule, 70 Fed. Reg. 118.

Van den Pol, R. A., Iwata, B. A., Ivancic, M. T., Page, T. J., Neef, N. A., & Whitley, F. P. (1981). Teaching the handicapped to eat in public places: Acquisition, generalization, and maintenance of restaurant skills. *Journal of Applied Behavioral Analysis, 14,* 61–70.

Vandever, T. R., Maggart, W. T., & Nasser, S. (1976). Three approaches to beginning reading. *Mental Retardation, 14*(4), 29–32.

Vandever, T. R., & Stubbs, J. C. (1977). Reading retention and transfer in TMR students. *American Journal of Mental Deficiency, 82,* 233–237.

Vaughn, S., Bos, C., & Schumm, J. S. (2007). *Teaching exceptional, diverse, and at-risk students in the general education classroom: IDEA 2004* (Updated ed.). Boston: Pearson, Allyn & Bacon.

Vaughn, S., & Klingner, J. K. (1999). Teaching reading comprehension through collaborative strategic reading. *Intervention in School and Clinic, 34,* 284–292.

Wagner, R., & Torgesen, J. (1987). The nature of phonological processing and its causal role in the acquisition of reading skills. *Psychological Bulletin, 101,* 191–212.

Weikle, B., & Hadadian, A. (2003). Can assistive technology help us not to leave any child behind? *Preventing School Failure, 47,* 181–187.

Whitehurst, G., & Lonigan, C. (2001). Emergent literacy: Development from pre-readers to readers. In S. Neuman & D. Dickson (Eds.), *Handbook for early literacy research* (pp. 11–20). New York: Guilford Press.

Witzel, B. S., Mercer, C. D., & Miller, M. D. (2003). Teaching algebra to students with learning difficulties: An investigation of an explicit instruction model. *Learning Disabilities Research and Practice, 18,* 121–131.

Writing with Symbols. (2000). [Computer software]. Solana Beach, CA: Mayer-Johnson.

WYNN. (2006). [Computer software]. Palo Alto, CA: Learning Systems Group, Freedom Scientific.

15

Social Interaction Interventions

*Promoting Socially Supportive Environments
and Teaching New Skills*

Erik W. Carter
Carolyn Hughes

Interacting socially with others can be one of the greatest sources of joy and satisfaction in our lives. Clearly, a primary incentive for students to attend school is the opportunity to spend time with their peers. As students age, they spend increasing amounts of time with their peers, and the roles that children play in each others' lives become more prominent (Gifford-Smith & Brownell, 2003). Through their relationships with each other, children learn critical social behaviors, peer norms, and values; they develop intellectually, emotionally, and academically; and they access important social, emotional, and instrumental supports (Rubin, Bukowski, & Parker, 1998; Sheridan, Buhs, & Warnes, 2003).

For children and youth with developmental disabilities, the potential benefits associated with peer interaction are equally apparent and may include skill acquisition, increased social competence, access to meaningful supports, attainment of educational goals, emergence of new friendships, and improved quality of life (e.g., Kraemer, McIntyre & Blacher, 2003; Ryndak & Fisher, 2001). Similarly, peers who interact with their classmates with disabilities frequently report substantial benefits emerging from these relationships, including personal growth, enhanced understanding of self, improved attitudes, greater appreciation of diversity, increased advocacy skills, and meaningful friendships (e.g., Carter, Hughes, Copeland, & Breen, 2001; Hughes et al., 2001).

Given such benefits, it is not surprising that improving the social participation of students with disabilities has remained a consistent and prominent focus of legislative, policy, and research initiatives. For example, the Individuals with Disabilities Education Improvement Act (2004) states that students with disabilities must be educated, to the maximum extent appropriate, with their general education peers. Moreover, teachers, administrators, parents, and students themselves have placed high value on creating opportunities for students with disabilities to develop meaningful relationships with their peers without disabilities (Copeland et al., 2004; Palmer, Fuller, Arora, & Nelson, 2001; Villa, Thousand, Meyers, & Nevin, 1996). Indeed, socially related goals are prominent on the individualized education programs (IEPs) of many students with disabilities (Gelzheiser, McLane, Meyers, & Pruzek, 1998).

For children and youth with developmental disabilities, however, opportunities to interact socially with their general education peers at school may be severely limited. Studies show that without intentional programming efforts, little interaction typically occurs between students with and without developmental disabilities, particularly in secondary schools (e.g., Dymond & Russell, 2004; Hughes et al., 1999; Orsmond, Krauss, & Seltzer, 2004). Further, even when special education students are physically included in classes with their general education peers, they are likely to remain socially isolated unless supportive measures are taken (Carter, Hughes, Guth, & Copeland, 2005).

Given these restricted opportunities to practice and refine their social interaction skills, it is not surprising that students with developmental disabilities typically have limited social skill repertoires. Moreover, speech or language impairments, challenging or stereotypical behaviors, or motor limitations may further hinder social skill development. Tragically, a "Catch-22" situation occurs for students who have not learned to effectively initiate or sustain conversation: Peers are less likely to engage in interactions with these students, and opportunities to learn conversational skills are further stifled. The substantial environmental barriers prevalent in many school settings, coupled with the presence of socially related skill limitations, have made meaningful and durable social relationships an elusive outcome for too many students with developmental disabilities. This social isolation can have a profound impact on the well-being of children and youth with developmental disabilities (Deater-Deckard, 2001).

IDENTIFYING EFFECTIVE INTERVENTION STRATEGIES

Social outcomes pose a significant challenge to researchers, educators, and others charged with providing an appropriate education for children and youth with developmental disabilities. Educators need effective strategies to promote meaningful social interaction among students with disabilities and their general education peers. Fortunately, a growing body of literature documents an increasing number of effective strategies that educators and others may use to promote social interaction opportunities and increase the social interaction skills of children and youth with developmental disabilities (e.g., Carter & Hughes, 2005; Goldstein, Kaczmarek, & English, 2002; McConnell, 2002; Paul, 2003).

In this chapter, we discuss and illustrate social interaction interventions by drawing on studies conducted during the past decade with students with developmental disabilities across an array of elementary, middle, and high school settings. Although the literature describes numerous examples of techniques for teaching new social skills and restructuring educational contexts, of ultimate importance is whether acquisition of these new skills and environmental changes translate into actual improvements in peer interactions. Thus this chapter focuses on intervention strategies that have been demonstrated to increase social interactions between students with and without developmental disabilities rather than on strategies found only to increase ratings of social skills or social status.

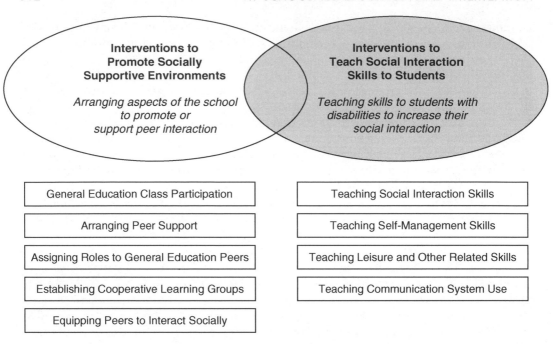

FIGURE 15.1. Interventions approaches for promoting social interaction.

Drawing on the organizational framework and review findings of Carter and Hughes (2005), we begin by reviewing effective intervention approaches that fall within two broad categories: (1) promoting socially supportive environments and (2) teaching social interaction skills (see Figure 15.1). Interventions designed to create socially supportive environments focus primarily on arranging classroom and school settings so that peer interactions are more actively prompted, promoted, and/or supported. Such interventions have variously been called "environmental arrangements," "ecological variations," and "support-based interventions." Interventions that focus primarily on teaching students with disabilities skills expected to increase their social interaction offer a second major approach to improving peer relationships. Within each category, we discuss individual intervention strategies and highlight key aspects of these interventions that may influence their effectiveness. To guide future research in this area, we discuss additional research needs related to participating students, interaction settings, outcome measures, analytic approaches, generalization, and social validity. Next, illustrative examples of intervention applications are provided, and implications are discussed for educators and families. We conclude this chapter with a brief discussion of future policy directions.

INTERVENTIONS TO PROMOTE SOCIALLY SUPPORTIVE ENVIRONMENTS

Environmental factors can have a profound influence on students' social development and opportunities for interaction. Context clearly matters when it comes to children's relationships (Gifford-Smith & Brownell, 2003; Sheridan et al., 2003). Unfortunately, many elementary, middle, and high school environments often do not support and, in fact, appear to hinder social interaction between students with developmental disabilities and their general education peers. To promote school environments that support social interaction among students with and without developmental disabilities, we present five intervention strategies found to be effective at increasing peer interaction: (1) supporting general education class participation, (2) arranging peer support, (3) assigning roles to general education peers, (4) establishing cooperative learning groups, and (5) equipping peers to interact socially with children with disabilities.

General Education Class Participation

The physical location in which educational services are provided undoubtedly affects students' opportunities for peer interaction. Although many students with developmental disabilities continue to receive much of their education in special education classrooms (U.S. Department of Education, 2003), increased inclusion in general education classes is strongly advocated. When it is implemented using recommended practices (see Hunt & McDonnell, Chapter 13, this volume), inclusion involves enrollment in general education classes supported by active collaboration between general and special educators, ongoing curricular adaptations and classroom modifications for students, and individually tailored classroom supports (e.g., supplementary aids and services, social facilitation by adults, partner systems). When these components are present, research suggests that the impact on social outcomes is quite promising. Relative to special education classrooms, Kennedy and colleagues found that general education class participation for students with moderate to severe disabilities was associated with more frequent interactions and social contacts, higher proportions of social support exchanged, and larger friendship networks for students with disabilities (e.g., Kennedy, Cushing, & Itkonen, 1997; Kennedy, Shukla, & Fryxell, 1997). Similar differences in interaction patterns have been identified in descriptive studies involving students with profound and multiple disabilities (e.g., Foreman, Arthur-Kelly, Pascoe, & King, 2004) and severe intellectual disabilities (e.g., Hunt, Farron-Davis, Beckstead, Curtis, & Goetz, 1994).

However, changes in the locations of educational service delivery are not, by themselves, sufficient to improve the social outcomes of students with disabilities. What actually happens in those inclusive environments—the specific interaction opportunities and supports provided to students—is of critical importance. For example, schools' heavy reliance on paraprofessionals to provide one-to-one support to students with disabilities in inclusive settings may inadvertently stifle peer interaction and friendship development (Giangreco, Halvorsen, Doyle, & Broer, 2004). Consequently, it is essential that general education class participation be coupled with additional changes and supports in those environments.

Arranging Peer Support

In recent years peer support interventions have been advocated as an effective approach to supporting the inclusion in general education classes of students with developmental disabilities and improving their peer relationships (Giangreco et al., 2004; Goldstein et al., 2002). Although these interventions may take various forms, peer support typically involves several features: (1) pairing one or more peers with a student with disabilities and teaching them to adapt class activities to facilitate the student's participation, (2) supporting the student's work toward attainment of IEP goals, (3) teaching and modeling normative social interaction skills, and/or (4) promoting communication between the student and his or her classmates. While providing this assistance to their classmates, the peers receive ongoing feedback and assistance from paraprofessionals, special education teachers, and/or general education teachers. Shukla, Kennedy, and Cushing (1998, 1999) examined the effects of peer-delivered support on social interactions among middle school students with moderate to profound disabilities and their general education peers. Peer-provided support, relative to one-to-one support provided by a paraprofessional or special education teacher, was associated with more frequent and longer durations of social interaction, as well as a greater variety of social support behaviors exchanged among students. Variations of peer support strategies have been implemented with younger children with developmental disabilities (e.g., Hunt, Alwell, Farron-Davis, & Goetz, 1996). For example, Laushey and Heflin (2000) paired kindergartners with and without autism together as part of a daily buddy system, teaching them how to play and interact together. Children with autism engaged in higher percentages of positive social interactions when paired with a buddy than when they were simply in physical proximity to their classmates but not paired together.

Because peer support interventions typically comprise multiple components related to selecting, training, monitoring, and providing feedback to peers, various intervention configurations might be expected to differentially affect students' social outcomes. For example, Carter, Cushing, Clark, and Kennedy (2005) documented higher levels of social interaction when middle and high school students with intellectual disabilities or autism were paired with two general education peers rather than with a single peer. Other salient variables may include the amount of monitoring and feedback provided by educators to participating students, the method used to pair students, the ages of participating students, and the social and academic skills of peers. Systematic study of these intervention components is needed to further enhance the effectiveness of peer support strategies.

Assigning Roles to General Education Peers

General education peers may be asked to assume a variety of different roles when interacting with their classmates with developmental disabilities, including that of friend, tutor, partner, advocate, or instructor. The specific approaches that educators take to facilitate interactions among students appear to influence the types of social exchanges and relationships that subsequently emerge. For example, Hughes, Carter, Hughes, Bradford, and Copeland (2002) compared dyadic peer interactions among high school students with and without severe intellectual disabilities as peers were assigned two alternating roles: an instructional role (i.e., students were asked to participate in an activity in which the classmate with disabilities required assistance) or a noninstructional role (i.e., students were asked engage in an activity in which a classmate with disabilities did not require assistance). Assigning a noninstructional role to a peer was associated with higher levels of socially related initiations and responses, greater variety of conversational topics, and higher observer ratings of interaction quality than assigning an instructional role. Similarly, McMahon, Wacker, Sasso, Berg, and Newton (1996) examined the interactions of third-grade students with mild to moderate intellectual disabilities as they were taught by general education peers to play various board games. Although interactions were initially task-related, socially related interactions increased as students with disabilities acquired greater competence in game play.

Indeed, simply prompting general education peers to interact with a classmate with disabilities "as a friend" may sometimes be a sufficient catalyst to facilitate peer interaction. Hughes, Copeland, et al. (2002) assessed the effects of delivering such a verbal directive to students engaged in leisure activities during lunch, in gym class, and in classrooms. Asking general education peers to interact as friends with children with disabilities was associated with increases in social interaction and communication behaviors, improvements in ratings of interaction quality, and greater variety of conversational topics discussed. When this directive was absent, negligible interaction among students was observed to occur, despite their being present in the same school setting.

The potential benefits and drawbacks associated with assigning different peer roles should be considered carefully by educators. Some educators have expressed concern that continuously placing peers in a tutorial role may impede the development of true friendships, arguing that such roles perpetuate stereotypes of students with disabilities and reinforce notions that students with developmental disabilities should always be the recipients of help (Van der Klift & Kunc, 2002). On the other hand, assuming an instructional role may actually contribute to peers' raised expectations and improved attitudes toward classmates with disabilities, as they become more aware of these children's strengths and capabilities (Carter et al., 2001; Copeland et al., 2004). Peer roles should be regularly examined and adjusted as needed to meet the social and instructional needs of students with disabilities and to match the classroom context.

Establishing Cooperative Learning Groups

In addition to supporting academic outcomes, the use of cooperative learning groups has been advocated as a promising instructional strategy for promoting interaction among students with and without developmental disabilities in general education classrooms (e.g., Demchak, 2005; Salisbury, Gallucci, Palombaro, & Peck, 1995). Such instructional groupings typically involve dividing the class into small groups of students, establishing common learning goals, delineating student roles within each group, and establishing interdependent contingencies. Dugan and colleagues (1995) investigated the impact of cooperative learning groups on the social outcomes of fourth graders with autism. Relative to traditional teacher-led instruction, participation in daily cooperative learning groups resulted in substantial increases in students' social initiations and responses. Piercy, Wilton, and Townsend (2002) documented similar outcomes in a study involving students with moderate to severe intellectual disabilities (kindergarten through second grade). Following participation in a cooperative learning program, children with disabilities were observed to engage in significantly more positive social interactions with their peers during unstructured play time. Less is known, however, about the impact of cooperative learning groups at the secondary level. Cushing, Kennedy, Shukla, Davis, and Meyer (1997) examined the impact of cooperative groupings in middle schools by comparing peer interactions in a combined cooperative group and a revised-curriculum condition with those in a revised-curriculum-only condition. Only minor differences on measures of social interaction were found between conditions, with one student receiving slightly higher levels of social support in the cooperative-group condition.

Cooperative learning groups, as with peer support arrangements, appear to offer a promising strategy for furthering the social goals of students with developmental disabilities in inclusive classrooms, settings within which social interaction might otherwise be discouraged by educators. Moreover, such instructional groups appear to provide frequent opportunities for students to practice and refine interaction skills among peers within a socially supportive context. The implementation requirements associated with these interventions, however, may make them less tractable in some middle and high school classrooms. Additional research is needed to understand effective methods for establishing (e.g., selecting group members, equipping peers for interactions) and maintaining (e.g., periodic monitoring by special educators, making adaptations) cooperative learning groups in secondary settings.

Equipping Peers to Interact Socially

Simply pairing students with and without disabilities often is not sufficient to produce meaningful, sustained peer interactions. General education peers sometimes report that, without some initial guidance from educators, they feel that they lack the skills and knowledge to initiate and maintain interactions with their classmates with developmental disabilities (e.g., Copeland et al., 2004; York & Tundidor, 1995). Early studies demonstrated that, by equipping peers with general information about disabilities, an understanding of communicative intent, strategies for promoting interaction, and structured and ongoing support, the social interactions and peer acceptance of students with developmental disabilities could be greatly improved (e.g., Haring & Breen, 1992; Staub & Hunt, 1993). These strategies continue to be refined further as researchers explore effective peer-mediated approaches for equipping general education students to interact meaningfully with their classmates with developmental disabilities.

For example, Garrison-Harrell, Kamps, and Kravits (1997) investigated the effects of a peer network intervention in which general education first graders were taught to use various interaction strategies (e.g., conversing, sharing, providing praise, providing instructions) with their classmates with autism. When coupled with communication system training for students with disabilities, these eight 30-minute social skill training sessions led to more frequent peer interactions and increased social acceptance for students with disabilities. Kamps et al. (2002) delivered a similar social skills curriculum to third-grade peers and noted substantial increases in the frequency and duration of interactions among students following the intervention. In a multicomponent intervention aimed at promoting interaction among elementary students with and without disabilities (i.e., cerebral palsy, intellectual disabilities, dual sensory impairments), Hunt et al. (1996) coupled ongoing provision of disability-related information (i.e., information about students' communication modes and adaptive equipment) to classmates with peer support strategies and communication system instruction. Following the intervention, students with disabilities substantially increased their reciprocal interactions with peers. Further, Weiner (2005) taught elementary-age peers strategies for requesting and reinforcing repair responses from their classmates with moderate to severe disabilities. Peers readily acquired and implemented these strategies, resulting in increases in their classmates' conversational repairs and turn taking, as well as improvements in their social relationships.

Although promising, these studies prompt important questions about how and where within the general curriculum such information and instruction might be provided to general education peers. Although general disability awareness efforts can readily be infused into the general curriculum and appear to reduce knowledge-related barriers to peer relationships, such efforts may be too broad to effect substantial increases in interaction. Providing child-specific information (e.g., interests, strengths, communication modes), coupled with modeling of specific interaction strategies, to likely interaction partners offers a more promising approach. Further research is needed to identify the best combination of intervention components that balance feasibility and effectiveness.

INTERVENTIONS TO TEACH SOCIAL INTERACTION SKILLS

Interventions aimed at increasing the social skills of children and youth with developmental disabilities have made up an active area of research for several decades. Acquisition of key social skills is not only critical to successful peer relationships but may also influence academic success. Yet, for many students with developmental disabilities, substantial limitations in social and communication skills are both prevalent and pervasive (de Bildt et al., 2005; Myles et al., 2001). In this section, we review four intervention approaches designed to increase students' social interaction skills: (1) teaching social interaction skills alone, (2) teaching self-management skills, (3) teaching leisure skills, and (4) teaching communication system use.

Teaching Social Interaction Skills Alone

Systematic instruction in various social and communication skills makes up an important instructional component for many students with disabilities. Although numerous studies have documented that students with developmental disabilities can acquire discrete social skills in intervention settings (e.g., Davies & Rogers, 1985; Haring, 1993), there is less evidence that use of those skills is maintained over time or that they generalize to interactions with their peers without disabilities (Gresham, Sugai, & Horner, 2001). Unless coupled with other intervention components, social skill instruction is unlikely to be sufficient by itself in promoting meaningful, sustained peer interactions among students with and without developmental disabilities. Consequently, researchers have recommended that social skill instruction be woven into more comprehensive intervention packages (e.g., Unified Plans of Support; Hunt, Soto, Maier, Muller, & Goetz, 2002).

Teaching Self-Management and Social Interaction Skills

Increasingly, researchers and educators are calling on students with disabilities to assume a more active and prominent role in educational interventions, including social interaction interventions. Teaching students to self-manage their own behavior is one effective approach to accomplishing this task. Self-management instruction involves teaching students to direct their own social behavior using strategies such as goal setting, self-prompting, self-monitoring, and self-evaluation. Actively involving students in managing their own social behavior may contribute to improved social outcomes by equipping students to deliver their own social prompts and reinforcement, thereby promoting greater student intervention buy-in and decreasing student reliance on educators. The portability of self-management strategies also appears to enhance generalization and maintenance of intervention effects, promoting more widespread improvements in peer interaction.

Hughes and colleagues (Hughes, Harmer, Killian, & Niarhos, 1995; Hughes, Killian, & Fischer, 1996) evaluated the efficacy of a self-instruction training package on the peer interactions of high school students with intellectual disabilities. Multiple peers volunteered to teach socially validated conversational initiations and self-instructional strategies to participants using systematic instructional procedures. Training was associated with substantial increases in students' initiations with familiar and unfamiliar peers, as well as greater eye contact. Hughes et al. (2000) asked peers to teach their classmates with disabilities to use a small picture booklet to prompt themselves to initiate conversation. Participants were taught to look at a peer, ask a question while pointing at the corresponding picture, wait for a response, expand on the response, and repeat the process with the next picture. Self-prompting instruction resulted in increases in participant initiations and peer responses, as well as a greater variety of conversational topics discussed by students.

Social interaction interventions that include self-management components also have been demonstrated to be effective with younger children with developmental disabilities and across school settings (e.g., Anctil & Degeneffe, 2003; Gilberts, Agran, Hughes, & Wehmeyer, 2001). For example, Morrison, Kamps, Garcia, and Parker (2001) found that teaching self-monitoring strategies to elementary and middle school students with autism had a substantial positive impact on their social skill use (i.e., requesting, commenting, sharing) and peer interactions, as well as decreases in their inappropriate behavior during game play. In addition to receiving social skill instruction, students were taught to record the number of times they used each social skill appropriately.

Teaching Leisure and Other Related Skills

Leisure and recreation activities provide a primary context for peers to engage together in mutually enjoyable activities, to interact socially, and to develop new friendships. Yet many students with developmental disabilities lack the skills to participate in such activities with their peers, thus restricting their opportunities for interaction within these contexts. Teaching students to participate competently in leisure activities commonly engaged in by their peers offers one effective approach to promoting social interaction. That is, student acquisition of these collateral skills appears to translate into related improvements in social outcomes. For example, Baker, Koegel, and Koegel (1998) taught elementary-age children with autism to play individually designed leisure games with their peers without disabilities. Each game was designed around a theme or topic on which the child with autism frequently perseverated. Instruction in game play was associated with increases in appropriate social interactions and positive student affect. Essential to the success of such interventions is the identification of age-appropriate, mutually reinforcing leisure activities that can be meaningfully adapted for children and youth with development disabilities. Physical education and related arts classes, extracurricular clubs, and inclusive community and after-school recreation programs all offer contexts for delivering such instruction.

Teaching Communication System Use and Social Interaction Skills

Many children and youth with developmental disabilities exhibit concomitant speech, language, and communication impairments that hinder their social interactions with their general education peers. To address these barriers to peer interaction, many students will benefit from instruction in using various augmentative and alternative communication systems (AAC; e.g., communication books, computerized devices).

Hunt and colleagues (2002) sought to increase the social participation of young children with cerebral palsy and severe speech impairments. As part of a comprehensive support plan (e.g., collaborative teaming, written support plans, provision of curricular adaptations, arrangement of peer supports), the students were taught to use communication boards and voice output devices during inclusive elementary classes. Increases in initiations, positive peer interactions, class engagement, and communication system use were noted for all participating students. Similarly, Hunt, Farron-Davis, Wrenn, Hirose-Hatae, and Goetz (1997) developed communication books for elementary students with severe disabilities (e.g., pervasive developmental disorder, intellectual disabilities, Asperger syndrome), which were made up of pictures depicting socially validated conversational topics with associated written labels. Students were taught to point to pictures and follow a specified conversational turn-taking structure when interacting with peers. Following the intervention, students with disabilities engaged in greater numbers of reciprocal interactions and spent less time alone.

Although numerous studies have evaluated the effects of aided and unaided communication systems on speech output and expressive language in clinical settings, researchers need to explore the value of and approaches to weaving AAC instruction into peer interaction interventions. Careful consideration must be given to the process of selecting meaningful communication systems, ensuring that they address a child's interaction needs, are appropriate matches for a variety of educational contexts, and offer enough flexibility to evolve as the child's needs change. In addition, attention should be given to the types of training that general education peers might need to interact effectively with someone who uses an AAC system.

REFINING SOCIAL INTERACTION INTERVENTIONS: IMPLICATIONS FOR RESEARCHERS

Unless intentional efforts are made to promote them, meaningful peer relationships will continue to elude many children and youth with developmental disabilities. The intervention strategies presented in this chapter offer promise for facilitating increased peer interaction, but additional research is required to understand how to improve students' social outcomes and to refine existing interventions. The following recommendations are offered to guide researchers in improving the effectiveness of these intervention strategies (Carter & Hughes, 2005).

Replicate across Students

Children with developmental disabilities are a heterogeneous population of students who exhibit diverse needs and who encounter a range of different barriers to peer interaction. Additional research with a broader range of students is needed to determine the parameters within which these intervention strategies remain effective and whether additional intervention components may be necessary. Previous research has focused most prominently on students with moderate to severe intellectual disabilities and/or autism. Less is known about intervention effectiveness for students who use AAC systems, students with multiple disabilities (e.g., cerebral palsy, physical disabilities, sensory impairments), and students with high-functioning autism (e.g., Asperger syndrome). It is likely that these students encounter additional barriers to peer interaction. Given the relatively small number of studies incorporating each intervention component, systematic replication of these findings is needed to determine the appropriateness of an intervention strategy for students who exhibit certain characteristics. Replication studies with less studied populations must include comprehensive, operational descriptions of participants (e.g., specific disability, functional assessments of limited social interaction, descriptions of speech mode and communication skill, study inclusion and exclusion selection criteria).

Additional research attention also should be focused on the conversational partners with whom students with developmental disabilities interact. Most students without disabilities participating in published interventions were involved in some type of peer support program (e.g., peer buddies, partner systems, circle of friends) or were specifically prompted by adults to interact with their classmates with disabilities. It seems probable that these students likely differ in important ways from students who were not involved in such programs or who chose not to volunteer for such interactions (e.g., Carter et al., 2001). To elucidate the role of general education peers in promoting improved social outcomes, researchers should explore the following questions: What factors influence peers' willingness to interact with their classmates with disabilities? What steps should educators take to identify potential interaction partners? How might students with developmental disabilities be more actively involved in determining who these peers are? If peer networks and reciprocal friendships are the ultimate goal of intervention strategies, it is essential that researchers examine the extent to which these interventions are indeed increasing interactions with peers whom students with disabilities judge to be socially important.

Expand Intervention Settings

Researchers have demonstrated that peer interaction can be increased across a wide range of elementary, middle, and high school environments, reflecting the array of settings encountered by students with developmental disabilities throughout a typical school day (U.S. Department of Education, 2003). In light of the growing emphasis placed on ensuring that students with disabilities are accessing and progressing within the general curriculum, additional research is needed to further our understanding of how social interaction intervention strategies might be implemented effectively and with fidelity in inclusive classrooms. For example, fewer interventions have been evaluated in core academic general education classrooms, in which lecture-dominated instructional arrangements and increased expectations for student independence sometimes results in diminished interaction opportunities.

Furthermore, significant changes in the school context take place as students progress through middle and high school. Whereas elementary students spend most or all of their school day in a single classroom accompanied by a consistent peer group, classmates in secondary schools often fluctuate from one period to the next as students rotate among classrooms. Moreover, the peer environment undergoes substantial transformation as students enter adolescence; peer affiliations assume greater importance, and social interactions take on increased complexity (Brown & Klute, 2003). Therefore, additional research is needed that examines how interventions found to be effective with younger children might be adapted for use with adolescents.

Broaden Social Interaction Measures

The diversity of social outcome measures utilized in research studies on social interaction speaks to the complexity of peer relationships. Although the range of potential social behaviors that might be addressed in intervention efforts is extensive, some tentative conclusions can be drawn from previous research in this area. Interventions involving social interaction skill instruction have been found to be effective at changing discrete social behaviors such as initiations, responses, and conversational turn taking. By contrast, interventions designed to promote socially supportive environments generally have been found to be effective at increasing outcomes, such as extended social contacts and interaction quality. Although all of these outcomes are important to capture, additional research is needed that explores how increases in students' interactions contribute to outcomes such as a greater sense of belonging, peer acceptance, the development of durable, meaningful friendships, and the maintenance and expansion of peer networks. Operationalizing these latter outcomes remains a continued challenge, and researchers should consider incorporating an expanded array of measures into future studies.

Refine Analytic Approaches

School-based social interaction interventions have consisted primarily of demonstration analyses, in which an intervention is shown to effect improvements in social interaction measures over and above preintervention or baseline levels. Indeed, positive effects have been found for all of the intervention strategies discussed in this chapter. To guide educators in selecting the most appropriate interventions, researchers should incorporate two additional types of analyses into future studies. First, direct comparisons of interventions would enable educators to discern which strategies are likely to be most effective under certain conditions (e.g., Odom et al., 1999; Schlosser & Sigafoos, 2006). Such comparative analyses would provide much needed information about the relative effectiveness of various interventions, facilitating more strategic decision making by educators. Second, most of the intervention strategies discussed in this chapter have been combined into multicomponent intervention packages. Component and parametric analyses would provide educators with information about which combinations of intervention components are necessary and/or sufficient to improve the social interactions of students with developmental disabilities. Indeed, refining these intervention packages to maximize effectiveness and reduce implementation requirements may offer one avenue for increasing educators' use of empirically validated intervention strategies (Snell, 2003).

Promote Maintenance and Generalization

Although each of the intervention strategies discussed in this chapter has demonstrated short-term increases in students' social outcomes, less is known about the durability of social improvements associated with these strategies and the impact of social improvements on social networks. In most research studies, the long-term effects of interventions have not been evaluated, highlighting the need for longitudinal evaluations that extend over the course of multiple semesters or school years. Moreover, as the peer environment shifts from an emphasis on dyadic friendships to associations with cliques and crowds, and as students move to new schools, more sophisticated intervention strategies will be needed to ensure that intervention effects spill over to and positively affect these changed relationships.

Ensuring Social Validity

The social interaction outcomes described in these studies are supported by evidence of strong social validity. Several intervention strategies (e.g., arranging peer support, equipping peers to interact socially) appear to be especially well received by students with and without disabilities (Kamps et al., 1998; Hughes et al., 2001). Less is known, however, about the extent to which the implementation requirements associated with these intervention strategies are feasible for educators and perceived to be effective. As more students with developmental disabilities are served in inclusive school settings, researchers should query educators about the extent to which these interventions align with instructional approaches and support strategies typically used in general education classrooms and should solicit their input about modifying interventions accordingly. Again, such refinements may play a role in diminishing the research-to-practice gap by ensuring that disseminated interventions couple high social validity with clear improvements in student outcomes.

IMPLICATIONS FOR EDUCATORS

As shown in Figure 15.1, we categorized social interaction interventions found in the literature into two groups: promoting socially supportive environments and teaching social interaction skills. In this section, we provide examples derived from the literature of educators applying these strategies to increase the social interactions of students with developmental disabilities.

Assessing Social Interaction Needs

Although considerable diversity exists among individuals who share the labels of intellectual disabilities, autism, and other developmental disabilities, limitations in social interaction skills are common and a key to definitional criteria. Assessing students' individual socially related needs and identifying the settings in which interventions should be delivered are essential first steps in intervention. A variety of assessment techniques is available to assist educators in (1) identifying which students might benefit from participation in these interventions, (2) establishing socially related educational goals, and (3) monitoring students' progress toward these goals throughout and following an intervention. For example, educators might directly observe students' social interaction patterns, complete rating scales (e.g., standardized social skill assessments, behavioral checklists, adaptive behavior assessments), utilize peer nomination techniques (e.g., sociometrics, peer ratings, social networks), and/or interview students with disabilities and/or their classmates (e.g., Black & Ornelles, 2001; Snell & Janney, 2000). To prioritize social outcomes for intervention, educators should consider querying students with disabilities about their own social goals, observing typical conversational skills used by classmates without disabilities, checking with family members, and asking other educators about their social expectations for given school settings and activities.

Applying the Intervention Strategies

Promoting Socially Supportive Environments

In this chapter, we have emphasized that including students with developmental disabilities in general education classes typically requires the application of support strategies to promote social interaction. Supports can include cooperative instruction groupings, such as having a student conduct an experiment in chemistry class with a group of peers, each of whom has a preassigned role to fulfill to complete the experiment. Or a teacher can assign pairs of students to complete instructional tasks, such as having a student and peer quiz each other on historical events and dates for an upcoming American history test. In either case, curricula or materials may need to be adapted to accommodate students' particular needs. Educators should note that verbal praise or other potential reinforcers may be required to maintain students' social interaction, at least initially. Peers may need to be taught and supported to increase their interactions with their peers with developmental disabilities, particularly if they have limited prior experience with people with disabilities. For example, peers who are supporting their classmates with disabilities can meet weekly with an adult sponsor (e.g., teacher, school counselor, parent). During meetings, they can receive instruction and feedback on their peer interactions and plan together ways to increase students' social networks and opportunities to interact in general education settings. Peers can also receive disability awareness instruction during the meetings, such as learning to use a pictorial communication system with a student with limited verbal skills. During social interaction opportunities, general education peers may also need to be told specifically to interact with their classmates with disabilities until patterns of social interaction are established in the environment. Finally, multiple support strategies may be required in concert, such as arranging peer supports, modifying classroom assignments, and providing reinforcement and instructional feedback, to achieve widespread and sustainable social interaction among students with developmental disabilities and their classmates in any general education setting.

Teaching Social Interaction Skills

Arranging an environment to promote social interaction may not be enough to support sufficient levels of interaction among students with developmental disabilities and their general education peers. Often, students with disabilities must be taught new skills to promote social interaction. Students who have had little opportunity to spend time with peers may simply need to be taught social skills, such as greeting or responding to their peers, through direct instruction. Educators may find that social skills taught by peers rather than by adults may generalize more effectively to other peers. In addition to social skills training, instruction in the use of communication systems may be necessary to increase the social interactions of students with limited verbal repertoires. Educators and family members should note that if newly acquired social behaviors are to be maintained, social skills or conversational topics taught must be socially valued and practiced within a setting. An effective strategy for promoting durable social interaction is to teach students to prompt and reinforce their own social behavior through self-management instruction. For example, peers can teach students to prompt themselves to initiate conversation and make eye contact with their classmates and then to praise themselves for doing so. Finally, teaching students recreation or leisure skills that are interactive, such as computer or board games, can promote social interaction between students with developmental disabilities and their general education peers.

Combining Approaches

A more balanced intervention approach may be to combine environmental and skill-building strategies into comprehensive intervention packages. Although skill instruction has the potential to increase students' independence, successful interaction, and overall social competence, no amount of instruction will increase interaction if classmates are not within physical proximity or if interaction is actively discouraged within a given school setting. Barriers such as self-contained classrooms, separate tables in the cafeteria, and hovering paraprofessionals prevent the needed proximity. Similarly, even when instructional activities and school environments are designed to provide frequent opportunities for peers to work together and converse with each other, interaction will remain limited if students with disabilities are not taught to converse with their peers. A focus on one approach to the exclusion of the other overlooks the important role that *both* social competence and environmental factors play in peer relationships.

Finally, educators must commit to frequent and systematic data collection to ensure that the social outcomes of students with developmental disabilities are improving as a result of intervention efforts. Many practical data collection tools are available to educators that can be adapted to document progress toward socially related goals (e.g., Kennedy, 2004). Intervention strategies can then be revised based on ongoing evaluation of student data.

IMPLICATIONS FOR FAMILY MEMBERS

Parents of children both with and without developmental disabilities recognize the importance of promoting peer relationships among their children (Overton & Rausch, 2002; Palmer et al., 2001; Peck, Staub, Gallucci, & Schwartz, 2004). Unfortunately, the school-based intervention strategies described in this chapter have not yet been shown to reliably promote relationships that extend beyond the school day. Encouraging such friendships among children with and without disabilities may require family members to actively support peer interactions in the afternoons and on weekends. For example, parents might identify shared community and home activities, set up play dates among children, provide transportation, and monitor children's interactions (Koegel, Werner, Vismara, & Koegel, 2005; Turnbull, Pereira, & Blue-Banning, 1999). Such efforts will require family members to establish creative partnerships and maintain ongoing communication with both educators and parents of general education classmates.

IMPLICATIONS FOR POLICY

The intervention strategies described in this chapter hold great promise for researchers, educators, and others wanting to increase peer interaction and social relationships among students with and without developmental disabilities. However, meaningful improvements in the social participation of children and youth with developmental disabilities are likely to come only when accompanied by broader, schoolwide efforts. Shifting from self-contained to inclusive service delivery models, devoting adequate resources to supporting the participation of students with disabilities in general education, designing efforts to improve staff perceptions regarding inclusion, and increasing general awareness of the needs and potential contributions of students with disabilities are all important to improving the culture of a school. Such efforts will require strong leadership from school and district administrators.

In addition, new professional development approaches are needed for delivering information concerning effective social interaction intervention strategies. As children and youth spend more time in inclusive school settings, a broader range of educators and other professionals will need to be fluent in effective strategies for improving the social participation of students with disabilities in their classrooms. Preservice teacher education programs offer one important avenue for equipping future general and special educators to employ these strategies. However, school districts must also identify creative approaches to providing their current educators with professional development in this critical area of students' lives. Although recent legislation (e.g., No Child Left Behind) places increased emphasis on improving academic outcomes for students with disabilities, this emphasis need not be at the expense of promoting enhanced social outcomes.

CONCLUSIONS

Peer relationships can have a strong and lasting influence on the lives of children and youth. Educators charged with meeting the instructional needs of students with developmental disabilities must be equipped to use interventions that will improve students' opportunities for and skills in interacting with their general education peers. The interventions discussed in this chapter offer considerable potential for improving the social lives of students with developmental disabilities. Still more research will elevate our understanding of the conditions under which these interventions are effective. The application of these findings by teachers in school settings will enable more children and youth with disabilities to access the benefits associated with meaningful peer relationships.

REFERENCES

Anctil, T. M., & Degeneffe, C. E. (2003). Self-management and social skills training for persons with developmental disabilities: A literature review. *Journal of Applied Rehabilitation Counseling, 34,* 17–24.

Baker, M. J., Koegel, R. L., & Koegel, L. K. (1998). Increasing the social behavior of young children with autism using their obsessive behaviors. *Journal of the Association for Persons with Severe Handicaps, 23,* 300–308.

Black, R. S., & Ornelles, C. (2001). Assessment of social competence and social networks for transition. *Assessment for Effective Intervention, 26,* 23–39.

Brown, B. B., & Klute, C. (2003). Friendships, cliques, and crowds. In G. R. Adams & M. D. Berzonsky (Eds.), *Blackwell handbook of adolescence* (pp. 330–348). Malden, MA: Blackwell.

Carter, E. W., Cushing, L. S., Clark, N. M., & Kennedy, C. H. (2005). Effects of peer support interventions on students' access to the general curriculum and social interactions. *Research and Practice for Persons with Severe Disabilities, 30,* 15–25.

Carter, E. W., & Hughes, C. (2005). Increasing social interaction among adolescents with intellectual disabilities and their general education peers: Effective interventions. *Research and Practice for Persons with Severe Disabilities, 30,* 179–193.

Carter, E. W., Hughes, C., Copeland, S. R., & Breen, C. (2001). Differences between high school students who do and do not volunteer to participate in peer interaction programs. *Journal of the Association for Persons with Severe Handicaps, 26,* 229–239.

Carter, E. W., Hughes, C., Guth, C., & Copeland, S. R. (2005). Factors influencing social interaction among high school students with intellectual disabilities and their general education peers. *American Journal on Mental Retardation, 110,* 366–377.

Copeland, S. R., Hughes, C., Carter, E. W., Guth, C., Presley, J., Williams, C. R., et al. (2004). Increasing access to general education: Perspectives of participants in a high school peer support program. *Remedial and Special Education, 26,* 342–352.

Cushing, L. S., Kennedy, C. H., Shukla, S., Davis, J., & Meyer, K. A. (1997). Disentangling the effects of curriculum revision and social grouping within cooperative learning arrangements. *Focus on Autism and Other Developmental Disabilities, 12,* 231–240.

Davies, R. R., & Rogers, E. S. (1985). Social skills training with persons who are mentally retarded. *Mental Retardation, 23,* 186–196.

Deater-Deckard, K. (2001). Annotation: Recent research examining the role of peer relationships in the development of psychopathology. *Journal for Child Psychology and Psychiatry, 42,* 565–575.

de Bildt, A., Serra, M., Luteijn, D., Sytema, S., & Minderaa, R. (2005). Social skills in children with intellectual disabilities with and without autism. *Journal of Intellectual Disability Research, 49,* 317–328.

Demchak, M. A. (2005). Teaching students with severe disabilities in inclusive settings. In M. L. Wehmeyer & M. Agran (Eds.), *Mental retardation and intellectual disabilities: Teaching students using innovative and research-based strategies* (pp. 57–77). Washington, DC: American Association on Mental Retardation.

Dugan, E., Kamps, D., Leonard, B., Watkins, N., Rheinberger, A., & Stackhaus, J. (1995). Effects of cooperative learning groups during social studies for students with autism and fourth-grade peers. *Journal of Applied Behavior Analysis, 28,* 175–188.

Dymond, S. K., & Russell, D. L. (2004). Impact of grade and disability on the instructional context of inclusive classrooms. *Education and Training in Developmental Disabilities, 39,* 127–140.

Foreman, P., Arthur-Kelly, M., Pascoe, S., & King, B. S. (2004). Evaluating the educational experiences of students with profound and multiple disabilities in inclusive and segregated classroom settings: An Australian perspective. *Research and Practice for Persons with Severe Disabilities, 29,* 183–193.

Garrison-Harrell, L., Kamps, D., & Kravits, T. (1997). The effects of peer networks on social–communicative behaviors for students with autism. *Focus on Autism and Other Developmental Disorders, 12,* 241–254.

Gelzheiser, L. M., McLane, M., Meyers, J., & Pruzek, R. M. (1998). IEP-specified interaction needs: Accurate but ignored. *Exceptional Children, 65,* 51–65.

Giangreco, M. F., Halvorsen, A. T., Doyle, M. B., & Broer, S. M. (2004). Alternatives to overreliance on paraprofessionals in inclusive schools. *Journal of Special Education Leadership, 17,* 82–90.

Gifford-Smith, M. E., & Brownell, C. A. (2003). Childhood peer relationships: Social acceptance, friendships, and peer networks. *Journal of School Psychology, 41,* 235–284.

Gilberts, G. H., Agran, M., Hughes, C., & Wehmeyer, M. (2001). The effects of peer-delivered self-monitoring strategies on the participation of students with severe disabilities in the general education classroom. *Journal of the Association for Persons with Severe Handicaps, 26,* 25–36.

Goldstein, H., Kaczmarek, L. A., & English, K. M. (2002). *Promoting social communication: Children with developmental disabilities from birth to adolescence.* Baltimore: Brookes.

Gresham, F. M., Sugai, G., & Horner, R. H. (2001). Interpreting outcomes of social skills training for students with high-incidence disabilities. *Exceptional Children, 67,* 331–344.

Haring, T. G. (1993). Strategies for teaching students with mild to severe mental retardation. In R. A. Gable & S. F. Warren (Eds.), *Strategies for teaching students with mild to severe mental retardation* (pp. 129–164). Baltimore: Brookes.

Haring, T. G., & Breen, C. G. (1992). A peer-mediated social network intervention to enhance the social integration of persons with moderate and severe disabilities. *Journal of Applied Behavior Analysis, 25,* 319–333.

Hughes, C., Carter, E. W., Hughes, T., Bradford, E., & Copeland, S. R. (2002). Effects of instructional versus non-instructional roles on the social interactions of high school students. *Education and Training in Mental Retardation and Developmental Disabilities, 37,* 146–162.

Hughes, C., Copeland, S. R., Guth, C., Rung, L. L., Hwang, B., Kleeb, G., et al. (2001). General education students' perspectives on their involvement in a high school peer buddy program. *Education and Training in Mental Retardation and Developmental Disabilities, 36,* 343–356.

Hughes, C., Copeland, S. R., Wehmeyer, M. L., Agran, M., Cai, X., & Hwang, B. (2002). Increasing social interaction between general education high school students and their peers with mental retardation. *Journal of Developmental and Physical Disabilities, 14,* 387–402.

Hughes, C., Harmer, M. L., Killian, D. J., & Niarhos, F. (1995). The effects of multiple-exemplar self-instructional training on high school students' generalized conversational interactions. *Journal of Applied Behavior Analysis, 28,* 201–218.

Hughes, C., Killian, D. J., & Fischer, G. M. (1996). Validation and assessment of a conversational interaction intervention. *American Journal of Mental Retardation, 100,* 493–509.

Hughes, C., Rodi, M. S., Lorden, S. W., Pitkin, S. E., Derer, K. R., Hwang, B., et al. (1999). Social interactions of high school students with mental retardation and their general education peers. *American Journal on Mental Retardation, 104,* 533–544.

Hughes, C., Rung, L. L., Wehmeyer, M., Agran, M., Copeland, S. R., & Hwang, B. (2000). Self-prompted communication book use to increase social interaction among high school students. *Journal of the Association for Persons with Severe Handicaps, 25,* 153–166.

Hunt, P., Alwell, M., Farron-Davis, F., & Goetz, L. (1996). Creating socially supportive environments for fully included students who experience multiple disabilities. *Journal of the Association for Persons with Severe Disabilities, 21,* 53–71.

Hunt, P., Farron-Davis, F., Beckstead, S., Curtis, D., & Goetz, L. (1994). Evaluating the effects of placement of students with severe disabilities in general education versus special classes. *Journal of the Association for Persons with Severe Handicaps, 19,* 200–214.

Hunt, P., Farron-Davis, F., Wrenn, M., Hirose-Hatae, A., & Goetz, L. (1997). Promoting interactive partnerships in inclusive educational settings. *Journal of the Association for Persons with Severe Handicaps, 22,* 127–137.

Hunt, P., Soto, G., Maier, J., Muller, E., & Goetz, L. (2002). Collaborative teaming to support students with augmentative communication needs in general education classrooms. *Augmentative and Alternative Communication, 18,* 20–35.

Individuals with Disabilities Education Improvement Act of 2004, Public Law 108-446, 118 Stat. 2647 (2004).

Kamps, D., Gonzalez-Lopez, A., Potucek, J., Kravits, T., Kemmerer, K., & Garrison-Harrell, L. (1998). What do peers think? Social validity of integrated programs. *Education and Treatment of Children, 21,* 107–134.

Kamps, D., Royer, J., Dugan, E., Travits, T., Gonzalez-Lopez, A., Garcia, J., et al. (2002). Peer training to facilitate social interaction for elementary students with autism and their peers. *Exceptional Children, 68,* 173–187.

Kennedy, C. H. (2004). Research on social relationships. In E. Emerson, C. Hatton, T. Parameter, & T. Thompson (Eds.), *International handbook of applied research in intellectual disabilities* (pp. 297–310). London: Wiley.

Kennedy, C. H., Cushing, L. S., & Itkonen, T. (1997). General education participation improves the social contacts and friendship networks of students with severe disabilities. *Journal of Behavioral Education, 7,* 167–189.

Kennedy, C. H., Shukla, S., & Fryxell, D. (1997). Comparing the effects of educational placement on the social relationships of intermediate school students with severe disabilities. *Exceptional Children, 64,* 31–47.

Koegel, R. L., Werner, G. A., Vismara, L. A., & Koegel, L. K. (2005). The effectiveness of contextually supported play date interactions between children with autism and typically developing peers. *Research and Practice for Persons with Severe Disabilities, 30,* 93–102.

Kraemer, B. R., McIntyre, L. L., & Blacher, J. (2003). Quality of life for young adults with mental retardation during transition. *Mental Retardation, 41,* 250–262.

Laushey, K. M., & Heflin, L. J. (2000). Enhancing social skills of kindergarten children with autism through the training of multiple peers as tutors. *Journal of Autism and Developmental Disorders, 30,* 183–193.

McConnell, S. R. (2002). Interventions to facilitate social interaction for young children with autism: Review of available research and recommendations for educational intervention and future research. *Journal of Autism and Developmental Disorders, 32,* 351–372.

McMahon, C. M., Wacker, D. P., Sasso, G. P., Berg, W. K., & Newton, S. M. (1996). Analysis of frequency and type of interactions in a peer-mediated social skills intervention: Instructional vs. social interactions. *Education and Training in Mental Retardation and Developmental Disabilities, 31,* 339–352.

Morrison, L., Kamps, D., Garcia, J., & Parker, D. (2001). Peer mediation and monitoring strategies to improve initiations and social skills for students with autism. *Journal of Positive Behavior Interventions, 3,* 237–250.

Myles, B. S., Barnhill, G. P., Hagiwara, T., Griswold, D. E., & Simpson, R. L. (2001). A synthesis of studies on the intellectual, academic, social/emotional and sensory characteristics of youth with Asperger syndrome. *Education and Training in Mental Retardation and Developmental Disabilities, 36,* 304–311.

Odom, S. L., McConnell, S. R., McEvoy, M. A., Peterson, C., Ostrosky, M., Chandler, L. K., et al. (1999). Relative effects of interventions supporting the social competence of young children with disabilities. *Topics in Early Childhood Special Education, 19,* 75–91.

Orsmond, G. I., Krauss, M. W., & Seltzer, M. M. (2004). Peer relationships and social and recreational activities among adolescents and adults with autism. *Journal of Autism and Developmental Disorders, 34,* 245–256.

Overton, S., & Rausch, J. L. (2002). Peer relationships as support for children with disabilities: An analysis of mothers' goals and indicators for friendship. *Focus on Autism and Other Developmental Disabilities, 17,* 11–29.

Palmer, D. S., Fuller, K., Arora, T., & Nelson, M. (2001). Taking sides: Parent views on inclusion for their children with severe disabilities. *Exceptional Children, 67,* 467–484.

Paul, R. (2003). Promoting social communication in high functioning individuals with autistic spectrum disorders. *Child and Adolescent Psychiatric Clinics of North America, 12,* 87–106.

Peck, C. A., Staub, D., Gallucci, C., & Schwartz, I. (2004). Parent perception of the impacts of inclusion on their nondisabled child. *Research and Practice for Persons with Severe Disabilities, 29,* 135–143.

Piercy, M., Wilton, K., & Townsend, M. (2002). Promoting the social acceptance of young children with moderate–severe intellectual disabilities using cooperative-learning techniques. *American Journal on Mental Retardation, 107,* 352–360.

Rubin, K. H., Bukowski, W., & Parker, J. G. (1998). Peer interactions, relationships, and groups. In W. Damon (Ed.), *Handbook of child psychology* (Vol. 1, pp. 619–700). New York: Wiley.

Ryndak, D. L., & Fisher, D. (Eds.). (2001). *The foundations of inclusive education: A compendium of articles on effective strategies to achieve inclusive education.* Baltimore: TASH.

Salisbury, C. L., Gallucci, C., Palombaro, M. M., & Peck, C. A. (1995). Strategies that promote social relations among students with and without disabilities in inclusive schools. *Exceptional Children, 62,* 125–137.

Schlosser, R. W., & Sigafoos, J. (2006). Augmentative and alternative communication interventions for persons with developmental disabilities: Narrative review of comparative single-subject experimental studies. *Research in Developmental Disabilities, 27,* 1–29.

Sheridan, S. M., Buhs, E. S., & Warnes, E. D. (2003). Childhood peer relationships in context. *Journal of School Psychology, 41,* 285–292.

Shukla, S., Kennedy, C. H., & Cushing, L. S. (1998). Component analysis of peer support strategies: Adult influence on the participation of peers without disabilities. *Journal of Behavioral Education, 8,* 397–413.

Shukla, S., Kennedy, C. H., & Cushing, L. S. (1999). Intermediate school students with severe disabilities: Supporting their social participation in general education classrooms. *Journal of Positive Behavior Interventions, 1,* 130–140.

Snell, M. E. (2003). Applying research to practice: The more pervasive problem? *Research and Practice for Persons with Severe Disabilities, 28,* 143–147.

Snell, M. E., & Janney, R. (2000). *Practices for inclusive schools: Social relationships and peer support.* Baltimore: Brookes.

Staub, D., & Hunt, P. (1993). The effects of social interaction training on high school peer tutors of schoolmates with severe disabilities. *Exceptional Children, 60,* 41–57.

Turnbull, A. P., Pereira, L., & Blue-Banning, M. J. (1999). Parents' facilitation of friendships between their children with a disability and friends without a disability. *Journal of the Association for Persons with Severe Handicaps, 24,* 85–99.

U.S. Department of Education. (2003). *Twenty-fifth annual report to Congress on the implementation of the Individuals with Disabilities Education Act*. Washington, DC: Author.

Van der Klift, E., & Kunc, N. (2002). Beyond benevolence: Supporting genuine friendship in inclusive schools. In J. Thousand, R. Villa, & A. Nevin (Eds.), *Creativity and collaborative learning: A practical guide to empowering students, teachers, and families* (2nd ed., pp. 21–28). Baltimore: Brookes.

Villa, R. A., Thousand, J. S., Meyers, H., & Nevin, A. (1996). Teacher and administrator perceptions of heterogeneous education. *Exceptional Children, 63*, 29–45.

Weiner, J. S. (2005). Peer-mediated conversational repair in students with moderate and severe disabilities. *Research and Practice for Persons with Severe Disabilities, 30*, 26–37.

York, J., & Tundidor, M. (1995). Issues raised in the name of inclusion: Perspectives of educators, parents, and students. *Journal of the Association for Persons with Severe Handicaps, 20*, 31–44.

16

Augmentative and Alternative Communication

Brenda Fossett
Pat Mirenda

This chapter focuses on the use of augmentative and alternative communication (AAC) to support persons with developmental disabilities whose speech is insufficient to meet their ongoing daily communication needs. We include only information about innovations and strategies that have empirical support or that are based on current research. We rely primarily on *Augmentative and Alternative Communication*, the official journal of the International Society for Augmentative and Alternative Communication (ISAAC), as well as on research cited in the third edition of *Augmentative and Alternative Communication: Supporting Children and Adults with Complex Communication Needs* (Beukelman & Mirenda, 2005). We focus on advancements between 1995 and 2005, with attention to developments specific to persons with developmental disabilities in general and individuals with intellectual and/or multiple disabilities in particular.

Historically, the field of AAC has focused on supporting individuals with severe expressive communication disorders only. However, in 2005, the American Speech–Language–Hearing Association (ASHA) issued a new definition defining AAC as both an area of research and a set of clinical and educational practices that

> attempts to study and, when necessary, compensate for temporary or permanent impairments, activity limitations, and participation restrictions of persons with severe disorders of speech–language production and/or comprehension, including spoken and written modes of communication. (p. 1)

The recent addition of "comprehension" to the definition of AAC draws attention to the unique communication needs of individuals who struggle to understand spoken language. This includes many people who experience significant intellectual and/or multiple disabilities in particular. By acknowledging the need for augmented comprehension, this definition helps to ensure that the broad-based needs of individuals with developmental disabilities are addressed.

There are two primary types of AAC techniques: aided and unaided. Aided AAC refers to techniques that require external equipment, such as nontechnical communication displays (e.g., picture books) or computerized speech-generating devices (SGDs). Unaided AAC refers to techniques that can be produced by a person's body alone, such as manual signs, gestures, and facial expressions. Most individuals use a combination of both aided and unaided techniques to communicate in various contexts across a range of communication partners (ASHA, 2004).

AAC ASSESSMENT

In many contexts, information derived from both formal and informal assessments is used to determine eligibility for specific types of service or support. For example, school-based assessments are often conducted to determine whether or not a student requires special education services. In the past, this was also the norm for assessments related to the provision of AAC supports. However, there is now increased awareness that assessment to determine AAC "eligibility" often impedes access to much-needed communication services and supports, especially for children and adults with severe disabilities. Thus one of the most notable advancements over the past 10 years relates to a number of official documents that address the inappropriateness of such eligibility criteria. For example, ASHA (2005) noted that, although there are no evidence-based procedures for determining whether or not a given individual is likely to benefit from AAC, "no individuals should be denied this right, irrespective of the type and/or severity of communication, linguistic, social, cognitive, motor, sensory, perceptual, and/or other disability[ies] they may present" (p. 1). ASHA's statement is aligned with that of the National Joint Committee (NJC) for the Communication Needs of Persons with Severe Disabilities (2003a, 2003b), which asserted that eligibility for communication services and supports should be based on communication needs alone, rather than on criteria such as discrepancies between cognitive and communication functioning, chronological age, diagnosis, absence of cognitive or other skills purported to be prerequisites, and other factors. Together, the ASHA and NJC statements are important advances in the AAC field, as they emphasize that assessment can no longer be used as a gatekeeping mechanism for determining who may or may not receive AAC services. The question to be addressed by AAC assessment is *how* AAC interventions and supports can best be applied to a given individual rather than *whether* an individual should have access to AAC intervention and support. This advancement is especially important for many individuals with significant or multiple disabilities who, as a result, may now have access to AAC assessment and intervention for the first time.

To develop and implement constructive individualized interventions, AAC assessment must be conducted with thoughtful precision. The purpose of an AAC assessment is to identify discrepancies between an individual's communication needs and his or her current capabilities and to use this information to identify AAC techniques that will result in improved receptive and expressive communication. AAC assessment is often quite challenging, given the effects of sensory, motor, intellectual, and/or language impairments commonly experienced by persons with developmental disabilities. It is critical that AAC assessments identify an individual's strengths, limitations, and needs in order to identify appropriate intervention techniques.

When conducting an AAC assessment, ASHA (2004) recommends the use of the Participation Model (Beukelman & Mirenda, 2005), which focuses on procedures aimed at identifying both current and potential strengths and needs to guide the development of AAC interventions for both the present and the future. Decisions related to AAC techniques for "today" are aimed at meeting an individual's current communication needs by utilizing existing capabilities. Decisions related to AAC for "tomorrow" are based on projections regarding potential capabilities, as established through assessment, instruction, and enhanced opportunities. This model of assessment and intervention views an individual's AAC system as dynamic and under continuous revision, based on current and projected capabilities, needs, and constraints.

Opportunity Assessment

Individuals with developmental disabilities often experience reduced opportunities to participate in age-appropriate, meaningful activities because of social, physical, and personal barriers. It is imperative to address these barriers to identify and neutralize their negative impact on communication. Beukelman and Mirenda (2005) described five types of opportunity barriers that may impede effective AAC assessment and intervention. First, *policy barriers* refer to legislative or regulatory policies that govern the environments in which persons who use AAC live, learn, and work. Such barriers may reduce an individual's opportunity to participate in activities with same-age peers, may restrict access to AAC equipment, and may limit funding for AAC services and equipment. Second, *practice barriers* refer to actions that take place in families, schools, or workplaces that, although not endorsed as policies, hinder participation nonetheless. Examples include the school district that restricts students from taking AAC equipment outside of the school building or the employer who will not hire an individual because he or she communicates differently. Third, *knowledge barriers* refer to support persons' lack of information regarding various aspects of AAC. For example, Sigafoos (1999) noted that untrained communication partners often (1) fail to recognize or make use of naturally occurring opportunities for or events related to communication; (2) preempt communication by anticipating individuals' wants and needs; and (3) unwittingly ignore the idiosyncratic or subtle communicative behaviors often used by individuals with physical and/or multiple disabilities. Fourth, *skill barriers* refer to a lack of ability to implement an AAC strategy, despite having sufficient knowledge. For example, support persons may acquire knowledge via courses, workshops, or readings but may still have difficulty putting their knowledge into practice. Finally, *attitude barriers* that result in reduced expectations for persons with developmental disabilities may restrict opportunities for participation. For example, both the speech–language pathologist who believes that people who do not speak are not his or her responsibility and the teacher who believes that students who cannot talk are unable to learn to read experience attitude barriers that impede communication.

Over the past decade, several research-based assessment tools have been developed to assess communication opportunities for people with developmental disabilities who use AAC. For example, *Time to Learn* (Rowland & Schweigert, 1999) is an environmental inventory designed to help teachers identify and create opportunities for active participation and learning in typical classroom activities for children who are deaf–blind or who have other severe or multiple disabilities. The *Communication Supports Checklist for Programs Serving Individuals with Severe Disabilities* (McCarthy et al., 1998) contains a number of self-assessment checklists for AAC teams to use in order to assess their current practices and plan related communication interventions. Finally, the *Social Networks Communication Inventory* (Blackstone & Hunt Berg, 2003) was designed for use by teams who are responsible for collecting and interpreting information toward the goal of dealing with limited opportunities and planning AAC interventions in inclusive settings.

Capability Assessment

Even when given access to environments and activities that afford opportunities for meaningful participation, many persons with developmental disabilities do not have access to the communication tools that are needed. The purpose of AAC capability assessment is to identify the strengths and needs of an individual toward the goal of identifying appropriate AAC interventions. Some of the most significant developments over the past decade relate to issues of capability assessment and are detailed in the following sections.

Assessment of Current Communication

When assessing an individual's current level of communication, it is essential to bear in mind that assessment is carried out to identify mismatches between an individual's current communication abilities and his or her communication needs. To ensure that assessment is tied to the context of communication, AAC specialists must determine (1) how an individual currently communicates, (2) what an individual needs to communicate, and (3) which communication modalities an individual is able to use when engaging in purposeful interactions with others. Rowland and Schweigert (2003) discussed six aspects of cognitive–communication development that affect the development of an individualized AAC system: awareness, communicative intent, world knowledge, memory, symbolic representation, and metacognition. In addition, Wilkinson and Jagaroo (2004) suggested that visual perceptual skills are relevant when making AAC decisions.

Presently, no empirically validated assessment tools are available to assess functioning across all seven of these areas. However, several research-based strategies can be used to assess many of these skills, using observational, interview, and direct assessment methods. For example, although not designed specifically for AAC assessment, the Communication and Symbolic Behavior Scales (Wetherby & Prizant, 1993) and its abbreviated version, the Communication and Symbolic Behavior Scales Developmental Profile (Wetherby & Prizant, 2002), include strategies for assessing current communicative functions and modalities, social–affective signaling and reciprocity, object use, and symbolic behavior. Rowland and Schweigert (2002a, 2002b) developed the School Inventory of Problem-Solving Skills and the Home Inventory of Problem-Solving Skills to assess basic skills with objects, the ability to gain access to objects, and the ability to use objects. The Communication Matrix[1] (Rowland, 1996) can be used to identify how a child currently communicates and to guide teams in identifying appropriate communication goals. The Inventory of Potential Communicative Acts (IPCA[2]; Sigafoos et al., 1998) was designed to assess prelinguistic communication behaviors and functions in

---

[1] A free, parent version of the Communication Matrix is available online at *www.designtolearn.com/pages/matrix2.html*.

[2] The IPCA is available from Dr. Jeff Sigafoos at *Jeff.Sigafoos@utas.edu.au*.

individuals with significant developmental and/or physical disabilities. Finally, the Social Networks Communication Inventory (Blackstone & Hunt Berg, 2003) can also be used to assess an individual's communication skills and abilities, modes of expression, representation strategies, and current selection techniques, among other things.

Assessment of Symbolic Understanding

Symbols are items that represent objects, actions, and concepts and may include such things as objects (e.g., a cup that represents drink), photographs (e.g., a photo of a slide that represents the playground), or commercially available black-and-white line drawings (e.g., a line drawing of a car that represents going for a drive). When planning an AAC intervention, it is important to select a system of representation that the individual is able to understand. Although symbol–referent relations may be apparent to adults without disabilities, these relationships may not be so obvious to young children or persons with significant cognitive and/or language impairments (Lund, Millar, Herman, Hinds, & Light, 1998). People who rely on AAC typically use a variety of symbol types across the lifespan; therefore, the goal of an initial symbol assessment is to select the type(s) of symbols that will meet an individual's current communication needs and that require minimal time for learning. Over time, additional symbol assessments may be conducted as well, to identify symbols that may be used in the future.

There is a rich research base regarding the relative ease with which individuals with developmental disabilities are able to learn and use symbols. In general, research has demonstrated the existence of a hierarchy of symbolic complexity. Tangible symbols (e.g., real objects, miniature objects, partial objects, and artificially associated and textured symbols) are among the easiest to learn (Beukelman & Mirenda, 2005). Research on the complexity of current commercially available symbol sets suggests that Picture Communication Symbols (PCS; Johnson, 1994) are easier to recognize without instruction than more abstract symbols such as Blissymbols (Mirenda & Locke, 1989). Research related specifically to symbol use in young children stresses the importance of using representations that reflect a child's understanding of emerging concepts and that represent meaningful contexts and experiences in the child's life (e.g., Lund et al., 1998).

None of the commonly used clinical approaches for assessing an individual's ability to understand symbols have been examined empirically. However, the Tangible Symbol Systems Levels of Representation Pre-Test (Rowland & Schweigert, 2000a) uses direct assessment of object–symbol matching capabilities to determine the appropriate level of symbolic representation when planning for AAC system development. In addition, Beukelman and Mirenda (2005) described a process of symbol assessment that involves selecting items with which an individual is familiar, gathering various types of symbols for the items (e.g., objects, photographs, and line drawings), and using specific tasks to assess the individual's ability to understand different levels of representation. Both of these symbol assessment methods are based on protocols developed for research studies related to symbol learnability and use (e.g., Mirenda & Locke, 1989).

Assessment of Literacy Skills

One area that is often overlooked when conducting AAC assessments for people with developmental disabilities is literacy. However, given that the ability to read, spell, and write affords maximum flexibility when communicating through AAC, it is important to identify and take advantage of any literacy skills an individual may possess. Recently,

Iacono and Cupples (2004) developed the Assessment of Phonological Awareness and Reading (APAR)[3] tool for determining phonological awareness and other reading skills in adults with physical and/or intellectual disabilities who are unable to speak and/or write. Because the test was designed specifically for individuals who are unable to speak, verbal responses are not required. The APAR includes tasks to assess phonological awareness, phonological recoding, single-word vocabulary, sentence comprehension, and text listening comprehension. Research on the APAR indicates that adults with complex communication needs demonstrate the same positive association between phonological awareness and reading as has been found in other groups of individuals, both with and without disabilities, and that the APAR tasks provide a valid means of assessing phonological awareness and single-word reading skills (Iacono & Cupples, 2004).

In addition, researchers at the Center for Literacy and Disability Studies are conducting research on the reliability and validity of a literacy assessment tool called *ABC-Link*[4] (Erickson, Clendon, Koppenhaver, & Spadorcia, 2004; Erickson, Spadorcia, Koppenhaver, Cunningham, & Clendon, 2004). This tool was designed to guide the development of individual literacy instruction plans for individuals with complex communication needs who rely on AAC. It is based on the whole-to-part model (WTP) of the constructs underlying silent reading comprehension, which asserts that word identification, language comprehension, and whole-text print processing are all part of silent reading comprehension ability (Erickson, Koppenhaver & Cunningham, 2006). Pilot testing of the instrument is ongoing.

Assessment of Cultural and Family Needs

Historically, most AAC assessment and intervention approaches have been based on Anglo-European values about disability in general and communication in particular. However, over the past decade, there has been an explosion of research related to AAC interventions with persons of diverse cultures. In North America, more than a dozen studies have been conducted since 1995 to examine the attitudes and preferences of individuals from a wide range of ethic and cultural backgrounds with regard to communication and AAC, including Americans of African, Mexican, Hispanic, Vietnamese, Filipino, Southeast Asian, and Chinese backgrounds; American Indians; and both Chinese and Indo-Canadians (see Beukelman & Mirenda, 2005). Similar work is under way in other parts of the world as well (see Alant & Lloyd, 2005). Such studies can be used to support the development of culturally sensitive assessment and intervention practices based on an understanding of the impact of diversity.

Building on this research, several resources have been developed for use by teams endeavoring to provide culturally and economically sensitive AAC services. For example, *Families, Cultures, and AAC* is an interactive, multimedia education tool that was designed to support practitioners and families involved in AAC assessment and intervention (VanBiervliet & Parette, 1999). It includes video segments of family members from a variety of cultural backgrounds whose children use AAC, as well as interactive learning games, links to websites, a glossary, and numerous printable documents. An edited book titled *Augmentative and Alternative Communication and Severe Disabilities: Beyond Poverty* (Alant & Lloyd, 2005) examines both the challenges faced by AAC service providers supporting individuals in socioeconomically adverse circumstances (e.g.,

---

[3]The APAR is available in both a print and a software version at *www.elr.com.au/apar/*.
[4]See *viper.med.unc.edu/abclink/home.cfm* for additional information about the ABC-Link.

those in developing countries, the unemployed), as well as a wide range of prospective solutions. Finally, Huer (1997) published the Protocol for Culturally Inclusive Assessment of AAC, which contains a self-assessment questionnaire, a communication partner inventory, a communication needs assessment interview, and a capability and technology assessment protocol.

Increased awareness of the importance of cultural sensitivity during the AAC assessment and intervention process has also resulted in changes to commercially available AAC products. For example, the Mayer–Johnson Company[5] now includes numerous languages in its updated version of the Boardmaker software program, which allows for multiple languages on both paper- and computer-based communication displays. In addition, modern SGDs can be programmed to speak in multiple languages, making devices available to individuals from a variety of linguistic backgrounds.

Self-Determination in AAC Assessment

Over the past decade, increasing emphasis has been placed on supporting self-determination of persons with developmental disabilities (e.g., Wehmeyer & Garner, 2003). Research evidence showing that individuals with developmental disabilities benefit from providing input on all aspects of their lives is beginning to affect how AAC assessment procedures are implemented. For example, Sigafoos, O'Reilly, Ganz, Lancioni, and Schlosser (2005) investigated the ability of two adolescents with significant developmental disabilities to (1) demonstrate their preference among three SGDs to communicate requests for "more" and (2) demonstrate their preference between an SGD and a communication board to request snack items. Both individuals demonstrated unique preferences for different SGDs when given choices between three options. Both also demonstrated clear preferences for their selected SGD over a communication board, choosing the SGD between 70 and 100% of the time. The results suggest that individuals with developmental disabilities can be empowered to participate in the AAC decision-making process and that strategies can be provided to support them in demonstrating their preferences for AAC systems and devices.

AAC INTERVENTION: PLANNING INTERVENTIONS FOR TODAY AND TOMORROW

As noted previously, the purpose of an AAC assessment is to identify and match an individual's strengths, needs, and constraints to particular AAC intervention techniques. On completion of the AAC assessment, an AAC team can begin to develop specific intervention techniques designed to maximize and expand on current skills, as well as develop additional skills to support the use of more advanced AAC intervention techniques in the future.

Development of Early Communication Skills

Individuals with developmental disabilities often experience difficulty understanding symbols and the rules of language. Often referred to as early or "beginning" communicators, they may express themselves using informal means such as vocalizations, facial

---

[5]The Mayer–Johnson Company: *www.mayer-johnson.com*.

expressions, and gestures. Interventions for these individuals should focus on enhancing the quality of their nonsymbolic expressions and on expanding their repertoires to include symbolic communication. A number of research-based programs and instructional approaches have been developed in the past decade for early or beginning communicators. For example, First Things First (Rowland & Schweigert, 2004) provides practical strategies for teaching children to request desired events, gain attention, and make choices using presymbolic behaviors such as gestures, facial expressions, vocalizations, or microswitches. The Hanen Centre[6] has also developed a number of tools specific to communication development in both children and adults with developmental disabilities. *Allow Me!* (Ruiter, 2000) is a guide for promoting nonsymbolic communication skills in adults with developmental disabilities. It provides facilitators with strategies for identifying, expanding, and adapting age-appropriate activities to encourage both general communication skills and AAC use during interactions. More Than Words (Sussman, 1999) is a parent/facilitator training program designed to teach parents to use research-based strategies with children at all stages of communication development. Two recent studies that examined More Than Words (McConachie, Randle, Hammal, & LeCouteur, 2005) and Child's Talk, a similar training program developed in the United Kingdom (Aldred, Green, & Adams, 2004), provide positive evidence of the potential impact of these parent-training approaches on young children with autism.

Tangible Symbol Systems

As individuals progress in their use of nonsymbolic behaviors for communication, it is important to support the development of symbolic forms of communication that may be more readily understood by a larger community of interaction partners. Whereas some individuals may readily use photographs or picture symbols to communicate, others experience difficulty in understanding and using these representations without systematic instruction. The Tangible Symbol Systems™ (Rowland & Schweigert, 2000a) instructional materials were developed in response to this difficulty. The effectiveness of this research-based instructional approach was examined in a report that studied 41 children with intellectual disabilities, sensory impairments, autism and other pervasive developmental disorders, and multiple disabilities over a 3-year period (Rowland & Schweigert, 2000b). Among other things, the results indicated that individuals who were already able to communicate effectively using gestures or vocalizations were more readily able to learn tangible symbols than were those without intentional presymbolic communication skills. In addition, whereas 15% of the participants did not acquire any tangible symbols, the remaining 85% acquired at least two tangible symbols each, and 24% moved on to acquire more abstract symbols, as well.

Picture Exchange Communication System

Like Tangible Symbol Systems, the Picture Exchange Communication System (PECS) is an instructional approach for teaching beginning symbol use (Frost & Bondy, 2002). It is unique in that individuals are taught to exchange (i.e., give) rather than simply point to symbols in order to request desired items or activities. PECS also emphasizes self-initiated rather than prompted or verbally cued communication from the outset of instruction. There are now a number of published studies documenting success of PECS

---

[6]The Hanen Centre: *www.hanen.org.*

instruction with both adults (Chambers & Rehfeldt, 2003) and children with developmental disabilities, especially autism (e.g., Charlop-Christy, Carpenter, Le, LeBlanc, &
Kellet, 2002). Some of these have also documented a concurrent decrease in problem
behavior and/or an increase in natural speech production (e.g., Charlop-Christy et al.,
2002; Frea, Arnold, & Vittimberga, 2001).

Microswitches

Another area of increased interest that pertains to beginning communicators involves
the use of microswitches to enable individuals with significant physical and cognitive
impairments to make choices among two or more options of foods, drinks, or activities.
For example, Singh et al. (2003) taught an adolescent with complex communication
needs to make choices between food and drink options using a series of microswitches.
Several studies have also focused on evaluating responses for microswitch use, on determining the feasibility of establishing multiple responses for use with multiple microswitches, on evaluating the maintenance of microswitch responses and positive expressions of mood, and on adapting microswitch programs to encourage word awareness
and associations (see Lancioni, Singh, O'Reilly, & Oliva, 2003, for a review).

Beyond Requesting

There is little question that the vast majority of AAC research with people with developmental disabilities has focused on two related communicative functions: requesting and
choice making (Sigafoos & Mirenda, 2002). The reason is probably that learning to ask
for or make choices between desired items and activities is not only one of the most
basic and essential communication skills but also one of the most motivating for the
learner and therefore easiest to teach. However, people with developmental disabilities
who rely on AAC, like all people, have much more to say than "I want" or "Give me,"
and they require instruction in other aspects of communication, as well. Acknowledgement of this is evident in the increased research related to functions other than requesting and choice making that has appeared over the past decade. This includes research
aimed at identifying instructional techniques to teach functions such as rejecting
(Sigafoos, Drasgow, Reichle, O'Reilly, & Tait, 2004), initiating and maintaining conversational interactions (e.g., Light & Binger, 1998), and conversational repairs (Halle,
Brady, & Drasgow, 2004). As empirically validated strategies are developed for teaching
communication skills that go beyond simple requesting, individuals with developmental
disabilities who rely on AAC will be increasingly able to participate in a wide array of
school- and community-based activities and interactions.

Speech-Generating Devices

The past decade has been marked by an increased research interest in the potential benefits of SGDs for individuals with intellectual disabilities, in particular. Schlosser,
Blischak, and Koul (2003) identified a number of studies that addressed the impact of
SGDs on both people who rely on AAC and their communication partners. Not surprisingly, they found that digitized or recorded speech enhances intelligibility for communication partners compared with synthetic speech, although some studies report
improved understanding of synthetic speech with repeated exposure. With regard to
the impact of SGDs on communication partners' attitudes, they noted that, whereas

some studies suggest that SGD use results in improved partner attitudes, others found no impact when SGDs were compared with nonelectronic techniques.

A growing body of research has also investigated the impact of SGDs on the functional communication abilities of individuals with varying degrees of intellectual disabilities. As is the case for AAC in general, most of these studies have focused on teaching communicative requesting using SGDs (e.g., Sigafoos, Didden, & O'Reilly, 2003; Van Acker & Grant, 1995). A few have also sought to teach SGD use for other purposes, including basic social interactions and conversational repairs (e.g., Schepis, Reid, Behrmann, & Sutton, 1998; Sigafoos, Drasgow, Halle, et al., 2004), as well as simple spelling (Schlosser, Blischak, Belfiore, Bartley, & Barnett, 1998). In addition to the acquisition of specific communication skills, several collateral effects of SGD use have also been documented, including increased receptive labeling skills, increased speech production, and decreased problem behavior (e.g., Brady, 2000; Durand, 1999; Sigafoos, Didden, & O'Reilly, 2003). It appears clear that SGD technologies, although still not in widespread use with people with intellectual disabilities, hold great promise.

Language Development

Recent research is also aimed at investigating the use of SGDs to promote language development in young children with developmental disabilities. Some research in this area is focused on the relative ease with which individuals learn to use SGDs that employ visual scene displays versus traditional grid displays (Fallon, Light, & Achenbach, 2003). A visual scene display (VSD) is a picture, photograph, or scanned image that represents a situation, place, or experience and that contains symbolic elements such as people, actions, or objects. When specific areas of the visual scene are activated (i.e., touched), a spoken message is produced. VSDs are different from traditional grid displays in that they display realistic-looking scenes in which symbols appear in context, whereas traditional grid displays contain symbols laid out in decontextualized rows and columns. Recent research suggests that VSDs arc casicr for young, typically developing children (as young as 2 years of age) to learn and use than traditional grid displays (Fallon et al., 2003). In addition, there is preliminary evidence that the use of VSDs to model language in play contexts can lead to rapid vocabulary and concept development in young children with such disabilities as severe cerebral palsy, Down syndrome, and autism (Drager et al., 2005; Light & Drager, 2005).

Including Students Who Use AAC in Inclusive Settings

To a greater extent than ever before, many students with developmental disabilities currently receive their education in inclusive settings. For inclusion to be successful, all students—including those who communicate and write using AAC—must be able to participate in the learning and social opportunities of the general education classroom. Research over the past decade has focused on understanding both the skills needed for participation and means of promoting participation in inclusive classrooms and other settings.

Young Children

The removal of eligibility criteria in AAC assessment and intervention has had a significant impact on the provision of AAC services to children ages birth to 5 years. Beliefs that AAC should be used only as a last resort, that AAC impedes spoken language development, that children must demonstrate numerous prerequisite skills in order to benefit from AAC, and that SGDs are appropriate only for older children or for those without cognitive disabilities have been refuted by accumulated research (Cress & Marvin, 2003; Romski & Sevcik, 2005). This marks the beginning of an important chapter in AAC: service delivery to infants and toddlers. Research in this area by Mary Ann Romski at Georgia State University[7] and by Janice Light at the Pennsylvania State University[8] is ongoing.

As increasing numbers of students are receiving AAC services at younger ages, more attention is being placed on strategies for supporting these students in preschool classrooms. For example, Von Tetzchner, Brekke, Sjothun, and Grindheim (2005) described numerous strategies for scaffolding communication and language development to support children using manual signs and graphic communication in inclusive preschool settings. In particular, they noted the importance of teaching nondisabled peers the skills required for successful interactions with classmates who rely on AAC in order to develop a shared language environment that enables all members of the class to communicate about self-determined topics with ease and efficiency.

School-Age Individuals

Research examining effective models for supporting students who use AAC in regular classrooms has also evolved over the past decade. For example, Schlosser et al. (2000) taught a school team to implement the assessment framework of the Participation Model with a student with cerebral palsy to enable him to participate in integrated literacy and math activities using AAC and other assistive technologies. Following student assessment and staff training, barriers to participation were reduced, and the student's participation approached the level of his nondisabled peers. Other authors have also described strategies for AAC assessment and for supporting the development of communication and literacy skills in general education classrooms. For example, Light, Roberts, Dimarco, and Greiner (1998) used Participation Model processes to design a multimodal communication system for a boy with autism in elementary school .

Currently, Beyond Access[9] is a 4-year model demonstration project being conducted by the Institute on Disability at the University of New Hampshire, with the goal of using accepted AAC principles and practices in novel ways to promote improved learning of the general education curriculum by students with significant disabilities. In a recent case study report, Sonnenmeier, McSheehan, and Jorgensen (2005) described use of the Beyond Access model to support Jay, a 10-year-old student with autism who was included in a general education classroom. This planning model emphasizes the assumption of student competence, focused strategies to support team collaboration, and the implementation of best-practice strategies for inclusive education. It was used to help Jay's team to identify the supports that were needed to fully include him in the general education curriculum. Throughout the process, Jay's team learned to have high expectations for him and to work together to plan and implement instructional supports. Concurrently, Jay developed an accurate and consistent "yes/no" response, learned to use a dynamic display SGD to participate in classroom activities, began to

---

[7]See *www2.gsu.edu/~wwwmar/index.html.*
[8]See *aac-rerc.org/pages/news/webcasts2005.htm#may1.*
[9]See *iod.unh.edu/projects/beyond_access.html.*

recognize printed words, and became increasingly involved as an active participant in regular classroom activities with his peers.

The provision of AAC interventions to adolescents in inclusive high school settings has also received attention. Downing (2005) addressed specific strategies that enabled students who rely on AAC to work on specific communication goals that were embedded within the academic curriculum (e.g., requesting a break, making choices, or saying "no" instead of engaging in problem behavior). Similarly, Hughes et al. (2000) provided evidence that self-prompted communication book training for four high school students with extensive support needs was associated with increases in participants' appropriate initiations and general education conversational partners' corresponding responses. Such approaches deal with one of the primary concerns regarding the educational inclusion of students with significant developmental disabilities in high schools: the belief that these students cannot address their unique learning goals within the context of an academic setting. Rather, evidence has accumulated to show that the inclusion of students who rely on AAC in general education settings ensures (1) a rich language environment in which they can develop language and communication skills, (2) increased opportunities for social interaction with nondisabled peers, and (3) increased opportunities for learning in the context of the general education curriculum.

AAC and Problem Behavior

Often, persons with developmental disabilities who do not have a reliable means of communication engage in problem behavior. Research has demonstrated that problem behavior may serve a number of functions, including (1) obtaining desired items, activities, or environments; (2) obtaining attention; (3) escaping a nonpreferred or nondesired activity, environment, or interaction; and (4) regulating levels of sensory arousal (Sigafoos, Arthur, & O'Reilly, 2003). Functional behavior assessment can be used to identify hypotheses regarding the functions (i.e., purposes) of problem behavior and to develop interventions based on this information (Bopp, Brown, & Mirenda, 2004).

Two types of AAC interventions are frequently used to address problem behavior in persons with developmental disabilities: functional communication training (FCT) and visual schedules. FCT involves teaching specific communication skills that are functionally equivalent to problem behavior, based on a behavior assessment. For example, if an individual engages in problem behavior in order to escape a nonpreferred task, FCT would involve teaching an alternative but appropriate means for achieving the same result. Just prior to the problem behavior occurring or as it begins, the individual might be taught to sign "break," to give a break card to a communication partner, or to activate a single-message SGD that has been programmed to say "I would like a break, please." Numerous research studies have demonstrated that FCT can be used successfully in school and home settings to address problem behavior that serves a variety of purposes (e.g., escape, attention, and access to desired items). FCT can be implemented with a variety of AAC modalities, including gestures, manual signs, picture symbols, printed words, and SGDs (Bopp et al., 2004).

Research has also demonstrated that, for many individuals with developmental disabilities, predictability is extremely important (Flannery & O'Neill, 1995). An AAC intervention intended to provide increased predictability is visual scheduling, which involves depicting a sequence of activities or steps using graphic symbols that are readily understood by the individual. The intention is to provide the individual with a way to understand upcoming events or a sequence of steps within an activity, in order to reduce problem behavior and increase independence (Mesibov, Browder, & Kirkland, 2002). More than a dozen research studies have provided evidence that visual schedules can be used successfully to reduce problem behavior dramatically and to increase independent, on-task performance (Bopp et al., 2004).

It is clear from the research that AAC interventions can have a profound impact on the resolution of problem behavior in persons with developmental disabilities. Understanding that problem behavior can be communicative in nature, using functional assessment to determine the function of problem behavior, and developing communication-based intervention strategies (including those that incorporate AAC) related to the identified function are all important strategies in this regard.

"Nothing about Me without Me"

As is the case in many other areas, people with developmental disabilities who rely on AAC have become increasingly outspoken as self-advocates over the past decade. This is evident in the publication of several edited books that feature stories and other media authored by these individuals (e.g., Fried-Oken & Bersani, 2000; Williams & Krezman, 2000). It is also evident in the increased focus on research in which augmented communicators and/or their families are actively involved in the research process, not as mere participants but as true collaborators (Krogh & Lindsay, 1999). For example, in two Australian studies, augmented communicators provided advice and guidance during the development phase (Balandin & Morgan, 2001; Balandin & Iacono, 1999). In another report, augmented communicators provided both feedback and guidance with regard to an ongoing large-scale project aimed at developing Web-based assessment and instructional supports for literacy development (Iacono, Balandin, & Cupples, 2001). Studies such as these are important in that they both acknowledge and incorporate the valuable insights of people who use AAC and their families (Bersani, 1999). They also remind us that, in the end, the outcomes of research must be aimed at enhancing the possibility that people who rely on AAC can become self-determined and autonomous. In the words of Michael Williams (1995), an advocate with cerebral palsy who communicates through AAC, "Whose outcome is it anyway?" (p. 2).

IMPLICATIONS

Implications for Practitioners

Advancements in the AAC field over the past decade have a number of implications for both preservice and in-service training of professionals who provide AAC supports. In light of "official" statements from organizations such as ASHA and the NJC regarding the inappropriateness of eligibility criteria, training is needed to provide information about assessment and intervention strategies for individuals across the ability range. Practitioners need to understand the impact of opportunity barriers on communication development and competence, as well as strategies for remediation of such barriers. Practitioners must also develop an awareness of how to frame AAC assessments and interventions to accommodate the diverse needs of families and augmented communicators from a wide range of cultural and linguistic backgrounds. As AAC interventions are increasingly shown to be effective for very young children, practitioners will require training on specific intervention strategies that are appropriate for this age group. In addition, as evidence continues to accumulate about the potential benefits of SGDs for persons with intellectual disabilities in particular, practitioners will need to develop the skills necessary to prescribe appropriate devices, secure funding for them, and implement effective SGD-based interventions. Finally, evidence on the effectiveness of AAC strategies for remediation of problem behavior means that practitioners must be prepared to conduct functional behavior assessment and to design AAC interventions based on this information.

Implications for Policy Makers

Perhaps the most significant implication of recent developments in the AAC field relates to the provision of SGDs for persons with developmental disabilities across the lifespan. In the United States, SGDs are now considered to be "durable medical equipment," and funding for SGDs can be accessed through Medicare by individuals who are eligible.[10] Those without Medicare coverage must apply for funding through private insurance companies or state-sponsored programs (e.g., the Division of Vocational Rehabilitation), depending again on eligibility. Assessment by a speech–language pathologist with background in AAC is required, regardless of the funding source. In Canada, each province has unique guidelines and programs related to SGD access. For example, school-age children in British Columbia with visual impairments, physical disabilities, and/or autism can access SGDs through a provincial resource program up to age 19; students with disabilities other than these (e.g., Down syndrome) cannot. In addition, a pilot project is currently in place in British Columbia to provide similar services to persons ages 19–27 with the same disabilities. However, in Alberta, the province directly to the east of British Columbia, none of these services are available on a province-wide basis. In both the United States and Canada, the variability of SGD access for individuals with developmental disabilities is a significant barrier at the present time and must be rectified in order to ensure that all individuals have equal access to such AAC interventions.

Implications for Researchers

The AAC research agenda over the next decade should be focused on a number of interrelated components that affect people with developmental disabilities. Research is needed to better understand how to involve persons with developmental disabilities more actively in AAC assessment and intervention planning, especially with regard to selecting specific components of an AAC system (Sigafoos et al., 2005). Empirically validated assessment tools are needed in areas such as symbol, literacy, and complex motor assessment. Research comparing the effectiveness of existing instructional techniques such as Tangible Symbols and PECS, as well as research aimed at developing new techniques for teaching communicative functions beyond simple requesting, are needed. Research aimed at identifying the impact of SGDs on natural speech development, language development, and functional communication skills is needed to guide both funding and intervention decisions. Research on the effectiveness of various AAC interven-

---

[10]For more information regarding Medicare funding of SGDs, go to *www.aac-rerc.com/pages/medicare/MCgeneral.htm.*

tions for very young children and on the development of child-friendly, readily learnable AAC devices is also crucial. Finally, focused research on efficient and effective models to include individuals who rely on AAC in inclusive school and community settings will serve to guide care providers and practitioners.

CONCLUSION

The past decade has seen an explosion of AAC research related to persons with developmental disabilities, including those with significant intellectual impairments. Research has been focused primarily on strategies for supporting functional communication development and increasing the social participation of persons with developmental disabilities across the lifespan. The Participation Model (Beukelman & Mirenda, 2005) has been widely used as a process for ongoing AAC assessment and intervention. Persons with developmental disabilities now have increased access to quality AAC interventions in inclusive environments; families have increasing access to AAC professionals who consider their unique cultural and linguistic needs; and educators are increasingly empowered to teach students who rely on AAC in general education classrooms. Recent emphasis on the importance of evidence-based research and on the evaluation of AAC intervention outcomes in natural contexts (Schlosser & Raghavendra, 2003) supports the development of a meaningful research agenda for the next decade. In particular, the AAC–Rehabilitation Engineering Research Center on Communication Enhancement[11] includes a number of research and development projects that pertain directly to individuals with developmental disabilities across the age range. The future for persons with developmental disabilities who experience communication challenges is promising as we continue to develop strategies for AAC assessment and intervention that enable them to fully participate in home, school, and community life.

REFERENCES

Alant, E., & Lloyd, L. L. (2005). *Augmentative and alternative communication and severe disabilities: Beyond poverty*. London: Whurr.

Aldred, C., Green, J., & Adams, C. (2004). A new social communication intervention for children with autism: Pilot randomized controlled treatment study suggesting effectiveness. *Journal of Child Psychology and Psychiatry, 45*, 1420–1430.

American Speech–Language–Hearing Association. (2004). Roles and responsibilities of speech–language pathologists with respect to augmentative and alternative communication: Technical report. *ASHA Supplement, 24*, 1–17.

American Speech–Language–Hearing Association. (2005). Roles and responsibilities of speech–language pathologists with respect to alternative communication: Position statement. *ASHA Supplement, 25*, 1–2.

Balandin, S., & Iacono, T. (1999). Crews, wusses, and whoppas: Core and fringe vocabularies of Australian meal-break conversations in the workplace. *Augmentative and Alternative Communication, 15*, 95–109.

Balandin, S., & Morgan, J. (2001). Preparing for the future: Aging and alternative and augmentative communication. *Augmentative and Alternative Communication, 17*, 99–108.

---

[11]See *www.aac-rerc.com/*.

Bersani, H., Jr. (1999). Nothing about me without me: A proposal for participatory action research in AAC. In F. T. Loncke, J. Clibbens, H. A. Arvidson, & L. L. Lloyd (Eds.), *Augmentative and alternative communication: New directions in research and practice* (pp. 278–289). London: Whurr.

Beukelman, D. R., & Mirenda, P. (2005). *Augmentative and alternative communication: Supporting children and adults with complex communication needs* (3rd ed.). Baltimore: Brookes.

Blackstone, S., & Hunt Berg, M. (2003). *Social networks: A communication inventory for individuals with complex communication needs and their communication partners: Manual.* Monterey, CA: Augmentative Communication.

Bopp, K. D., Brown, K. E., & Mirenda, P. (2004). Speech–language pathologists' roles in the delivery of positive behavior supports for individuals with developmental disabilities. *American Journal of Speech–Language Pathology, 13,* 5–19.

Brady, N. (2000). Improved comprehension of object names following voice output communication aid use: Two case studies. *Augmentative and Alternative Communication, 16,* 197–204.

Chambers, M., & Rehfeldt, R. A. (2003). Assessing the acquisition and generalization of two mand forms with adults with severe developmental disabilities. *Research in Developmental Disabilities, 24,* 265–280.

Charlop-Christy, M., Carpenter, M., Le, L., LeBlanc, L., & Kellet, K. (2002). Using the Picture Exchange Communication System (PECS) with children with autism: Assessment of PECS acquisition, speech, social–communicative behavior, and problem behavior. *Journal of Applied Behavior Analysis, 35,* 213–232.

Cress, C., & Marvin, C. (2003). Common questions about AAC services in early intervention. *Augmentative and Alternative Communication, 19,* 254–272.

Downing, J. E. (2005). Inclusive education for high school students with severe intellectual disabilities: Supporting communication. *Augmentative and Alternative Communication, 21,* 132–148.

Drager, K., Light, J., Angert, E., Finke, E., Larson, H., Venzon, L., et al. (2005, November). *AAC and interactive play: Language learning in children with autism.* Paper presented at the annual conference of the American Speech–Language–Hearing Association, San Diego, CA.

Durand, V. M. (1999). Functional communication training using assistive devices: Recruiting natural communities of reinforcement. *Journal of Applied Behavior Analysis, 32,* 247–267.

Erickson, K. A., Clendon, S. A., Koppenhaver, D. A., & Spadorcia, S. A. (2004, October). *The reliability of a written language comprehension assessment measure.* Seminar presented at the biennial conference of the International Society for Augmentative and Alternative Communication (ISAAC), Natal, Brazil.

Erickson, K. A., Koppenhaver, D. A., & Cunningham, J. W. (2006). Balanced reading intervention in augmentative communication. In R. McCauley & M. Fey (Eds.), *Treatment of language disorders in children: Conventional and controversial interventions.* Baltimore: Brookes.

Erickson, K. A., Spadorcia, S., Koppenhaver, D., Cunningham, J., & Clendon, S. (2004, December). *Establishing the construct validity of a universally accessible word recognition assessment.* Paper presented at the annual meeting of the National Reading Conference, San Antonio, TX.

Fallon, K. A., Light, J., & Achenbach, A. (2003). The semantic organization patterns of young children: Implications for augmentative and alternative communication. *Augmentative and Alternative Communication, 19,* 74–85.

Flannery, B., & O'Neill, R. E. (1995). Including predictability in functional assessment and individual program development. *Education and Treatment of Children, 18,* 499–509.

Frea, W., Arnold, C., & Vittimberga, G. (2001). A demonstration of the effects of augmentative communication on the extreme aggressive behavior of a child with autism within an integrated preschool setting. *Journal of Positive Behavior Interventions, 3,* 194–198.

Fried-Oken, M., & Bersani, H., Jr. (Eds.). (2000). *Speaking up and spelling it out.* Baltimore: Brookes.

Frost, L., & Bondy, A. (2002). *Picture Exchange Communication System training manual* (2nd ed.). Newark, DE: Pyramid Education.

Halle, J., Brady, N., & Drasgow, E. (2004). Enhancing socially adaptive communicative repairs of beginning communicators with disabilities. *American Journal of Speech–Language Pathology, 13,* 43–54.

Huer, M. B. (1997). Culturally inclusive assessments for children using augmentative and alternative communication. *Journal of Children's Communication Development, 19,* 23–34.

Hughes, C., Rung, L., Wehmeyer, M., Agran, M., Copeland, S., & Hwang, B. (2000). Self-prompted communication book use to increase social interaction among high school students. *Journal of the Association for Persons with Severe Handicaps, 25,* 153–166.

Iacono, T., Balandin, S., & Cupples, L. (2001). Focus group discussions of literacy assessment and World Wide Web-based reading intervention. *Augmentative and Alternative Communication, 17,* 27–36.

Iacono, T., & Cupples, L. (2004). Assessment of phonemic awareness and word reading skills of people with complex communication needs. *Journal of Speech, Language, and Hearing Research, 47,* 437–449.

Johnson, R. (1994). *The Picture Communication Symbols combination book.* Solana Beach, CA: Mayer-Johnson.

Krogh, K. S., & Lindsay, P. H. (1999). Including people with disabilities in research: Implications for the field of augmentative and alternative communication. *Augmentative and Alternative Communication, 15,* 222–233.

Lancioni, G. E., Singh, N. N., O'Reilly, M. F., & Oliva, D. (2003). Some recent research efforts on microswitches for persons with multiple disabilities. *Journal of Child and Family Studies, 12,* 251–256.

Light, J., & Binger, C. (1998). *Building communicative competence with individuals who use augmentative and alternative communication.* Baltimore: Brookes.

Light, J., & Drager, K. (2005, November). *Maximizing language development with young children who require AAC.* Paper presented at the annual conference of the American Speech–Language–Hearing Association, San Diego, CA.

Light, J., Roberts, B., Dimarco, R., & Greiner, N. (1998). Augmentative and alternative communication to support receptive and expressive communication for people with autism. *Journal of Communication Disorders, 31,* 153–180.

Lund, S., Millar, D., Herman, M., Hinds, A., & Light, J. (1998, November). *Children's pictorial representations of early emerging concepts: Implications for AAC.* Paper presented at the annual convention of the American Speech–Language–Hearing Association, San Antonio, TX.

McCarthy, C., McLean, L., Miller, J., Paul-Brown, D., Romski, M. A., Rourk, J., et al. (1998). *Communication supports checklist for programs serving individuals with severe disabilities.* Baltimore: Brookes.

McConachie, H., Randle, V., Hammal, D., & LeCouteur, A. (2005). A controlled trial of a training course for parents of children with suspected autism spectrum disorder. *Journal of Pediatrics, 147,* 335–340.

Mesibov, G. B., Browder, D. A., & Kirkland, C. (2002). Using individualized schedules as a component of positive behavioral support for students with developmental disabilities. *Journal of Positive Behavior Interventions, 4,* 73–79.

Mirenda, P., & Locke, P. A. (1989). A comparison of symbol transparency in nonspeaking persons with intellectual disabilities. *Journal of Speech and Hearing Disorders, 54,* 131–140.

National Joint Committee for the Communicative Needs of Persons with Severe Disabilities. (2003a). Position statement on access to communication services and supports: Concerns regarding the application of restrictive "eligibility" policies. *ASHA Supplement, 23,* 19–20.

National Joint Committee for the Communicative Needs of Persons with Severe Disabilities. (2003b). Supporting documentation for the position statement on access to communication services and supports: Concerns regarding the application of restrictive "eligibility" policies. *ASHA Supplement, 23,* 73–81.

Romski, M. A., & Sevcik, R. A. (2005). Augmentative communication and early intervention. *Infants and Young Children, 18,* 174–185.

Rowland, C. (1996). *Communication matrix.* Portland, OR: Design to Learn Projects.

Rowland, C., & Schweigert, P. (1999). *Time to learn.* Portland, OR: Design to Learn Projects.

Rowland, C., & Schweigert, P. (2000a). *Tangible Symbol Systems: Making the right to communicate a reality for individuals with severe disabilities.* Portland, OR: Design to Learn Projects.

Rowland, C., & Schweigert, P. (2000b). Tangible symbols, tangible outcomes. *Augmentative and Alternative Communication, 16,* 61–78.

Rowland, C., & Schweigert, P. (2002a). *The home inventory of problem-solving skills (HIPSS).* Portland, OR: Design to Learn Projects.

Rowland, C., & Schweigert, P. (2002b). *The school inventory of problem-solving skills (SIPSS).* Portland, OR: Design to Learn Projects.

Rowland, C., & Schweigert, P. (2003). Cognitive skills and AAC. In J. C. Light, D. R. Beukelman, & J. Reichle (Eds.), *Communicative competence for individuals who use AAC: From research to effective practice* (pp. 241–275). Baltimore: Brookes.

Rowland, C., & Schweigert, P. (2004). *First things first: Early communication for the pre-symbolic child with severe disabilities*. Portland, OR: Design to Learn Projects.

Ruiter, I. (2000). *Allow me!* Toronto, Ontario, Canada: Hanen Centre.

Schepis, M., Reid, D., Behrmann, M., & Sutton, K. (1998). Increasing communicative interactions of young children with autism using a voice output communication aid and naturalistic teaching. *Journal of Applied Behavior Analysis, 31,* 561–578.

Schlosser, R., Blischak, D., Belfiore, P., Bartley, C., & Barnett, N. (1998). Effects of synthetic speech output and orthographic feedback in a student with autism: A preliminary study. *Journal of Autism and Developmental Disorders, 28,* 309–319.

Schlosser, R., Blischak, D., & Koul, R. (2003). Roles of speech output in AAC. In R. Schlosser (Ed.), *The efficacy of augmentative and alternative communication: Toward evidence-based practice* (pp. 472–532). New York: Elsevier.

Schlosser, R., McGhie-Richmond, D., Blackstien-Adler, S., Mirenda, P., Antonius, K., & Janzen, P. (2000). Training a school team to integrate technology meaningfully into the curriculum: Effects on student participation. *Journal of Special Education Technology, 15,* 31–44.

Schlosser, R., & Raghavendra, P. (2003). Toward evidence-based practice in AAC. In R. Schlosser (Ed.), *The efficacy of augmentative and alternative communication: Toward evidence-based practice* (pp. 260–297). New York: Elsevier.

Sigafoos, J. (1999). Creating opportunities for augmentative and alternative communication: Strategies for involving people with developmental disabilities. *Augmentative and Alternative Communication, 15,* 183–190.

Sigafoos, J., Arthur, M., & O'Reilly, M. (2003). *Challenging behavior and developmental disability*. Baltimore: Brookes.

Sigafoos, J., Didden, R., & O'Reilly, M. (2003). Effects of speech output on maintenance of requesting and frequency of vocalizations in three children with developmental disabilities. *Augmentative and Alternative Communication, 19,* 37–47.

Sigafoos, J., Drasgow, E., Halle, J., O'Reilly, M., Seely-York, S., Edrisinha, C., et al. (2004). Teaching VOCA use as a communicative repair strategy. *Journal of Autism and Developmental Disorders, 34,* 411–422.

Sigafoos, J., Drasgow, E., Reichle, J., O'Reilly, M., & Tait, K. (2004). Tutorial: Teaching communicative rejecting to children with severe disabilities. *American Journal of Speech–Language Pathology, 13,* 31–42.

Sigafoos, J., & Mirenda, P. (2002). Strengthening communicative behaviors for gaining access to desired items and activities. In J. Reichle, D. Beukelman & J. Light (Eds.), *Exemplary practices for beginning communicators: Implications for AAC* (pp. 123–156). Baltimore: Brookes.

Sigafoos, J., O'Reilly, M. F., Ganz, J. B., Lancioni, G. E., & Schlosser, R. (2005). Supporting self-determination in AAC interventions by assessing preference for communication devices. *Technology and Disability, 17,* 1–11.

Sigafoos, J., Woodyatt, G., Tucker, M., Roberts-Pennell, D., Keen, D., Tait, K., et al. (1998). *Inventory of Potential Communicative Acts (IPCA)*. Queensland, Australia: University of Queensland.

Singh, N., Lancioni, G., O'Reilly, M., Molina, E., Adkins, A., & Oliva, D. (2003). Self-determination during mealtimes through microswitch choice-making by an individual with complex multiple disabilities and profound mental retardation. *Journal of Positive Behavior Interventions, 5,* 209–215.

Sonnenmeier, R. M., McSheehan, M., & Jorgensen, C. M. (2005). A case study of team supports for a student with autism's communication and engagement within the general education curriculum: Preliminary report of the beyond access model. *Augmentative and Alternative Communication, 21,* 101–115.

Sussman, F. (1999). *More than words: The Hanen program for parents of children with autism spectrum disorder*. Toronto, Ontario, Canada: Hanen Centre.

Van Acker, R., & Grant, S. (1995). An effective computer-based requesting system for persons with Rett syndrome. *Journal of Childhood Communication Disorders, 16,* 31–38.

VanBiervliet, A., & Parette, P. (1999). *Families, cultures, and AAC* [CD-ROM]. Little Rock, AR: Southeast Missouri State University and University of Arkansas.

Von Tetzchner, S., Brekke, K. M., Sjothun, B., & Grindheim, E. (2005). Constructing preschool communities of learners that afford alternative language development. *Augmentative and Alternative Communication, 21,* 82–100.

Wehmeyer, M., & Garner, N. (2003). The impact of personal characteristics of people with intellectual and developmental disability on self-determination and autonomous functioning. *Journal of Applied Research in Intellectual Disabilities, 16,* 255–265.

Wetherby, A., & Prizant, B. M. (1993). *Communication and Symbolic Behavior Scales (CSBS).* Baltimore: Brookes.

Wetherby, A., & Prizant, B. M. (2002). *Communication and Symbolic Behavior Scales Developmental Profile (CSBS DP).* Baltimore: Brookes.

Wilkinson, K. M., & Jagaroo, V. (2004). Contributions of principles of visual cognitive science to AAC system display design. *Augmentative and Alternative Communication, 20,* 123–136.

Williams, M. (1995, March). Whose outcome is it anyway? *Alternatively Speaking, 2*(1), 1–2, 6.

Williams, M., & Krezman, C. (Eds.). (2000). *Beneath the surface: Creative expressions of augmented communicators.* Toronto, Ontario, Canada: ISAAC Press.

17

Physical Activity and Youth with Developmental Disabilities

Georgia C. Frey

Physical activity is a leading health indicator that has received significant attention in the research literature over the past 20 years. The Healthy People documents have prompted a concerted effort to better understand the association between physical activity and various health outcomes, dose–response relationships, and activity determinants in both adults and children, including those with developmental disabilities (DD; U.S. Department of Health and Human Services [USDHHS], 2000). The importance of physical activity to physiological, emotional, cognitive, and social development of all youth is well accepted (U.S. Department of Health and Human Services and Department of Education [USDHHSDE], 2000); however, little is known about physical activity behaviors, determinants, and outcomes in youth with DD. Regular physical activity may be even more vital to the development of children with DD because secondary conditions and complications that stem from inactivity can negatively affect global health, personal functioning, and independence (Heath & Fentem, 1997).

The incidence of childhood disability and life expectancies of people with disabilities are increasing, and even those with severe disabilities are living into adulthood (Ayyangar, 2002). The ability of children with DD to enjoy their youth and to become and remain confident and contributing adult members of society largely depends on their physical health, which is directly influenced by participation in regular physical activity. Therefore, the purpose of this chapter is to review the extant literature on physical activity and school-age youth with DD. The goal is to provide academics, practitioners, and families with the knowledge necessary to enhance physical activity in the target population by: (1) increasing the quantity and quality of empirical research and

(2) developing policies and practices that will increase the quantity and quality of activity opportunities.

Before proceeding, I must clarify basic terminology used throughout this document. "Physical activity" is defined as bodily movement that produces muscle contractions resulting in energy expenditure; "exercise" is a subcategory of physical activity that is planned, structured, and repetitive and undertaken for the purpose of improving fitness; and "physical fitness" is a set of attributes related to the ability to perform activity (Caspersen, 1989). The terms "physical fitness" and "physical activity" are frequently used interchangeably, but they represent distinct, albeit related, health indicators, with somewhat different applications in children and adults. The term "developmental disability" will include those with physical, mental, and health conditions that could contribute to a developmental delay, according to the Developmental Disabilities Assistance and Bill of Rights Act (2000).

Physical activity is the current focus of public health and school-based interventions because it is viewed as a modifiable behavior, whereas physical fitness is an attribute that may be more difficult to alter (USDHHSDE, 2000). This chapter focuses primarily on published research in which *physical activity* is the variable of interest. Exercise, physical fitness, play, motor behavior, recreation, and sports are discussed as they relate to physical activity, but the terms are not used interchangeably.

STATUS OF PHYSICAL ACTIVITY IN YOUTH WITH DEVELOPMENTAL DISABILITIES

Physical activity in children without disabilities has been the topic of significant inquiry over the past 10 years. Similar research in children with DD is relatively limited, but there appears to be an increased interest in this area as evidenced by recent government publications (USDHHS, 2005; U.S. Public Health Service [USPHS], 2002). The following section presents a general summary of the research on activity levels and determinants in children with and without DD.

Physical Activity Levels

Unlike adults, elementary-age children typically acquire physical activity intermittently and sporadically through play (Bailey et al., 1995) and seldom engage in formal exercise with the intention to lose weight or become physically fit (National Association for Sport and Physical Education [NASPE], 1998). Physical activity in adolescents tends to be more prolonged and organized, similar to that of adults (Malina, Bouchard, & Bar-Or, 2004). Obvious fundamental movement differences and global developmental disparities required the creation of separate health-related activity recommendations for children and adults. Children should accumulate at least 30–60 minutes of physical activity on all or most days of the week, including 10–15 minutes of continuous moderate to vigorous activity. Up to several hours of activity each day is encouraged, and periods of inactivity are discouraged (NASPE, 1998). During adolescence, the recommendations begin to approximate those for adults, with an increased emphasis on activity duration, specifically daily or almost daily moderate activity and 20 or more minutes of continuous moderate to vigorous activity at least three times per week (USDHHSDE, 2000).

Despite the public health emphasis on the importance of regular activity, many children across age groups are not meeting the basic guidelines, which undoubtedly contributes to the dramatic rise in childhood obesity and other health problems over the past 15 years (Rosenbloom, Young, Joe, & Winter, 1999). Most adolescents do not engage in five or more bouts of moderate activity per week (Gordon-Larsen, Nelson, & Popkin, 2004). The data on physical activity in preadolescent youth indicates that whereas on average children meet activity guidelines, many engage in minimal levels of regular physical activity (Simons-Morton et al., 1997). Low activity levels have also recently been observed in preschool-age children (Pate, Pfeiffer, Trost, Ziegler, & Dowda, 2004), and a possible trend toward sedentary behavior at this young age poses particularly disturbing health and educational concerns.

Whereas extensive research exists on the physical activity behaviors, patterns, and determinants in youth without DD, there is a paucity of similar data on children with DD. The available research is primarily descriptive, and only a few published exercise or activity intervention studies have included youth with DD, with most designed to improve physical fitness, not physical activity (Eiholzer et al., 2003; Klepper, 1999; Lotan, Isakov, & Merrick, 2004). There is a general consensus that children with DD are less active than nondisabled peers, but this is not uniformly substantiated by research. Several studies report that youth with intellectual disabilities (Suzuki et al., 1991), physical disabilities (Longmuir & Bar-Or, 2000), visual impairments (Kozub & Oh, 2004; Longmuir & Bar-Or, 2000), and other health impairments (Fredriksen, Ingjer, & Thaulow, 2000) are less active than nondisabled peers. Conversely, there are reports that children with other health impairments (Nixon, Orenstein, & Kelsey, 2001), intellectual disabilities (Faison-Hodge & Porretta, 2004), and autism spectrum disorders (Rosser Sandt & Frey, 2005) exhibit activity levels similar to those of peers without DD. The few studies that have interpreted physical activity levels of youth with DD according to published guidelines indicate that, although this population is less active than peers, minimum recommendations are being met (Kozub, 2003; Pan & Frey, 2006; Rosser Sandt & Frey, 2005). However, because there is no consistency in study designs or instrumentation, and in absence of a large-scale national study, it is premature to draw conclusions about physical activity levels in youth with DD across age levels, gender, ethnicity, or disability categories.

Physical Activity Determinants

Youth physical activity determinants are difficult to ascertain and vary greatly according to complex and dynamic biological, environmental, psychosocial, and cultural influences. The data are fairly consistent that (1) activity levels are highest during childhood and decline dramatically during adolescence, (2) girls are less active than boys, and (3) ethnic minorities are less active than European Americans (Sallis, Prochaska, & Taylor, 2000). Fox and Riddoch (2000) maintain that physical activity in youth is decreasing due to parental safety fears, reduction in time designated for physical education in schools, overreliance on automobiles for transportation, and excessive use of technology for entertainment. Because physical activity is a multidimensional and dynamic behavior that varies among diverse groups, it is unlikely that research will pinpoint stable and generalizable psychosocial or environmental determinants.

Information is lacking about factors that influence activity in youth with DD. Functional abilities and severity of disabling condition appear to have a greater influence on activity participation than actual diagnosis (Schenker, Coster, & Parush, 2005); however, those whose needs are less physical (e.g., who are deaf) are more active than those with mental or physical disabilities (Longmuir & Bar-Or, 2000; Suzuki et al., 1991). Other social and environmental activity determinants in youth with DD that have been studied include parent influence and participation in sedentary activities. Pan, Frey, Longmuir, and Bar-Or (2005) observed no concordance in activity levels of children with physical disabilities and their parents, regardless of child gender, age, or disabling condition. Pan and Frey (2005) also found that neither parent modeling of activity nor support were strong predictors of activity in youth with autism spectrum disorders. Activity was primarily influenced by age and participation in sedentary activities (i.e., computer games, reading). The lack of parental influence on the activity of children with DD is surprising for two reasons. First, previous reports indicate that activity of youth with DD primarily occurs with family members (Levinson & Reid, 1991; Margalit, 1981). Second, parent factors, particularly parent support (e.g., driving children to activities, paying fees), are significant predictors of activity in youth without DD (Trost et al., 2003). Pan and Frey (2006) used the social model of disability (Llewellyn & Hogan, 2000) to propose that parent influences were not potent enough to overcome societal barriers to physical activity in youth with autism spectrum disorders. That is, the lack of available programs and supports within existing programs negatively influenced both the child's ability to engage in physical activity and parents' ability to support active pursuits.

Media use (television and computer) may also be an activity determinant common to youth with and without DD, but the relationship between this factor and physical activity is reportedly too small to be of clinical significance (Marshall, Biddle, Gorely, Cameron, & Murdey, 2004). Regardless, television viewing and computer games are highly reinforcing and more likely to be selected over available activity options (Vara & Epstein, 1993), which could result in excessive sedentary behavior. There is a dearth of information regarding media use time in youth with DD, but there is evidence that youth with autism spectrum disorders (Pan & Frey, 2005) and physical disabilities (Brown & Gordon, 1987) do not watch more television than peers without DD.

Of concern is the use of technology for educational and behavioral interventions, as well as for leisure. Rosser Sandt and Frey (2005) reported that children with and without autism spectrum disorders primarily engaged in media-based sedentary activities, such as video games or TV, after school. Technology is a valuable intervention tool that promotes a variety of positive behavioral and psychosocial outcomes in youth with DD, but parents and practitioners are cautioned not to justify excessive time in technology-based sedentary pursuits for educational purposes to the exclusion of activity participation, particularly outside of scheduled instructional periods.

OPPORTUNITIES TO PROMOTE PHYSICAL ACTIVITY

Interactions between functional limitations associated with disabling conditions and environmental and sociocultural factors dictate the extent to which youth with DD can participate in physical activity. Many structural barriers to participation are being reduced, but individuals with DD may be prevented from engaging in activity programs due to a complex combination of personal factors (e.g., low self-efficacy, overprotective parents) or external societal factors (e.g., liability concerns, lack of trained personnel, lack of specialized programs; Rimmer, Riley, Wang, Rauworth, & Jurkowski, 2004), even though these latter exclusions are legally prohibited (Block, 1995). Children with DD participate in recess (Rosser Sandt & Frey, 2005), physical education (Lieberman & Cruz, 2001), and extracurricular activities such as youth sports (Simeonsson, Carlson, Huntington, McMillen, & Brent, 2001) at lower rates than do peers without DD, usually because there are not enough strong supports to facilitate involvement. The next section addresses the extant research on activity opportunities for youth with DD in school- and community-based settings.

Recess

Recess is one of the most opportune times for children to engage in physically active play, which is a necessary component of normal growth and development (Pellegrini & Smith, 1998). This time is more than just a break to expend excess energy; it is one of the few opportunities to engage in activities that combine the social, physical, emotional, and cognitive domains in a setting children find meaningful (National Association of Early Childhood Specialists in State Departments of Education [NAECS], 2001). Unfortunately, and without a basis in empirical research, recess is being increasingly eliminated from the school day to allow more time for academics (NAECS, 2001). In fact, it is well established that taking breaks from tasks, rather than continuous task practice, facilitates learning and retention (Willingham, 2002). Besides the potentially negative academic outcomes of less recess time, findings indicate that children lose a valuable opportunity to engage in physical activity and that this is not compensated for by engaging in more activity after school (Dale, Corbin, & Dale, 2000).

Recess play of children with DD has been studied primarily from a social-cognitive viewpoint, with less attention given to the physically active component (Rosenbaum, 1998). Various physical or behavior limitations may reduce their ability to engage in physically active play, but to date only a handful of researchers have explored this issue. Studies of youth with intellectual disabilities (Faison-Hodge & Porretta, 2004) and autism spectrum disorders (Rosser Sandt & Frey, 2005) reported no differences in recess activity levels compared with peers without DD. Interestingly, Lorenzi, Horvat, and Pellegrini (2000) found that youth with intellectual disabilities were more active than peers without DD during recess, a result that has not been reported elsewhere.

Of concern is the potential reduction in recess time for youth with DD. For example, the highest levels of physical activity exhibited by youth with autism spectrum disorders occurred during recess, but allotted time was slightly less compared with peers without DD, and some children in the sample were removed early to ease transitions (Rosser Sandt & Frey, 2005). The opportunity to attend recess is not available in middle and high school, and because children with DD are primarily inactive after school (Rosser Sandt & Frey, 2005), it is important to maximize use of this time to facilitate activity in elementary-age children with DD. In addition, compensatory activity times must be identified for those at middle and high school levels.

Although recess presents an optimal time for physically active play, children do not always choose to be active during this time (Kraft, 1989). For example, Simeonsson et al. (2001) found that although about 67% of youth with DD reported attending recess, only 33% actually participated in playground games, and this percentage varied according to student and school environment characteristics. Quality of the playground structure, area size and type, equipment availability, and presence of adult supervision all affect physical activity levels during recess (Sallis et al., 2001). The advent of universal playground design will help facilitate physically active play of children with DD during recess, but it is unclear how many schools have modified existing structures to accommodate all users, and more research is needed on this topic.

Physical Education

Physical education (PE) is a direct service and the only required curricular area specified in the Individuals with Disabilities Education Improvement Act of 2004 (IDEIA; Sec. 300.38). The law clearly states that PE means the development of physical and motor fitness, fundamental motor skills and patterns, and skills in aquatics, dance, and individual and group games and sports, including intramural and lifetime sports; adapted physical education is identified as a service option (IDEIA, 2004, Sec. 300.38). The importance of PE to physical activity and health for youth is strongly emphasized for all children (USDHHSDE, 2000); however, similar to recess, PE is being eliminated or reduced to allow time for more "academic" subjects. Physical education requirements decline significantly across grade levels, and only 8% and 6% of elementary and middle/high schools, respectively, provide full-year, daily PE (Burgeson, Wechsler, Brener, Young, & Spain, 2001).

Physical education should be an opportune time for youth to participate in physical activity, but the time for activity is insufficient, most children are not active during PE, and most classes are not taught by trained physical educators (Sallis & McKenzie, 1991). Simeonsson et al. (2001) documented that almost 70% of youth with disabilities regularly attend PE, but 42% of the sample was composed of elementary school teacher reports, which biased findings. Rosser Sandt and Frey (2005) and Pan and Frey (2006) reported that elementary-age youth with autism spectrum disorders attended PE 2–3 days per week and that 52% of older youth with autism spectrum disorders regularly attended PE. Burgeson et al. (2001) surveyed state, district, and local education agencies across the United States to assess PE services. Numbers varied according to government agency, so only the school-level findings are discussed here. Of the almost two-thirds of schools that reported enrolling children with permanent cognitive or physical disabilities, approximately 85% of those included PE on individualized education plans (IEPs), and over 95% had students with DD participating in required PE, although there were no data to suggest that PE teachers were contributing to the IEP. The majority of students with DD participated in regular PE (84.5%), and others were involved in a combination of regular and adapted PE (37.7%) or adapted PE (27.5%). A large number of middle/junior and senior high schools (> 60%) allowed PE exemptions, and most of these were due to physical disabilities, whereas exemptions for students with cognitive disabilities ranged from 28 to 36%. Reasons for blanket medical excuses may range from overprotective parents and medical professionals to children requesting exemptions due to negative experiences in PE (Lieberman & Cruz, 2001). Teachers and coaches may require medical releases for youth with certain disabilities in PE classes, despite the absence of an increased health risk compared with nondisabled peers (Nixon et al., 2001). Some physical educators allow youth with disabilities to choose whether or not to participate, which is inappropriate as such decisions are not allowed in other curricular areas (Lightfoot, Wright, & Sloper, 1998). Failure to provide appropriate PE services not only violates federal law but also deprives youth with DD opportunities to engage in physical activity that enhances all aspects of development.

Children should be physically active more than 50% of the time in PE, and it appears that not all youth are meeting this criterion (USDHHS, 2000). Low physical activity levels during elementary PE classes have been documented in children with intellectual disabilities (Faison-Hodge & Porretta, 2004) and autism spectrum disorders (Rosser Sandt & Frey, 2005), similar to findings of low PE activity levels in youth without DD. Children and adolescents with mild intellectual disabilities are less engaged in motor activity during integrated PE than peers without DD, despite no actual differences in allotted time devoted to content (Temple & Walkley, 1999). Youth with physical disabilities reported that activity participation during PE was limited because adaptations to allow full involvement were not made, and these students were often relegated to nonmovement roles such as line judges or boundary markers (Blinde & McCallister, 1998). Physical education days perceived as "bad" by youth with physical disabilities reflect these practices and occur due to social isolation, questioning of competence by peers, and restricted participation, all of which can be attributed to lack of teacher support, scarce engagement with classmates, and environmental constraints (Goodwin & Watkinson, 2000). Consequences of such exclusion and marginalization are anger, sadness, embarrassment, and feelings of being an outsider (Blinde & McCallister, 1998).

Successful PE experiences occur when the curriculum creates a sense of belonging, allows children to understand the benefits of activity, and provides opportunities for skillful participation, particularly in inclusive settings (Goodwin & Watkinson, 2000). Activities administered in segregated placements are not viewed as stimulating and are recognized by youth with DD as being different from those of peers without DD (Goodwin & Watkinson, 2000). Enjoyment of PE, but not free play or sports, was associated with self-perceptions of adequacy in and predilection for physical activity in youth with health impairments, and the reason was that instructors made efforts to modify the curriculum to enhance participation (Wright, Galea, & Barr, 2003).

Thus it is clear that successful involvement in PE can have a powerful, positive effect on physical, emotional, cognitive, and social development in youth with DD; conversely, negative PE experiences can have equally powerful effects on the same variables. As a result, it is important to identify best practices in PE service delivery for youth with DD. The National Association of State Directors of Special Education (1999) suggested that the failure to provide appropriate PE services was due to a lack of several key elements: (1) a philosophical commitment by public education systems to deliver services, (2) implementation of the least restrictive environment, (3) qualified personnel, (4) curricula, (5) inclusion of PE on IEPs, and (6) understanding among parents, teachers, and administrators regarding the differences between services (e.g., therapy vs. athletics vs. PE).

A lack of qualified personnel to provide PE services is an area of particular concern. Recent revisions to the Individuals with Disabilities Education Act (IDEA) clarify the term "qualified personnel" in special education, but the term "qualified physical educators" was not addressed. Many undergraduate PE teacher-preparation programs require one survey course in adapted PE, which may be sufficient to modify activities for someone with minimal constraints included in regular classes; however, this is not enough preparation to enable a professional to address the PE needs of those with more significant conditions in other least-restrictive-placement options (Hardin, 2005). Advanced training in adapted PE is required for individuals to better meet the diverse needs of youth with DD in PE. The National Adapted Physical Education Standards certification is not required by most education agencies, and only 14 states require adapted PE certifications or endorsements (Zhang, Kelly, Berkey, Joseph, & Chen, 2000). Zhang et al. (2000) reported that 22,000 additional qualified teachers are required to address the PE needs of youth with DD. Burgeson et al. (2001) found that most students with DD receive PE from regular PE teachers, whereas only 23% of schools utilized adapted PE teachers, which calls into question the quality of services. Unfortunately, PE services for youth with DD are often provided by special educators, therapists, or classroom teachers without proper training in this area. Effective teaching behaviors and expertise are associated with higher activity levels in PE (McKenzie, Sallis, Faucette, Roby, & Kolody, 1993); thus it is clear that more teachers with training in adapted PE are needed to provide quality services in this curriculum area. Physical education presents an important opportunity to engage in physical activity, and more emphasis should be placed on delivery of quality instruction by teachers with proper certification and experience working with youth with DD.

Another area of concern in the provision of quality PE services is curriculum. In general, PE has not been successful at increasing or promoting activity for the majority of children due to a traditional emphasis on sports, performance, fitness, and skill that has discouraged activity participation (Corbin, 2002). As such, a quality PE curriculum for youth with DD should be designed to help people engage in lifetime physical activity (Jobling, 1997). Regular PE teachers typically simplify instructional content and provide more skill modeling and practice, but only 55% actually modify equipment or facilities (Burgeson et al., 2001). In addition, there is little collaboration between PE and special education teachers to develop optimal instructional strategies. PE curricula designed to address the needs of youth with DD (Dunn, Morehouse, & Fredericks, 1986; Wessel & Zittel, 1995) are available, and several school districts have developed adapted PE curricula that are available through electronic resources. However, the focus should be on adapting the existing regular PE curriculum to include children with DD with peers to the maximum extent possible. Curricular adaptations must also emphasize participation in physical activity, and there are excellent resources to assist practitioners in this matter (Kasser, 1995; Lieberman & Houston-Wilson, 2002).

Extracurricular Activities, Sport, and Recreation

Participation rates in extracurricular activity, sports, and recreation are strongly associated with emotional well-being and health in youth (Steptoe & Butler, 1996); however, there are large disparities between youth with and without DD in this area. Simeonsson et al. (2001) found that only 17.5% and 13.6% of youth with disabilities participated in after-school programs and organized sports, respectively. In contrast, about 84% of elementary age and 37% of high school age youth without DD participate in at least one community-based physical activity or sport team (Kann, Warren, & Harris, 1999).

Although sport and active recreation participation rates of youth with DD are much lower than those of nondisabled peers, the importance of these activities to overall development of this population cannot be overstated. Research has demonstrated that participation in sport activities has a significant, positive effect on various aspects of social and emotional functioning of youth with various disabilities (Kristen, Patriksson, & Fridlund, 2002; Riggen & Ulrich, 1993), but the impact on physical and fitness parameters is less promising. Riggen and Ulrich (1993) found that Special Olympics participants in both integrated and segregated programs improved their basketball skills but not their cardiovascular fitness. These findings have also been observed in adults with intellectual disabilities (Pitetti, Jackson, Stubbs, Campbell, & Battar, 1989) and are largely attributed to inadequate frequency, intensity, and duration of the training needed to improve physical fitness.

The contribution of sport participation to overall physical activity in youth with DD is not well known, and the limited existing data are variable. Pan and Frey (2005) found that extracurricular physical activities in youth with autism spectrum disorders usually occurred once per week and accounted for little total activity. Factors influencing the extracurricular activity participation of youth with DD have not been thoroughly studied, but certainly a lack of quality programs, disability-related variables, and sociocultural attitudes can be implicated. Laws provide equal access for youth with DD to sport and recreation opportunities and the reader is referred to Block (1995) and Goedert (1995) for further information on this topic. Field and Oates (2001) stated that youth with cystic fibrosis and spina bifida had fewer extracurricular outlets than peers without DD and that access to programs was lowest for those with spina bifida and greater physical needs. The high skill level required for participation, behavioral expectations, the competitive nature of many extracurricular activity programs, and lack of trained personnel may also inhibit involvement of youth with DD.

Conaster, Block, and Gansneder (2002) found that aquatic instructors had less favorable attitudes toward teaching students with severe disabilities in inclusive swim classes, but it was not clear whether this finding reflected negative attitudes regarding disability or inclusion. Public school coaches agreed that youth with disabilities had a right to sport opportunities, yet most felt inadequately trained to facilitate integration into interscholastic sports, and many had no prior experience coaching athletes with disabilities (Kozub & Porretta, 1998). There is a paucity of data on the impact of training on attitudes or intentions toward coaching or instructing youth with DD in extracurricular activities, but there is evidence that the willingness to coach youth with certain disabilities increases in accordance with increases in perceived coaching competence, which suggests that the issue is related less to negative attitudes about disability and more to personal feelings of inadequacy or uncertainty (Rizzo, Bishop, & Tobar, 1997). Therefore, time devoted to appropriate instructor training is crucial to the successful administration and maintenance of extracurricular activity programs for youth with DD (Fennick & Royle, 2003).

Most communities embrace Special Olympics, which clearly has the highest visibility of all specialized extracurricular physical activity outlets. Special Olympics is an excellent resource, yet it is somewhat limited because the presence of an intellectual disability is required for participation. As such, many youth with physical, communication, or sensory disabilities do not qualify and do not have access to other opportunities. There is less general knowledge about other opportunities offered through specialized sport organizations affiliated with the Paralympics. Disability sport/recreation associations exist for many different activities, such as golf and rock climbing, and there are disability-specific sport organizations such as the United States Association for Blind Athletes and the Dwarf Athletic Association of America. Other programs aimed at providing activity opportunities for youth with various DD exist and are gaining momentum, such as the American Association of Adapted Sports Programs and Blaze Sports. These segregated organizations provide opportunity for higher level competition, and all youth with DD should have access to these options in order to meet activity needs and interests.

A main obstacle is finding a critical mass of participants, as well as a stable volunteer and financial base to maintain operations over the long term. In addition, awareness of such programs is low, even among well-informed parents and school personnel (Kozub & Porretta, 1998), and improving communication regarding these opportunities is the responsibility of PE, sport, and recreation professionals. Both segregated programs that offer equitable competition and integrated extracurricular activity venues with appropriate modifications that allow maximal participation should be made available to youth with DD.

Therapy

Physical and occupational therapists are health professionals who are responsible for administering treatments that are designed to improve many physical factors, such as mobility, and that contribute to the ability to become and remain physically active (Shapiro & Sayers, 2003). According to IDEIA (2004), such therapies are related services and should not be confused with PE, which is a direct service that must be included in the IEP. This point needs to be emphasized because therapies are often substituted or provided in place of, rather than to augment, PE, in violation of federal law (Shapiro & Sayers, 2003).

Any therapeutic intervention must be based on established or supported theory. Theories used are generated from neuroscience perspectives on motor control (nature and cause of movement) and motor learning (acquisition and modification of movement). Within these domains, there are many specific theories to explain movement, and each possesses strengths and weaknesses. The most current, accepted understanding is that movement occurs due to multiple, interactive processes such as the qualities and experiences of the individual, the environment, and the task (Shumway-Cook & Woollacott, 1995).

Quality therapeutic interventions are integral to the optimal development of youth with DD, but the availability of strong, empirical, controlled research on the efficacy of approaches is limited. Recent reviews have concluded that the effectiveness of therapies commonly used to remediate or ameliorate symptoms associated with various DD, such as neurodevelopmental treatment (NDT, or Bobath technique), sensory integration (SI), conductive education, and patterning (also known as the Doman and Delacato method), varies depending on the outcome measure, type of disability, and practitioner's skill. However, none of these therapies are uniformly supported as evidence-based practices (Brown & Patel, 2005). Most studies have been conducted with youth with cerebral palsy and are weakened due to small sample sizes, subject heterogeneity, lack of information on statistical power, and lack of appropriate controls (Butler & Darrah, 2001). In particular, patterning is a therapeutic approach that has received significant criticism from the scientific community because it is based on unsound theory and is not supported with well-controlled empirical studies (American Academy of Pediatrics, 1999). It is of greater concern that these therapeutic interventions do not take into account the dynamic interaction between individual, task, and environment, which ultimately dictates movement responses. As such, it is unlikely that any one therapy will be a panacea for the symptoms associated with DD.

IMPLICATIONS

Families and Practitioners

It is well documented that the presence of a disability significantly alters family functioning (Brown, Anand, Isaacs, Baum & Fung, 2003). Parents of youth with DD report less participation in social activities (Barnett & Boyce, 1995), reduced participation in hobbies, and devotion of more time to child care activities (Taanila, Syrjälä, Kokkonen,

& Järvelin, 2002) compared with parents of youth without DD. However, few data exist on how these factors affect family physical activity participation.

Studies have demonstrated that physical activity in youth with DD is primarily family directed. Mactavish and Schleien (2000, 2004) reported that physical activities in families of youth with physical disabilities were informal and family initiated and occurred both in the home and in the community. Parents of children with cerebral palsy reported more limitations that apparently influenced the recreational pursuits of other family members. These parents were primarily sedentary during leisure time, engaging in activities such as watching television, playing board games, or going to movies. Additional research supports findings that leisure pursuits of youth with DD occur in the home and are family oriented and that family members are the most common leisure companions (Levinson & Reid, 1991; Margalit, 1981).

Families are critical in shaping activity experiences (USDHHSDE, 2000), but families of youth with DD may face greater challenges than the general population due to a variety of factors. For example, these families may not perceive physical activity/recreation/leisure to be a priority when there are so many other basic needs to be met. An expressed need for help in recreation has not been consistently reported by parents of youth with DD, but it is unclear whether this is an issue of priority or values (Bailey, Blasco & Simeonsson, 1992).

Other parent factors that may affect the physical activity of youth with DD, and that are somewhat more difficult to assess, are expectations and overprotection. Children with various DDs often feel or are overprotected by parents, which may negatively affect activity participation, particularly attempts to experiment with novel activities or situations (Holmbeck et al., 2002; Kortering & Braziel, 1999). The issue of overprotection is further complicated by lower expectations, and the dearth of research indicates that parents' movement expectations for youth with DD are low (Edwards-Beckett, 1995). Overprotection and low expectations with regard to physical abilities and activity are also displayed by health professionals, teachers, and coaches. Frey, Buchanan, and Rosser Sandt (2005) found that throughout their lives adults with intellectual disabilities were cautioned in terms of engaging in activity by doctors, PE teachers, parents, and coaches and that these messages undermined positive health behaviors. For example, obesity-related health problems were sometimes not addressed by physicians, and consequently they were not seen as a concern by parents. Coaches often oversimplified activities based on the rationale that the individuals were incapable of performing the task, and people with intellectual disabilities were often told by physical educators not to "overdo it" or "they might burn out." Pervasive messages of incompetence and instilling fear of physical danger had a negative impact on the perceived physical activity competency in the sample. As such, there needs to be a concerted effort among support systems to avoid transferring personal fears to children with DD. Low expectations and overprotection serve only to further disable these individuals and to compound the effects of the actual condition.

Researchers

Physical activity in youth with DD is a complex topic that has not been well researched but is an identified health priority (USDHHS, 2005; USPHS, 2002). Available findings indicate that children with DD are generally less active than nondisabled peers, which could have a significant impact on overall growth and development. Multiple dynamic factors influence activity in this population, and, although many are similar to those observed in youth without DD, there are unique issues related to the nature of the disability, as well as to physical and programmatic access. Caution is warranted when attempting to draw general conclusions about physical activity in youth with DD based on the existing literature. There are large inconsistencies in research methodology, terminology, and samples, but greater concerns are the lack of theory-driven research, flawed research designs, and inappropriate application of certain techniques. For example, surveys and motion sensors are commonly used and acceptable methods to assess youth physical activity in field-based settings. Many of these tools can be reasonably applied with youth with DD without further validation; for instance, pedometers can be used as a measure of activity in populations without significantly altered gait patterns or age-appropriate questionnaires in populations without cognitive delays. However, several published reports of activity in youth with DD are based on instrumentation with questionable validity for the intended purposes and subject population (Eiholzer et al., 2003; van den Berg-Emons et al., 2001; Visser, Geuze, & Kalverboer, 1998), which compromises the trustworthiness of the knowledge base. There is a clear need for collaboration among scholars across such disciplines as exercise science, special education, and psychology to better address the aforementioned research issues and improve the quality of research on this topic.

Most studies on physical activity and youth with DD are based on the medical or deficit model; that is, that the presence of a disabling condition alone is sufficient to cause low levels of physical activity. Current thought does not prescribe to this narrow view of disability (Llewellyn & Hogan, 2000), but only a handful of studies have used alternate theoretical approaches to examine physical activity behavior in youth with DD, such as family systems theory and the social model of disability (Pan et al., 2005; Pan & Frey, 2006). Advances in understanding activity behavior in youth with DD can occur only when researchers extend beyond the confines of the medical model to include both standard behavioral and disability theories as a basis of inquiry.

A clearly established need exists for well-controlled empirical research in all areas related to physical activity and youth with DD. This is best accomplished through the multidisciplinary effort of scholars, practitioners, and parents. An increase in the quality and quantity of data will assist policy makers in developing specific physical activity goals and objectives to ultimately influence health and functional ability outcomes. Further, practitioners will have access to evidence-based strategies that will allow achievement of these goals.

Policy Makers

Of the 22 objectives used to track the leading 10 health indicators in the United States, only 12 include people with disabilities. The reason for this exclusion is the existence of inadequate data on this large, heterogeneous population (USDHHS, 2000). Children with DD are mentioned in only 2 of the 13 goals specified for people with disabilities: reducing the proportion of youth with DD who are reportedly sad, unhappy, or depressed (item 6-2) and increasing the proportion of youth with DD ages 6–21 who spend at least 80% of the time in regular education (item 6-9). The federal government recently published reports specifically aimed at improving the health of people with disabilities (USPHS, 2002; USDHHS, 2005). Although these are extremely important and timely documents, the unique needs of children with DD receive little attention.

Children with DD are included in strategies for promoting participation in physical activity and sport (USDHHSDE, 2000), but because no national data exist on activity participation rates, appropriate targets cannot be established. A coalition of physicians, educators, researchers, policy makers, and families is needed to (1) outline research needs, (2) establish reasonable physical activity participation targets, (3) provide recommendations on research-based best practices, and (4) develop achievable procedures aimed at meeting the targets for appropriate levels of health-related physical activity in youth with DD. An initial step in this process has been the creation of the National Center on Physical Activity and Disability (NCPAD), which is funded by the Centers for Disease Control. NCPAD provides a comprehensive information dissemination resource to assist parents, professionals, and researchers in locating and accessing not only opportunities for activity, but also the latest research findings, advocacy issues, and other topics of interest surrounding physical activity for people with disabilities across the lifespan. In addition, the Inclusive Fitness Coalition (*www.incfit.org*) was launched in January 2007 to promote physical activity, sport, recreation, and fitness participation among people with disabilities by facilitating agency collaboration, advocacy, and public awareness. These initiatives and resources must be supported by professionals, families, and people with disabilities to ensure that physical activity remains recognized as a critical health need for all individuals.

Assigning importance and value to promoting health through participation in regular activity will help dispel the pervasive belief that a disabling condition condemns someone to an unhealthy life. Attention must be diverted from a singular focus on treating symptoms of the disability only, to an emphasis on healthy living with a disability. Positive behaviors, such as regular physical activity participation, should be established during childhood in order to promote healthy lifestyles in people with DD. Research on adults with disabilities indicates that physical activity participation is a vital component of overall health and well-being (Blinde & McClung, 1997). Therefore, it is critical that youth with DD be encouraged to participate in high levels of activity as soon as possible, and this behavior must be nourished and facilitated throughout childhood to increase the probability that this population will become lifelong movers.

REFERENCES

American Academy of Pediatrics. (1999). The treatment of neurologically impaired children using patterning. *Pediatrics, 104,* 1149–1151.

Ayyangar, R. (2002). Health maintenance and management in childhood disability. *Physical Medicine and Rehabilitation Clinics of North America, 13,* 793–821.

Bailey, D. B., Blasco, P. M., & Simeonsson, R. J. (1992). Needs expressed by mothers and fathers of young children with disabilities. *American Journal on Mental Retardation, 97,* 1–10.

Bailey, R. C., Olson, J., Pepper, S. L., Porszasz, J., Barstow, T. J., & Cooper, D. M. (1995). The level and tempo of children's physical activities: An observational study. *Medicine & Science in Sports & Exercise, 27,* 1033–1041.

Barnett, W. S., & Boyce, G. (1995). Effects of children with Down syndrome on parents' activities. *American Journal on Mental Retardation, 99,* 115–127.

Blinde, E. M., & McCallister, S. G. (1998). Listening to the voices of students with physical disabilities. *Journal of Physical Education, Recreation, & Dance, 69,* 64–68.

Blinde, E. M., & McClung, L. R. (1997). Enhancing the physical and social self through recreational activity: Accounts of individuals with physical disabilities. *Adapted Physical Activity Quarterly, 14,* 327–344.

Block, M. E. (1995). Americans with Disabilities Act: Its impact on youth sports. *Journal of Physical Education, Recreation, & Dance, 66,* 28–32.

Brown, I., Anand, S., Isaacs, B., Baum, N., & Fung, W. L. A. (2003). Family quality of life: Canadian results from an international study. *Journal of Developmental and Physical Disabilities, 15,* 207–230.

Brown, K. A., & Patel, D. R. (2005). Complementary and alternative medicine in developmental disabilities. *Indian Journal of Pediatrics, 72*, 949–952.

Brown, M., & Gordon, W. A. (1987). Impact of impairment on activity patterns of children. *Archives of Physical and Medical Rehabilitation, 68*, 828–832.

Burgeson, C. R., Wechsler, H., Brener, N. D., Young, J. C., & Spain, C. G. (2001). Physical education and activity: Results from the School Health Policies and Programs Study 2000. *Journal of School Health, 71*, 279–293.

Butler, C., & Darrah, J. (2001). Effects of neurodevelopmental treatment (NDT) for cerebral palsy: An AACPDM evidence report. *Developmental Medicine & Child Neurology, 43*, 778–790.

Caspersen, C. J. (1989). Physical activity epidemiology: Concepts, methods, and applications to exercise science. *Medicine & Science in Sports & Exercise Reviews, 17*, 423–461.

Conaster, P., Block, M., & Gansneder, B. (2002). Aquatic instructor's beliefs toward inclusion: The theory of planned behavior. *Adapted Physical Activity Quarterly, 19*, 172–187.

Corbin, C. B. (2002). Physical activity for everyone: What every physical educator should know about promoting lifelong physical activity. *Journal of Teaching in Physical Education, 21*, 128–144.

Dale, D., Corbin, C. B., & Dale, K. S. (2000). Restricting opportunities to be active during school time: Do children compensate by increasing physical activity levels after school? *Research Quarterly for Exercise and Sport, 71*(3), 240–248.

Developmental Disabilities Assistance and Bill of Rights Act of 2000, Public Law 106-402 S. 1809, 42 U.S.C. §15001.

Dunn, J. M., Morehouse, J. W., & Fredericks, H. D. B. (1986). *Physical education for the severely handicapped: A systematic approach to a data based gymnasium.* Austin, TX: PRO-ED.

Edwards-Beckett, J. (1995). Parental expectations and child's self-concept in spina bifida. *Children's Health Care, 24*(4), 257–267.

Eiholzer, U., Nordmann, Y., L'Allemand, D., Schlumpf, M., Schmid, S., & Kromeyer-Hauschild, K. (2003). Improving body composition and physical activity in Prader–Willi syndrome. *Journal of Pediatrics, 142*, 73–79.

Faison-Hodge, J., & Porretta, D. L. (2004). Physical activity levels of students with mental retardation and students without disabilities. *Adapted Physical Activity Quarterly, 21*, 139–152.

Fennick, E., & Royle, J. (2003). Community inclusion for children and youth with developmental disabilities. *Focus on Autism and Other Developmental Disabilities, 18*, 20–27.

Field, S. J., & Oates, R. K. (2001). Sport and recreation activities and opportunities for children with spina bifida and cystic fibrosis. *Journal of Science and Medicine in Sport, 4*, 71–76.

Fox, K. R., & Riddoch, C. (2000). Charting the physical activity patterns of contemporary children and adolescents. *Proceedings of the Nutrition Society, 59*, 497–504.

Fredriksen, P. M., Ingjer, E., & Thaulow, E. (2000). Physical activity in children and adolescents with congenital heart disease: Aspects of measurements with an activity monitor. *Cardiology in the Young, 10*, 98–106.

Frey, G. C., Buchanan, A. M., & Rosser Sandt, D. D. (2005). "I'd rather watch TV": An examination of physical activity in adults with mental retardation. *Mental Retardation, 43*, 241–254.

Goedert, J. G. (1995). Schools, sports and students with disabilities: The impact of federal laws protecting the rights of students with disabilities on interscholastic sports. *Journal of Law & Education, 24*, 403–421.

Goodwin, D. L., & Watkinson, E. J. (2000). Inclusive physical education from the perspective of students with physical disabilities. *Adapted Physical Activity Quarterly, 17*, 144–150.

Gordon-Larsen, P., Nelson, M., & Popkin, B. M. (2004). Longitudinal physical activity and sedentary behavior trends: Adolescence to adulthood. *American Journal of Preventive Medicine, 27*, 277–283.

Hardin, B. (2005). Physical education teachers' reflections on preparation for inclusion. *Physical Educator, 62*, 44–56.

Heath, G. W., & Fentem, P. H. (1997). Physical activity among persons with disabilities: A public health perspective. *Exercise and Sport Sciences Reviews, 25*, 195–234.

Holmbeck, G. N., Johnson, S. Z., Wills, K. E., McKernon, W., Rose, B., Erklin, S., et al. (2002). Observed and perceived parental overprotection in relation to psychosocial adjustment in preadolescents with a physical disability: The mediational role of behavioral autonomy. *Journal of Consulting and Clinical Psychology, 70*, 96–110.

Individuals with Disabilities Education Improvement Act of 2004, Public Law 108-446, 118 Stat. 2647. Retrieved January 15, 2006, from *http://thomas.loc.gov/cgi-bin/query/z?c108:h.r.1350.enr:%20.*

Jobling, A. (1997). "Quality" in physical education for children with disabilities: Are there opportunities to learn? *Brazilian International Journal of Adapted Physical Education Research, 4,* 33–46.

Kann, L., Warren, W., & Harris, W. A. (1999). Youth risk behavior surveillance—United States, 1995. *Journal of School Health, 66,* 365–377.

Kasser, S. L. (1995). *Inclusive games: Movement for everyone.* Champaign, IL: Human Kinetics.

Klepper, S. E. (1999). Effects of an eight-week physical conditioning program on disease signs and symptoms in children with chronic arthritis. *Arthritis Care and Research, 12,* 52–60.

Kortering, L. J., & Braziel, P. M. (1999). Staying in school: The perspective of ninth-grade students. *Remedial and Special Education, 20,* 106–113.

Kozub, F. M. (2003). Explaining physical activity in individuals with mental retardation: An exploratory study. *Education and Training in Developmental Disabilities, 38,* 302–313.

Kozub, F. M., & Oh, H.-K. (2004). An exploratory study of physical activity levels in children and adolescents with visual impairments. *Clinical Kinesiology, 58,* 1–7.

Kozub, F. M., & Porretta, D. L. (1998). Interscholastic coaches' attitudes toward integration of adolescents with disabilities. *Adapted Physical Activity Quarterly, 15,* 328–344.

Kraft, R. E. (1989). Children at play: Behavior of children at recess. *Journal of Physical Education, Recreation, & Dance, 60,* 21–24.

Kristen, L., Patriksson, G., & Fridlund, B. (2002). Conceptions of children and adolescents with physical disabilities about their participation in a sports programme. *European Physical Education Review, 8,* 139–156.

Levinson, L., & Reid, G. (1991). Patterns of physical activity among youngsters with developmental disabilities. *Canadian Association for Health, Physical Education, and Recreation, 56,* 24–28.

Lieberman, L. J., & Cruz, L. (2001). Blanket medical excuses from physical education: Possible solutions. *Teaching Elementary Physical Education, 12,* 27–30.

Lieberman, L. J., & Houston-Wilson, C. (2002). *Strategies for inclusion: A handbook for physical educators.* Champaign, IL: Human Kinetics.

Lightfoot, J., Wright, S., & Sloper, P. (1998). Supporting pupils in mainstream school with an illness or disability: Young people's views. *Child: Care, Health and Development, 25,* 267–283.

Llewellyn, A., & Hogan, K. (2000). The use and abuse of models of disability. *Disability & Society, 15,* 157–165.

Longmuir, P. E., & Bar-Or, O. (2000). Factors influencing the physical activity levels of youths with physical and sensory disabilities. *Adapted Physical Activity Quarterly, 17,* 40–53.

Lorenzi, D. G., Horvat, M., & Pellegrini, A. D. (2000). Physical activity of children with and without mental retardation in inclusive recess settings. *Education and Training in Mental Retardation and Developmental Disabilities, 35,* 160–167.

Lotan, M., Isakov, E., & Merrick, J. (2004). Improving functional skills and physical fitness in children with Rett syndrome. *Journal of Intellectual Disability Research, 48,* 730–735.

Mactavish, J. B., & Schleien, S. J. (2000). Exploring family recreation activities in families that include children with developmental disabilities. *Therapeutic Recreation Journal, 34,* 132–153.

Mactavish, J. B., & Schleien, S. J. (2004). Re-injecting spontaneity and balance in family life: Parents' perspectives on recreation in families that include children with developmental disability. *Journal of Intellectual Disability Research, 48,* 123–141.

Malina, R. M., Bouchard, C., & Bar-Or, O. (2004). *Growth, maturation, and physical activity* (2nd ed.). Champaign, IL: Human Kinetics.

Margalit, M. (1981). Leisure activities of cerebral palsied children. *Israel Journal of Psychiatry and Related Science, 18,* 209–214.

Marshall, S. J., Biddle, S. J. H., Gorely, T., Cameron, N., & Murdey, I. (2004). Relationships between media use, body fatness and physical activity in children and youth: A meta-analysis. *International Journal of Obesity, 28,* 1238–1246.

McKenzie, T. L., Sallis, J. F., Faucette, N., Roby, J. J., & Kolody, B. (1993). Effects of a curriculum and inservice program on the quantity and quality of elementary physical education classes. *Research Quarterly for Exercise and Sport, 64,* 178–187.

National Association for Sport and Physical Education. (1998). NASPE releases first ever physical activity guidelines for preadolescents. *Journal of Physical Education, Recreation and Dance, 69,* 8.

National Association of Early Childhood Specialists in State Departments of Education. (2001). *Recess and the importance of play: A position statement on young children and recess.* Denver: Colorado State Department of Education.

National Association of State Directors of Special Education. (1999). Physical education and sports: The unfulfilled promise for students with disabilities. *Liaison Bulletin, 17,* 1–10.

Nixon, P. A., Orenstein, D. M., & Kelsey, S. F. (2001). Habitual physical activity in children and adolescents with cystic fibrosis. *Medicine & Science in Sports & Exercise, 33,* 30–35.

Pan, C.-Y., & Frey, G. C. (2005). Identifying physical activity determinants in youth with autism spectrum disorders. *Journal of Physical Activity and Health, 2,* 412–422.

Pan, C.-Y., & Frey, G. C. (2006). Physical activity patterns in youth with autism spectrum disorders. *Journal of Autism and Developmental Disorders, 36,* 587–606.

Pan, C.-Y., Frey, G. C., Longmuir, P. E., & Bar-Or, O. (2005). Concordance of physical activity among parents and youth with physical disabilities. *Journal of Developmental and Physical Disabilities, 17,* 395–407.

Pate, R., Pfeiffer, K. A., Trost, S. G., Ziegler, P., & Dowda, M. (2004). Physical activity among children attending preschools. *Pediatrics, 114,* 1258–1263.

Pellegrini, A. D., & Smith, P. K. (1998). Physical activity play: The nature and function of a neglected aspect of play. *Child Development, 69,* 577–598.

Pitetti, K. H., Jackson, J. A., Stubbs, N. B., Campbell, K. D., & Battar, S. S. (1989). Fitness levels of adult Special Olympic participants. *Adapted Physical Activity Quarterly, 6,* 354–370.

Riggen, K., & Ulrich, D. (1993). The effects of sport participation on individuals with mental retardation. *Adapted Physical Activity Quarterly, 10,* 42–51.

Rimmer, J. H., Riley, B., Wang, E., Rauworth, A., & Jurkowski, J. (2004). Physical activity participation among persons with disabilities: Barriers and facilitators. *American Journal of Preventive Medicine, 26,* 419–425.

Rizzo, T. L., Bishop, P., & Tobar, D. (1997). Attitudes of soccer coaches toward youth players with mild mental retardation: A pilot study. *Adapted Physical Activity Quarterly, 14,* 238–251.

Rosenbaum, P. (1998). Physical activity play in children with disabilities: A neglected opportunity for research. *Child Development, 69,* 607–608.

Rosenbloom, A. L., Young, R. S., Joe, J. R., & Winter, W. E. (1999). Emerging epidemic of type 2 diabetes in young. *Diabetes Care, 22,* 345–354.

Rosser Sandt, D. D., & Frey, G. C. (2005). Comparison of physical activity levels between children with and without autistic spectrum disorders. *Adapted Physical Activity Quarterly, 22,* 146–159.

Sallis, J. F., Conway, T. L., Prochaska, J. J., McKenzie, T. L., Marshall, S. J., & Brown, M. (2001). The association of school environments with youth physical activity. *American Journal of Public Health, 91,* 618–620.

Sallis, J. F., & McKenzie, T. L. (1991). Physical education's role in public health. *Research Quarterly for Exercise and Sport, 62,* 124–137.

Sallis, J. F., Prochaska, J. J., & Taylor, W. C. (2000). A review of correlates of physical activity of children and adolescents. *Medicine & Science in Sports & Exercise, 32,* 963–975.

Schenker, R., Coster, W. J., & Parush, S. (2005). Neuroimpairments, activity performance, and participation in children with cerebral palsy mainstreamed in elementary schools. *Developmental Medicine & Child Neurology, 47,* 808–814.

Shapiro, D. R., & Sayers, K. L. (2003). Who does what on the interdisciplinary team regarding physical education for students with disabilities? *TEACHING Exceptional Children, 35,* 32–38.

Shumway-Cook, A., & Woollacott, M. (1995). *Motor control: Theory and practical applications.* Baltimore: Williams & Wilkins.

Simeonsson, R. J., Carlson, D., Huntington, G. S., McMillen, J. S., & Brent, J. L. (2001). Students with disabilities: A national survey of participation in school activities. *Disability and Rehabilitation, 23,* 49–63.

Simons-Morton, B. G., McKenzie, T. J., Stone, E., Mitchell, P., Osganian, V., Strikmiller, P. K., et al. (1997). Physical activity in a multiethnic population of third graders in four states. *American Journal of Public Health, 87,* 45–50.

Steptoe, A., & Butler, N. (1996). Sports participation and emotional well-being in adolescents. *Lancet, 347,* 1789–1792.

Suzuki, M., Saitch, S., Tasaki, Y., Shimomura, Y., Makishima, R., & Hosoy, N. (1991). Nutritional status and daily physical activity of handicapped students in Tokyo metropolitan schools for deaf, blind, mentally retarded and physically handicapped individuals. *American Journal of Clinical Nutrition, 54,* 1101–1111.

Taanila, A., Syrjälä, L., Kokkonen, J., & Järvelin, M. R. (2002). Coping of parents with physically and/or intellectually disabled children. *Child: Care, Health and Development, 28,* 73–86.

Temple, V. A., & Walkley, J. W. (1999). Academic learning time–physical education (ALT-PE) of students with mild intellectual disabilities in regular Victorian schools. *Adapted Physical Activity Quarterly, 16,* 64–74.

Trost, S. G., Sallis, J. F., Pate, R. R., Freedson, P. S., Taylor, W. C., & Dowda, M. (2003). Evaluating a model of parental influence on youth physical activity. *American Journal of Preventive Medicine, 25,* 277–282.

U.S. Department of Health and Human Services. (2000). *Healthy people 2010: Understanding and improving health* (2nd ed). Washington, DC: U.S. Government Printing Office.

U.S. Department of Health and Human Services. (2005). *The Surgeon General's call to action to improve the health and wellness of persons with disabilities.* Washington, DC: U.S. Government Printing Office.

U.S. Department of Health and Human Services and Department of Education. (2000). *Promoting better health for young people through physical activity and sports.* Silver Spring, MD: Author.

U.S. Public Health Service. (2002). *Closing the gap: A national blueprint for improving the health of individuals with mental retardation.* Washington, DC: U.S. Government Printing Office.

van den Berg-Emons, H. J., Bussmann, J. B., Brobbel, A. S., Roebroeck, M. E., van Meeteren, J., & Stam, H. J. (2001). Everyday physical activity in adolescents and young adults with meningomyelocele as measured with a novel activity monitor. *Journal of Pediatrics, 139,* 880–886.

Vara, L. S., & Epstein, L. H. (1993). Laboratory assessment of choice between exercise or sedentary behaviors. *Research Quarterly for Exercise and Sport, 64,* 356–360.

Visser, J., Geuze, R. H., & Kalverboer, A. F. (1998). The relationship between physical growth, the level of activity and the development of motor skills in adolescence: Differences between children with DCD and controls. *Human Movement Science, 17,* 573–608.

Wessel, J. A., & Zittel, L. L. (1995). *Smart start: Preschool movement curriculum designed for children of all abilities.* Austin, TX: PRO-ED.

Willingham, D. T. (2002). Allocating student study time: "Massed" versus "distributed" practice. *American Educator, 26,* 37–39, 47.

Wright, M. J., Galea, V., & Barr, R. D. (2003). Self-perceptions of physical activity in survivors of acute lymphoblastic leukemia in childhood. *Pediatric Exercise Science, 15,* 191–201.

Zhang, J., Kelly, L., Berkey, D., Joseph, D., & Chen, S. (2000). The prevalence-based need for adapted physical education teachers in the United States. *Adapted Physical Activity Quarterly, 17,* 297–309.

V

POSTSCHOOL AND ADULT ISSUES

All students face challenges when they leave school behind and enter the adult world. The transition for youth with developmental disabilities, however, often differs greatly from that of their peers. Successful transition into adulthood for youth with developmental disabilities often requires (1) systematic planning over several years, (2) careful attention to the development of essential skills, (3) assistance in the transition process, and (4) ongoing support in adulthood. Successful outcomes are more likely when planning defines sources of support and links individuals and their families to service-providing agencies. When young adults do not seek services or their communities do not provide them with appropriate supports, the outcomes can be grim. Unemployment rates for people with disabilities have hovered around 60–70% for years, community supports for independent living lag behind the needs, and leisure and social opportunities are often minimal or segregated from the cross-section of the community. Adults with developmental disabilities predictably will need support that meets specific issues in their lives, and it is wise that practitioners anticipate these needs and plan for regular or occasional support. In this section five chapters address what we know about meeting the challenges of adulthood for individuals with developmental disabilities.

The transition from high school to adulthood is particularly significant for youth with developmental disabilities. In Chapter 18, Bambara, Wilson, and McKenzie review the research on effective transition services for youth with developmental disabilities with the intent of identifying evidence-based transition practices. One such practice is the involvement of students with disabilities in community-based work experiences

367

while they are still in school. Research has shown that school work experience is related to postschool job success. Research also indicates the crucial role families play in the transition-to-work process: finding jobs, negotiating with agencies for supports, helping to design career and living plans, and informing the educational team. These authors argue that successful transition depends on how well multiple factors come together to address the needs of youth with developmental disabilities.

Mank focuses on employment for youth and adults with developmental disabilities. He outlines the core role of employment in adulthood, in our society, and in a complex, rich pattern of life. Employment is more than a wage-earning activity. Employment is a framework for daily living. It is a structure for social relationships and a strategy for continued skill development, and it often defines the "contribution" that individuals make to their community. Current research suggests that individuals with developmental disabilities are more capable of employment contributions, can benefit from a large array of supports, and are more likely to become sustainable members of their community when there is an investment in employment assistance. Mank offers a vision of ways in which future policy, research, and practice can better support employment opportunities for youth and adults with developmental disabilities.

Postschool outcomes often shift attention from traditional skill building to larger quality-of-life concerns. Felce and Perry emphasize the core importance of quality of life in their chapter on community living supports. Among the major advances in the field of developmental disabilities has been the attention now given to the quality of life a person experiences. The support received by an individual and his or her family can have dramatic effects on activity patterns, social networks, independence, productivity, and general life quality. Felce and Perry trace the history of both social policy and systematic scholarship, as questions about (1) location of living settings, (2) size and staffing models for residential support, (3) strategies for individualizing support, and (4) systematic measurement of lifestyle quality have been debated. The authors offer a perspective for examining personal, material, social, productive, and emotional and civic well-being—all of which act to frame a rich adult lifestyle. Felce and Perry help us avoid a simplistic vision of adulthood, emphasize the complex interrelationships that we all depend on, and provide the framework for new research that is committed to linking adult supports to quality of life.

Stancliffe and Lakin tackle the topic of independent living. Their review of research deals with adults with developmental disabilities and lower support needs who live in community settings outside the family home and receive little or no regular paid staff support. These people typically reside in homes that they own or rent—described as *independent living, semi-independent living, supported living,* or *consumer-directed services.* These individuals face problems of affordable housing, ongoing employment, transportation, and health services and medications, and they require some level of intermittent support. The fact that informal or natural supports are crucial to independent living is well established by research, yet there is little research evidence on sustaining and enhancing natural supports. The authors conclude from their understanding of the literature that individuals with developmental disabilities, when given the needed supports, can enjoy self-determined lives in the community.

It is not surprising that people with disabilities, like the rest of us, report the central role that friends and social relationships play in their lives. Most of the research on these relationships, as set forth by Janis Chadsey, has been conducted either in employment settings or community contexts, and a majority of this work is nonexperimental quantitative research. These studies also indicate that the professional field states a preference for friendships between people with and without disabilities over relationships that people with disabilities have with each other or relationships between adults with disabilities and their caregivers. The literature Chadsey reviews suggests that adults with disabilities do form satisfying relationships with others but that their relationships may not be with individuals endorsed by the field. She argues that service provision should extend to social relationships with the goal of fostering community connectedness and relationship with others, not merely to achieve physical integration into the community.

The chapters in this section integrate a wealth of information about (1) instructional strategies that can be applied in work, community, and home contexts; (2) social policy that affects the opportunities for individuals with developmental disabilities to be active, contributing members of society; and (3) the interlinking supports from family, friends, colleagues, and paid staff that may be needed for a rich and successful adulthood. A theme that weaves through these chapters and ties their messages together is the ongoing need to attend to the individual preferences, talents, and challenges of each adult. We each have different ways of fulfilling similar needs, and it is the honoring of individualization that often results in more successful and efficient support.

18

Transition and Quality of Life

Linda M. Bambara
Barbara A. Wilson
Molly McKenzie

Marked with both excited anticipation and uncertainty about the future, the transition from high school to adulthood is significant for everyone. Yet, for youth with developmental disabilities this transition looks very different than it does to those without disabilities, in terms of both outcomes and the services and supports needed to achieve a desirable postschool life. Fortunately, beginning with federal initiatives during the mid-1980s, the past 20 years have been marked by a substantial interest in improving school-based transition services and outcomes through numerous research, policy, and practice initiatives. Mandated by the Individuals with Disabilities Act of 1990 (IDEA) and later reaffirmed and strengthened in IDEA amendments of 1997 and 2004, federal legislation requires schools to identify needed in-school and postschool transition services and to establish linkages with postschool agencies for all youth with disabilities beginning at age 16 or younger. These transition services are to be accomplished through a coordinated set of activities among school personnel, community representatives, parents, and students for the purpose of promoting movement from school to postschool activities, including employment, vocational training, postsecondary education, community participation, or independent living.

Spurred by federal legislation, research has focused on evaluating the most effective school-based transition practices, but not without challenges. Like transition itself, research on effective transition practices is exceedingly complex, as a myriad of factors, not all identified through research, must come together to effect positive outcomes for individual students (Kohler & Field, 2003). Moreover, recent educational reform initiatives, such as No Child Left Behind (NCLB), create new challenges that schools must face in addressing the transition needs of secondary education students (Johnson, Stodden, Emanuel, Luecking, & Mack, 2002).

In this chapter, we review state-of-the-art research with regard to effective transition services for youth with developmental disabilities. Our purpose is to identify best and promising transition practices, challenges and barriers to transition, and future directions for research, policy, and practice based on our analysis of the literature. As a framework to guide and evaluate transition practices, we begin with a brief discussion of quality of life and the concept of adulthood.

TRANSITION TO ADULTHOOD: QUALITY OF LIFE AS KEY INDICATOR

Our cultural understanding of adulthood goes well beyond chronological age and the simple act of completing secondary school. According to Ferguson and Ferguson (2006), adulthood consists of *autonomy*, or the assertion of individuality and independence; *membership*, including affiliation and acceptance by some community group or organization; and *change*, or the ongoing capacity for continued personal growth. Quality of life, a construct closely related to adulthood, shares similar characteristics. Although no single definition or taxonomy of quality of life exists (Hughes, Hwang, Kim, Eisenman, & Killian, 1995), Schalock (2000) offers a useful taxonomy consisting of eight quality-of-life domains frequently used in disability research. These domains include: material well-being (e.g., ownership, employment), emotional well-being, physical well-being, self-determination (e.g., personal control, choices), rights (e.g., privacy, due process, barrier-free environments), social inclusion (e.g., participation, integrated environments), interpersonal relationships (e.g., affiliations, friendships, intimacy), and personal development (e.g., competence, education).

Historically, quality of life has been used as a conceptual framework for evaluating transition outcomes and for guiding the development of transition services for youth with disabilities (Halpern, 1993). Indeed, much of the rationale for transition services is based on poor postschool outcomes for all youth with disabilities as monitored by two national databases. The National Longitudinal Transition Study (NLTS) (NTLS2; n.d.), sponsored by the Office of Special Education Programs (OSEP), tracks the experiences of large cohorts of transition-age youth in special education and as they exit high school. As a follow-up to the initial NTLS1 study, conducted from 1985–1993, NTLS2 currently tracks a second cohort of approximately 12,000 youth with disabilities, starting in 2000 and continuing through 2010. NTLS2 promises comparisons regarding postschool outcomes for young adults with disabilities based on school program components, disability category, and other demographic factors (gender, household income, race) within and across NTLS cohorts (Wagner, Newman, Cameto, & Levine, 2005). Similarly, the National Organization on Disability (NOD) conducts periodic surveys of individuals with and without disabilities to determine whether, and in what ways, life experiences differ for adults with disabilities (NOD, 2004). Currently reporting results of the fifth survey, the NOD provides a comparative picture of the quality of life of adults with disabilities since the initial survey in 1986.

These two national databases consistently reveal that on almost all measures involving aspects of adult living, those with disabilities fare less well than their nondisabled peers. Specifically with regard to material well-being and personal development, individuals with disabilities are less likely to be competitively employed (Blackorby & Wagner, 1996; NOD, 2004; Wagner et al., 2005), to be enrolled in postsecondary education (Blackorby & Wagner, 1996; Wagner et al., 2005), and to live independently or own a home; they are more likely to live in poverty and to worry about their futures (NOD, 2004). Further, with regard to emotional well-being and social inclusion, individuals with disabilities are less likely to socialize and to access their communities (NOD, 2004), and they report fewer friendships and social activities (Johnson et al., 1996; NOD, 2004), less autonomy (Johnson et al., 1996), and lower rates of overall life satisfaction (NOD, 2004) than individuals without disabilities. In the few studies that report data by disability level and type (e.g., Blackorby & Wagner, 1996; Heal, Khoju, Rusch, & Harnish, 1999; Johnson et al., 1996), individuals with "severe" disabilities (including moderate to severe mental retardation and multiple disabilities) experience poorer outcomes on almost all measures than do those with "mild" disabilities (learning disabilities, speech and language impairments). Preliminary findings from the NTLS2, however, paint a somewhat brighter future for young adults with mental retardation, showing an increased percentage holding paying jobs since leaving high school, earning more than minimum wage, and attending postsecondary education over the first cohort group (Wagner et al., 2005).

RESEARCH ON EFFECTIVE TRANSITION PRACTICES

Fueled by this information on poor postschool outcomes, research, for over two decades, has focused on two important questions: What transition practices influence or are predictive of postschool success? How successful have schools been with implementing IDEA transition requirements and "quality" transition services?

With regard to the first question, numerous comprehensive follow-up or follow-along studies of youth with disabilities have linked certain school-based practices with desirable postschool outcomes (e.g., Benz, Lindstrom, & Yovanoff, 2000; Benz, Yovanoff & Doren, 1997; Halpern, Yovanoff, Doren, & Benz, 1995, Hasazi, Furney & Destefano, 1999; Fabian, Lent, & Willis, 1998; Wehmeyer & Schwartz, 1997). These practices include:

- Vocational education, especially actual and paid work experiences while in school.
- Individualized programming based on student needs and interests, emphasizing independent living and self-determination skills.
- Active student and family involvement in the transition planning process.
- Inclusive educational opportunities.
- Interagency collaboration among schools, employers, and adult service providers.

Because these factors are linked to successful outcomes, they serve as the basis for "best practices" in transition education; however, they are not without limitations, especially with regard to students with developmental disabilities. First, competitive employment and, to a lesser extent, postsecondary education predominate the outcome measures used in this predictor-variable research. Although, arguably, financial well-being and postsecondary education are gateway variables to a good life, we know very little about what school-based practices are associated with other outcomes, such as community inclusion, social relationships, and satisfaction with one's quality of life. Second, with the exception of a few studies that focus on youth with mental retardation (e.g., Wehmeyer & Schwartz, 1997), individuals with developmental disabilities often make up a small proportion of the studies' participants. Thus what is not certain is whether these predictor variables hold true for the full range and characteristics of individuals with developmental disabilities, especially those with severe cognitive disabilities. More important, it is not certain what *other* program variables are needed to support these students' unique transition needs. Third, as with all correlational research, causality between predictor variables and postschool outcomes cannot be assumed, as there may be a myriad of other unidentified variables, including student competence (e.g., Heal et al., 1999), that contribute to the variance. Thus what remains uncertain is what specific variables, and in what combinations, produce the most successful adult outcomes for all youth with developmental disabilities.

With regard to the second question, research has revealed that full procedural compliance with transition requirements has not been achieved by schools (deFur, 2003), despite substantial federal and state training initiatives provided to school personnel (National Center on Secondary Education and Transition [NCSET], 2004). Recent data from NLTS2 revealed that 10% of all individualized education plans (IEPs) for transition-age students do not identify transition services (Cameto, Levine, & Wagner, 2004), a figure that remains unchanged over the past decade (Baer, Simmons, & Flexer, 1996). Additionally, for plans that are developed, research has documented numerous procedural violations, including failure to comply with mandated timelines, to invite students to attend the meeting, to invite or otherwise ensure that adult service providers attend the meeting in which interagency linkages would be discussed, and to have a general education teacher attend the meeting (e.g., Baer et al., 1996; Grigal, Test, Beattie, & Wood, 1997; Williams & O'Leary, 2001).

Quality of transition plans is also problematic. For example, in a recent analysis of transition plans contained in 399 IEPs, Powers et al. (2005) found that the majority of the goals (61%) contained little detail on the expected student outcomes, that less than 20% indicated that they were linked to student interests or preferences, and that many did not identify who was responsible for implementing the goals. Once transition plans were written, Baer et al. (1996) found little indication that IEP teams reconvened if the plans were unable to be implemented, and Grigal et al. (1997) found a dearth of annual reviews and revisions of developed plans. Interestingly, some variation in transition planning exists among students with disabilities. Recently, using NTLS2 data, Katsiyannis, Zhang, Woodruff, and Dixon (2005) found that plans for students with developmental disabilities tend to link more detailed instruction to their transition goals and to prescribe more contact with outside agencies than those for students with learning disabilities or emotional disturbance; but the students with developmental disabilities were less likely to participate in the development of their plans than these other students. These variations again remind us to be cautious about generalizing the findings of transition research to all students with disabilities.

Our brief review of these two research foci on effective transition practices illustrates the challenges in interpreting transition research for students with developmental disabilities. First, and simply stated, our knowledge about what practices result in successful outcomes for young adults with developmental disabilities is far from complete. Second, despite tremendous federal effort, compliance with transition mandates is far from satisfactory. Thus it is difficult to define exactly what "effective" transition practices means. Nevertheless, substantial research activity, model demonstration projects, and program evaluation studies continue to unravel pieces of the puzzle both at the program and at the individual student levels. In the next section, we review six best thematic practices in transition education frequently discussed in the literature for all students with disabilities. These practices are research based (linked to postschool outcomes), policy influenced, and/or expert driven, stimulated by critical challenges posed by both policy and practice. Wherever possible, we discuss research and unique challenges for students with developmental disabilities and suggest promising practices for these youth based on emerging research.

BEST AND PROMISING PRACTICES

Create a Student-Centered Transition Plan

Both IDEA mandates and expert-recommended practices emphasize the student-centered nature of the transition process. Transition planning should be a comprehensive and outcome-driven process that takes into consideration all aspects of adult living, as well as individual student and family preferences and needs. Although IDEA does not specify how transition planning should proceed, several key elements have been recommended for keeping the transition process student centered and outcome oriented.

Articulating a vision for postschool life through person-centered planning (PCP) is the first key element recommended by numerous professionals (e.g., deFur, 2003; Morningstar, Kleinhammer-Tramill, & Lattin, 1999). Although several different models of PCP exist, all utilize a group-planning format involving the student, the student's family, and significant professionals. The group identifies and plans for an inclusive vision for the target student based on the student's strengths, preferences, and dreams (Morningstar et al., 1999). The vision then serves as the focal point around which all subsequent transition planning activities develop (e.g., conducting assessments, generating goals and outcomes, collaborating with adult service agencies). Articulating a vision unrestricted by programmatic constraints may be an especially useful activity for students with moderate and severe mental retardation, because both parental (Kraemer & Blacher, 2001) and professional (Hagner, Helm, & Butterworth, 1996) goals for these students tend to be influenced by what is typically made available—segregated living and employment options (e.g., sheltered workshops, group homes)—rather than by inclusive options that might be obtained through strategic planning and advocacy. Research assessing the impact of PCP on postschool outcomes is limited (see Test et al., 2004); however, Flannery and colleagues (2000) provide initial evidence that PCP strategies can result in improved goals for postschool life based on student preferences and strengths, increased student and parent participation, and better parent, student, and educator satisfaction with transition planning meetings.

A second key element of student-centered transition planning is ensuring that the transition plan actually drives all aspects of the student's secondary education. Referred to by Kohler and Field (2003) as "transition-focused education," transition planning is viewed not as an "add-on" activity for students once they reach age 16 but rather as the foundation for which all educational activities and secondary student experiences are developed. In other words, transition planning becomes the action agenda or strategic plan for guiding subsequent IEP goals and the student's educational curriculum, resulting in one integrated plan focused on the student's vision for postschool life (deFur, 2003).

Finally, ensuring that transition practices are implemented flexibly (Benz, Lindstrom, Unruh, & Waintrup, 2004; deFur, 2003; Kohler, 1996) is the third key element of student-centered transition planning. To implement a truly student-centered transition plan, the document must be reviewed annually to reflect the changing skills, needs, and priorities of the transitioning student and his or her family (deFur, 2003). Unfortunately, the biggest threat to implementing these three student-centered transition practices is the general failure of schools to view transition planning as an integral and meaningful series of activities. Viewing the transition plan *as the IEP document* rather than as an additional requirement tacked on to an already developed IEP may help to address the fundamental disconnection between the students' overall educational curriculum and the transition plan, while also increasing compliance with the mandated transition requirements.

Align the School Curriculum with Visions for Postschool Life

The newest challenge facing schools is to prepare students with developmental disabilities for postschool life within the current context of standards-based reform. Brought about by the requirements of NCLB and the 1997 and 2004 amendments to IDEA, standards-based reform requires students with disabilities to "access the general education curriculum" and participate in state and district testing that measures their progress toward achieving the standard outcomes for *all students* in core academic areas defined by their states. The intended consequence of having students with disabilities participate in rigorous academic curriculum is to promote higher levels of learning and increased opportunity to learn grade-level material that will result in a standard high school diploma needed for postschool employment or postsecondary education (Johnson et al., 2002; Stodden, Galloway, & Stodden, 2003). However, a chief concern with the standards-reform movement is that the current emphasis on single-dimension testing on statewide achievement tests will narrow the students' curriculum to the academic content being measured (Turnbull, Turnbull, Wehmeyer, & Park, 2003). Thus nonacademic, functional curriculum domains and vocational work experiences that have been shown to enhance transition outcomes for students with disabilities (e.g., Benz et al., 2000) may be increasingly deemphasized or overlooked. Reviewing the findings of transition research within the context of recent national policy changes, Johnson et al. (2002) concluded that IEP teams must work to ensure that students with disabilities are accessing the general education curriculum while also developing the skills needed for postschool life through a range of curriculum options offered through secondary education settings. The challenge is not to view standards-based reform and transition practices in competition with one another but rather to align transition goals with the general education curriculum while maintaining nonacademic curriculum options shown to enhance transition outcomes. At the same time, transition models are desperately needed to show how effective transition practices can be integrated into general education secondary programs rather than being offered in distinct special education programs only (Kochlar-Bryant & Basset, 2003). To meet these challenges, a number of practices are recommended.

• *Promote high expectations for student learning while making the general education curriculum accessible to learners with developmental disabilities* (Kochlar-Bryant & Basset, 2003; Johnson, et al., 2002; Stodden et al., 2003). High expectations for achievement by students with disabilities in core academic subjects must be maintained. Yet, at the same time, curricular accommodations and adaptations through the use of universal design, differentiated instruction, and assistive technology must be made available in secondary education programs if students with disabilities are to succeed. Unfortunately, our knowledge of and experience with making accommodations at the secondary level is critically limited (Stodden et al., 2003).

• *Ensure that students have access to a full range of secondary education programs and functional curricula* (Johnson et al., 2002). In order to link transition goals to secondary education, a full range of secondary program options is necessary, including those shown to produce successful outcomes for students with disabilities, such as career guidance and work-based learning experiences (Phelps & Hanley-Maxwell, 1997). To avoid the potential narrowing of curriculum options and to ensure that a range of options is made available to *all* students, special educators must be at the table with general educators.

• *Support the use of alternative measures to determine graduation requirements* (Johnson et al., 2002; National Center on Secondary Education and Transition, 2004; Stodden et al., 2003; Thurlow & Johnson, 2000). If the intended goal of the standards-based reform movement is to reduce the disproportionately high dropout rate among students with disabilities (National Center for Education Statistics, 2001) and to increase graduation rates, then standard high school diplomas must be made more achievable by students with disabilities. Consistent with the principles of universal design and differentiated instruction, this may include using alternative and multiple sources of information to document student learning, such as portfolios and other authentic performance-based measures.

• *Establish functional postsecondary programs.* For many students with developmental disabilities, achieving a standard high school diploma will not be a viable option. Developed for students with severe and moderate cognitive disabilities who require educational support to age 21, postsecondary education programs offer a promising solution to meeting both academic and functional transition preparation requirements. The essential characteristics of these programs entail collaborative partnerships between high schools and postsecondary institutions, such as 2- and 4-year colleges, to offer students between ages 18 and 21 continued education and training for postschool life, including employment, independent living, community participation, and lifelong learning (Stodden & Whelley, 2004). Housed in college settings, program models range from "substantially separate," in which high school students with disabilities primarily receive community-based instruction and employment training separate from the curriculum offered to other students in the postsecondary institution, to integrated and highly individualized programs that provide a range of options that include access to typical college classes, as well as community-based instruction and vocational training (Stodden & Whelley, 2004).

The primary purported benefit of the postsecondary education programs is to enhance employability (Hart, Mele-McCarthy, Pasternack, Zimbrich, & Parker, 2004), not only through direct employment training but by also making postsecondary education possible for students with developmental disabilities who have been historically denied this opportunity. Further, postsecondary programs make it possible for students who require a functional curriculum to pursue age-appropriate inclusive high school experiences to the greatest extent possible by postponing employment and community-based instruction until after age 18 or older. Recent research (White & Weiner, 2004) suggests that combined community-based instruction and integrated experiences with age-appropriate nondisabled peers are critical factors leading to the postschool employability of students with severe disabilities.

Research evaluating the outcomes of postsecondary education programs for students with severe and moderate disabilities is in its infancy. Zaft, Hart, and Zimbrich (2004) found that students with severe disabilities who participated in a model demonstration postsecondary education program were more likely to be employed in competitive work and less likely to need employment supports than a matched set of cohorts who did not attend the program. Surveying teachers across 17 postsecondary education settings, Nuebert, Moon, and Grigal (2004) reported that 87% of the students with disabilities served by the programs were employed on campus or in the community, but few participated in college courses for credit or noncredit. Clearly, future research must continue to address the barriers, as well as the outcomes, to postsecondary education programs, including the extent to which students are fully integrated with age-appropriate peers.

Cultivate Student Involvement and Self-Determination

More than just a requirement of IDEA, fostering students' active involvement in their own educational planning and enhancing their self-determination appear paramount to fostering empowerment, lifelong learning, and personal satisfaction with one's life. Although the rationale for promoting self-determination is largely philosophical (Wehmeyer, Field, Doren, Jones, & Mason, 2004) several studies (e.g., Wehmeyer & Palmer, 2003; Wehmeyer & Schwartz, 1997) demonstrate a relationship between self-determination and quality of life. For example, measuring the self-determination levels of 94 high school students with learning disabilities and mental retardation, Wehmeyer and Palmer (2003) found that students who were more self-determined, regardless of their disability classification, fared better on several postschool outcomes, including employment, access to health care, financial independence, and independent living.

Increase IEP Participation

The most promising practices for enhancing self-determination center on teaching skills for self-determination directly, as it can never be assumed that students with developmental disabilities will acquire these critical skills without planned intervention. First, in order for students to take an active role in transition and IEP planning, they not only must be adequately prepared with knowledge of their future goals but also know how to assert and conduct themselves during professional meetings. Test et al. (2004) reviewed 16 studies designed to increase students' participation in their IEP or transition planning meetings. Taken together, these studies show that students with disabilities, including those with mild mental retardation, can be taught the skills needed to participate in their IEP planning and that, when they are prepared to participate through direct instruction, they will increase their level of involvement. Several studies cited in the review also reported increases in self-determination as evaluated by self-determination scales and other measures of self-efficacy as a result of students' participation in IEP training curriculum.

Teach Self-Advocacy

Teaching skills for self-advocacy is another promising practice for promoting positive adult outcomes. Viewed as a subcomponent of self-determination, self-advocacy involves (1) knowledge of oneself, including strengths, limitations, interests, and disability; (2)

knowledge of rights, including general citizenship and disability rights; and (3) effective communication skills for negotiating, persuading, and compromising concerning one's rights and interests (Test, Fowler, Wood, Brewer, & Eddy, 2005). Self-advocacy is needed not only during transition planning but also to ensure that one's rights to appropriate accommodations and services are met in college and employment situations. For example, in one study, college students with disabilities reported that understanding their disabilities and knowing about needed accommodations for academic achievement were essential to their college success; however, they claimed that they were largely unprepared with this knowledge when they entered college and only learned about themselves through trial and error (Thoma & Getzel, 2005).

Research demonstrating the effectiveness of various self-advocacy curricula for students with disabilities, including those with mental retardation, is just beginning to emerge (for a review, see Test, Fowler, Brewer, & Wood, 2005). Although this research shows that students with disabilities can acquire self-advocacy skills through direct instruction, the research base is limited by its exclusive focus on IEP participation. To encourage lifelong self-advocacy, greater attention needs to be paid to teaching students (1) about their own disabilities, (2) general rights and disability law, and (3) general applications of self-advocacy beyond IEP and transition planning meetings.

Infuse Instruction

A third promising practice for enhancing students' self-determination is to infuse self-determination teaching strategies throughout the day. Proponents of self-determination have long held that self-determination is developmental—that is, that instructional opportunities for enhancing self-determination skills such as choice making, decision making, goal setting, problem solving, self-regulation and self-management must start at an early age and be infused throughout the day if learners with developmental disabilities are to acquire the critical skills needed to self-direct during their adult lives. Whereas teaching skills for self-determination has typically fallen under the auspices of special education, the current challenge is figuring out how to infuse self-determination instruction within the current context of standards-based reform (Wehmeyer et al., 2004). The self-determined learning model of instruction (SDLMI), which teaches students to set educational goals, develop action plans to achieve those goals, and self-evaluate goal achievement, is one empirically supported strategy that can be applied to learning situations in the general education curriculum (Wehmeyer, Palmer, Agran, Mithaug, & Martin, 2000). Several studies involving students with developmental disabilities, including those with mild mental retardation, autism, and severe cognitive disabilities, showed that when students were involved in the SDLMI model, they attained self-selected academic and social goals related to their participation in the general education curriculum (Agran, Blanchard, Wehmeyer, & Hughes, 2002; Palmer & Wehmeyer, 2003; Palmer, Wehmeyer, Gipson, & Agran, 2004) and attained self-selected transition goals (Agran, Blanchard, & Wehmeyer, 2000) at or beyond teacher expectations for their performance. Further, Palmer et al. (2004) reported improved problem-solving and study-planning skills related to academic content, as well as general increases in student self-determination for middle and high school students with intellectual disabilities as a result of SDLMI.

Perhaps one the biggest obstacles to enhancing students' self-determination and involvement in their educational planning is supporting teachers in implementing these practices routinely. Recent surveys revealed that many teachers (both general and special educators) were unfamiliar with the concept of self-determination and, that those who were familiar with the concept reported few opportunities for students to practice their self-determination skills or to be involved in IEP planning despite teachers' views that self-determination is important (e.g., Grigal, Nueber, Moon, & Graham, 2003; Mason, Field, & Sawilowsky, 2004; Wehmeyer, Agran, & Hughes, 2000). This suggests that a greater focus on teacher preparation and systems-change research is needed to better understand and eliminate the barriers to promoting student self-determination in schools.

Establish Interagency Collaboration

Interagency collaboration is one transition practice that has a long history of empirical support (e.g., Benz, et al, 2000; Kohler, 1993). As required by IDEA, IEP teams are responsible for identifying and engaging responsible agencies, needed resources, and accommodations required for successful postschool outcomes before students exit high school. Despite this requirement, recent NLTS2 data collected on transition-age youth during 2001–2002 revealed moderate to poor collaboration between schools and adult service providers (NCSET, 2005). As reported, school contacts with adult service providers and other community agencies for students ranged from fewer than 5% to 38%, depending on the postschool program, with the greatest number of contacts made with state vocational rehabilitation agencies (VR; 38%), followed by contacts with vocational and postsecondary schools (both at 24%). With regard to interagency participation in student transition planning, school personnel reported that about only 30% of the students with transition plans had had representatives from outside agencies actively participate. Again, VR representatives were more likely to be involved than all other adult providers or organizations.

Barriers to interagency collaboration are numerous, including: (1) lack of information sharing about students across agencies, making it impossible to develop needed service plans that support students in achieving postschool goals; (2) ineffectual contract agreements between schools and outside agencies; (3) lack of systematic planning across agencies; (4) difficulties projecting needed postschool services; and (5) inefficient practices for establishing interagency collaboration (Johnson et al., 2002). Families report that poor coordination creates undue stress and frustration as they try to secure needed services for their children (Benz, Johnson, Mikkelsen, & Lindstrom, 1995). Perhaps the single factor contributing most to poor interagency collaboration is the fact that schools, vocational providers, and other adult disability service organizations operate as distinct and separate systems, each constrained by its own priorities, policies, and challenges, especially financial, that inhibit their ability to act flexibly and coordinate with others (Certo et al., 2003). Additionally, although adult service providers may be committed to providing the best services to their consumers, they are not obligated to participate in transition planning.

Multilevel interagency transition teams offer one promising solution to establishing long-term and effective collaborations among key transition stakeholders (Blalock, 1996; Stodden, Brown, Galloway, Mrazek, & Noy, 2005). Originally proposed by Blalock (1996), interagency transition teams comprise coordinated levels of service that include: (1) an individualized student team that develops and implements a student's transition plan; (2) a schoolwide transition team that develops and monitors schoolwide practices; (3) a community or regional transition team that establishes key partnerships among schools, adult provider agencies, postsecondary institutions, and future employers; and (4) a state-level transition team that functions to create policy and a state infra-structure needed for community-level agencies to collaborate and improve services. Both program evaluation (Aspel, Bettis, Quinn, Test, & Wood, 1999; Benz, Linstrom, & Halpern, 1995), and qualitative case data (Collet-Klingenberg, 1998) offer evidence that a multilevel approach can improve student and family satisfaction, transition services, and outcomes for students.

To overcome the challenges inherent in different systems serving youth with dis-abilities, NCSET (2004) recommends that agencies pool their resources to enhance coordination and to financially support needed services. Certo et al. (2003) described an integrated transition model designed for students with severe and moderate cogni-tive disabilities in which local area school districts, VR, and developmental disabilities providers pooled their finances and expertise to create a "hybrid" agency that served as a bridge from high school to the adult service system. Certo and colleagues (2003) reported impressive outcomes, considering the often interrupted services and the low employment rates experienced by youth with severe disabilities. Of the 224 graduates of the program, 88% transitioned into the adult service system without a lapse of service. Further, 71% were competitively employed 3 years after completing the program.

Facilitate Work-Based Learning Experiences

For more than two decades, numerous research and model demonstration projects stimulated by federal initiatives, such as the School-to-Work Opportunities Act (e.g., Kohler & Hood, 2000; Phelps & Hanley-Maxwell, 1997) have documented the impor-tance of involving students with disabilities in community-based work experiences while they are still in school. Research continues to show a strong link between school work experience and postschool job success for all students with disabilities (e.g., Baer et al., 2003) including those with severe intellectual disabilities (e.g., White & Weiner, 2004). In addition to fostering critical employment skills needed for postschool success (Lueking & Gramlich, 2003), work experiences, when structured around social inclu-sion, can serve as the gateway to other quality-of-life outcomes, including friendships, job satisfaction, and community participation for youth with developmental disabilities (Wehman, 2003).

Built around activities that provide actual work experiences or connect classroom learning to work, examples of work-based learning include: career awareness and explo-ration activities, workplace mentoring, and direct work experience through volunteer and community service; paid work and on-the-job training; and youth apprenticeships and school-based enterprises (Sitlington & Clark, 2006). Quality indicators for success-ful programs include clear training plans geared specifically to individual student out-comes, connections between work and classroom-based learning, clear expectations of student performance in the workplace, clearly defined roles between teachers and work-place supervisors, and continued, well-structured feedback on student performance (Lueking & Gramlich, 2003). In addition, effective work-based learning programs incor-porate "connecting activities" that provide continuous support for students at risk for work failure during high school and through their early postsecondary transition years (Benz et al., 1997), such as Certo et al.'s (2003) hybrid agency, as previously described.

Many work-based models exist (Kohler & Hood, 2000), but one widely replicated model that incorporates many of the quality features already identified is the bridge from school to work model (Luecking & Fabian, 2000; Luecking & Gramlich, 2003). The bridge model features paid internships with local employers for students with disabilities in their last year of high school. Follow-up studies of over 3,000 students served by the program across seven program sites revealed a high rate of postschool employment regardless of gender, race, or primary disability (Luecking & Fabian, 2000).

Clearly, successful work-based learning depends on establishing strong partnerships between schools, prospective employers, and adult service providers. Although the emphasis of transition research has been on school practice, employers and the adult service system also play a critical role. One challenge to address is the negative perceptions that employers may have about hiring youth with disabilities. Luecking and Mooney (2002) recommend that work-based learning programs develop marketing strategies that emphasize "return of investment" for employers who hire students with disabilities. Another challenge is coordinating long-term employment supports with overtaxed and underfunded adult service providers. In order to maintain competitive employment, many students with developmental disabilities will need the ongoing services of supported employment. Unfortunately, although the number of supported-employment programs continues to grow nationally, funding for these programs has not kept pace with that for segregated adult day programs and sheltered workshops. Rusch and Braddock (2004) report that funding for segregated programs is more than four times that provided for supported employment and, further, that enrollment in segregated adult programs continues to grow at the same rate as that in supported employment. These data suggest that opportunities for competitive employment are limited for youth with significant support needs, despite federal disability employment initiatives (e.g., Ticket-to-Work and Work Improvement Act) that are intended to empower individuals with disabilities to choose and purchase their own employment supports.

Promote Family Involvement and Partnerships

Research has shown that both immediate and extended family members influence and facilitate adult living and employment opportunities by assisting in identifying and obtaining community employment (Hasazi, Gordon, & Roe, 1985), by negotiating with social agencies for needed services (Devlieger & Trach, 1999), by helping to formulate students' personal career and living plans (Morningstar, Turnbull & Turnbull, 1995), and by providing critical information to professionals regarding the preferences and abilities of their children (Cooney, 2002). For many individuals with developmental disabilities, the family constitutes the most reliable source of support throughout their lives (Kim & Morningstar, 2005). Although parents of students with disabilities have been mandated members of the transition team since 1990, parents are not consistently invited to transition planning meetings (Baer et al., 1996), and, when they do attend, they are often not treated as valued members (deFur, Todd-Allen, & Getzel, 2001).

Families state that barriers to their participation include: (1) not being perceived as meaningful participants in the IEP meeting or transition process, (2) lack of empathy or understanding of cultural and family differences by professionals, and (3) lack of specific supports or recommendations for meeting the unique needs of the student and family. For example, parents participating in qualitative investigations that focused on their transition planning experiences (Cooney, 2002; deFur et al., 2001) report feelings of powerlessness within the planning team. Culturally diverse parents indicate that the general lack of understanding of and respect for their family's culture, as well as specific challenges they face when attending meetings (language differences, child care, work hours, etc.) hinders their participation in their child's transition planning (Kim & Morningstar, 2005). Additionally, Rueda, Monzo, Shapiro, Gomez, and Blacher (2005) point out that the typical desired outcomes of transition planning, especially those that emphasize individualism and independent living, are not necessarily representative of the goals that some (e.g., Latino) cultures have for their adult children, further contributing to the alienation some parents feel. Finally, across disability and cultural groups, parents express frustration with the lack of information about adult services and postschool options received from school personnel (see, e.g., deFur et al., 2001; Kim & Morningstar, 2005; Rueda et al., 2005). In fact, some parents believe that information is consciously withheld to discourage their participation (Rueda et al., 2005).

Maximizing the unique contribution of family members to the transition planning process requires specific attention to the needs of families and removal of the barriers identified by parents as limiting their participation. No one best-practice model exists to facilitate parental involvement; however, researchers and transition experts recommend the following research-based practices. First, professionals involved in the transition planning process must work to develop a trusting relationship with families characterized by open and respectful communication. Parental support has been identified as perhaps the primary factor contributing to student achievement (deFur et al., 2001), and establishing a trusting relationship is considered a critical component in building a meaningful family–school partnership (Hanley-Maxwell, Pogoloff, & Whitney-Thomas, 1998). In fact, parents report increased participation in transition/IEP meetings when a relationship with school and adult service personnel has been established prior to the meeting (Salembier & Furney, 1997). Although there may be many reasons why families elect not to participate in formal meetings (deFur et al., 2001), parents consistently identify communication difficulties as barriers to partnering with school staff (deFur et al., 2001; Salembier & Furney, 1997). As identified by parents, strategies for enhancing parent–professional relationships include listening to the contributions of the parents, maintaining frequent communication, and ensuring that the communication reflects both honesty and respect (Pruitt, Wandry, & Hollums, 1998).

Second, school personnel must be made more aware of the impact that various cultural and family differences have on the transition planning process and must adjust the process to meet family values, priorities, and needs. The transition to adulthood affects not only the student but also the whole family in terms of its impact and outcomes (Kim & Morningstar, 2005). Specific recommendations for increasing professional responsiveness to families include increasing the cultural awareness of school personnel, as well as developing an understanding of and empathy for the uniqueness of each family's situation, including language and support needs and differences in family structures (Kim & Morningstar, 2005).

Third, information on the transition process should be made available to parents through both formal and informal means. Parent training and information centers can serve as valuable resources for information relating to the transition requirements and services available to parents and can provide transition-related information specific to the geographic area in which the student lives (Aspel et al., 1999; Johnson et al., 2002). In addition, informal information sharing through parent-to-parent support groups is another way for families to obtain relevant information (Rueda et al., 2005). Finally, NCSET (2004) recommends extending parent involvement beyond the individual level by providing opportunities for families to be involved in defining transition practices at the policy level.

SUMMARY AND IMPLICATIONS FOR FUTURE DIRECTIONS

In the final analysis, successful transition to adulthood will depend on how well multiple factors can come together to address the needs of youth with developmental disabilities and whether we can structure the educational and service systems that surround them to provide for and maintain what is needed for postschool success. Toward this end, our field has made substantial progress toward identifying research-based practices and understanding what works; yet numerous challenges exist. To summarize some of the key points made in this chapter and to identify the issues we believe are most critical to the future development and implementation of transition education, we offer the following implications for policy makers, researchers, and practitioners and families.

For Policy Makers

- *Facilitate stronger linkages between schools and various adult-serving systems, including postsecondary institutions, community employers, and vocational and developmental disabilities providers.* Improved collaboration across systems cannot happen without increased federal incentives and established statewide and local infrastructures of support.

- *Work toward the unification of general and special education.* As long as a dual system of education continues to exit, conflicting priorities between general and special education will threaten transition services for youth with developmental disabilities. The longevity of sustainable transition practices seems dependent on the commitment of one single educational system with shared priorities that will benefit all children.

- *Transform the adult developmental disabilities service system to better align with transition education.* Looking beyond interagency collaboration, an infrastructure of continued resources and support must be in place to enable a seamless transition in the adult service system for youth who will require lifelong assistance. Positive long-term outcomes for these individuals will not be possible unless the adult service system shares the same priorities as transition education and is empowered financially to provide integrated employment and community living supports.

For Researchers

- *Focus transition research on identifying and addressing implementation barriers.* Identifying and mandating best and research-based practices are hollow efforts unless we figure out how to implement these practices in meaningful and sustainable ways within existing and emerging educational systems. Sustainable practice will largely depend on how well transition can be aligned with typical school procedures and on how it is valued by both school administrators and the general school community.

- *Expand quality-of-life outcome measures of postschool success; consider individual variations, preferences, and cultural influences.* Outcome measures in transition research are largely competency based, overly focused on employment, and fail to take into account individual and family preferences that are influenced by culture and needs. To the extent that outcome measures drive transition policy, research, and practice, our understanding of what it takes to promote a good life beyond "normative" views of employment and independent living is greatly underdeveloped. Increased attention needs to be paid to fostering community participation, social inclusion, friendships, personal satisfaction, and self-determination in culturally responsive ways.

• *Focus transition research on the support needs of students with moderate and severe developmental disabilities.* Certainly, all students with disabilities will benefit from the common core of transition practices identified in this chapter; however, students with more significant challenges are likely to require long-term supports and accommodations through supported living, supported employment, and natural social networks that are not typically addressed in the mainstream school-based transition literature. At issue here is a greater need to focus on the environmental and social support needs of students, not just on the skills needed for adult life.

For Practitioners and Families

• *Foster shared information and collaborative partnerships among families and practitioners.* In order for families to be empowered to advocate for their children, they need to be knowledgeable about existing resources and opportunities. Practitioners should focus on how to best engage families to establish true partnerships.

• *Improve the quality of teacher/practitioner preparation and training.* To develop a qualified workforce of transition-age youth, consideration must be given to strengthening preservice and in-service training that implements best transition practices.

REFERENCES

Agran, M., Blanchard, C., & Wehmeyer, M. L. (2000). Promoting transition goals and self-determination through student and self-directed learning: The self-determined learning model of instruction. *Education and Training in Mental Retardation and Developmental Disabilities, 35*, 351–364.

Agran, M., Blanchard, C., Wehmeyer, M., & Hughes, C. (2002). Increasing the problem-solving skills of students with developmental disabilities participating in general education. *Remedial and Special Education, 23*, 279–288.

Aspel, N., Bettis, G., Quinn, P., Test, D. W., & Wood, W. M. (1999). A collaborative process for planning transition services for students with disabilities. *Career Development for Exceptional Individuals, 22*, 21–42.

Baer, R., Simmons, T., & Flexer, R. (1996). Transition practice and policy compliance in Ohio: A survey of secondary special educators. *Career Development for Exceptional Individuals, 19*, 61–71.

Baer, R. M., Flexer, R. W., Beck, S., Hoffman, L., Brothers, J., Stelzer, D., et al. (2003). A collaborative follow-up study on transition service utilization and postschool outcomes. *Career Development for Exceptional Individuals, 26*, 7–25.

Benz, M. R., Johnson, D. K., Mikkelsen, K. S., & Lindstrom, L. E. (1995). Improving collaboration between schools and vocational rehabilitation: Stakeholder identified barriers and strategies. *Career Development for Exceptional Individuals, 18*, 133–144.

Benz, M. R., Lindstrom, L. E., & Halpern, A. S. (1995). Mobilizing local communities to improve transition services. *Career Development for Exceptional Individuals, 18*, 21–32.

Benz, M. R., Lindstrom, L., Unruh, D., & Waintrup, M. (2004). Sustaining secondary transition programs in local schools. *Remedial and Special Education, 25*, 39–50.

Benz, M. R., Lindstrom, L., & Yovanoff, P. (2000). Improving graduation and employment outcomes of students with disabilities: Predictive factors and student perspectives. *Exceptional Children, 66*, 509–529.

Benz, M. R., Yovanoff, P., & Doren, B. (1997). School to work components that predict postschool success for students with and without disabilities. *Exceptional Children, 63*, 151–165.

Blackorby, J., & Wagner, M. (1996). Longitudinal postschool outcomes of youth with disabilities: Findings from the National Longitudinal Transition Study. *Exceptional Children, 62*, 399–413.

Blalock, G. (1996). Community transition teams as the foundation for transition services for youth with learning disabilities. *Journal of Learning Disabilities, 29,* 148–159.

Cameto, R., Levine, P., & Wagner, M. (2004). *Transition planning for students with disabilities: A special topic report of findings from the National Longitudinal Transition Study-2 (NLTS2).* Retrieved October 10, 2005, from *www.nlts2.org/pdfs/transitionplanning_execsum.pdf.*

Certo, N. J., Mautz, D., Pumpian, I., Sax, C., Smalley, K., Wade, H. A., et al.. (2003). Review and discussion of a model for seamless transition to adulthood. *Education and Training in Developmental Disabilities, 38,* 3–17.

Collet-Klingenberg, L. L. (1998). The reality of best practices in transition: A case study. *Exceptional Children, 65,* 67–78.

Cooney, B. F. (2002). Exploring perspectives on transition of youth with disabilities: Voices of young adults, parents, and professionals. *Mental Retardation, 40,* 425–435.

deFur, S. (2003). IEP transition planning: From compliance to quality. *Exceptionality, 11,* 115–128.

deFur, S. H., Todd-Allen, M., & Getzel, E. E. (2001). Parent participation in the transition planning process. *Career Development for Exceptional Individuals, 24,* 19–36.

Devlieger, P. J., & Trach, J. S. (1999). Mediation as a transition process: The impact on postschool employment outcomes. *Exceptional Children, 65,* 507–524.

Fabian, E. S., Lent, R. W., & Willis, S. P. (1998). Predicting work transition outcomes for students with disabilities: Implications for counselors. *Journal of Counseling and Development, 76,* 311–316.

Ferguson, P., & Ferguson, D. (2006). The promise of adulthood. In M. E. Snell & F. Brown (Eds.), *Instruction of students with severe disabilities* (6th ed., pp. 610–637). Upper Saddle River, NJ: Pearson/ Merrill Prentice Hall.

Flannery, B., Newton, S., Horner, R., Slovic, R., Blumberg, R., & Ard, W. R. (2000). The impact of person-centered planning on the content and organization of individualized supports. *Career Development for Exceptional Individuals, 23,* 123–137.

Furney, K. S., Hasazi, S. B., & Destephano, L. (1997). Transition policies, practices, and promises: Lessons from three states. *Exceptional Children, 63,* 343–355.

Grigal, M., Neubert, D. A., Moon, M. S., & Graham, S. (2003). Self-determination for students with disabilities: Views of parents and teachers. *Exceptional Children, 70,* 97–112.

Grigal, M., Test, D. W., Beattie, J., & Wood, W. M. (1997). An evaluation of transition components of individualized education programs. *Exceptional Children, 63,* 357–372.

Hagner, D., Helm, D. T., & Butterworth, J. (1996). "This is your meeting": A qualitative study of person-centered planning. *Mental Retardation, 34,* 159–171.

Halpern, A. S. (1993). Quality of life as a conceptual framework for evaluating transition outcomes. *Exceptional Children, 59,* 486–498.

Halpern, A. S., Yovanoff, P., Doren, B., & Benz, M. R. (1995). Predicting participation in postsecondary education for school leavers with disabilities. *Exceptional Children, 62,* 151–164.

Hanley-Maxwell, C., Pogoloff, S. M., & Whitney-Thomas, J. (1998). Families: The heart of transition. In F. R. Rusch & J. G. Chadsey (Eds.), *Beyond high school: Transition from school to work* (pp. 234–264). Belmont, CA: Wadsworth.

Hart, D., Mele-McCarthy, J., Pasternack, R. H., Zimbrich, K., & Parker, D. R. (2004). Community college: A pathway to success for youth with learning, cognitive, and intellectual disabilities in secondary settings. *Education and Training in Developmental Disabilities, 39,* 54–66.

Hasazi, S. B., Furney, K. S., & Destefano, L. (1999). Implementing the IDEA transition mandates. *Exceptional Children, 65,* 555–566.

Hasazi, S. B., Gordon, L. R., & Roe, C. A. (1985). Factors associated with the employment status of handicapped youth exiting high school from 1979 to 1983. *Exceptional Children, 6,* 455–469.

Heal, L. W., Khoju, M., Rusch, F. R., & Harnish, D. L. (1999). Predicting quality of life of students who have left special education high school programs. *American Journal on Mental Retardation, 104,* 305–319.

Hughes, C., Hwang, B., Kim, J., Eisenman, L. T., & Killian, D. J. (1995). Quality of life in applied research: A review and analysis of empirical measures. *American Journal on Mental Retardation, 99,* 623–641.

Johnson, D. R., McGrew, K., Bloomberg, L., Bruininks, R. H., & Lin, H. (1996). *Postschool outcomes and community adjustment of young adults with severe disabilities.* Minneapolis, MN: Center on Residential

Services and Community Living, University of Minnesota. (ERIC Document Reproduction Service No. ED392209).

Johnson, D. R., Stodden, R. A., Emanuel, E., Luecking, R., & Mack, M. (2002). Current challenges facing secondary education and transition services: What research tells us. *Exceptional Children, 68,* 519–531.

Katsiyannis, A., Zhang, D., Woodruff, N., & Dixon, A. (2005). Transition supports to students with mental retardation: An examination of data from the National Longitudinal Transition Study-2. *Education and Training in Developmental Disabilities, 40,* 109–116.

Kim, K., & Morningstar, M. E. (2005). Transition planning involving culturally and linguistically diverse families. *Career Development for Exceptional Individuals, 28,* 92–103.

Kochlar-Bryant, C. A., & Basset, D. S. (2003). *Aligning transition and SBE: Beyond square pegs and round holes.* Retrieved October 17, 2005, from *www.ncset.org/summit03/ppts/NCSET2003Align.ppt.*

Kohler, P. D. (1993). Best practices in transition: Substantiated or implied? *Career Development for Exceptional Individuals, 16,* 107–121.

Kohler, P. D. (1996). *Taxonomy for transition programming: Linking research and practice.* Champaign: University of Illinois at Urbana-Champaign, Transition Research Institute.

Kohler, P. D., & Field, S. (2003). Transition-focused education: Foundation for the future. *Journal of Special Education, 37,* 174–182.

Kohler, P. D., & Hood, L. (2000). *Improving student outcomes: Promising practices and programs for 1999–2000.* Champaign: University of Illinois at Urbana-Champaign, Transition Research Institute.

Kraemer, B. R., & Blacher, J. (2001). Transition for young adults with severe mental retardation: School preparation, parent expectations, and family involvement. *Mental Retardation, 39,* 423–435.

Luecking, R. G., & Fabian, E. S. (2000). Paid internships and employment success for youth in transition. *Career Development for Exceptional Children, 23,* 205–221.

Luecking, R., & Gramlich, M. (2003, September). Quality work-based learning and postschool employment success. *Issue Brief: Examining Current Challenges in Secondary Education and Transition, 2*(2), 1–5.

Luecking, R. G., & Mooney, M. (2002, December). Tapping employment opportunities for youth with disabilities by engaging effectively with employers. *Research to Practice Brief: Improving Secondary Education and Transition Services through Research, 1*(3), 3–7.

Mason, C., Field, S., & Sawilowsky, S. (2004). Implementation of self-determination activities and student participation in IEPs. *Exceptional Children, 70,* 441–451.

Morningstar, M. E., Kleinhammer-Tramill, P. J., & Lattin, D. L. (1999). Using successful models of student-centered transition planning and services for adolescents with disabilities. *Focus on Exceptional Children, 31*(9), 1–19.

Morningstar, M. E., Turnbull, A. P., & Turnbull, H. R. (1995). What do students with disabilities tell us about the importance of family involvement in the transition from school to adult life? *Exceptional Children, 62,* 252–260.

National Center for Education Statistics. (2001). *Dropout rates in the United States: 2000* (NCES No. 2002114). Washington, DC: U.S. Department of Education, Office of Educational Research and Improvement.

National Center on Secondary Education and Transition. (2004). *Current challenges facing the future of secondary education and transition services for youth with disabilities in the United States.* Retrieved January 11, 2006, from *www.ncset.org/publications/discussionpaper.pdf.*

National Center on Secondary Education and Transition. (2005). *NTLS2 data brief: The transition planning process.* Retrieved August 9, 2005, from *www.ncset.org/publications/printresource.asp?id=2130.*

National Longitudinal Transition Study-2. (n.d.). *NTLS2 home and news.* Retrieved February 12, 2006, from *www.nlts2.org/gindex.html.*

National Organization on Disability. (2004). *N.O.D./Harris survey of Americans with disabilities.* New York: Harris International.

Neubert, D. A., Moon, M. S., & Grigal, M. (2004). Activities of students with disabilities receiving services in postsecondary settings. *Education and Training in Developmental Disabilities, 39,* 16–25.

Palmer, S. B., & Wehmeyer, M. L. (2003). Promoting self-determination in early elementary school: Teaching self-regulated problem solving and goal setting skills. *Remedial and Special Education, 24,* 115–126.

Palmer, S. B., Wehmeyer, M. L., Gipson, K., & Agran, M. (2004). Promoting access to the general curriculum by teaching self-determination skills. *Exceptional Children, 70*, 427–439.

Phelps, L. A., & Hanley-Maxwell, C. (1997). School-to-work transitions for youth with disabilities: A review of outcomes and practices. *Review of Educational Research, 67*, 197–226.

Powers, K. M., Gil-Kashiwabara, E., Geenen, S. I., Powers, L. E., Balandran, J., & Palmer, C. (2005). Mandates and effective transition planning practices reflected in IEPs. *Career Development for Exceptional Individuals, 28*, 47–59.

Pruitt, P., Wandry, D., & Hollums, D. (1998). Listen to us! Parents speak out about their interactions with special educators. *Preventing School Failure, 42*, 161–166.

Rueda, R., Monzo, L., Shapiro, J., Gomez, J., & Blacher, J. (2005). Cultural models of transition: Latina mothers of young adults with developmental disabilities. *Exceptional Children, 71*, 401–414.

Rusch, F. R., & Braddock, D. (2004). Adult day programs versus supported employment (1998–2004): Spending and service practices of mental retardation and developmental disabilities state agencies. *Research and Practice for Persons with Severe Disabilities*, 237–242.

Salembier, G., & Furney, K. S. (1997). Facilitating participation: Parents' perceptions of their involvement in the IEP/transition planning process. *Career Development for Exceptional Individuals, 20*, 29–42.

Schalock, R. (2000). Three decades of quality of life: Mental retardation in the 21st century. In M. L. Wehmeyer & J. R. Patton (Eds.), *Mental retardation in the year 2000* (pp. 335–355). Austin, TX: PRO-ED.

Sitlington, P., & Clark, G. M. (2006). *Transition education and services for students with disabilities.* Boston: Pearson/Allyn & Bacon.

Stodden, R. A., Brown, S. E., Galloway, L. M., Mrazek, S., & Noy, L. (2005). *Essential tools: Interagency transition team development and facilitation.* Minneapolis, MN: University of Minnesota, Institute on Community Integration, National Center on Secondary Education and Transition.

Stodden, R. A., Galloway, L. M., & Stodden, N. J. (2003). Secondary school curricula issues: Impact on postsecondary students with disabilities. *Exceptional Children, 70*, 9–25.

Stodden, R. A., & Whelley, T. (2004). Postsecondary education and persons with intellectual disabilities: An introduction. *Education and Training in Developmental Disabilities, 39*, 6–15.

Test, D. W., Fowler, C. H., Brewer, D. M., & Wood, W. (2005). A content and methodological review of self-advocacy intervention studies. *Exceptional Children, 72*, 101–125.

Test, D. W., Fowler, C. H., Wood, W. M., Brewer, D. M., & Eddy, S. (2005). A conceptual framework of self-advocacy for students with disabilities. *Remedial and Special Education, 26*, 43–54.

Test, D. W., Mason, C., Hughes, C., Konrad, M., Neale, M., & Wood, W. M. (2004). Student involvement in individualized education program meetings. *Exceptional Children, 70*, 391–412.

Thoma, C. A., & Getzel, E. E. (2005). "Self-determination is what it's all about": What postsecondary students with disabilities tell us are important considerations for success. *Education and Training in Developmental Disabilities, 40*, 234–242.

Thurlow, M. L., & Johnson, D. R. (2000). High stakes testing of students with disabilities. *Journal of Teacher Education, 51*, 305–314.

Turnbull, H. R., Turnbull, A. P., Wehmeyer, M. L., & Park, J. (2003). A quality of life framework for special education outcomes. *Remedial and Special Education, 24*, 67–74.

Wagner, M., Newman, L., Cameto, R., & Levine, P. (2005). *Changes over time in the early postschool outcomes of youth with disabilities.* Retrieved October 10, 2005, from *www.nlts2.org/pdfs/str6_completereport.pdf.*

Wehman, P. (2003). Workplace inclusion: Persons with disabilities and coworkers working together. *Journal of Vocational Rehabilitation, 18*, 131–141.

Wehmeyer, M. L., Agran, M., & Hughes, C. (2000). A national survey of teachers' promotion of self-determination and student-directed learning. *Journal of Special Education, 34*, 58–68.

Wehmeyer, M. L., Field, S., Doren, B., Jones, B., & Mason, C. (2004). Self-determination and student involvement in standards-based reform. *Exceptional Children, 70*, 413–425.

Wehmeyer, M. L., & Palmer, S. B. (2003). Adult outcomes for students with cognitive disabilities three years after high school: The impact of self-determination. *Education and Training in Developmental Disabilities, 38*, 131–144.

Wehmeyer, M. L., Palmer, S. B., Agran, M., Mithaug, D. E., & Martin, J. (2000). Teaching students causal agents in their lives: The self-determining learning model of instruction. *Exceptional Children, 66,* 439–453.

Wehmeyer, M. L., & Schwartz, M. (1997). Self-determination and positive adult outcomes: A follow-up study of youth with mental retardation or learning disabilities. *Exceptional Children, 63,* 245–255.

White, J., & Weiner, J. S. (2004). Influence of least restrictive environment and community based training on integrated employment outcomes for transitioning students with severe disabilities. *Journal of Vocational Rehabilitation, 21,* 149–156.

Williams, J. M., & O'Leary, E. (2001). What we've learned and where we go from here. *Career Development for Exceptional Individuals, 24,* 51–71.

Zaft, C., Hart, D., & Zimbrich, K. (2004). College career connection: A study of youth with intellectual disabilities and the impact of postsecondary education. *Education and Training in Developmental Disabilities, 39,* 45–53.

Employment

David Mank

Meaningful choices and quality of life become possible with discretionary income. Having discretionary income means being able to: pay your expenses in life, choose where you live, choose whom you live with, make choices about how you spend your free time, give a gift to a friend or to a favorite social cause, plan a vacation, choose whether to buy an entertainment system or a golf membership, buy a home, or indulge an interest in a hobby of woodworking or piano lessons. For the vast majority of people in almost any culture, discretionary income is the product of working. Some people have discretionary income because they live with someone who earns enough money to provide discretionary income in the household, and choices can be made about how to contribute in life through raising children, maintaining a household, or doing volunteer work or other activities of one's choosing. A few people are simply wealthy and have many choices and opportunities for quality of life because they have the resources to support those choices. For most, contributing in life and creating discretionary resources are the results of the income generated from working.

In addition, having life choices and discretionary income also makes it much more likely that people who are employed will have a social network. Social networks bring a sense of belonging and participation in the culture of a workplace and in the flow of community life. The alternative is having fewer friends and a greater probability of isolation. Further, as those who are employed know, employment provides a structure for day-to-day life and the benefits of contributing to society.

For people with developmental disabilities, gainful employment and the choices of everyday life have been limited, to say the least. Choosing where and with whom one lives, as well as other choices in life, is difficult if one has little money and lives on Social Security benefits. People with developmental disabilities have historically had very limited access to the gainful employment that results in making contributions to life and in possessing discretionary income.

Remarkably, or perhaps not so, the possibilities and expectations for employment for people with developmental disabilities are approaching those of others in society. Although the unemployment and underemployment rates for people with developmental disabilities remain unacceptably high in the late 2000s (as high as 75%), it is becoming increasingly clear that people with developmental disabilities have the ability to be gainfully employed.

In part, this change in employment possibilities for people with developmental disabilities reflects a change in expectations. And, in part, this change in expectations is the result of discovering the employment potential of people with developmental disabilities and of the discovery of interventions and methods to create and support their long-term employment goals. Initially, a focus on employment was intended to emphasize the value of working and to create opportunities for real work for people with developmental disabilities. This emphasis on creating opportunity is now giving way to an expectation of gainful employment for people with developmental disabilities (e.g., Wehman, Revell, & Brooke, 2003; Mank, Cioffi, & Yovanoff, 2003; Callahan & Garner, 1997; Hagner, 2000).

The number of people with developmental disabilities in community employment has grown from just a few thousand in 1984 to more than 150,000 in 2005 (Wehman et al., 2003). Despite the gains that have been made, fewer than 30% of people with developmental disabilities are employed in community settings. For example, data from the State of Indiana shows that about 25% of people with developmental disabilities hold jobs in the community (e.g., Grossi & Mank, 2005). Even fewer are working full time or nearly full time, acquiring company-paid benefits, and earning a living wage. This reality of unemployment and underemployment remains at odds with the interventions well known to be effective, the clear capabilities of people with developmental disabilities, and the policy framework that encourages gainful employment.

The purpose of this chapter is to explore the history of, research on, and implications of several decades of innovation, research, values clarification, and policy development related to the future of employment for people with developmental disabilities.

HISTORICAL CONTEXT

The path to changing the employment status of people with developmental disabilities is rich in the history of several decades of discovery through research, and the evolving mission of community rehabilitation agencies, along with policy and legal changes over time. The research related to employment began with the discovery of teaching strategies that demonstrated that people with developmental disabilities, even the most significant ones, could work productively on tasks. This research evolved into interventions and demonstrations of people working in regular community jobs. At the same time, the organizations that provided day services to people with developmental disabilities evolved to take advantage of this newfound potential and the focus on community jobs, rather than services in congregate and segregated settings increased. Along with this community-scale evolution, the policy and legal structure of states and the United States evolved to emphasize independence, productivity, and integration (Developmental Disabilities Assistance and Bill of Rights Act, 2000). Together, the research and the evolving mission of community agencies, along with policy and funding changes, are combining to create a focus on significant earnings, along with benefits management and building of assets, through work.

EVOLVING RESEARCH

Through the 1960s, little was expected of people with developmental disabilities in any way, including learning skills of daily living or vocational tasks. The advent of applied behavior analysis and new instructional approaches resulted in the discovery of the ability of people with developmental disabilities to learn and maintain skills. Initially, this research focused on the skills of daily living: doing laundry, cooking, handling money, and so forth. Over time, these new interventions were applied to work tasks, albeit in segregated settings (e.g., Gold, 1973; Bellamy, Horner, & Inman, 1979).

The 1970s brought an expansion of research on interventions applied to work tasks, including self-management skills, attention to environmental cues, and generalization and maintenance of learned behaviors (e.g., Bellamy et al.,, 1979; Wehman, 1981). Increasingly, these interventions were applied in community job settings rather than segregated work activity centers and sheltered workshops. In addition, methods emerged to address behavioral challenges and to improve social skills in community settings (e.g., Greenspan & Schoultz, 1981).

Research in the 1980s brought the emergence of strategies for applying employment supports in integrated jobs, rejecting the assumption that employment supports could be only applied in segregated vocational settings (Taylor, 1988). Initially, this research included delivering job supports for small crews of four to six people with a supervisor, engaged in such tasks as groundskeeping or janitorial work. In addition, "enclaves" were created of small groups of people—often five to eight—working together in a company setting with a full-time supervisor assigned to provide employment supports (Mank, Rhodes, & Bellamy, 1986). Increasingly, research on employment interventions emphasized individualized employment, recognizing that crews and enclaves maintained some of the less-than-desirable characteristics of segregation found in sheltered workshop settings (Mank, Cioffi, & Yovanoff, 1997). In addition, data clearly show that people in individual employment are much more likely to earn more and to be better integrated in the workplace (e.g., Butterworth, Hagner, Kiernan, & Schalock, 1996). Research also began to focus on the benefits of job experiences for young people still in high school and during the transition from school to adult life (Leucking, Fabian, Tilson, Donovan, & Fabian, 2004; Hanley-Maxwell, Whitney-Thomas, & Pogoloff, 1995; Butterworth, Hagner, Helm, & Whelley, 2000).

The 1990s brought research that showed the capacity of coworkers and supervisors to provide employment supports for people in individualized settings. This discovery of "natural supports" in the workplace, along with studies of employer leadership in employing people with developmental disabilities, meant that any barriers to employment were likely to be barriers of funding and systems rather than any assumed inability of individuals. Research emerged in the 1990s showing that people with developmental disabilities were more likely to earn high wages and to be more fully integrated in typical workplace cultures when coworkers received information about and assistance in supporting people with disabilities, when job arrangements reflected what is typical in a given workplace, and when individuals were well matched in jobs that mirror their interests and unique talents (Nisbet & Callahan, 1987; Mank, Cioffi, & Yovanoff, 1998, 2000; Storey, 2002; Fillary & Pernice, 2006; Jordan de Urries, Verdugo, Jenaro, Crespo, & Caballo, 2005). Methods of assessment, now called "discovery," have emerged to better uncover individual talents and preferences (Callahan & Garner, 1997). Methods of applying technology and assistive technology to employment settings emerged to the benefit of people with physical and multiple disabilities, in addition to assisting people with intellectual disabilities (e.g., Gilmore, Schuster, Timmons, & Butterworth, 2000; Cooper & Mank, 1990; Sowers, McLean, & Owens, 2002).

After the year 2000, research shifted in part toward interventions of a more systemic or structural nature. The ability of people with developmental disabilities could hardly be questioned anymore. Nonetheless, the perplexing chronic unemployment and underemployment has continued. The gap between knowledge and policies, when compared with practice, is notable. Thus research began to emphasize "customized" employment, meaning specific tailoring of jobs to the talents, interests, and accommodation needs of the individual (Luecking et al., 2004). Demonstrations of self-employment, such as small businesses owned and run by people with developmental disabilities, emerged as another way to tailor work to individual abilities and circumstances while maintaining a focus on earning significant wages (Griffin & Hammis, 2003; Callahan, Shumpert, & Mast, 2002). In addition, demonstrations of employer initiatives from the 1990s expanded in hospitality industries, technology companies, the health care industry, and public-sector employment (Luecking, 2003; Mank, O'Neill, & Jensen, 1998; Wehman, 2001; Hagner & Cooney, 2003).

Research in the late 1990s and the 2000s also emphasized the importance of choice and self-determination by people with developmental disabilities. This line of innovation has focused on having decisions made by people with disabilities rather than by professionals—who have begun to assume the role of advisors—and on those decisions being supported by individual goals rather than by professionals who determined the next step in employment (West, 1995; Harkin, 1998; Griffin & Hammis, 1996; Callahan & Mank, 1998). Increasingly promising, is a focus on careers and employment advancement rather than on simply having a job at the moment (Taylor, 2004; Wehman & Kregel, 1998; Arksey, 2003).

Table 19.1 provides a summary of notable interventions in recent decades, along with the possible result of the intervention for people with developmental disabilities.

This research has also provided clarity about strategies for maximizing the employment outcomes of earnings and integration. That is, people with more individualized jobs, who are well matched to their duties, and who have natural supports in the workplace are more likely to earn more money, to be more integrated into the work culture, to work more hours, and to have greater job stability (Murphy, Rogan, Handley, Kincaid, & Royce-Davis, 2002; Mank, Cioffi, & Yovanoff, 1999). The potential of self-employment has also emerged as an employment opportunity with earning potential (e.g., Callahan, Shumpert, & Mast, 2002).

Nonetheless, despite numerous research studies and demonstration projects even into the late 2000s, the unemployment and underemployment rates have remained remarkably unchanged for 15 years. This reality of a lack of broad implementation of community employment strategies is not the result of inability on the part of people with developmental disabilities. Instead, the continuing unemployment and underemployment are clearly the result of the lack of broad-scale implementation strategies and

TABLE 19.1. Summary of Employment Interventions

Intervention	Result for people with developmental disabilities
Instructional technology	Demonstration of ability to work productively
Generalization and maintenance	Demonstration of ability to work productively in community settings
Behavior supports	Demonstration that behavioral issues need not preclude community employment
Self-management	Increased independence in community settings
Job analysis and job matching	Benefit of understanding and matching individual to specific jobs
Environmental management	Importance of arranging job environment and natural cues for employment success
Natural supports	Ability of coworkers and supervisors to support successful employees with developmental disabilities
Technology supports	Inclusion of people in community employment who have physical disabilities, multiple disabilities, or severe intellectual disabilities
Choice and self-determination applied to employment	Increased choices and self-direction of employment goals, supports, and outcomes.

of a new kind of research on implementation of known strategies and interventions that have resulted in successful employment of a relatively small percentage of people with developmental disabilities.

At the same time that research on individual interventions, teaching, and support strategies was evolving, the mission and emphasis of community agencies that support people with developmental disabilities has changed.

EVOLVING MISSION

At the same time that research on employment was evolving, so was the mission of community agencies that support people with developmental disabilities. This was a change from a lack of expectation of employment potential to a belief and demonstration of the ability of people with developmental disabilities to work productively. In addition, it was an evolution from segregation to integration.

In the 1960's and early 1970's, community agencies emerged based on funding paradigms that were designed primarily to provide a place for people with developmental disabilities to go during the day. Families often started these programs in the interest of giving their sons and daughters something to do during the day (e.g., West, Revell, & Wehman, 1998; Chambless, 1996) other than staying at home. At that time there was little expectation of people learning work tasks of any kind.

As the intervention and instructional research evolved to show that people with developmental disabilities could learn effectively, the mission of community agencies changed to take advantage of the results of research. Instruction technology allowed agencies to declare their mission as a place for people to go to learn daily living skills, such as doing household chores, riding public transportation, and handling money.

As research focused more and more on vocational tasks, the mission of many agencies changed again. That is, segregated day service settings became places for people to go in order to prepare for work. And, before research results that emphasized integration were well established, community agencies also focused on creating sheltered settings where people could go to work alongside others with disabilities.

As the notion of supported employment emerged, many community agencies developed, or more often added to their services, an emphasis on supporting people in working in community job settings. Although few long-established agencies have eliminated their delivery of segregated services, an increasing number of agencies have been created in every state whose mission is entirely supporting people in community job settings without providing services in any congregate or segregated setting (e.g., Rogan, Held, & Rinne, 2001; Albin, Rhodes, & Mank, 1994; Butterworth, Fesko, & Ma, 2000; DiLeo & Rogan, 1999).

Most recently, more progressive community agencies are emphasizing individual outcomes and choices. As such, the mission of newer organizations is focused on supporting people in making choices about their employment and on helping them to prosper over time in employment (Sowers, McLean, & Owens, 2002).

Table 19.2 provides a summary of the evolution of day-service approaches in recent decades, a description of the services, and the impact and outcomes for people with developmental disabilities.

The research of more than three decades has made it possible to make certain statements. People with developmental disabilities, including those with the most significant disabilities:

TABLE 19.2. Summary of Employment Approaches

Approach	Description	Impact/outcomes
Work activity	Day program for daily living skills and limited exposure to work tasks	• Access to some instruction • A place to go during the day
Sheltered work	Segregated work setting in which the majority of employees have disabilities	• Access to work tasks with limited earnings
Supported employment • Crews • Enclaves • Individualized jobs	Employment in integrated settings with individualized support	• Increased earnings and integration compared with work activity and sheltered work
Customized employment	Employment roles negotiated carefully and specifically related to the interests and abilities of the person	• Employment tailored to the person—including people with the most severe disabilities
Self-employment	Small business owned or run by a person with a disability	• Potential for individualized work role and asset building as a business owner
Transition from school to work	Employment emphasis while in middle school and high school	• Increased probability of entering workforce soon after completing formal education

- Can be productive on work tasks.
- Can work productively in integrated job settings.
- Can be supported in community job settings with a combination of paid supports and natural supports.
- Can earn significant money and be fully integrated into the culture of the workplace.
- Can own or run income-producing businesses.

Another way to show the changes in the purpose and focus of community support agencies is to display the evolution, or expansion of the missions of provider agencies across the United States. In some instances, new organizations have been created, beginning with the more progressive missions. More often, long-standing organizations that provide supports to people have expanded their missions to include, if not emphasize, innovations in employment (e.g., Butterworth, Fesko, & Ma, 2000).

Table 19.3 provides a summary of the evolution that took place in thousands of organizations over the past three decades and of the missions of newer organizations as they were created during these decades. It is important to note that the missions listed first have not necessarily been replaced. Instead, new missions have evolved even as older ones fade away slowly.

Despite research results and numerous successful demonstrations of employment for people with developmental disabilities, arguments linger against full implementation of community employment for all people with developmental disabilities. These arguments include the following:

- Many people choose to congregate.
- Many people are happy where they are in segregated settings.
- Community employment is too expensive.
- The community is not a friendly place.
- Some people are not ready for community employment.
- Some people have disabilities that are too severe for community employment

Research and demonstration projects counter these arguments. Although it should be noted that each argument has an element of truth, they are largely perceptions, which can be real enough in their consequences. Nonetheless, studies show that the

TABLE 19.3. Evolving Missions of Community Agencies

Mission	Time period in which mission evolved
A safe place for people to go during the day	1950s
A place for people to go to learn daily living skills	1960s
A place for people to go to prepare for work	1970s
A place for people to go to work with others who have disabilities	1970s
Support for people to work in the community	1980s
Support for people with disabilities to choose and prosper in community employment	Mid-1990s

majority of people will not choose segregation when presented with multiple alternatives, even if they indicate some level of satisfaction with their current segregated state (Migliore, 2006; Rogan, Banks, & Howard, 2000; Butterworth, Fesko, & Ma, 2000). Limited exposure to alternatives means limited experiences, which translates into limited understanding of possibilities and choices. The cost issues may appear important in the short term, inasmuch as an early investment is required to create integrated employment. Longer term studies clearly demonstrate, however, that the overall economic benefits to individuals and to social service systems accrue when people work in jobs and earn more substantial wages. Finally, the issue of whether people are "ready" for work was resolved by research some years ago (e.g., Wehman & Revell, 1996). That is, when people are well matched in job duties in light of their interests and skills, everyone is capable of some kind of employment, including those with the label of "most severe" disabilities (e.g., Rogan, Grossi, Mank, Haynes, & Thomas, 2001).

Table 19.4 provides a summary of these arguments, along with evidence-based and alternative perspectives.

Another question surfaces in the discussion of people "choosing" to work in a segregated setting: Should people not have the choice? Choice is both an important and an often misused notion. That is, from a public policy standpoint, choices are limited in every walk of life. Seat belts are required in cars. Some medical treatments are not covered by insurance. In a number of states, it is no longer a choice to send a family member to a state institution. These circumstances are related in part to public-sector and social benefits and costs. They are also related to data about individual benefits over time and to a social policy obligation to deliver better ideas and interventions. One can

TABLE 19.4. Arguments against Community Employment

Argument	Response
Many people choose to congregate.	People have had few experiences and limited opportunity to make choices (West, 1995; Callahan & Mank, 1998).
Many people are happy where they are in segregated settings.	People have had few experiences and limited opportunity to make choices (West, 1995; Callahan & Mank, 1998).
Community employment is too expensive.	Data indicate the upfront cost may be higher, but community employment has a better cost benefit over time (Wehman, Revell, & Brooke, 2003).
The community is not a friendly place.	Some places in a community may not be "friendly" to people with disabilities, but data show multiple places and businesses that are welcoming to people with disabilities (Wehman, 2001; Hagner & Cooney, 2003).
Some people are not ready for community employment.	Supported employment demonstrates that readiness is not a requirement for successful employment (Sowers et al., 2002; Wehman et al., 2005).
Some people have disabilities that are too severe for community employment.	Studies show methods of successful employment for people labeled with the most severe disabilities (Callahan et al., 2002; Mank, Cioffi, & Yovanoff, 1998; Griffin & Hammis, 2003).

hardly imagine checking into a hospital that practices medicine as it was known in 1980.

In addition to the continuing debate about the need for community employment (and despite data about benefits and advocacy that promotes employment), local agencies nationwide struggle to find, keep, and train sufficient support personnel to assist in the employment goals of people with developmental disabilities. Low wages, high turnover, and a lack of preservice and in-service training make it difficult to invest the needed human resources to improve employment outcomes. With high turnover, the training that is provided is focused on basic skills rather than on implementation of the best practices. As a result, implementation has been outstripped by the evolving policy and legal framework that is described next.

EVOLVING POLICY AND LEGAL FRAMEWORK

Parallel developments have occurred along with the development of research and implementation. Closely related to these has been the evolving policy and legal framework that emphasizes independence, productivity, and integration. This section relies heavily on Wehman and colleagues' description of the policy and legal framework of employment for people with disabilities (Wehman et al., 2005). This section describes the triangulating themes from the Rehabilitation Act of 1973, the Developmental Disabilities Assistance and Bill of Rights Act of 2000, the Americans with Disabilities Act of 1990, the Workforce Investment Act of 1998, the Individuals with Disabilities Education Act of 1990, and the Ticket to Work and Workforce Incentives Improvement Act of 1999.

The Rehabilitation Act

The Rehabilitation Act (Rehab Act) of 1973 and its amendments (1998) support local authorities in serving the employment needs of people with disabilities and focus on their transition from secondary education to adult life. It is the primary employment-support resource for adults with disabilities. The Rehabilitation Act Amendments of 1998 provide federal dollars, matched by state dollars, to all states to give people with developmental disabilities the opportunity to obtain employment and independent living assistance as needed. This Act also provides opportunities for people with disabilities to gain access to vocational services and to choose the specific services needed for them to achieve individualized employment goals. Also, recipients of vocational rehabilitation services have control over the contents of their individualized plans for employment (IPEs) and have information made available so they may make informed choices about specific services they will receive. As of 1999, the Rehab Act emphasizes community-integrated employment. The vocational rehabilitation system no longer recognizes (nor will pay for) an outcome of segregated employment. This is a very important position of the nation's employment policy for people with disabilities overall and for people with developmental disabilities in particular.

The Developmental Disabilities Act

In the Developmental Disabilities Assistance and Bill of Rights Act (DD Act) of 2000, Congress observed that national policy for people with disabilities should be characterized by independence, productivity, and integration. This built on the 1984 amendment, which for the first time focused on employment as an important hallmark of services for people with developmental disabilities. In fact, supported employment for people with developmental disabilities was first defined in the 1984 amendment.

The Americans with Disabilities Act

The intent of the Americans with Disabilities Act (ADA) of 1990 was to end discrimination toward people with disabilities throughout society, and it emphasized decent jobs with decent incomes. The ADA supports the rights of persons with disabilities to be in the community. This act was followed exactly 1 year later by a comprehensive set of regulations that provided for accessibility, nondiscrimination, and greater access to workplaces, community facilities, public transportation, and telecommunications. Employment is a central focus of the ADA. The law went on to state that individuals with disabilities continually encounter various forms of discrimination, including outright intentional exclusion; discriminatory effects of architectural, transportation, and communication barriers; overprotective rules and policies; failure to make modifications to existing facilities and practices; exclusionary qualification standards and criteria; segregation; and relegation to lesser services, programs, activities, benefits, jobs, or other opportunities.

The Workforce Investment Act

In the Workforce Investment Act (WIA) of 1998, Congress established a requirement that states and localities fully include and provide for appropriate accommodation for persons with disabilities. WIA is the first major reform of the nation's job training system since 1982. WIA includes the following key components:

- Streamlining services through a one-stop service-delivery system.
- Empowering job seekers with information and access to training resources through individual training accounts.
- Providing universal access to core services.
- Ensuring a strong role for local workforce investment boards and the private sector in the workforce investment system.
- Improving youth programs.

With the passage of the WIA, local service delivery areas across the country began teaming with other employment and workforce development partners to establish a one-stop career center system.

The Individuals with Disabilities Education Act

The Individuals with Disabilities Education Act (IDEA) of 1990, 1997, and 2004 established clear expectations that the secondary school programs of adolescents with disabilities, including those with substantial disabilities, would include the explicit statement that special education and related services are intended to prepare students for employment and independent living; this makes it clear that educators, parents, and students must consider adult outcomes as they plan for students' school experiences. A key element of IDEA related to employment is stated in §300.29:

As used in this part, transition services means a coordinated set of activities for a student with a disability that

(1) Is designed within an outcome oriented process, that promotes movement from school to post-school activities, including post-secondary education, vocational training, integrated employment (including supported employment), continuing and adult education, adult services, independent living, or community participation

(2) Is based on the individual student's needs, taking into account the student's preferences and interests

(3) Includes:

- Instruction
- Related services
- Community experiences
- The development of employment and other post-school adult living objectives
- If appropriate, acquisition of daily living skills and functional vocational evaluation

Transition services for students with disabilities may consist of special education, if provided as specially designed instruction, or related services, if required, to assist a student with a disability to benefit from special education.

At a minimum, the individualized education plan (IEP) team should address each of the areas, including instruction, community experiences, and development of employment and other postschool adult living objectives. In many cases, each of these areas, and possibly some others, will be included in students' IEPs; however, transition services may be provided by the education agency or, as outlined in §300.248 of the IDEA regulations, by agencies outside the school.

The Ticket to Work and Workforce Incentives Improvement Act

The Ticket to Workforce and Work Incentives Improvement Act (TWWIIA) of 1999 is designed to ensure that many of the country's 9 million adults with disabilities who receive Medicare and Medicaid keep their benefits after they obtain remunerative jobs. Until the law went into effect, many people with disabilities were faced with losing federal benefits needed to cover their medical costs if they went to work. Some feared that, by taking any jobs that paid even a minimal income, they would be cut off from access to these benefits, which are vital to maintaining their lives.

With the passage of the TWWIIA, a dramatic new era of work opportunities for persons with disabilities has been ushered in. Often people with disabilities have been determined to be ineligible for Medicaid and Medicare if they work, thus putting thousands of individuals in the position of having to choose between health care coverage and work. When Congress passed the TWWIIA, people with disabilities were able to join the workforce without fear of losing their Medicare or Medicaid coverage. In recent years, Medicaid waivers have included an emphasis on employment outcomes.

States' Policy

Employment policy in a number of states is now being reconsidered for people with developmental disabilities. Such states as Washington, New Mexico, Georgia, and Indiana are now emphasizing an "employment first" policy for day-services funding. These policies affirm a recognition of the abilities of people with developmental disabilities to work successfully in community jobs and point out the personal and public-sector benefits of community employment compared with unemployment, underemployment, and segregated employment. In fact, in the state of Washington, a 2004 policy of the Division of Developmental Disabilities creates an expectation of employment in community jobs. This policy goes well beyond encouraging community employment as a valuable outcome and clearly states that people with developmental disabilities, like other citizens, are expected to work in integrated jobs.

The Olmstead Decision

The ADA and its subsequent interpretation by the U.S. Supreme Court in *Olmstead v. L.C., et al.* (1999) makes it clear that discrimination against persons with disabilities is illegal. That is, people choosing to leave institutions are entitled to have financial resources follow them to the services of their choice in community settings. The Olmstead decision embraced not only the importance of community inclusion but also the value of productive activity and employment.

In the state of Wisconsin, a lawsuit (*Schwartz v. Jefferson County*, 2005), has been filed and is progressing, that cites the Olmstead decision and the ADA as a basis for having resources follow individuals to integrated supported employment rather than into a segregated setting. This landmark case provides a most recent example of the incremental challenge to segregation and an expectation of individual rights to integrated employment.

IMPLICATIONS

The research, successes, problems, and opportunities of employment for people with developmental disabilities present important implications for these people and their families, for practitioners, for policy makers, and for researchers. For all of these stakeholders, a few things are clear and largely agreed: Employment is preferable to unemployment; greater earnings are preferable to lesser earnings; integration is preferable to segregation; free choice in employment among multiple options is preferable to limited or forced choices. Even critics will agree to these statements in at least a general sense regarding the majority of people with developmental disabilities. The following implications are offered with this in mind.

Implications for People with Disabilities and Families

Foremost in present and future discussions of employment of people with developmental disabilities are the viewpoint, knowledge, and choices of people with disabilities and their family and personal allies in life—much the same as for any family in the Western world. Professionals bring knowledge, research, ideas, and possibilities. Individuals and the people who care about them make the decisions. Acknowledging this creates a number of implications for people with disabilities and the people around them.

Investigating the Possibilities of Employment

If individuals do actually have a choice in employment, it is often presented as the choice between a place in the workshop or day center and a job in the community.

This kind of choice can suggest that the choice is between limited options. In reality, the choices are much broader. Choosing a job in the public or private sector is a matter of choice among hundreds, if not thousands, of jobs (including self-employment). A choice about how to spend one's time for economic benefit that is presented as a choice between segregation and integration is a simple, if inaccurate, representation of the possibilities. For people with disabilities, dealing with a forced choice or a free choice requires some knowledge of possibilities for employment. This means that people with disabilities and their families need and should expect information about employment possibilities, about research results, and about examples of what is possible and real for people with developmental disabilities in their own states or elsewhere in the country.

Creating an Expectation of Contribution and Employment

Most parents expect their children to work when they become adults. This expectation has often not been applied to people with developmental disabilities; or, at best, the expectation has been, and remains, severely compromised. Now, in the face of clear demonstrations of the ability of people with developmental disabilities, this expectation is changing. Any survey of adults with disabilities indicates a clear desire for employment and discretionary income. At this point, most older adults with disabilities have not grown up with an expectation of working. This can change with the generation of young people and those still in schools. Migliore (2006) provides information about the expectations of people with developmental disabilities and their families in a study of people in sheltered settings.

Pursuing Asset Building

Only recently has the discussion of working and generating income included the broader context of asset building. Regrettably, qualifying for social security benefits defines a life near or below the poverty line. Even working part time provides very limited discretionary income. Social Security Administration rules make it difficult to build more than minimal financial assets. Only recently have ideas begun to emerge to address the need to build financial assets over time.

Pursuing Careers beyond the Current Circumstance

Success in working should allow any adult to consider the kind of job he or she wishes to do beyond the current job situation. Pursuit of careers can begin with a new expectation, not only of employment but also of a sequence of work situations that involve improvement and advancement. Families and people with disabilities should be at the center of this discussion.

Participating in Research and Public Policy Developments

The emergence of self-advocacy organizations, on both a national and state basis, creates new opportunity for people with developmental disabilities and families to participate in the public policy discussion of supports and services, as well as to help guide research interests for improvements in quality of life. This participation is important for ensuring that innovations and the implementation of public policy reflect the interests and support needs of individuals and their families.

Implications for Practitioners

Practitioners who provide the employment supports for people with developmental disabilities play a critical role in helping to improve employment outcomes. It has typically been community nonprofit organizations that have provided day and employment services to adults with developmental disabilities. The quality of employment outcomes will surely be related to the quality of the employment supports provided.

Understanding and Investing in the Implementation of Innovations in Employment for People with Developmental Disabilities

The past three decades of research and innovation have generated proven methods for developing jobs and for providing employment supports. Along with public policy makers and training personnel, providers of services must understand and pursue quality innovations, especially those related to individual and work assessments, natural supports, customized employment, and so forth. As the number of people with developmental disabilities who have jobs grows, it will also be necessary to create a greater focus on career development over time. This will require improved methods and structures for personnel preparation and mentoring of direct support professionals. This investment in personnel is required in order for local agencies and businesses to fully implement the policy and legal developments of the past several decades.

Participating in the Public Process of Policy, Funding, and Expansion of Employment

Because of their key role in delivering employment outcomes, practitioners are needed in the ongoing discussion and creation of public policy for implementation of improved employment outcomes. This includes work with local, state, and federal governments to establish and maintain creative and productive funding models, address personnel preparation issues, and create incentives for people with developmental disabilities, as well as for the providers of services.

Investing in Employer Relations That Emphasize Including People with Developmental Disabilities in Community Employment

Even as the possibilities for self-employment and new businesses owned by people with developmental disabilities emerge, the clear majority of jobs will be found, developed, or created in existing businesses, large and small. As such, the relationship between the business community, people with developmental disabilities, and practitioners is worthy of investment. Even though the unemployment rates continue at a remarkably high level, people with developmental disabilities are nonetheless more visible in typical community jobs than they were two decades ago. Partnerships are needed with the business community that show the contributions people with disabilities can make in the changing local and national workforce context of the next decade.

Working with Schools and Families in the Transition of Young People from School to Work

Research has shown that when young people with developmental disabilities have work experiences and leave school employed, they are more likely to be employed years later. This knowledge creates an obvious opportunity to greatly reduce unemployment and underemployment rates by ensuring that these young adults go to work after high school or to postsecondary education, rather than to nonemployment activities or to segregated employment. This imperative calls for new partnerships with schools, especially high schools, to create employment opportunities during the school years of young adults.

Implications for Policy Makers

Creating Clarity in Policy and Funding about the Value and Expectation of Employment for People with Developmental Disabilities

Despite the emerging federal policies and funding guidelines that emphasize productivity, independence, and integration, the vast majority of funding for day services for people with developmental disabilities is paying for segregation and nonemployment activities. Following the federal government's leadership in policy statements, states will need to create their own policy directions that align accordingly, not unlike recent initiatives in Washington, Indiana, Georgia, and New Mexico. These states are now creating their own "employment first" priorities and working to align funding and incentives with integrated employment outcomes.

Investing in Innovations and Personnel Preparation with Community Agencies for Implementation of Best Practices

Policy makers and funding agents are needed in the development of personnel preparation structures that train the employment support workforce and that make available information and assistance for implementation of known best practices and emerging innovations. The primary tool for increasing employment outcomes is the time and talent of the direct-support professionals in local communities, and it is incumbent on state-level policy makers to provide leadership to invest in this workforce in partnership with practitioners and people with disabilities. This investment in human resources for implementation of best practices will be a necessity in improving employment outcomes for people with developmental disabilities and in improving quality of life.

Investing in Training for People with Disabilities and Families to Participate in Public Policy Development and Implementation

The self-advocacy movement of the past 15 years provides an unprecedented opportunity for a new kind of relationship between government and people with developmental disabilities. For the first time, expectations are emerging that people with developmental disabilities can and should be involved in policy and implementation decisions about community supports overall and about employment specifically. This calls for investment in the leadership and participation skills of people with developmental disabilities.

Collecting, Publicizing, and Using Data in Decision Making for Improvement of Employment Outcomes

Few states have accurate and reliable data systems to show with precision the employment status of all adults with developmental disabilities. In an era of public accountability for taxpayer resources, information is needed about the precise outcomes of the present, as well as of improvements, as they emerge. Accurate data should be used to better inform policy makers, people with disabilities, and practitioners in decision making about strategies to improve outcomes. Specific employment outcomes that should be collected include such things as wages, access to company benefits, hours worked weekly, the percentage of people with developmental disabilities with earnings above the poverty line, degree of integration with nondisabled coworkers, and improvement in wages and career advancement over time.

Implications for Researchers

Researchers have a continuing responsibility regarding the employment outcomes of people with developmental disabilities. Research to date has clearly shown capability and the possibility of community employment. Expansion of this kind of research is needed.

Organizing Known Research Findings into Usable Best-Practice Strategies for Practitioners, People with Disabilities, Their Families, and the Business Community

Research has delivered methods that can improve employment outcomes. These findings should be translated from research reports into best-practice strategies and training that can be fully implemented in community settings. Researcher's knowledge will be needed in a partnership with practitioners, people with disabilities, and the business community.

Increasing Research on New Interventions, Especially Related to People with Multiple Disabilities and Dual Diagnoses and Those Considered to Have the Most Severe Disabilities

The research noted in this chapter shows the employment potential of many people with developmental disabilities. Nonetheless, the available data also show that people with multiple disabilities, people with dual diagnoses of developmental disability and mental illness, and people considered to have more severe intellectual disabilities are clearly underrepresented in the employment successes that have been realized. This fact points to the ongoing need for research exploring methods of successful employment for people with these labels. Research is needed at the level of individual interventions, as well as in the community-scale implementation of emerging research findings.

Conducting Research on Methods of Wide-Scale Implementation of Community Employment

Many innovative practices and organizations are producing valuable employment outcomes. And yet rarely are these practices widely implemented in an entire community or across a state. This situation calls for researchers to invest in studies aimed specifically at wide-scale implementation of best practices beyond demonstration projects. Demonstrations of employment and transition have been impressive in their creativity and their outcomes for a small percentage of people with developmental disabilities. A different kind of research on structural and organizational change strategies is needed to investigate local agency and state structures for transforming an entire system of day services well beyond the creation of demonstration projects. We need systems-level research on transforming investment and outcomes in entire geographic areas, rather than in communities scattered across states.

Conducting Policy and Funding Analyses

In partnership with governments and advocates, research is needed on the ongoing analyses of public policy and funding structures that promote employment outcomes. Such research is needed at both the state and federal level. If outcomes are to become more aligned with federal legislation and litigation, then policy and funding within states will need attention. This should include assisting local, state, and national government in the collection, analysis, and use of data for decisions on improvement in employment outcomes.

CONCLUSIONS

The history of employment of people with developmental disabilities has evolved in a number of important ways. Three decades ago, it was largely assumed that people with this label could not work in community jobs. Research and implementation strategies clearly show that people can work successfully if provided with appropriate and individualized supports. In the same decades, community agencies have been increasingly adopting a mission of supporting employment. Policy and funding are moving toward providing such opportunities for employment. The emerging societal expectation is the same for everyone—that people should work and contribute.

Employment provides the opportunity to pay one's way, at least in part, in life, to contribute, to be a part of the natural community, to develop relationships, and to see the benefits of individual choices in life that come from having discretionary income. The coming decades will witness the extent to which this becomes a reality for the majority of people with developmental disabilities.

REFERENCES

Albin, J. M., Rhodes, L., & Mank, D. (1994). Realigning organizational culture, resources, and community roles: Changeover to community employment. *Journal of the Association for Persons with Severe Handicaps, 19*(2), 105–115.

Americans with Disabilities Act of 1990, Public Law 101-336, 42 U.S.C. § 12101 *et seq.* (2000).

Arksey, H. (2003). People into employment: Supporting people with disabilities and carers into work. *Health and Social Care in the Community, 11*(3), 283–292.

Bellamy, G. T., Horner, R. H., & Inman, D. P. (1979). *Vocational habilitation of severely retarded adults: A direct service technology.* Austin, TX: PRO-ED.

Butterworth, J., Fesko, S. L., & Ma, V. (2000). Because it was the right thing to do: Changeover from facility-based services to community employment. *Journal of Vocational Rehabilitation, 14*(1), 23–35.

Butterworth, J., Hagner, D., Helm, D. T., & Whelley, T. A. (2000). Workplace culture, social interactions, and supports for transition-age young adults. *Mental Retardation, 38*(4), 342–353.

Butterworth, J., Hagner, D., Kiernan, W. E., & Schalock, R. L. (1996). Natural supports in the workplace: Defining an agenda for research and practice. *Journal of the Association for Persons with Severe Handicaps, 21*(3), 103–113.

Callahan, M., & Mank, D. (1998). *Choice and control of employment for people with disabilities.* Paper prepared for the Robert Wood Johnson Foundation Self-Determination Initiative. Indiana Institute on Disability and Community, Indiana University.

Callahan, M., Shumpert, N., & Mast, M. (2002). Self-employment, choice and self-determination. *Journal of Vocational Rehabilitation, 17*(2), 75–85.

Callahan, M. J., & Garner, J. B. (1997). *Keys to the workplace: Skills and supports for people with disabilities.* Baltimore: Brookes.

Chambless, C. E. B. (1996). The relationship between natural supports and social integration in supported employment. *Dissertation Abstracts International, 57*(2A), 746.

Cooper, A., & Mank, D. (1990). Integrated employment for people with severe physical disabilities: Five case studies. *American Rehabilitation, 15*(3), 16–23.

Developmental Disabilities Assistance and Bill of Rights Act of 2000, Public Law No. 106-402, 42 U.S.C. § 15001 *et seq.* (2000).

DiLeo, D., & Rogan, P. M. (1999). *Towards integrated employment for all: APSE's position on segregated services for people with disabilities.* Richmond, VA: The Association for Persons in Supported Employment.

Fillary, R., & Pernice, R. (2006). Social inclusion in workplaces where people with intellectual disabilities are employed: Implications for supported employment professionals. *International Journal of Rehabilitation Research, 29*(1), 31–36.

Gilmore, D. S., Schuster, J. L., Timmons, J. C., & Butterworth, J. (2000). An analysis of trends for people with mental retardation, cerebral palsy, and epilepsy receiving services from state vocational rehabilitation agencies: Ten years of progress. *Rehabilitation Counseling Bulletin, 44*(1), 30–38.

Gold, M. (1973). Research on the vocational rehabilitation of the retarded: The present, the future. In N. Ellis (Ed.), *International review of research in mental retardation* (Vol. 6, pp. 97–147). New York: Academic Press.

Greenspan, S., & Schoultz, B. (1981). Why mentally retarded adults lose their jobs. Social competence as a factor in work adjustment. *Applied Research in Mental Retardation, 21*(1), 23–38.

Griffin, C., & Hammis, D. (1996). *Streetwise guide to person-centered career planning.* Denver, CO: Center for Technical Assistance and Training Denver Options.

Griffin, C., & Hammis, D. (2003). *Making self-employment work for people with disabilities.* Baltimore: Brookes.

Grossi, T. A., & Mank, D. (2005). *Indiana day and employment outcomes systems report.* Bloomington: Indiana University, Indiana Institute on Disability and Community.

Hagner, D. C. (2000). Supporting people as part of the community: Possibilities and prospects for change. In J. Nisbet & D. Hagner (Eds.), *Part of the community: Strategies for community membership.* Baltimore: Brookes.

Hagner, D., & Cooney, B. (2003). Building employer capacity to support employees with severe disabilities in the workplace. *Work, 21*(1), 77–82.

Hanley-Maxwell, C., Whitney-Thomas, J., & Pogoloff, S. M. (1995). The second shock: Parental perspectives of their child's transition from school to adult life. *Journal of the Association for Persons with Severe Handicaps, 20*(1), 3–16.

Harkin, D. (1998). *Are we swimming in the right direction?: From dependency to self-determination for Idahoans with developmental disabilities.* Boise: Idaho Council on Developmental Disabilities.

Individuals with Disabilities Education Act of 1990, Public Law No. 101-476, 20 U.S.C. §§ 1400 *et seq.* (2000).

Jordan de Urries, F. B., Verdugo, M. A., Jenaro, C., Crespo, M., & Caballo, C. (2005). Supported employment and job outcomes. Typicalness and other related variables. *Work, 25*(3), 221–229.

Luecking, R. G. (2003). *Doing it the company way: Employer perspectives on workplace supports.* Rockville, MD: George Washington University HEALTH Resource Center.

Luecking, R. G., Fabian, E. S., Tilson, G., Donovan, M., & Fabian, E. S. (2004). *Working relationships: Creating career opportunities for job seekers with disabilities through employer partnerships.* Baltimore: Brookes.

Mank, D., Cioffi, A., & Yovanoff, P. (1997). Analysis of the typicalness of supported employment jobs, natural supports, and wage and integration outcomes. *Mental Retardation, 35*(3), 185–197.

Mank, D., Cioffi, A., & Yovanoff, P. (1998). Employment outcomes for people with severe disabilities: Opportunities for improvement. *Mental Retardation, 36*(3), 205–216.

Mank, D., Cioffi, A., & Yovanoff, P. (2000). Direct support in supported employment and its relation to job typicalness, coworker involvement, and employment outcomes. *Mental Retardation, 38*(6), 506–516.

Mank, D., Cioffi, A., & Yovanoff, P. (2003). Supported employment outcomes across a decade: Is there evidence of improvement in the quality of implementation? *Mental Retardation, 41*(3), 188–197.

Mank, D., O'Neill, C. T., & Jensen, R. (1998). Quality in supported employment: A new demonstration of the capabilities of people with severe disabilities. *Journal of Vocational Rehabilitation, 11*(1), 83–95.

Mank, D. M., Cioffi, A. R., & Yovanoff, P. (1999). The impact of coworker involvement with supported employees on wage and integration outcomes. *Mental Retardation, 37*(5), 383–394.

Mank, D. M., Rhodes, L. E., & Bellamy, G. T. (1986). Four supported employment alternatives. In W. Kiernan & J. Stark (Eds.), *Pathways to employment for developmentally disabled adults* (pp. 139–153). Baltimore: Brookes.

Migliore, A. (2006). *Job retention, performance, and attributional styles of employment specialists.* Unpublished doctoral dissertation, Indiana University, Bloomington.

Murphy, S. T., Rogan, P. M., Handley, M., Kincaid, C., & Royce-Davis, J. (2002). People's situations and perspectives eight years after workshop conversion. *Mental Retardation, 40*(1), 30–40.

Nisbet, J., & Callahan, M. (1987). Achieving success in integrated workplaces: Critical elements in assisting persons with severe disabilities. In S. J. Taylor, D. Biklen, & J. Knoll (Eds.), *Community integration for people with severe disabilities* (pp. 184–201). New York: Teachers College Press.

Olmstead et al. v. L.C. et al. 527 U.S. 581,119 S. Ct. 2176 (1999).

Rehabilitation Act Amendments of 1998, Public Law No. 105-220, 29 U.S.C. § 701 *et seq.* (2000).

Rehabilitation Act of 1973, Public Law No. 93-112, 29 U.S.C. §§ 701 *et seq.* (2000).

Rogan, P., Banks, B., & Howard, M. (2000). Workplace supports in practice: As little as possible, as much as necessary. *Focus on Autism and Other Developmental Disabilities, 15*(1), 2–11.

Rogan, P., Grossi, T., Mank, D., Haynes, D., & Thomas, F. (2001). *Report for the President's Task Force on the Employment of Adults with Disabilities: A comparison of wages, hours, benefits, and integration between former sheltered workshop participants who are now in supported employment.* Bloomington: The University Affiliated Program of Indiana, Indiana University, Indiana Institute on Disability and Community.

Rogan, P., Held, M., & Rinne, S. (2001). Organizational change from sheltered to integrated employment for adults with disabilities. In P. Wehman (Ed.), *Supported employment in business: Expanding the capacity of workers with disabilities* (pp. 215–226). St. Augustine, FL: Training Resource Network.

Schwartz, et al. v. Jefferson County et al. Case No. 04-CV-91. Milwaukee, WI (2005).

Sowers, J. A., McLean, D., & Owens, C. (2002). Self-directed employment for people with developmental disabilities: Issues, characteristics, and illustrations. *Journal of Disability Policy Studies, 13*(2), 97–104.

Storey, K. (2002). Strategies for increasing interactions in supported employment settings: An updated review. *Journal of Vocational Rehabilitation, 17*(4), 231–237.

Taylor, S. (2004). *Commentary: Workers with disabilities deserve real choices, real jobs.* Retrieved August 20, 2004, from *www.thearclink.org/news/article.asp?ID=318.*

Taylor, S. J. (1988). Caught in the continuum: A critical analysis of the principle of the least restrictive environment. *Journal of the Association for Persons with Severe Handicaps, 13*(1), 41–53.

Ticket to Work and Workforce Incentives Improvement Act of 1999, Public Law No. 106-170, 42 U.S.C. §§ 1305 *et seq.* (2000).

Wehman, P. (1981). *Competitive employment: New horizons for severely disabled individuals.* Baltimore: Brookes.

Wehman, P. (2001). *Supported employment in business: Expanding the capacity of workers with disabilities.* St. Augustine, FL: TRN.

Wehman, P., & Kregel, J. (1998). *More than a job: Securing satisfying careers for people with disabilities.* Baltimore: Brookes.

Wehman, P., Mank, D., Rogan, P., Luna, J., Kregel, J., Kiernan, W., et al. (2005). Employment and productive life roles. In K. C. Lakin & A. Turnbull (Eds.), *National goals and research for people with intellectual and developmental disabilities* (pp. 149–178). Washington, DC: American Association on Mental Retardation.

Wehman, P., Revell, W. G., & Brooke, V. (2003). Competitive employment: Has it become the "first choice" yet? *Journal of Disability Policy Studies, 14*(3), 163–173.

Wehman, P., & Revell, W. G. (1996). Supported employment from 1986 to 1993: A national program that works. *Focus on Autism and Other Developmental Disabilities, 11*(4), 235–242.

West, M. D. (1995). Choice, self-determination and vocational rehabilitation services: Systemic barriers for consumers with severe disabilities. *Journal of Vocational Rehabilitation, 5*(4), 281–290.

West, M., Revell, G., & Wehman, P. (1998). Conversion from segregated services to supported employment: A continuing challenge to the vocational rehabilitation service system. *Education and Training in Mental Retardation and Developmental Disabilities, 33*(3), 239–247.

Workforce Investment Act of 1998, Public Law No. 105-220, 29 U.S.C. §§ 2801 *et seq.* (2000).

Living with Support in the Community

Factors Associated with Quality-of-Life Outcome

David Felce
Jonathan Perry

Homes have a fundamental place in human society. They serve multiple functions. They provide shelter, comfort, and an environment for maintaining personal health and self-care. They often constitute a social space, where people live with intimate friends or family, raise children, and entertain visitors. They provide a place for organizing interests and pursuits and a base from which individuals transact relationships with the people and amenities that constitute their community. Homes are central to the way people live. The characteristics of people's homes and the nature of their home lives are, therefore, likely to have a significant influence on their overall quality of life.

Adults with mild mental retardation may develop homes and home lives independent of formal agency support once the time comes for them to live separately from their families. However, the majority of adults with moderate, severe, or profound mental retardation at that stage of their lives will live with some level of staff support in accommodations arranged through or in association with service agencies. The arrangements that such agencies make will greatly influence the quality of life of their service users. This chapter discusses what is known about how such arrangements affect quality-of-life outcomes for service users.

Those countries that have experienced deinstitutionalization have seen a corresponding expansion of community-based support arrangements (Braddock, Emerson, Felce, & Stancliffe, 2001). Overall, this reform has brought significant improvements in material standards, personal development, choice, participation in activities of daily living, and involvement in activities in the community (Emerson & Hatton, 1996; Felce, 2000; Kim, Larson, & Lakin, 2001; Young, Sigafoos, Suttie, Ashman, & Grevell, 1998).

However, considerable variation has been reported in the quality of community services and the lifestyle outcomes that residents experience (Emerson & Hatton, 1996; Felce, 2000), even among settings that are ostensibly examples of a similar class or model. Although the research literature on deinstitutionalization may satisfactorily demonstrate the superiority of community settings as a general class over institutional settings as another general class, it tells us little about the factors that may predict outcome within community settings. For this, one must look to research that has investigated how inputs and processes within community living arrangements may affect outcome. This chapter reviews research that sheds light on such relationships. The particular emphasis is on individual or small-group living.

THE LIMITATIONS OF MUCH EXISTING RESEARCH WITH RESPECT TO IDENTIFYING PREDICTORS OF OUTCOME

Before progressing further, it is important to explain why the majority of studies concerned with residential arrangements provide little guidance as to which specific arrangements influence outcome and in what ways. Generally, evaluation of the impact of deinstitutionalization has involved comparative research that has contrasted the outcomes of fairly crudely dichotomized service models. Setting descriptors have tended to reflect the focus of reform, which in turn has reflected popular assumptions concerning the critical variables that influence outcome (e.g., "community" vs. "campus" location, "small" vs. "large" resident groupings, "group homes" vs. "supported living") or administrative policy (e.g., governmental agency vs. independent sector, Intermediate Care Facilities for the Mentally Retarded (ICF-MR) group homes vs. state-funded community living arrangements). Unfortunately, there has been no agreement between researchers on how to classify settings and no standardization of the relevant setting variables that should be measured or described when characterizing the settings being researched.

As a result, setting description in evaluative studies is idiosyncratic and often provides limited detail. Although a research study may be characterized as comparing settings that differ in certain defined ways, and although compared settings may differ in outcome, one cannot necessarily conclude that the differences between the settings described are the reasons for the differences in outcome. For example, based on the general superiority of outcome in small community homes compared with large institutions, it would be tempting to conclude that the comparative research literature provides evidence to support the proposition that small size was linked to better outcome. However, this variable may be only a proxy for the many functional differences that might similarly divide the two types of settings (e.g., in location, in proximity to salient people and amenities, in architecture and equipment, in nature and number of staff, in staff orientation, in staff working methods). Within small community settings that may be similar in many other respects, resident group size may have little effect on outcome.

Differences between residential support models are typically multifaceted, and it is not a straightforward matter to determine the precise reasons that a certain outcome may be superior in one type of arrangement compared with another. Separating the impact of single variables within a complex package calls for research with a particular focus. Scientific investigation needs to typify the environmental, staffing, procedural, and staff performance variables associated with particular support arrangements and to associate these with outcome. Comparative research between broadly similar models that differ in particular arrangements (i.e., where the differences between alternative options are closely constrained) has potential to illuminate the impact of such specific arrangements. However, ensuring that settings are similar in other respects may not always be possible, particularly where staff attitudes, experience, knowledge, and performance are concerned. More generally, research employing some form of multivariate statistical analysis that is capable of partitioning variance in the dependent variable among putative independent variables has the potential to identify factors that have an apparent association with outcome. In addition, experimental research has a role to play whereby the impact of changing one variable at a time is evaluated, although its utility may be limited to such issues as staff training and working methods because of ethical and contractual constraints that would prevent direct manipulation of many other provision arrangements.

This chapter is based on a literature that has employed either of the first two approaches: comparison between distinct community models and multivariate analysis of association between arrangements made and outcome. It is beyond the scope of this chapter to review the experimental staff training and performance literature to identify methods that might improve the quality of residential support arrangements.

QUALITY-OF-LIFE OUTCOME

Contemporary mission statements that underpin the provision of support arrangements for people with mental retardation often refer to helping service users lead typical lives that involve community integration, social relationships, skill development, choice, self-determination, and the opportunities to work and lead a socially valued lifestyle. Generally, the term "quality of life" is employed as an encapsulation of an outcome that encompasses the breadth of lived experience. It is a multidimensional construct that reflects outcomes across important domains of life. How researchers have categorized life domains in conceptualizing quality of life differs in detail, but, at a broad level of generality, what is important to people is well known, and this common ground is reflected in the literature (e.g., Felce, 1997; Schalock et al., 2002). Physical well-being (e.g., health, fitness, safety), material well-being (e.g., income, wealth, housing, neighborhood), social well-being (e.g., interpersonal relationships, community activity, community acceptance), productive well-being (e.g., personal development, self-determination, constructive occupation), emotional well-being (e.g., happiness, contentment with self, freedom from stress) and civic well-being (e.g., state of the nation, civil rights) are part of an overall assessment of quality of life.

Quality-of-life assessment may be objective or subjective in nature. Both approaches have strengths and weaknesses (see Cummins, 2005; Schalock & Felce, 2004). Space precludes a detailed exposition of these differences here. However, for the purposes of this chapter, we describe what is known about how community living arrangements affect objective measures of quality of life in the six domains listed and review their impact on reported life satisfaction. A summary of the findings of the studies reviewed is given in Table 20.1.

TABLE 20.1. Comparative and Multivariate Studies of the Association between Setting Characteristics and Objective Quality-of-Life Outcome

Domain	Outcome	Study	Method	Association with . . .	No association with . . .	Comment
Physical well-being	Health	Heller et al. (2002)	Multivariate		Service model, setting size or attractiveness, choice-making opportunities, family involvement	Controlled for age, level of MR, adaptive behavior, baseline health
	Health	Emerson et al. (2001)	Comparative		Service model, setting size	Controlled for adaptive behavior
	Risk: accidents in home, traffic accidents, danger out of home, abuse by community, exploitation by coresidents	Emerson et al. (2001)	Comparative		Service model, setting size	Controlled for adaptive behavior
	Risk: abuse by coresidents	Emerson et al. (2001)	Comparative	Setting size	Service model	Controlled for adaptive behavior Large > small
	Risk: exploitation by community	Emerson et al. (2001)	Comparative	Service model	Setting size	Controlled for adaptive behavior Supported living > large group homes
	Health care, healthy lifestyle, safety	Stancliffe & Keane (2000)	Comparative		Service model, staffing level, setting size	Controlled for adaptive behavior and range of disabilities
	Risk of obesity or smoking	Robertson et al. (2000)	Multivariate		Range of unspecified setting variables	Risks related to participant characteristics

(continued)

TABLE 20.1. *(continued)*

Domain	Outcome	Study	Method	Association with . . .	No association with . . .	Comment
Physical well-being (*cont.*)	Risk of inactivity	Robertson et al. (2000)	Multivariate	Senior staff holding qualification	Range of other unspecified setting variables	Controlled for participant characteristics Risk also related to participant characteristics
	Risk of poor diet	Robertson et al. (2000)	Multivariate	Resident holding a tenancy	Range of other unspecified setting variables	Controlled for participant characteristics Risk also related to prior residence in family home
Material well-being	Deprivatization (concept including home-likeness)	Tossebro (1995)	Multivariate	Setting size	Staff characteristics	Among settings for 1–5 people Controlled for adaptive behavior and age
	Home-likeness	Emerson et al. (2001)	Comparative	Service model–setting size interaction		Controlled for adaptive behavior Supported living > large group homes
Social well-being	Size of social network	Emerson et al. (2001)	Comparative	Setting size	Service model	Controlled for adaptive behavior Supported living and small group homes > large group homes
	People in social network other than family, staff, other people with MR	Emerson et al. (2001)	Comparative	Setting size	Service model	Controlled for adaptive behavior Small group homes > large group homes
		Robertson et al. (2001a)	Multivariate	Setting size Social climate	Service model, architecture, staffing/	Controlled for adaptive and challenging behavior and other

Measure	Study	Design	Predictor	Setting	Participant characteristics
	Stancliffe & Keane (2000)	Comparative		staff characteristics, working practices, cost Fully staffed larger settings vs. partially staffed smaller settings	Matched groups controlling for adaptive and challenging behavior
Variety of community activities Frequency of community activities Frequency of activities with others Variety of activity partners	Howe et al. (1998)	Comparative	Service model[a]		Matched groups controlling for age and MR level Supported living > group homes
Variety of community activities Frequency of social activities Personal integration Family contact	Stancliffe & Lakin (1998)	Multivariate		Setting size	Controlled for adaptive behavior
Variety and frequency of social activities	Stancliffe & Keane (2000)	Comparative		Fully staffed larger settings vs. partially staffed smaller settings	Matched groups controlling for adaptive and challenging behavior
Frequency and independence of community activities	Stancliffe & Keane (2000)	Comparative	Staffing level (service model) interacting with setting size		Matched groups controlling for adaptive and challenging behavior Partially staffed smaller settings > fully staffed larger settings

(continued)

TABLE 20.1. *(continued)*

Domain	Outcome	Study	Method	Association with . . .	No association with . . .	Comment
Social well-being *(cont.)*	Frequency of community activities	Emerson et al. (2001)	Comparative	Service model	Setting size	Controlled for adaptive behavior Supported living > small and large group homes
		Egli et al. (2002)	Multivariate	Staff interaction Home-likeness Staff attitudes		Home-likeness and attitudes mediated by staff-initiated interactions
		Felce et al. (2002a)	Multivariate	Staffing level Social climate	Setting size, staff qualification and experience, working methods, extent of planned activities, presence of key workers, attention from staff	Controlled for adaptive and challenging behavior and presence of autism More with higher staffing and more individualized social climate
	Frequency of social activities	Felce et al. (2002a)	Multivariate	Presence of key workers Social climate Extent of day activities	Setting size, staffing level, staff qualification and experience, working methods, attention from staff	Controlled for adaptive and challenging behavior and presence of autism More with higher % with key workers, more with less individualized social climate and lower organized day activities
	Frequency of community activities	Heller et al. (2002)	Multivariate	Choice making opportunities Family involvement	Service model, setting size or attractiveness	Controlled for age, level of MR, adaptive behavior, baseline integration
	Variety of social and community activities	Perry & Felce (2005)	Multivariate	Setting size Attention from staff	Provider agency, home-likeness,	Controlled for adaptive and challenging behavior

416

					staffing level, physical integration, social climate, working methods	More with larger size (within range 1–5) and more attention from staff
	Frequency of social and community activities	Perry & Felce (2005)	Multivariate	Provider agency Assessment and teaching	Setting size, home-likeness, staffing level, physical integration, social climate, other working methods, attention from staff	Less with private proprietor who lived separately and with greater emphasis on assessment and teaching
Productive well-being	Growth in adaptive behavior	Heller et al. (2002)	Multivariate	Setting attractiveness Choice-making opportunities	Service model, setting size, family involvement	Controlled for age, level of MR, baseline adaptive behavior
	Self-determination	Tossebro (1995)	Multivariate	Setting size	Staff characteristics	Among settings for 1–5 people Controlled for adaptive behavior and age
	Choice	Stancliffe (1997)	Multivariate	Staff level Setting size[b]	Setting size[b]	Controlled for IQ & adaptive & challenging behavior
		Stancliffe & Lakin (1998)	Multivariate		Setting size	Controlled for adaptive behavior
		Emerson et al. (2001)	Comparative	Service model	Setting size	Controlled for adaptive behavior Supported living > small and large group homes
		Robertson et al. (2001b)	Multivariate	Setting size Home-likeness Activity planning	Service model, staffing/staff characteristics, other working practices, cost	Controlled for adaptive and challenging behavior and other participant characteristics More with smaller size, more home-like, better activity planning

(continued)

417

TABLE 20.1. (continued)

Domain	Outcome	Study	Method	Association with . . .	No association with . . .	Comment
Productive well-being (cont.)	Personal control	Stancliffe et al. (2000)	Comparative	Service model	Setting size[c]	Controlled for adaptive and challenging behavior Semi-independent > supported living > ICF/MR
		Stancliffe et al. (2000)	Multivariate	Supportive policies Social climate Level of discretionary spending	Staffing level Staff autonomy, attitudes, skills, and knowledge	Controlled for adaptive and challenging behavior and self-determination competencies More with more supportive policies, more individualized social climate and more money
	Staff-reported choice Adult autonomy	Perry & Felce (2005)	Multivariate	Individual planning Assessment and teaching Physical integration Attention from staff	Setting size, home-likeness, staffing level, physical integration, other working methods, social climate	Controlled for adaptive and challenging behavior More with greater emphasis on individual planning and less emphasis on assessment and teaching; more with better physical integration and more attention from staff
	Self-reported choice	Perry & Felce (2005)	Multivariate	Provider agency Setting size	Home-likeness, staffing level, physical integration, working methods, social climate, attention from staff	Controlled for adaptive and challenging behavior More with voluntary rather than private provider agency and with smaller setting
	Occupation: engagement in activity	Emerson et al. (2000)	Multivariate	Assistance from staff		Controlled for adaptive behavior More with more assistance from staff
		Felce et al. (2002a)	Multivariate	Setting size Assistance from staff	Staffing level, staff qualification and experience, social	Controlled for adaptive and challenging behavior and presence of autism

418

Outcome	Study	Design	Factor	Variables controlled	Findings
				climate, extent of planned activities, presence of key workers	More with larger setting and more assistance from staff
	Felce et al. (2003)	Multivariate	Attention from staff	Setting size, staffing level, provider agency, working methods, social climate	Controlled for adaptive behavior More with more attention from staff
	Perry & Felce (2005)	Multivariate	Attention from staff	Setting size, home-likeness, staffing level, physical integration, working methods, social climate	Controlled for adaptive and challenging behavior More with more attention from staff
Occupation: participation in domestic activities	Felce et al. (2002a)	Multivariate	Staffing level Staff qualifications Attention from staff	Setting size, staff experience, working methods, social climate, extent of planned activities, presence of key workers	Controlled for adaptive and challenging behavior and presence of autism More with lower staffing, less qualified staff, and more attention from staff
	Stancliffe & Keane (2000)	Comparative	Staffing level (service model) interacting with setting size		Matched groups controlling for adaptive and challenging behavior Partially staffed smaller settings > fully staffed larger settings
	Perry & Felce (2005)	Multivariate	Physical integration	Setting size, home-likeness, staffing level, working methods, social climate, attention from staff	Controlled for adaptive and challenging behavior More with better physical integration

Notes. MR, mental retardation; ICF/MR, Intermediate Care Facilities for the Mentally Retarded.
[a]Setting size confounded with service model.
[b]Setting size significant only for staff report.
[c]Absence of linear association with setting size.

THE INFLUENCE OF PERSONAL CHARACTERISTICS

Measures of developmental status, such as intelligence quotient (IQ) assessments, mental-age assessments, or normed scales of adaptive behavior, characterize the skills that individuals possess to meet the demands of the environment. It would not be surprising, therefore, if such quality-of-life issues as the degree of self-determination exercised and the extent and range of social, community, and household activities undertaken were to be strongly related to assessed skills. There is now a sizable body of evidence that a range of objective quality-of-life indicators are positively related to IQ or adaptive behavior, including: home-likeness (Thompson, Robinson, Dietrich, Farris, & Sinclair, 1996a; Tossebro, 1995), range and frequency of social and community activities (Emerson & McVilly, 2004; Felce & Emerson, 2001; Felce, Lowe, & Jones, 2002a; Heller, Miller, & Hsieh, 2002; Perry & Felce, 2005; Stancliffe & Lakin, 1998), contact with family members (Stancliffe & Lakin, 1998), autonomy or personal control (Perry & Felce, 2005; Stancliffe, Abery, & Smith, 2000), self-determination or choice (Perry & Felce, 2005; Stancliffe, 1997), and engagement in constructive activity (Felce & Emerson, 2001; Felce et al., 2002a; Perry & Felce, 2005; Thompson, Robinson, Dietrich, Farris & Sinclair, 1996b) or in household activity (Felce & Emerson, 2001; Perry & Felce, 2005). It is, therefore, important that investigations should control for the disability characteristics of participants before seeking to uncover any association between environmental arrangements and outcome, either by closely matching groups in comparative research or by first removing variance in outcome attributable to personal characteristics in multivariate research.

There is a similar need to consider controlling for other participant characteristics such as age, gender, challenging behavior, or mental health status. Although such characteristics have generally not been found to have a strength of association with outcome similar to adaptive behavior, a minority of studies have found independent associations between these other characteristics and certain outcomes. Therefore, rigor would suggest that the need to control for a range of participant characteristics should be empirically determined and undertaken where necessary. Analyses included in this chapter have at minimum controlled for adaptive behavior and usually other characteristics, as well, before any conclusion has been reached about the association between a provision arrangement and outcome (see Table 20.1).

PHYSICAL WELL-BEING

Whether specific community support arrangements influence health, fitness, and safety has been little studied. Those studies that have been conducted have tended to find little association between residential arrangements and outcome after controlling for participant characteristics. Heller et al. (2002) found no significant relation between type of residence, residence size, architectural attractiveness, choice-making opportunities, or family involvement and a measure of health. Emerson et al. (2001) found no significant differences among three types of community support arrangements on a number of health indicators: supported-living arrangements (1–3 residents, not registered under U.K. legislation as either a residential care home or nursing home and described by the provider agency as "supported living"), small group homes (1–3 residents), and large group homes (4–6 residents). There were also no differences in five categories of reported risks. However, exploitation by people in the local community was reported for a higher proportion of residents in supported living compared with large group homes, and abuse by coresidents was reported for a higher proportion of residents in large compared with small group homes. Stancliffe and Keane (2000) found no differences in staff-reported health care, healthy lifestyle, or safety between matched samples living in group homes that were either fully staffed (3–7 residents, mean 42.1 hours paid support per person per week) or partially staffed (1–4 residents, mean 10.5 hours paid support per person per week).

Further analysis of the Emerson et al. (2001) community sample using multivariate logistic regression (Robertson et al., 2000) showed that, after controlling for adaptive behavior, predictors of risk factors for poor health were mainly unrelated to current residential support arrangements. There were two exceptions: risk of inactivity was positively related to having senior staff with relevant qualifications, and risk of poor diet was related to being the named tenant within the accommodation, as opposed to being a resident of a registered care home.

MATERIAL WELL-BEING

Income and wealth will be influenced more by benefit regulations and working situation than by residential arrangements, although the latter could have an impact on the former (e.g., in the U.K., whether a person lives in his or her own home or a registered care home affects welfare benefit entitlements). However, little research has investigated this. In contrast, the quality of the home environment is clearly dependent on the residential arrangements made. Thompson, Egli, and Robinson (2000) found that perceived home-likeness was correlated with certain architectural features, typically clustered in combinations. Some architectural features negatively correlated with home-likeness were associated with the number of residents living together. Overall, home-likeness was inversely correlated with setting size. Consistent with this, Tossebro (1995) found that living-unit size was a significant predictor of a measure of deprivatization, which is described as reflecting markers of private territory, disposition of territory, and home-likeness. Emerson et al. (2001) also found a trend toward reduced home-likeness across supported living schemes, small group homes, and large group homes, although differences in post hoc comparison reached significance only between supported living schemes and large group homes.

Surprisingly, given the emphasis on community location in the deinstitutionalization reform movement, there has been little research on the quality of neighborhoods in which people in supported accommodations live and how these might vary according to the accommodation arrangements made.

SOCIAL WELL-BEING

There is considerable evidence that the social networks of people with mental retardation are limited in size and restricted mainly to family members, staff, and other people with mental retardation (see Robertson, Emerson, Gregory, et al., 2001). In addition, there is little evidence that friendship patterns expand with length of time living in the community. Emerson et al. (2001) found that residents in supported-living arrangements and small group homes had larger social networks than those in large group homes. Residents in small group homes had more people in their social networks other than family members, staff, and other people with mental retardation than did residents in large group homes. In a further analysis, Robertson, Emerson, Gregory, et al. (2001) found that the presence of people in social networks other than family members, staff, and other people with mental retardation was predicted by a less institutional social climate and living in a setting for three or fewer people (note that these results were mistakenly omitted from Table 5 in Robertson, Emerson, Gregory, et al.'s article and have been supplied by the authors). However, Stancliffe and Keane (2000) found no differences between fully and partially staffed group homes in the proportions of residents with friends who were not family, staff, or fellow residents despite the fact that the settings also differed with respect to size of setting.

Community integration has also been measured by the variety and frequency of social and community activities. Howe, Horner, and Newton (1998) found that residents in supported-living arrangements (defined by 12 operational criteria) took part in a significantly greater variety of community activities and participated in community activities overall more frequently than did residents in traditional group homes. They also performed more activities with other people and with a significantly greater variety of other people. However, setting types varied in a variety of respects other than those defining the distinction between supported living and traditional (e.g., in their size), and it is not possible to link outcome to any particular environmental characteristic with any certainty. Stancliffe and Lakin (1998) found that various measures of social or community activity were unrelated to size of residence. Stancliffe and Keane (2000) found no difference between small, partially staffed and larger, fully staffed group homes in the distribution and frequency of social activities but did find an increased frequency of community activities among residents in the former. Emerson et al. (2001) found more frequent community activities among residents in supported living compared with equivalently small group homes and large group homes.

Egli, Feurer, Roper, and Thompson (2002) used path analysis to model the possible influence on community activities of the home-likeness of the setting, staff attitudes toward community inclusion, and staff-initiated interactions. In one model, setting home-likeness had direct and indirect effects (via staff-initiated interactions) on community activities, and positive attitudes also had an indirect impact via staff-initiated interactions. In the second model, both setting home-likeness and positive staff attitudes had indirect effects via staff-initiated interactions. Felce et al. (2002a) found that the frequency of community activities was predicted by living in a setting with a more individualized social climate and higher staff-to-resident ratios and that the frequency of social activities was predicted by living in a setting in which a higher proportion of residents had staff named as a key worker[1], the social climate was less individualized, and residents had a lower attendance at day services. Heller et al. (2002) found that greater community integration was predicted by greater opportunities to make choices and greater family involvement. Perry and Felce (2005) found that a greater variety of integrative activities was predicted by larger setting size and greater receipt of attention from staff and that a greater frequency of integrative activities was predicted by less emphasis on assessment and teaching and by not living in a setting operated by a private proprietor who lived separately.

In summary, there is some evidence linking social and community integration to reduced setting size, but results are inconsistent, and most studies did not substantiate a

---

[1]A key worker is a member of staff nominated to have a particular responsibility for ensuring that individual plans and programs are completed and that the resident is a party to all decision making.

link. Rather, service model and staff orientation (staff attitudes, social climate, staff interactions) appear to be more significant factors, possibly reinforced by greater home-likeness and smaller scale. Greater presence of staff members appeared to have a positive impact in a study involving people with more severe disabilities but a negative impact among people with sufficient skills to live semi-independently. Whether community acceptance is influenced by the nature of the community residential arrangements made and the nature of neighborhoods has not been studied.

PRODUCTIVE WELL-BEING

Overviews of the deinstitutionalization literature cited previously have concluded that the move from institutional to community-based residential services has generally but not always been accompanied by significant increases in adaptive behavior. However, studies focusing on the longer-term development of adults with mental retardation once they have moved into the community tend to report a "plateau effect," which suggests that the reported improvements in adaptive behavior on moving may simply reflect the impact of increased opportunities to display existing skills. Community settings may not be inherently better environments for promoting developmental growth than the institutions that they have replaced. Although an extensive experimental literature exists about the types of technical and educational support that may accelerate behavioral development, very little is known about the types of general environmental conditions, including varieties of residential support arrangements, that are associated with developmental growth (Felce & Emerson, 2001). Heller et al. (2002) found that a more attractive physical environment and greater opportunities for making choices were associated with higher adaptive behavior at follow-up assessment after controlling for adaptive behavior at baseline.

The factors associated with self-determination within community settings have been more extensively studied. Tossebro (1995) showed that setting size predicted self-determination within the range of 1 to 5 residents but not 5 to 16. Stancliffe (1997), also studying community settings varying in size from 1 to 5 residents, showed that greater choice was predicted by lower staff presence (for both self-report and staff report measures) and smaller setting size (staff report measure only). However, Stancliffe and Lakin (1998) found no effect for setting size across residences for 2–4, 5–6, and 7–15 people. Emerson et al. (2001) found that the total score on a scale measuring choice was significantly greater in supported-living arrangements compared with both equally small and larger group homes. In a further analysis, Robertson, Emerson, Hatton, et al. (2001) showed that greater choice was predicted by smaller size, more home-like architectural features, and better activity planning.

After controlling for adaptive and challenging behavior, Stancliffe et al. (2000) found that personal control differed across service types (with people living semi-independently having greater control than people living in supported-living arrangements, who, in turn, had more control than people living in ICF-MR facilities). They also found that personal control differed according to setting size, but nonsystematically (i.e., control in one- and three-person residences was greater than in two- and four-person residences). In addition, hierarchical regression showed that greater personal control was predicted by settings with policies supporting service user autonomy and more individualized social climate. Individuals with more money available for discretionary spending also exercised greater personal control. Perry and Felce (2005) found that greater staff-reported choice was predicted by living in settings with a greater emphasis on individual planning, less emphasis on behavioral assessment and skill teaching, greater receipt of attention from staff, and better physical integration in the community. Greater choice among a reduced sample capable of completing the self-report version of the measure was predicted by settings having fewer residents and living in a setting operated by a voluntary body rather than a private proprietor. Greater scores on a staff-completed index of autonomy were predicted by a greater emphasis on individual planning, greater receipt of attention from staff, and better physical integration in the community.

In summary, there is some evidence from more than one study that greater self-determination is associated with smaller size, certain aspects of service model or staff orientation, and settings that are more home-like or physically integrated.

Whether residential support arrangements provide an environment that allows residents to be occupied within the home (e.g., in self-help, household, or leisure activities) is another facet of their day-to-day quality of life. After controlling for subject and setting characteristics, Thompson et al. (1996b) found that residents in more home-like community settings were more likely to engage in household tasks and other individual activities. They also found that home-likeness and the orientation of staff toward supporting resident choice and participation in activities were intertwined. Hence it is possible that home-likeness was both an influence on and influenced by the orientation of staff. Consistent with this interpretation, a growing body of evidence demonstrates the strength of association between engagement in activity and the receipt of either attention or assistance from staff (Emerson et al., 2000; Felce et al. 2002a; Felce, Jones, Lowe, & Perry, 2003; Perry & Felce, 2005). In addition, higher scores on an index of participation in household tasks have been shown to be associated with receipt of staff attention, lower staff-to-resident ratios and a lower proportion of formally qualified staff (Felce et al., 2002a), living more independently of staff support (Stancliffe & Keane, 2000), and living in settings that have better physical integration (Perry & Felce, 2005).

EMOTIONAL AND CIVIC WELL-BEING

These are underresearched areas. There are no studies that link specific residential support arrangements to the emotional and civic well-being of residents.

PERSONAL LIFE SATISFACTION

The observation is long-standing that expressions of subjective well-being, or satisfaction with life, tend to have trait-like stability. As such, measured satisfaction may be insensitive to environmental differences unless these are so great as to prevent adaptation (see Cummins, 2005, for a summary of this position). Even when very different environments have been compared, such as institutions and supported housing in the community, resident satisfaction has rarely been shown to differ (Emerson & Hatton, 1996; Felce, 2000). Consistent with these results, Stancliffe and Keane (2000) found no significant differences between the satisfaction of residents living in fully and in partially staffed group homes; Emerson et al. (2001) found none between residents living in supported-living arrangements, small group homes, and large group homes; and Perry and Felce (2005) found no environmental predictors of satisfaction in five out of six subjective aspects measured. There are no robust findings to link residential support arrangements and resident life satisfaction.

CONCLUSIONS

The environmental determinants of outcome are incompletely understood. There is little evidence in relation to some areas (e.g., health, safety, income, skill development, and emotional or civic well-being), and, even where evidence does exist, it is not consistent. Moreover, even though the studies selected have merit in relation to isolating links between environmental arrangements and outcome, they are not without their methodological limitations. One general criticism would be that the selection of independent variables considered as potentially influencing outcome varies between studies. Those considered by any one study cannot be regarded as comprehensive, given this variability. This gives rise to the problem in comparative studies of different service models that setting differences described may be confounded with those that have not been described.[2]

In multivariate research, whether a variable remains in a predictive model depends on which other variables have been considered. For example, in one of our own studies of the influences on staff activity in community group homes (Felce, Lowe & Jones, 2002b), the final regression model for predicting resident receipt of attention changed after the data were reanalyzed following a referee's suggestion that range in resident adaptive behavior should be included as an independent variable. Some of the variability in findings across the studies documented herein inevitably arises from the fact that investigators have considered different sets of potential environmental influences.

In this regard, it is, therefore, important that more attention be given to reaching an international consensus about the important variables to be described when doing research on residential support arrangements, so that relationships between environmental characteristics and outcome can be identified with greater confidence. It is understandable that evaluation in such a policy-related area as this should have highlighted administrative distinctions or variables commonly thought to be important. However, research in the postdeinstitutionalization era needs to become more sophisticated. The issue of the integrity of the independent variable is as important to this research endeavor as it is to intervention or treatment research. A more consistent approach to analyzing setting characteristics is required for further progress to be made.

Before summarizing existing knowledge, we must emphasize that our concern here was to address the determinants of outcome within community residential support arrangements, not to revisit the institution–community divide. The range of certain environmental variables is constrained by this focus. For example, in a particular study, the sizes of settings investigated might only vary between one and five residents. The fact that variation within this range might not be found to have a significant influence on outcome should not be interpreted as suggesting that greater size differences would

---

[2]Actually, confounding of variables exists to some extent even among those for which information is available, such as between service model and size of setting, in both Howe et al., 1998, and Stancliffe & Keane, 2000).

be equally insignificant. So with due caution in mind, we can make the following broad conclusions from the existing literature about the features of community residential support arrangements that are important to outcome:

- Although some studies found that certain outcomes were associated with setting size, its absence of influence in others suggests that size is not such a strong influence on quality of life as it is commonly regarded to be. Its strongest link appears to be with home-likeness and choice.
- Home-likeness and physical integration are desirable properties. Achieving these is likely to constrain setting size to groupings that can be accommodated within architecturally typical, normatively located homes.
- Little is known about the characteristics of community neighborhoods, if any, that influence community acceptance and integration.
- Resource inputs (e.g., staff-to-resident ratios), although considered as potentially influential variables in many of the studies, were rarely found to be significant. The fact that improved outcome in a minority of studies was linked to both greater and less intensive staffing reinforces the conclusion that staff presence needs to be closely matched to the support needs of residents and not seen as necessarily linked to quality of life. Those studies that considered the extent to which staff possessed formal qualifications as an influence on outcome either found no effect or a negative effect.
- The "operational culture" of the setting has a significant influence on outcome, whether this is reflected in the orientation embraced by "supported living," in staff attitudes toward inclusion, in social climate or individualization of approach, in the focus and degree of organization of planning and other working methods, or in the level of staff–resident interaction. Further research is required to identify desirable social and operational processes more precisely. A greater emphasis probably needs to be given by service providers to these aspects of support arrangements.
- Support arrangements can have mixed beneficial and adverse effects. For example, in the Emerson et al. (2001) and Robertson et al. (2000) set of studies, living in a supported-living arrangement (holding a tenancy) predicted having both greater choice and poorer diet. It is important to recognize that outcomes associated with a particular service model may not be universally superior to those associated with an alternative. Two implications follow. One is that providers may need to make particular efforts to create an organizational culture that compensates for a tendency toward poor outcome. In relation to the preceding example, effective encouragement of healthy living may need to be developed in situations in which people have greater personal control. Second, consumer choice is important in matching preferred lifestyle to the outcomes that alternative residential arrangements support. People differ in the quality of life that they want. Better information on the outcomes associated with particular support arrangements will help individuals to make more informed choices based on how they want to live.

REFERENCES

Braddock, D., Emerson, E., Felce, D., & Stancliffe, R. J. (2001). The living circumstances of children and adults with mental retardation in the United States, Canada, England and Wales, and Australia. *Mental Retardation and Developmental Disabilities Research Reviews, 7*, 115–121.

Cummins, R. A. (2005). Caregivers as managers of subjective well-being: A homeostatic perspective. *Journal of Applied Research in Intellectual Disabilities, 18*, 335–344.

Egli, M., Feurer, I., Roper, T., & Thompson, T (2002). The role of residential homelikeness in promoting community participation by adults with mental retardation. *Research in Developmental Disabilities, 23*, 179–190.

Emerson, E., & Hatton, C. (1996). Deinstitutionalization in the UK and Ireland: Outcomes for service users. *Journal of Intellectual and Developmental Disability, 21*, 17–37.

Emerson, E., & McVilly, K. (2004). Friendship activities of adults with intellectual disabilities in supported accommodation in Northern England. *Journal of Applied Research in Intellectual Disabilities, 17*, 191–197.

Emerson, E., Robertson, J., Gregory, N., Hatton, C., Kessissoglou, S., Hallam, A., et al. (2001). Quality and costs of supported living residences and group homes in the United Kingdom. *American Journal on Mental Retardation, 106*, 401–415.

Emerson, E., Robertson, J., Gregory, N., Kessissoglou, S., Hatton, C., Hallam, A., et al. (2000). The quality and costs of community-based residential supports and residential campuses for people with severe and complex disabilities. *Journal of Intellectual and Developmental Disability, 25*, 263–279.

Felce, D. (1997). Defining and applying the concept of quality of life. *Journal of Intellectual Disability Research, 41*, 126–143.

Felce, D. (2000). *Quality of life for people with learning disabilities in supported housing in the community: A review of research.* Exeter, UK: University of Exeter, Centre for Evidence-Based Social Services.

Felce, D., & Emerson, E. (2001). Living with support in a home in the community: Predictors of behavioral development and household and community activity. *Mental Retardation and Developmental Disabilities Research Reviews, 7*, 75–83.

Felce, D., Jones, E., Lowe, K., & Perry, J. (2003). Rational resourcing and productivity: Relationships among staff input, resident characteristics, and group home quality. *American Journal on Mental Retardation, 108*, 161–172.

Felce, D., Lowe, K., & Jones, E. (2002a). Association between the provision characteristics and operation of supported housing services and resident outcomes. *Journal of Applied Research in Intellectual Disabilities, 15*, 404–418.

Felce, D., Lowe, K., & Jones, E. (2002b). Staff activity in supported housing services. *Journal of Applied Research in Intellectual Disabilities, 15*, 388–403.

Heller, T., Miller, A., & Hsieh, K. (2002). Eight-year follow-up of the impact of environmental characteristics on the well-being of adults with developmental disabilities. *Mental Retardation, 40*, 366–378.

Howe, J., Horner, R., & Newton, J. (1998). Comparison of supported living and traditional residential services in the state of Oregon. *Mental Retardation, 36*, 1–11.

Kim, S., Larson, S. A., & Lakin, K. C. (2001). Behavioural outcomes of deinstitutionalisation for people with intellectual disability: A review of studies conducted between 1980 and 1999. *Journal of Intellectual and Developmental Disability, 26*, 35–50.

Perry, J., & Felce, D. (2005). Factors associated with outcome in community group homes. *American Journal on Mental Retardation, 110*, 121–135.

Robertson, J., Emerson, E., Gregory, N., Hatton, C., Kessissoglou, S., Hallam, A., et al. (2001). Social networks of people with mental retardation in residential settings. *Mental Retardation, 39*, 201–214.

Robertson, J., Emerson, E., Gregory, N., Hatton, C., Turner, S., Kessissoglou, S., et al. (2000). Lifestyle related risk factors for poor health in residential settings for people with intellectual disabilities. *Research in Developmental Disabilities, 21*, 469–486.

Robertson, J., Emerson, E., Hatton, C., Gregory, N., Kessissoglou, S., Hallam, A., et al. (2001). Environmental opportunities and supports for exercising self-determination in community-based residential settings. *Research in Developmental Disabilities, 22*, 487–502.

Schalock, R., & Felce, D. (2004). Quality of life and subjective well-being; Conceptual and measurement issues. In E. Emerson, C. Hatton, T. Thompson, & T. Parmenter (Eds.), *International handbook of applied research in intellectual disabilities* (pp. 261–279). Chichester, UK: Wiley.

Schalock, R. L., Brown, I., Brown, R., Cummins, R. A., Felce, D., Matikka, L., et al. (2002). Conceptualization, measurement, and application of quality of life for persons with intellectual disabilities: Report of an international panel of experts. *Mental Retardation, 40*, 457–470.

Stancliffe, R. (1997). Community living-unit size, staff presence, and residents' choice-making. *Mental Retardation, 35*, 1–9.

Stancliffe, R., Abery, B., & Smith, J. (2000). Personal control and the ecology of community living settings: Beyond living-unit size and type. *American Journal on Mental Retardation, 105*, 431–454.

Stancliffe, R., & Keane, S. (2000). Outcomes and costs of community living: A matched comparison of group homes and semi-independent living. *Journal of Intellectual and Developmental Disability, 25*, 281–305.

Stancliffe, R., & Lakin, K. (1998). Analysis of expenditures and outcomes of residential alternatives for persons with developmental disabilities. *American Journal on Mental Retardation, 102*, 552–568.

Thompson, T., Egli, M., & Robinson, J. (2000). Architecture and behavior of people with intellectual disabilities: Observational methods and housing policy. In T. Thompson, D. Felce, & F. J. Symons (Eds.), *Behavioral observation: Technology and applications in developmental disabilities* (pp. 101–114). Baltimore: Brookes.

Thompson, T., Robinson, J., Dietrich, M., Farris, M., & Sinclair, V. (1996a). Architectural features and perceptions of community residences for people with mental retardation. *American Journal on Mental Retardation, 101*, 292–314.

Thompson, T., Robinson, J., Dietrich, M., Farris, M., & Sinclair, V. (1996b). Interdependence of architectural features and program variables in community residences for people with mental retardation. *American Journal on Mental Retardation, 101*, 315–327.

Tossebro, J. (1995). Impact of size revisited: Relation of number of residents to self-determination and deprivatization. *American Journal on Mental Retardation, 100*, 59–67.

Young, L., Sigafoos, J., Suttie, J., Ashman, A., & Grevell, P. (1998). Deinstitutionalisation of persons with intellectual disabilities: A review of Australian studies. *Journal of Intellectual and Developmental Disability, 23*, 155–170.

21

Independent Living

Roger J. Stancliffe
K. Charlie Lakin

This chapter focuses on adults with intellectual and developmental disabilities (ID/DD) who live in community settings outside the family home, with relatively little or no regular paid staff support, usually in homes they own or rent. Such individuals typically have lower support needs and milder intellectual disability (ID) than people served in settings with 24-hour staffing such as group homes (Burchard, Hasazi, Gordon, & Yoe, 1991; Stancliffe, 2005). Our coverage of independent living errs toward inclusiveness by examining research on what is described as *independent living, semi-independent living, supported living,* or *consumer-directed services*. We have not looked in detail at important matters such as employment (except as it relates to poverty) or behavior support and mental health, because these issues are dealt with in other chapters in this volume. The support needs of people with ID/DD living independently who are parents were not considered for reasons of space.

This chapter begins with a brief look at research on independent living throughout the 20th century. Next, we discuss principles of supported living to give a values context to the research findings. In the third section and thereafter, attention is given to contemporary studies, mostly published after 1994. Our intent is to distill contemporary research findings, but to do so within a broader context of issues that impinge on the lives of adults with ID/DD living independently and that therefore also affect those who support them. These issues take account of the opportunities and constraints imposed by the environment, including the economic, social, service provision, legislative, and regulatory environments. In so doing, we also focus on public policy and service provision issues to an extent.

HISTORICAL STUDIES THAT CHANGED EXPECTATION OF DEPENDENCE

Historically, public facilities for people with ID/DD were intended to provide asylum and care for those seen as unable to care for themselves. The perceived need for such facilities resulted in expectations of dependence and failure to recognize the capacities of people with ID/DD. Early follow-up studies, such as Fernald (1919), showed that individuals released from state institutions with no continuing formal community supports fared better than most people had expected. In his meta-analysis of the first 50 years of follow-up studies, Cobb (1972) observed that "the most consistent and outstanding finding of all follow-up studies is the high proportion of the adult retarded who achieve satisfactory adjustments, by whatever criteria are employed" (p. 145). Cobb noted that about three in four avoided reinstitutionalization or incarceration, but that most found it difficult to attain permanent employment, marriage, their own homes, and other signs of stable community life.

Looking at people released from state institutions in California living without specialized formal supports, Edgerton (1967) reported that, for many, survival in the community depended on the support of family and friends ("benefactors"). Edgerton (1967, 1981, 1990) made clear that, although most persons with mild ID/DD adjust to the demands of community life, their lives are modest, with a constant risk of losing employment, housing, or basic social and personal supports and that those outcomes, in turn, threaten individual health, safety, independence, and quality of life.

Seminal Research on (Semi-)Independent Living

An important development from the late 1970s was the rise of services offering *part-time* community-living training, habilitation, and support to people with ID/DD living "independently." These include semi-independent living services (Halpern, Close, & Nelson, 1986) and independent living services (Lozano, 1993), which may provide long-term, regular part-time support and/or episodic support for problems that arise. Seminal studies (Burchard et al., 1991; Edgerton, 1967; Halpern et al., 1986; Lozano, 1993; Schalock & Harper, 1978; Schalock, Harper, & Carver, 1981) have documented the ability of many people with ID to live reasonably successfully in the community with relatively modest formal support from such services. Factors associated with success include living skills, friendship, family involvement, community access, employment and finances, and access to independent living with appropriate supports. Success was often defined in terms of not returning to full-time care. One crucial systemic factor in the breakdown of independent living was the inability of service systems to provide needed increases in supports during periods of interpersonal, financial, psychiatric, or behavioral distress, with substantially higher levels of support being offered only via other living arrangements, such as group homes or institutions.

Lozano (1993) showed that the very experience of independent living is associated with the development and maintenance of living skills. She questioned the notion that access to independent living should be earned through living-skill acquisition and stated that the issue for people with ID/DD "should not be whether they have the skills to live on their own, but rather, how the systems created to serve them can provide the necessary supports to enable them to do so" (Lozano, 1993, p. 261).

Commitments by and to Persons with Disabilities to Live with Independence: Supported Living

As noted, early studies of community living generally found that people with relatively mild ID/DD wanted an integrated community life and that, with proper support, they were able to achieve it. Like other community members, people with ID/DD want homes of their own, jobs that they like, control over the basic decisions of their lives, support from people who care about them, and opportunities to participate in their communities. People with ID/DD seek self-determination, independence, inclusion, and typical, valued social roles. These values have been a defining aspect of a growing commitment to the concept of "supported independent living," which may be contrasted with more *traditional* community living arrangements, such as small group homes and host family arrangements in which the providers of the needed support also control the home in which the individual lives. In addition to differences regarding in whose home the people with disabilities are living, supported living and traditional community living services tend to differ in household composition, staffing and support arrangements, regulations and funding, as well as flexibility, individualization, and the degree to which people have control over their own services and supports. In traditional congregate, facility-based services, individual service users have little control over where and with whom they live, who provides support, or the nature and timing of specific support services. Their support staff, services, and living arrangements are managed by a service provider that operates within the constraints of a funding and regulatory system that tends to be rigid, uniformly applied, and relatively unresponsive to individual preferences in its provision of a standard package of services that varies little from individual to individual.

The principles of supported community living are intended to produce a fundamental shift not just in the places where people live but in the balance of power in how people live, work, and participate. These principles acknowledge and respect what people with ID/DD share in common with their neighbors. They reflect a commitment to listen carefully, to share in the struggles, and to assist people to live their lives as much on their own terms as possible given their needs, their circumstances, and the resources available to them (Bradley, Ashbaugh & Blaney, 1994; Lakin & Smull, 1995). Increasingly, the quality of services and the effectiveness of service systems for persons with ID/DD are defined by the achievement of outcomes that reflect supported community living principles (see Howe, Horner, & Newton, 1998; Racino & Taylor, 1993). These six principles are described next.

1. *Separation of housing from supports.* As noted, traditional disability services bundle housing and support into a single, provider-controlled package. An individual must live in a setting operated by the service and receive the amount and type of support defined by the service, regardless of what is needed or desired by the individual. To change service providers, one must also change where and with whom one lives. In supported living, individuality is respected above program considerations. One's home, community, and lifestyle are chosen first, then the services and supports needed to achieve the desired lifestyle are considered. This can be achieved only when the selection of housing and the selection of supports needed to live in that home are independent decisions.

2. *Living in one's own home.* A major way that people with disabilities can gain control over their own lives is by living in their own homes. This may be a place owned or

rented by the individual with disabilities or by his or her family. It may mean continuing to live in one's family home. Consistent with the separation of housing and supports, living in one's home changes the dynamics of service delivery, because the home is not dependent on a continuing relationship with a service provider, and the individual decides who crosses the threshold of his or her own home. However, no specific research has evaluated the relationship between living in one's own home and having control over services and supports.

3. *Supported living manifests differently for each individual.* Supported living is a not a program but an individually focused approach to providing support. Therefore, specific living arrangements and paid and natural supports manifest differently for each individual.

4. *Supported living requires choice making among competing desires.* In supported living, people trade off competing priorities, as other citizens do. They must find affordable housing and balance the cost of housing against other economic decisions they would like to make. The budgets available to accomplish what one wishes are not budgets for a group; they are budgets for an individual. As such, they usually are zero sums in that one choice affects other choices.

5. *Supported living involves more participation in instrumental activities.* People participate more fully in their own lives, and support providers assist the person with activities and participation rather than taking over and doing it for the person.

6. *Supported living integrates informal support.* A key feature in supported living is fostering natural supports (Howe et al., 1998; Racino & Taylor, 1993). The growing understanding of the importance of natural supports or benefactors to independent living has led to efforts to structure such assistance within "circles of support": a group of people with an organized collective commitment to assist the person in achieving personal life goals. Circles of support assist people not only with independence through work and home life but also with identifying and participating in community activities (Bradley, Agosta, & Kimmich, 2001; Ducharme, Beeman, DeMarasse, & Ludlum, 1994). The efforts of people with disabilities to live as independently and free from formal, paid supports as they can are often greatly assisted by the quality and commitment of the "natural supports" in their lives.

ABILITY, IMPAIRMENT, ACCOMMODATION, AND OTHER CONCEPTS IN INDEPENDENT LIVING

Proposed definitions of disability, conceptual frameworks, and related classification systems (e.g., Luckasson et al., 2002; World Health Organization, 2001) share an understanding that an individual's opportunity to perform an activity is dependent on both that individual's characteristics (abilities, limitations) and environmental factors. Environmental factors include the expectations, demands, and accommodations available in the social and physical environment that transform impairments (mental or physical conditions) and functional limitations (inability to perform typical activities with normally expected proficiency) into disability (inability to fulfill typical social roles).

By definition, people identified as having ID/DD have functional limitations in areas associated with independent living (self-care, communication, mobility, economic self-sufficiency, etc.). These limitations can contribute to disability, but their effects may also be negated by "accommodations" within the environment that change demands and expectations so that the individual can fulfill a typical social role, such as living in his or her own home without full-time care and supervision. Such accommodations include physical modifications (e.g., ramps, redesigned kitchens and bathrooms), technologies (e.g., alerting systems, one-touch dial phones), modified supports (e.g., phone calls, training in independent living skills rather than personal care), or carefully selected environments (e.g., choosing housing near shops, family, and/or work to decrease travel demands for a person without independent public transportation skills).

Discussion of these issues may seem academic, but they are at the heart of the contemporary supports model for assisting people to live independently with the support they need to minimize the effects of their limitations. This approach is not unique to persons with disabilities. Hiring experts such as plumbers or tax specialists is common practice in overcoming individual limitations for people with and without disabilities alike. Most people, including people with ID/DD, strive for a balance of independence and focused dependence on others, as abilities and disabilities necessitate. Individuals with ID/DD likely need more accommodations than most people. Help with needed accommodations may come from paid staff or unpaid individuals, referred to as "natural supports," who often include family, neighbors, friends (Schalock & Genung, 1993), and benefactors (Edgerton, 1967).

NEED FOR SUPPORT IN VARIOUS SOCIAL ROLES AND SETTINGS

What Proportion of People with Intellectual Disability Live Independently?

This section examines contemporary research on the proportion of people with ID who live independently. Some studies present this information for a sample of people with ID (Blackorby & Wagner, 1996; Luftig & Muthert, 2005; Maughan, Collishaw, & Pickles, 1999; Richardson & Koller, 1996). Other studies examine broader populations, including individuals with ID, such as former special education students (Gardner & Carran, 2005; Heal, Rubin, & Rusch, 1998; Seltzer et al., 2005). Some of these studies did not report on independent living per se but provided data on marital status that could serve as a rough proxy for independent living.

Nationally representative U.S. comparison data from the early 1980s on age peers from the general population showed independent living rates of 37% (0–2 years after school) and 60% (3–5 years after school; Center for Human Resource Research, 1988, cited in Blackorby & Wagner, 1996). Several conclusions emerge from the studies examined.

1. In early adulthood, the percentage of adults with ID living independently increases with age. This has been shown directly in some longitudinal studies (Blackorby & Wagner, 1996) and may be inferred by comparison of findings between cross-sectional studies that examine different age ranges. Presumably the percentage plateaus at some point, but the age at which this occurs is unknown. Seltzer et al. (2005) reported no change in the percentage of people who were married by age 36 and by age 55.

2. Adults with ID have lower rates of independent living than the general community (Blackorby & Wagner, 1996; Maughan et al., 1999; Richardson & Koller, 1996). The difference seems most marked in the first few years after school.

3. Adults with ID have lower rates of independent living than people with other disabilities, such as learning disability (Blackorby & Wagner, 1996; Luftig & Muthert, 2005).

4. There are higher rates of independent living among women with ID than among men with ID, related to the higher rate of marriage among women with ID than among men with ID (Blackorby & Wagner, 1996; Maughan et al., 1999; Richardson & Koller, 1996).

5. Gardner and Carran's (2005) data on disability service users show a low rate of independent living compared with population-based studies (Blackorby & Wagner, 1996; Heal et al., 1998; Maughan et al., 1999; Richardson & Koller, 1996; Seltzer et al., 2005). This implies that there may be substantial numbers of people with ID living independently who do not use formal disability services. It may also suggest that people in the formal service system live in more supervised environments than peers with similar abilities who are outside this system (see Stancliffe, 2005; Stancliffe & Keane, 2000).

It is important to note that Seltzer et al.'s (2005) findings may contradict the conclusions in points 2, 4 and 5, but Seltzer et al.'s study included a substantial majority of people in the "low IQ" sample with IQs above the ID range.

The absolute incidence of independent living varies considerably between studies, seemingly related to sampling, to participants' age (or years since leaving school), high school graduation status, type of disability, gender, ethnic group, and use of disability services; and to the time period when the data were gathered (due to changes in service availability, housing costs, etc.).

As noted, Gardner and Carran (2005) reported quite low rates of independent living among disability service users. This finding may be attributed to individuals with greater needs for support utilizing formal services and/or to risk avoidance by service providers. It may be easier to continue to support an individual in a group home rather than to risk changing to semi-independent living. For example, Stancliffe and Keane (2000) found it relatively easy to locate group-home residents whose abilities matched those of people living semi-independently.

Environments and Expectations

Contemporary research that compares different types of community living arrangements shows that smaller, more normalized community living settings, such as (semi-)independent living and supported living, are associated with better outcomes.

Semi-Independent and Independent Living

Comparisons of outcomes for individuals living in group homes (with full-time staffing) or semi-independently (i.e., with drop-in staff support) reveal better outcomes for semi-independent settings on the following factors: choice, self-determination, autonomy, satisfaction, independence, lifestyle normalization, physical and social integration, domestic participation, community participation, and personal well-being (Burchard et al., 1991; Stancliffe, 1995, 1997, 2005; Stancliffe, Abery, & Smith, 2000; Stancliffe & Keane, 2000; Stancliffe & Wehmeyer, 1995; Wehmeyer & Bolding, 1999). Loneliness, self-care, domestic management, personal safety, money management, and health are potential areas of concern for semi-independent residents, but Stancliffe (2005) and Stancliffe and Keane (2000) reported that these outcomes did not differ from those experienced by group-home residents, even though the former group received much less staff support.

Supported Living

Howe et al. (1998) found that supported-living residents experienced a greater variety and frequency of community-based and social activities, more participation in preferred activities, better compatibility with living companions, and greater self-determination than participants in "traditional" community services. Emerson et al. (2001) reported similar findings in the United Kingdom. Although this chapter focuses on people with milder disabilities and less need for support, it is important to recognize that the benefits of supported living have also been shown for people with severe disability, although they receive more support (Gardner & Carran, 2005).

Individuals in supported-living settings do exercise greater control over choice of living companions than residents of more traditional community settings (Emerson et al., 2001; Howe et al., 1998). Gardner and Carran (2005) found a consistent and significant relation between the outcome "people chose where and with whom to live" and a number of other important outcomes, such as safety and freedom from abuse and neglect. This result suggests that choosing where and with whom to live—a defining feature of supported living (see Howe et al., 1998)—may also be related to achieving other outcomes. Possible reasons may include greater likelihood of friendship among chosen living companions, plus a reduction in incompatibility and in associated client-to-client abuse evident when people have not chosen to live together.

Support and Everyday Opportunities for Participation

Independence and competence are supported by regular opportunities to apply one's skills. Levine and Langness (1985) found that competence at supermarket shopping was unrelated to age, sex, IQ, or amount of training. The most competent shoppers were those whose circumstances required them to shop independently as adults. Likewise, Lozano (1993) found that the experience of independent living, not the amount of independent living skills training, accounted for improvement or maintenance of skills. Suto, Clare, Holland, and Watson (2005) showed that basic financial understanding *and* everyday decision-making opportunities were both crucial for maximizing financial decision-making abilities. Stancliffe (2005) found better outcomes in semi-independent settings than in group homes and argued that because of frequent staff absence, semi-independent living not only *provided* opportunities for independent participation but also it *demanded* such participation. Similarly, Stancliffe (1997) found that individuals living in settings with less staff presence (i.e., having periods with no staff present) exercised more choice.

These studies suggest that environmental demands, such as routine opportunities to undertake tasks independently (due, in part, to the absence of continuous support), are important in achieving superior outcomes in (semi-)independent living. However, almost all of the studies cited involved people with lower support needs. People with severe disabilities are likely to do poorly when given little support (better seen as *neglect*). Gardner and Carran (2005) found that individuals with mild to moderate ID living independently attained the highest personal outcomes (80%) but that those with severe to profound disability achieved the *lowest* outcomes (52%) for independent living and did better in living arrangements with more support, such as supported living. Low levels of staff support in independent living may facilitate independence and better outcomes for people with milder disabilities, but independent living provides insufficient support for people with more severe disabilities to attain personal outcomes.

Regularly undertaking activities independent of (staff) support is associated with skill development and achievement of personal outcomes for people with lower support needs, but not for those with severe disability, who instead require active support from caregivers for successful participation in meaningful activities. This provides one explanation of why people with milder disabilities typically enjoy better outcomes when living (semi-)independently. The issue seems to be one of *matching* support to the person's support needs: that is, providing enough assistance in areas where it is needed without infringing on autonomy by interfering in matters with which the person needs no help. Too much and too little support can both be detrimental.

Economic and Social Factors and Independent Living

Poverty and Disability

Household income of families with a member with ID/DD is much lower than for the general community, and dramatically so for single-parent households (Fujiura, 1998, 2003; Lewis & Johnson, 2005). Fujiura (2003) showed that people with mild ID share a comparable need for supports and experience similar functional limitations and exposure to poverty as people identified as having more severe ID. For example, four times as many households containing a person with ID were below the poverty level compared with the U.S. general population. Fujiura (1998) found that the people with ID/DD living in their own households (alone or with roommates) had a mean monthly earned income of $983, vastly below the income of other households. These individuals are often simply too poor to afford even the most modest rental housing (O'Hara & Cooper, 2005).

Housing Affordability

Independent living typically involves renting or owning one's own home, so cost is a fundamental barrier. Federal housing affordability guidelines specify that households should pay no more than 30% of income toward housing costs, because money is also needed for other basic needs such as food, clothing, utilities, and transportation. Rental affordability has become markedly worse in recent years for people on Supplemental Security Income (SSI; O'Hara & Cooper, 2005). Federal SSI payments in 2004 were $564 per month. Adding state SSI supplements available to individuals with disabilities living independently raised the national monthly average to $617, or $7,404 annually. In 2004 nationally, average annual rent for a one-bedroom unit represented 110% of this combined amount (ranging from 71.1% in West Virginia to 185.3% in the District of Columbia), and rent for a studio/efficiency apartment was 96% of SSI (ranging from 61.7% in North Dakota to 162.2% in the District of Columbia; O'Hara & Cooper, 2005).

Effective, flexible supports for housing affordability do exist, such as the rental assistance available under the Section 8 voucher programs funded by the Department of Housing and Urban Development, but waiting lists are long, and the burdensome regulations make applying to this program very challenging for individuals with mild ID who do not have advocacy support (Galbraith, 2001). People with disabilities who receive SSI are priced out of rental housing unless they obtain a subsidy, such as a Section 8 voucher. The lower rates of independent living among people with ID/DD noted previously are consistent with the reality that few can afford this option. Consequently, people with disabilities who depend on SSI are forced to remain living with aging parents, in (frequently substandard) board and care facilities, or, for those with access to Medicaid-funded mental retardation/developmental disability (MR/DD) services, in costly nursing homes, institutions, or group homes. If they do gain access to homes of their own, economic necessity may force them to share the homes with others, and there may be frequent changes of residence interspersed with periods in shelters or motels or of homelessness (Tymchuk, 2001). Clearly, much more needs to be done regarding housing affordability if adults with ID/DD are ever going to be able to join their fellow citizens in meaningful numbers in having homes of their own.

Employment and Poverty

Chapter 19 in this volume provides more detailed consideration of employment issues than is appropriate here. Even so, it is important to understand the relation between employment, income, poverty, and lifestyle. The income, sense of self-worth, and social connections provided by work are all important contributors toward quality of life.

Wages are substantially higher in competitive and supported employment than in segregated employment and day programs (e.g., Stancliffe & Lakin, 1999). Those living independently or in partially supervised settings are more likely to be employed than those in supervised settings (McDermott, Martin, & Butkus, 1999). Individuals with milder ID and fewer challenging behaviors are more likely to gain competitive employment, receive higher wages, enjoy better integration outcomes, and experience more typical features of employment (Braddock, Rizzolo, & Hemp, 2004; Mank, Cioffi, & Yovanoff, 1998; Moore, Harley, & Gamble, 2004).

Does this mean that people with mild ID living independently are doing well in employment? Relative to people with more severe ID, this is true, but compared with the general population, pervasive concerns remain. Many supported employees work in entry-level service jobs, are underemployed, and receive low wages (Yamaki & Fujiura, 2002). Even basic issues, such as transportation to and from work, remain major problems (Conley, 2003).

Yamaki and Fujiura's (2002) national profile of the employment and income status of U.S. adults with DD living in community households (not in the formal residential service system) found an employment rate (27.6%) that was vastly lower than that of the general community (75.1%), with a much higher proportion of part-time work. Typical jobs involved basic service occupations (such as janitor) or unskilled labor jobs. Taking benefits into account, the median total income of people with DD was 20% below the poverty threshold and about one-third of the median total income of the general population. Even those who were employed did not generally achieve economic self-sufficiency. Such poverty-level incomes have a pervasive effect on the person's lifestyle and impact strongly on the affordability of housing, health services, transportation, clothing, and leisure. Extremely low incomes mean that people with DD will continue to rely on family and/or public support, resulting in continuing financial strain on the family (Lewis & Johnson, 2005) and on the capacity of publicly funded services.

Other systemic issues also interfere with employment and wages. Medicaid reimbursement policies and state policies on allowable income have been cited as serious barriers (Stancliffe & Lakin, 1999), and Braddock et al. (2004) noted that disincentives to work arose because of the possibility of losing access to publicly funded health services once becoming employed.

Transportation

Lack of transportation can be a significant barrier to community participation, employment, and social activities (Conley, 2003). Many individuals with ID have not obtained a driver's license and/or cannot afford to own and run a car. In areas where public transportation is limited or nonexistent, they are forced to stay home, walk, use a bicycle, or rely on support people for transportation. Even when public transportation is available, people may need to be taught how to use it safely. Careful selection of where to live (near family, friends, work, and shopping) can reduce the need for transportation.

Access to Benefits

People with ID/DD living independently face challenges when trying to access benefits. On the one hand, people may not be seen to be eligible for Medicaid-funded disability services because, by virtue of their independent-living status, they are seen not to need a 24-hour plan of care. This circumstance may have consequent effects on eligibility for other benefits and services. For example, many people with mild ID are ineligible for SSI payments and, consequently, may not have access to Medicaid (Galbraith, 2001). On the other hand, some people may choose to avoid stigma by shunning disability services and disability benefits for which they may be eligible.

Finally, there is the practical difficulty of dealing with complex application processes and regulatory requirements in gaining access to benefits. Without significant support, people with ID/DD may find this task extremely challenging. People with mild ID are frequently invisible to mainstream services and welfare, and their needs for support in dealing with the welfare bureaucracy go unrecognized. This can result in their not being able to take full advantage of available benefits or even being "punished" by the system because they did not report income or employment that can affect benefits.

Health Services

Health outcomes for people with ID/DD are poorer than for the general community (U.S. Department of Health & Office of the Surgeon General, 2002). Taanila, Rantakallio, Koiranen, von Wendt, and Järvelin (2005) reported that people with mild ID were hospitalized more often and for much longer than people with borderline ID or no intellectual impairment. Yamaki (2005) reported that a significantly larger proportion of U.S. young adults and women with ID were obese compared with the general population, with the majority of adults with ID being overweight or obese. For most individuals, these issues are directly related to lifestyle, in particular to nutrition and physical activity, and people with ID living independently may need support to understand and pursue good nutrition and healthy lifestyles.

Poorer health outcomes can interfere with employment and lifestyle. For example, McDermott et al. (1999) showed that good physical and mental health are important predictors of employment. Appropriate support from (semi-)independent living agencies or natural supports in accessing health services, communicating with health professionals, following up treatment recommendations, and pursuing healthy lifestyles likely could benefit the individual's lifestyle and employment.

Social/Economic Responsibilities (Paying Bills, Managing Money, etc.)

Maughan et al. (1999) found that, relative to a non-ID comparison group, over four times as many people with mild ID reported having practical difficulties with literacy and numeracy skills. One way such difficulties are manifested is in relation to financial management. Money management was considered by service users to be the hardest aspect of living independently, the most needed skill, and an area in which the majority felt that they needed to improve their skills (Halpern et al., 1986). Indeed, Halpern et al. reported that running out of money was a frequent problem for 43% of their participants living semi-independently. Likewise, Schalock and Genung (1993) reported that help with money management was the most frequent support function provided by natural supports. These findings indicate that long-term support in managing finances will likely be needed by many people living independently.

Social Opportunities, Social Networks, and Relationships

Natural supports often contribute to the success of independent living. For example, Schalock and Genung (1993) found that people with ID who lived independently received more support from family, advocates, and neighbors, whereas those receiving formal disability services obtained more support from paid staff and fellow service users. Schalock and Genung (1993) also found that some individuals who had lived independently now needed longer-term paid staff support and that some clients moved in and out of the formal service system over time.

Loneliness can be an important issue for people with ID. Almost half of Halpern et al.'s (1986) semi-independent respondents reported feeling lonely a lot. Superficially, it might be thought that people living independently, with few living companions and little or no contact from staff, might be worse off than those living in group homes with constant staff presence. However, Stancliffe and Keane (2000) and Stancliffe (2005) found no difference in loneliness between group-home residents and people living semi-independently, whereas Stancliffe et al. (2007) found that people living in community households of one or two people with ID/DD were significantly less lonely than residents in community settings of seven to 15 people. Having other people around most or all of the time is not necessarily a protection against loneliness. Rather, it is the quality of the interaction with others and contact with specific important people that seems to be important in alleviating loneliness. Effective supports may include helping people learn how to respond constructively to feelings of loneliness and to develop the amount and quality of contact with friends. This may involve support and training about how to phone a friend and reconnect with old friends or assistance in resolving conflicts with friends (McVilly, Parmenter, Stancliffe, & Burton-Smith, 2006).

Individual Training and Learning as a Key Element of Accommodation

In the preceding section, we examined various areas of life in which people living independently may need support and accommodations. Support provision was discussed largely in terms of assistance from paid caregivers or from natural supports (unpaid). However, there is another alternative. Individual training and learning, combined with opportunities to utilize the new skill, can result in the individual being able to do things for him- or herself without the need for frequent support from others (a notion that applies to people with severe disability, as well). For example, a person who previously received supervision when taking medication can learn to take medication without supervision (Harchik, 1994). This approach may be combined with accommodations to simplify skills, such as using individualized blister packs containing predispensed oral medication ("Webster packs").

MODELS OF ASSISTANCE IN SUPPORTING LIVES WITH ROLES THAT ARE DESIRED AND VALUED

Identifying Formal and Informal Supports

Securing and Funding Needed Assistance

Formal (paid) supports have traditionally been provided through the facility-based, regulated service systems, in which funding is often based on the costs of providing services to a certain size group of people in a particular setting. Such funding is rarely flexible, individually tailored, or portable, because it is not associated with specific individuals or their needs (Stancliffe & Lakin, 1998, 2004). Under these circumstances, individual service users have little control over where, by whom or about what formal supports are provided; these matters are dictated by funding regulations and the provider and are often presented as a package.

Developments in supported living, needs-based funding, and individual budgets have opened the way for more flexible, individualized formal supports, all intended to provide a much greater degree of consumer control. Needs-based resource allocation is founded on the notion that individuals with greater support requirements should receive more resources. Various approaches are available to identify support needs and to link them to resource allocation, with resources usually provided in the form of individual budgets used to pay for formal supports (Fortune et al., 2005; Moseley, Gettings, & Cooper, 2005; Stancliffe & Lakin, 2004).

Stancliffe and Lakin (2004) examined approaches to needs-based funding in several states and found that some approaches were substantially more needs-based than others. They concluded that, in addition to employing data-based assessment of support needs and costs, needs-based individual funding should (1) be applied to *all* recipients, not just those entering the system for the first time; (2) be provided as continuous *individualized* funding amounts (rather than a small number of discrete funding levels); (3) allocate a specific amount to pay for services to be received *by the individual* rather than it being infused into an overall pool to be managed by an intermediate agency for multiple service recipients; and (4) reflect different circumstances in variations in allocated amounts (e.g., people living with family members vs. in residential settings; children who are enrolled in public schools). Funding arrangements based on individual assessment of support needs appear to offer a rational and equitable basis for allocation of public money. Challenges remain in assessing support needs reliably (see Fortune et al., 2005).

Consumer-Directed Supports

Parallel to individual budgets and needs-based funding is a move toward consumer-directed supports (CDS), in which the consumer and his or her family or advocates exercise control over their individual budget and direct the nature of formal support and who provides it (Head & Conroy, 2005; Moseley et al., 2005). Available research suggests that consumers experience better outcomes with individual budgets and CDS (Head & Conroy, 2005), but this research is limited. To understand the impact of CDS more fully, we need to understand not only whether service users have access to a consumer-controlled individual budget but also what support service users choose to purchase with these funds, as well as the way in which formal supports and living arrangements under CDS differ from more traditional arrangements. In addition, it is important to identify how much control consumers and families actually exercise.

In supported living and CDS, the person with a disability and his or her chosen advocates are supposed to have control over the amount and type of support received. However, several studies suggest that this is not necessarily achieved in practice to any greater extent than in traditional community living services (Conroy & Yuskauskas, 1996; Emerson et al., 2001; Howe et al., 1998). Head and Conroy (2005), however, did show substantial increases in control over services and supports following implementation of CDS in a "self-determination" project in Michigan funded by the Robert Wood Johnson Foundation. Taken together, these findings suggest that it cannot be assumed that control over services and supports will necessarily pass to consumers just because support is claimed to involve supported living or "self-determination" or utilizes an individual budget. Further research is needed on the impact of consumer control on consumer outcomes and on the factors that result in greater or lesser degrees of consumer control over formal services. A further issue is distinguishing between control by the individual consumer and control by family or advocates (see Stancliffe & Lakin, 2005).

Informal Supports

The importance of informal supports (family, benefactors) to successful independent living is long established (Edgerton, 1967; Schalock & Genung, 1993). What is less well understood is how informal supports for independent living can be provided, maintained, and enhanced when formal services are part of the picture. As compared with group homes, several studies of supported and/or semi-independent living have shown no difference in family contact (Conroy & Yuskauskas, 1996; Emerson et al., 2001; Stancliffe, 2005; Stancliffe & Keane, 2000), availability of an unpaid advocate (Stancliffe, 2005; Stancliffe & Keane, 2000), implementation of natural support networks (Howe et al., 1998), and having a "circle of friends" (Conroy & Yuskauskas, 1996). On the other hand, following implementation of CDS in New Hampshire, Conroy and Yuskauskas (1996) found an increase in the size of the "circle of friends" for those with such a circle, as well as increased participation in planning teams by chosen and unpaid people. The assumption that "progressive" approaches to support will inevitably be accompanied by higher levels of natural support is not necessarily supported by the literature. Identifying effective ways to maintain and enhance informal supports remains a challenge.

Training Support Workers

Living in one's own home with control over who provides support and in what way is at the heart of contemporary thinking about services and supports. Kennedy (2004) noted the practical challenges involved, including high staff turnover, difficulty recruiting suitable people (with gaps between staff members), and staff members who do not do as they are asked. Such challenges remind us of the need to establish a sustainable staffing infrastructure of support for individualized services.

High staff turnover has been consistently related to low pay, which for disability support workers averages about 55% of average pay for U.S. workers (Lakin, Polister, & Prouty, 2003). Larson, Hewitt, and Lakin (2004) found that ratings of poorer overall residential service quality and poorer quality of life were associated with lower staff wages. These systemic workforce issues have largely been left to individual provider agencies to deal with. Growing numbers of families and consumers are involved in recruiting support workers but have no background in recruitment, training, or supporting workers. Structures are needed to recruit and train support workers and to match them with consumers (Lakin & Stancliffe, 2005). Without a sufficiently large, stable, and well-prepared workforce, the quality of independent living will be tenuous.

Vulnerabilities and Challenges

Without the protection provided by 24-hour staff or family support, people with ID/DD living independently and semi-independently are exposed to the usual risks faced by other members of society. Areas of potential vulnerability include medication, household safety, substance abuse, and dealings with the legal system. Support may be needed regarding such matters and may involve teaching the person to manage the situation independently, with some degree of specific assistance as needed.

Medication

Harchik (1994) described a detailed approach to assessing and teaching self-medication skills to people with ID. Although it is clear that some individuals with ID can acquire these skills, available research tends to focus on other populations, such as people with a psychiatric disability. Harchik (1994) concluded that structured teaching, specific prompting systems (reminders to take medication at the appropriate time), a well-organized medication regimen, and ongoing monitoring can all promote accurate and safe self-medication.

Household Safety

Juracek (1994) reviewed the literature on fire safety training and concluded that people with milder ID can be successfully taught to evacuate during emergencies, to call 911, and to extinguish contained fires, although the teaching and maintenance of nighttime fire drills was not particularly effective. Limited success has been reported for fire safety training involving individuals with more severe disability. Appropriate alarms, assistive devices, and fire prevention skills are also important.

Safety and risk in (semi-)independent or supported living have generally been found to be no different from those in group homes (Emerson et al., 2001; Stancliffe & Keane, 2000). However, Emerson et al. (2001) found a higher reported risk of exploitation by people in the neighborhood of those in supported living.

The Legal System

People with severe ID are often considered to lack legal capacity and so have little involvement with the legal system. However, those with mild ID frequently fare poorly at all levels of the justice system, often because their disability is not detected and appropriate supports are not provided to enable them to navigate the system's complexities. Thus persons with ID living in the community, particularly independently, are vulnerable as alleged perpetrators of crimes (Luckasson, 2001), as witnesses (Kebbell & Hatton, 1999), and as victims (Luckasson, 2001).

Substance Abuse

Available evidence shows a lower prevalence of drug and alcohol use by people with ID as compared with the general community (Christian & Poling, 1997; Degenhardt, 2000; Halpern et al., 1986). Even so, some people with ID, including individuals living independently, experience serious problems with alcohol and other drugs. Christian and Poling (1997) noted barriers in accessing generic substance abuse treatment programs for people with ID, with the result that people may not receive needed treatment. Barriers include lack of knowledge of ID by program staff, the complexity of the material used, and cost. Likewise, ID service providers are frequently not equipped to deal with drug and alcohol problems. Modifications of generic substance abuse programs have been implemented in an attempt to meet the needs of people with ID, but no controlled evaluations have been reported (Christian & Poling, 1997).

CONCLUSIONS: IMPLICATIONS FOR PRACTITIONERS, POLICY MAKERS, AND RESEARCHERS

Our examination of independent living has identified a number of issues with important implications for practitioners, policy makers, and researchers.

Implications for Practitioners

People with ID/DD living "independently" predictably will need support in relation to specific issues. Practitioners should plan independent-living supports on the assumption that regular or occasional support is needed. Like many people living in poverty, people with ID/DD living independently face difficulties obtaining affordable housing, stable employment, and transportation, as well as purchasing health services and medications and accessing health insurance or publicly funded health services. They will require intermittent support in these areas.

With functional limitations in literacy and numeracy, many people with ID/DD need regular assistance with financial management, plus as-needed help with complex bureaucracies (e.g., when obtaining benefits). In addition, particular challenges face those in certain circumstances—substance abuse or dealing with the legal system—in which skilled, trusted support is invaluable.

The challenge for practitioners is to effectively provide needed support without being overintrusive, infringing unnecessarily on independence, or displacing existing natural supports. This can be difficult when a crisis develops (loss of natural support, physical or mental health problems, loss of housing) that requires substantial support for a period. The formal service system is often inflexible, with little capacity to respond to sudden changes in support needs. All too often, the person is simply placed in an available service "slot," such as a group home, which can be disabling, creating dependency and bringing about loss of skills and self-determination. Finding ways to help the person through a crisis, while maintaining his or her independent lifestyle, appears likely to be more beneficial, both for the person and for resources within the formal long-term care system. However, these are issues that have received little research attention, and careful follow-along studies are needed to test these propositions.

Funding such flexible formal support is more difficult without federal cost sharing, because many people with ID/DD living independently may not meet the current eligibility requirements for Medicaid. Of necessity, specialist disability practitioners may need to work with generic agencies that provide community supports for housing, employment, or substance abuse and to assist those agencies in providing effective services to community members with ID/DD. Controlled evaluations of such initiatives are rare, so the research literature is not especially helpful in guiding such endeavors.

Implications for Policy Makers

Workforce issues continue to be crucial for disability services, which are struggling with basic matters such as recruitment, retention, and training of direct-support workers. These issues provide even greater challenges to families and people with ID/DD who take a direct role in staffing issues. Policy responses are needed to provide individuals, families, and service providers with access to a qualified, stable workforce.

Poverty and unemployment have pervasive effects on the lifestyles of people living independently. Expanding access to a reasonable income through stable employment, lessening restrictive social service regulations, and dealing with the crisis in housing affordability remain fundamental priorities. Other policy concerns include providing specific support for individuals with ID caught up in the justice system, as well as education for judges, lawyers, and police regarding, for example, accommodations needed for fair questioning.

Policy makers must find ways to ensure health and safety for independent living without compromising self-determination and rights. Traditional quality assurance systems have not met the needs of dispersed community residential settings. With the increased freedom comes a degree of risk that must be attended to carefully.

Implications for Researchers

There remain many basic issues on which research on independent living is poorly developed. The strong research focus on formal services has seen a corresponding lack of attention to less formal arrangements. Knowledge is limited about basic issues, such as how many people with ID/DD are living independently, in what circumstances, and with what supports. Likewise, little is known about the pathways into and out of independent living and the events that shape a change in this status.

Independent living, semi-independent living, supported living, and CDS all remain substantially underresearched. Cross-sectional and longitudinal research is needed to describe in detail how these services operate and who uses them; to identify the crucial features that are related to desired outcomes; to evaluate outcomes (relative both to other ID/DD services and to typical lifestyles in the general community); and to account for variability in outcomes among service users. Likewise, there has been little detailed description or evaluation of the ways in which such services differ from traditional services and the effect of these differences on outcomes. For example, Stancliffe and Lakin (2005) found that having access to an individual budget in itself had a modest relation to individual outcomes. To understand the impact of CDS more fully, we need to evaluate not only whether service users have access to a consumer-controlled individual budget but also what supports they purchase with these funds and how these differ from more traditional services.

The importance of informal (natural) supports for independent living is well established by research, but there is little research evidence about how natural supports can be maintained and enhanced. All of the issues mentioned should form part of our future agenda for research on independent living to help guide policy and practice in a direction in which the scientific evidence shows that people with ID/DD can enjoy self-determined lives with quality support as needed.

REFERENCES

Blackorby, J., & Wagner, M. (1996). Longitudinal postschool outcomes of youth with disabilities: Findings from the National Longitudinal Transition Study. *Exceptional Children, 62*, 399–413.

Braddock, D., Rizzolo, M. C., & Hemp, R. (2004). Most employment service growth in developmental disabilities during 1988–2002 was in segregated settings. *Mental Retardation, 42*(4), 317–320.

Bradley, V. J., Agosta, J. M., & Kimmich, M. (2001). Social and community participation: How to enhance supports for people with mild cognitive limitations. In A. J. Tymchuk, K. C. Lakin, & R. Luckasson (Eds.), *The forgotten generation: The status and challenges of adults with mild cognitive limitations* (pp. 169–189). Baltimore: Brookes.

Bradley, V. J., Ashbaugh, J. W., & Blaney, B. C. (Eds.). (1994). *Creating individual supports for people with developmental disabilities: A mandate for change at many levels.* Baltimore: Brookes.

Burchard, S. N., Hasazi, J. S., Gordon, L. R., & Yoe, J. (1991). An examination of lifestyle and adjustment in three community residential alternatives. *Research in Developmental Disabilities, 12*(2), 127–142.

Christian, L., & Poling, A. (1997). Drug abuse in persons with mental retardation: A review. *American Journal on Mental Retardation, 102*(2), 126–136.

Cobb, H. (1972). *The forecast of fulfillment: A review of research on predictive assessment of the adult retarded for social and vocational adjustment.* New York: Teachers College Press.

Conley, R. W. (2003). Supported employment in Maryland: Successes and issues. *Mental Retardation, 41*(4), 237–249.

Conroy, J. W., & Yuskauskas, A. (1996). *Independent evaluation of the Monadnock self-determination project.* Ardmore, PA: Center for Outcome Analysis.

Degenhardt, L. (2000). Interventions for people with alcohol use disorders and an intellectual disability: A review of the literature. *Journal of Intellectual & Developmental Disability, 25*(2), 135–146.

Ducharme, G., Beeman, P., DeMarasse, R., & Ludlum, C. (1994). Building community one person at a time. In V. J. Bradley, J. W. Ashbaugh, & B. C. Blaney (Eds.), *Creating individual supports for people with developmental disabilities: A mandate for change at many levels* (pp. 347–360). Baltimore: Brookes.

Edgerton, R. B. (1967). *The cloak of competence: Stigma in the lives of the mentally retarded.* Berkeley: University of California Press.

Edgerton, R. B. (1981). Crime, deviance and normalization. In R. H. Bruininks, C. E. Meyers, B. B. Sigford, & K. C. Lakin (Eds.), *Deinstitutionalization and community adjustment of mentally retarded persons* (pp. 145–166). Washington, DC: American Association on Mental Retardation.

Edgerton, R. B. (1990). Quality of life from a longitudinal perspective. In R. L. Schalock (Ed.), *Quality of life: Perspectives and issues* (pp. 149–160). Washington, DC: American Association on Mental Retardation.

Emerson, E., Robertson, J., Gregory, N., Hatton, C., Kessissoglou, S., Hallam, A., et al. (2001). Quality and costs of supported living residences and group homes in the United Kingdom. *American Journal on Mental Retardation, 106*(5), 401–415.

Fernald, W. E. (1919). After care study of the patients discharged from Waverley for a period of twenty-five years. *Ungraded, 5*(1), 25–31.

Fortune, J. R., Smith, G. A., Campbell, E. M., Clabby, III, R. T., Heinlein, K. B., Lynch, R. M., et al. (2005). Individual budgets according to individual needs: The Wyoming DOORS system. In R. J. Stancliffe & K. C. Lakin (Eds.), *Costs and outcomes of community services for people with intellectual disabilities* (pp. 241–262). Baltimore: Brookes.

Fujiura, G. T. (1998). Demography of family households. *American Journal on Mental Retardation, 103*(3), 225–235.

Fujiura, G. T. (2003). Continuum of intellectual disability: Demographic evidence for the "forgotten generation." *Mental Retardation, 41*(6), 420–429.

Galbraith, S. (2001). A home of one's own. In A. J. Tymchuk, K. C. Lakin, & R. Luckasson (Eds.), *The forgotten generation: The status and challenges of adults with mild cognitive limitations* (pp. 141–167). Baltimore: Brookes.

Gardner, J. F., & Carran, D. T. (2005). Attainment of personal outcomes by people with developmental disabilities. *Mental Retardation, 43*(3), 157–174.

Halpern, A. S., Close, D. W., & Nelson, D. S. (1986). *On my own: The impact of semi-independent living programs for adults with mental retardation.* Baltimore: Brookes.

Harchik, A. E. (1994). Self-medication skills. In M. Agran, N. E. Marchand-Martella, & R. C. Martella (Eds.), *Promoting health and safety: Skills for independent living* (pp. 55–69). Baltimore: Brookes.

Head, M. J., & Conroy, J. W. (2005). Outcomes of self-determination in Michigan: Quality and costs. In R. J. Stancliffe & K. C. Lakin (Eds.), *Costs and outcomes of community services for people with intellectual disabilities* (pp. 219–240). Baltimore: Brookes.

Heal, L. W., Rubin, S. S., & Rusch, F. R. (1998). Residential independence of former special education high school students: A second look. *Research in Developmental Disabilities, 19*(1), 1–26.

Howe, J., Horner, R. H., & Newton, J. S. (1998). Comparison of supported living and traditional residential services in the state of Oregon. *Mental Retardation, 36*(1), 1–11.

Juracek, D. B. (1994). Fire safety skills. In M. Agran, N. E. Marchand-Martella, & R. C. Martella (Eds.), *Promoting health and safety: Skills for independent living* (pp. 103–119). Baltimore: Brookes.

Kebbell, M. R., & Hatton, C. (1999). People with mental retardation as witnesses in court: A review. *Mental Retardation, 37*(3), 179–187.

Kennedy, M. J. (2004). Living outside the system: The ups and downs of getting on with our lives. *Mental Retardation, 42*(3), 229–231.

Lakin, K. C., Polister, B., & Prouty, R. W. (2003). Wages of non-state direct support professionals lag behind those of public direct support professionals and the general public. *Mental Retardation, 41*(2), 178–182.

Lakin, K. C., & Smull, M. (1995). Supported living. *IMPACT, 8*(4).

Lakin, K. C., & Stancliffe, R. J. (2005). Expenditures and outcomes: Directions in financing, policy, and research. In R. J. Stancliffe & K. C. Lakin (Eds.), *Costs and outcomes of community services for people with intellectual disabilities* (pp. 313–337). Baltimore: Brookes.

Larson, S. A., Hewitt, A. S., & Lakin, K. C. (2004). Multiperspective analysis of workforce challenges and their effects on consumer and family quality of life. *American Journal on Mental Retardation, 109*(6), 481–500.

Levine, H. G., & Langness, L. L. (1985). Everyday cognition among mildly mentally retarded adults: An ethnographic approach. *American Journal of Mental Deficiency, 90*, 18–26.

Lewis, D. R., & Johnson, D. R. (2005). Costs of family care for individuals with developmental disabilities. In R. J. Stancliffe & K. C. Lakin (Eds.), *Costs and outcomes of community services for people with intellectual disabilities* (pp. 63–89). Baltimore: Brookes.

Lozano, B. (1993). Independent living: Relation among training, skills, and success. *American Journal on Mental Retardation, 98*(2), 249–262.

Luckasson, R. (2001). The criminal justice system and people with mild cognitive limitations. In A. J. Tymchuk, K. C. Lakin, & R. Luckasson (Eds.), *The forgotten generation: The status and challenges of adults with mild cognitive limitations* (pp. 347–356). Baltimore: Brookes.

Luckasson, R., Borthwick-Duffy, S., Buntinx, W. H. E., Coulter, D. L., Craig, E. M., Reeve, A., et al. (2002). *Mental retardation: Definition, classification, and systems of supports.* Washington, DC: American Association on Mental Retardation.

Luftig, R. L., & Muthert, D. (2005). Patterns of employment and independent living of adult graduates with learning disabilities and mental retardation of an inclusionary high school vocational program. *Research in Developmental Disabilities, 26*(4), 317–325.

Mank, D., Cioffi, A., & Yovanoff, P. (1998). Employment outcomes for people with severe disabilities: Opportunities for improvement. *Mental Retardation, 36*(3), 205–216.

Maughan, B., Collishaw, S., & Pickles, A. (1999). Mild mental retardation: Psychosocial functioning in adulthood. *Psychological Medicine, 29*, 351–366.

McDermott, S., Martin, M., & Butkus, S. (1999). What individual, provider, and community characteristics predict employment of individuals with mental retardation? *American Journal on Mental Retardation, 104*(4), 346–355.

McVilly, K. R., Parmenter, T. R., Stancliffe, R. J., & Burton-Smith, R. M. (2006). "I get by with a little help from my friends": Adults with intellectual disability discuss loneliness. *Journal of Applied Research in Intellectual Disabilities, 19*, 191–203.

Moore, C. L., Harley, D. A., & Gamble, D. (2004). Ex-post-facto analysis of competitive employment outcomes for individuals with mental retardation: National perspective. *Mental Retardation, 42*(4), 253–262.

Moseley, C. R., Gettings, R. M., & Cooper, R. E. (2005). Having it your way: A national study of individual budgeting practices within the states. In R. J. Stancliffe & K. C. Lakin (Eds.), *Costs and outcomes of community services for people with intellectual disabilities* (pp. 263–288). Baltimore: Brookes.

O'Hara, A., & Cooper, E. (2005). *Priced out in 2004: The housing crisis for people with disabilities.* Retrieved November 22, 2005, from *www.c-c-d.org/priced_out_2004.htm*.

Racino, J. A., & Taylor, S. J. (1993). "People First." Approaches to housing and support. In J. A. Racino, P. Walker, S. O'Connor, & S. J. Taylor (Eds.), *Housing, support and community: Choices and strategies for adults with disabilities* (pp. 33–56). Baltimore: Brookes.

Richardson, S. A., & Koller, H. (1996). *Twenty-two years: Causes and consequences of mental retardation.* Cambridge, MA: Harvard University Press.

Schalock, R. L., & Genung, L. T. (1993). Placement from a community-based mental retardation program: A 15-year follow-up. *American Journal on Mental Retardation, 98*(3), 400–407.

Schalock, R. L., & Harper, R. S. (1978). Placement from community-based mental retardation programs: How well do clients do? *American Journal of Mental Deficiency, 83*, 240–247.

Schalock, R. L., Harper, R. S., & Carver, G. (1981). Independent living placement: Five years later. *American Journal of Mental Deficiency, 86*, 170–177.

Seltzer, M. M., Floyd, F., Greenberg, J., Lounds, J., Lindstromm, M., & Hong, J. (2005). Life course impacts of mild intellectual deficits. *American Journal on Mental Retardation, 110*(6), 451–468.

Stancliffe, R. J. (1995). *Choice and decision making and adults with intellectual disability.* Unpublished doctoral thesis, Macquarie University, Sydney, Australia.

Stancliffe, R. J. (1997). Community living-unit size, staff presence, and residents' choice-making. *Mental Retardation, 35*(1), 1–9.

Stancliffe, R. J. (2005). Semi-independent living and group homes in Australia. In R. J. Stancliffe & K. C. Lakin (Eds.), *Costs and outcomes of community services for people with intellectual disabilities* (pp. 129–150). Baltimore: Brookes.

Stancliffe, R. J., Abery, B. H., & Smith, J. (2000). Personal control and the ecology of community living settings: Beyond living-unit size and type. *American Journal on Mental Retardation, 105*(6), 431–454.

Stancliffe, R. J., & Keane, S. (2000). Outcomes and costs of community living: A matched comparison of group homes and semi-independent living. *Journal of Intellectual & Developmental Disability, 25*(4), 281–305.

Stancliffe, R. J., & Lakin, K. C. (1998). Analysis of expenditures and outcomes of residential alternatives for persons with developmental disabilities. *American Journal on Mental Retardation, 102*(6), 552–568.

Stancliffe, R. J., & Lakin, K. C. (1999). A longitudinal comparison of day program services and outcomes of people who left institutions and those who stayed. *Journal of the Association for Persons with Severe Handicaps, 24*(1), 44–57.

Stancliffe, R. J., & Lakin, K. C. (2004). Costs and outcomes of community services for persons with intellectual and developmental disabilities. *Policy Research Brief (University of Minnesota, Minneapolis, Institute on Community Integration), 15*(1), 1–10.

Stancliffe, R. J., & Lakin, K. C. (2005). Individual budgets and freedom from staff control. In R. J. Stancliffe & K. C. Lakin (Eds.), *Costs and outcomes of community services for people with intellectual disabilities* (pp. 203–218). Baltimore: Brookes.

Stancliffe, R. J., Lakin, K. C., Taub, S., Doljanac, R., Byun, S., & Chiri, G. (2007). *Loneliness and living arrangements*. Manuscript submitted for publication.

Stancliffe, R. J., & Wehmeyer, M. L. (1995). Variability in the availability of choice to adults with mental retardation. *Journal of Vocational Rehabilitation, 5*, 319–328.

Suto, W. M. I., Clare, I. C. H., Holland, A. J., & Watson, P. C. (2005). Capacity to make financial decisions among people with mild intellectual disabilities. *Journal of Intellectual Disability Research, 49*(3), 199–209.

Taanila, A., Rantakallio, P., Koiranen, M., von Wendt, L., & Järvelin, M. R. (2005). How do persons with intellectual disability manage in the open labour markets? A follow-up of the Northern Finland 1966 birth cohort. *Journal of Intellectual Disability Research, 49*(3), 218–227.

Tymchuk, A. J. (2001). Family life. In A. J. Tymchuk, K. C. Lakin & R. Luckasson (Eds.), *The forgotten generation: The status and challenges of adults with mild cognitive limitations* (pp. 249–274). Baltimore: Brookes.

U.S. Department of Health & Office of the Surgeon General. (2002). *Closing the gap: A national blueprint to improve the health of persons with mental retardation*. Rockville, MD: Author.

Wehmeyer, M. L., & Bolding, N. (1999). Self-determination across living and working environments: A matched samples study of adults with mental retardation. *Mental Retardation, 37*(5), 353–363.

World Health Organization. (2001). *The international classification of function, disability and health*. Geneva, Switzerland: Author.

Yamaki, K. (2005). Body weight status among adults with intellectual disability in the community. *Mental Retardation, 43*(1), 1–10.

Yamaki, K., & Fujiura, G. T. (2002). Employment and income status of adults with developmental disabilities living in the community. *Mental Retardation, 40*(2), 132–141.

22

Adult Social Relationships

Janis Chadsey

Social relationships are essential to happiness. Within studies of subjective well-being (e.g., Diener, Oishi, & Lucas, 2003) and positive psychology (e.g., Seligman, Steen, Park, & Peterson, 2005), positive social relationships with others are consistently identified as being important predictors of happiness. In a study conducted by Diener and Seligman (2002), the 10% of the 222 undergraduates who were the very happiest were also highly social and had strong romantic and other close social relationships with others, compared with less happy groups. Similarly, when young people with disabilities leave high school for adulthood, social relationships have been cited as an essential outcome (Halpern, 1993). Most important, people with disabilities have mentioned how critical friends and social relationships are to their lives (O'Connor, 1983).

The purpose of this chapter is to discuss empirical work that has been conducted with adults with disabilities in the area of social relationships. Because of the nature of the literature, the term "social relationships" will be used in a broad sense to reflect the many ways researchers have defined and measured this outcome. Consequently, studies are included that measure a range of dependent variables, such as social interactions, friendships, social integration, and social inclusion. In a sense, we can think of social relationships as connections between individuals and groups that include how they behave, feel, and communicate with one another. In this chapter, whenever a study is discussed, the dependent variable is explicitly labeled (e.g., social integration) so that the outcome is apparent to the reader.

Most of the studies in the area of adult social relationships and developmental disabilities have been conducted in two contexts: employment and community. Representative studies from these two contexts are reviewed. Additionally, the majority of studies examined can be classified as nonexperimental quantitative research designs, such as correlational, descriptive, or causal–comparative. Although not experimental, these studies are reviewed because they have important implications for the design and conduct of experimental work.

Experimental work is sparse; however, this literature reflects the current state of knowledge and leads to implications for practice, policy, and future research directions. Before this literature is considered, it is important first to examine research on the perceptions of adults with disabilities about their social relationships.

PERCEPTIONS OF SOCIAL RELATIONSHIPS OF ADULTS WITH DISABILITIES

Social Relationships with Individuals with and without Disabilities

It is crucial to hear from adults with disabilities about their own perceptions of social relationships in order to understand the meaning of their relationships and how they are constructed. Although few in number, these studies suggest that relationships are formed between people with and without disabilities (such as coworkers) and between people who both have disabilities. In an early study conducted by Neumayer and Bleasdale (1996), 30 individuals with mild to moderate levels of intellectual disability and a mean age of 33 years were interviewed about their personal lifestyle preferences; several of the questions asked about relationships. When participants were asked who their friends were, the majority (14) answered that their friends came from work, whereas the remaining participants indicated that friends were neighbors, staff members, girlfriends or boyfriends, housemates, old school friends, or friends who came from church or their day program. When the respondents were asked whether they preferred doing activities with people with disabilities or people without disabilities, 63% preferred doing activities with both groups or felt it did not matter, but 17% chose people without disabilities and 10% selected people with disabilities.

In a more recent qualitative study on individual's views on supported employment and social inclusion (Wistow & Schneider, 2003), 30 individuals (ranging in age from 16 to 65 years) were interviewed, with the majority (80%) feeling supported, involved, and treated as equals by colleagues and coworkers. The majority of the respondents felt that they got along well with people at work, but 40% reported that they did not have close friends at work. Wistow and Schneider (2003) noted that physical integration does not necessarily result in social integration and that some of the individuals in their sample reported feeling alienated from the rest of the workforce. Future research is needed to determine whether the lack of close social relationships in some settings, for example, work settings, is really problematic. It is quite possible that individuals with disabilities have friends in other contexts and that the lack of close social relationships at work may not be considered difficult for them. However, it is also possible that the converse is true and that those adults with disabilities who are working desire more friends at work.

In a more revealing study, Knox and Hickson (2001) conducted interviews with four people with intellectual disabilities about relationships they had with other people with disabilities, which were described as being close friendships. The adults ranged in age from 26 to 58, and each had from one to three close friends. The results from the interviews revealed that there were two types of close social relationships: the "good mate" and the girlfriend or boyfriend. Good mates did lots of things together (e.g., lived together, watched videos), had a sense of shared history (e.g., had known each other a long time), liked doing the same things, and helped each other. These adults stated that their relationships were maintained by making definite times to see one another and planning activities that were mutually enjoyable, but they also recognized the need to balance their time with other people, too.

Knox and Hickson (2001) reported that the boyfriend–girlfriend relationship was characterized by intimacy, physical attraction, and an expectation that the relationship might change in the future (e.g., result in marriage). Dating, spending time alone, and having a commitment to the future maintained the romantic relationships.

Knox and Hickson's research (2001) is important not only because it highlights the meaning of close social relationships from the perspective of adults with disabilities but also because it focuses on relationships that people with disabilities can have with one another. They note that only the research field seems to prefer friendships between people with and without disabilities and gives less value to relationships that people with disabilities have with each other.

Social Relationships with Caregivers

Friendships between adults with disabilities and their caregivers also seem to be less valued by researchers. However, Pottie and Sumarah (2004) described just this type of friendship relationship that existed within the L'Arche community—a community designed to be inclusive, where people with and without disabilities live, work, and share their lives. In this qualitative study, four friendship dyads were interviewed. The friendships, which had been ongoing from 7 to 15 years, were described as being reciprocal and characterized by trust, respect, support, fidelity, and sharing of lives. The individuals without disabilities provided physical care and help with daily tasks, but the relationship went further and was deeper than just providing care. The adult with disabilities helped to maintain the relationship by extending dinner invitations, telephoning, remembering important occasions, and offering and asking for support. The long duration of the relationships was felt to be due to the frequency of contact in the L'Arche community and the intentional choice on the part of both members to be faithful to the relationship. Thus Pottie and Sumarah (2004) stated that caregiving relationships that are reciprocal and supported by a community could evolve into friendships.

Summary and Future Research

Who should make the decision about our friendships and other close social relationships? The answer is obvious: We should, and so should adults with disabilities. The literature just reviewed suggests that adults with disabilities do form relationships with others but that the relationships may not always be with people who are endorsed by researchers (Knox & Hickson, 2001). Most would probably agree that the goal of service provision should be to foster community connectedness and relationship with others, not merely physical integration into the general community (Cummins & Lau, 2003). Some have even suggested that this connectedness may be more likely to occur with other people with disabilities than with people without disabilities (Cummins & Lau, 2003). Certainly, research is needed to determine whether closer social connections are more likely to occur between individuals with disabilities than with people without disabilities, while also controlling for such factors as opportunities to interact with others who do not have disabilities. In addition, researchers should explore how physical integration is beneficial to adults with disabilities, even if social integration is not achieved. There is a need for public policy based on research findings that can guide the field in establishing and supporting the many different types of social relationships for adults with disabilities.

THE FORMATION OF CLOSE SOCIAL RELATIONSHIPS

Although adults can form a wide range of relationships, friendships are regarded as being among the most important. How are friendships formed? The literature involving adults without disabilities is consistent in identifying the variables that are associated with friendship formation. In her book, Fehr (1996) discusses four factors that need to converge in order for friendships to be formed: (1) environmental, (2) individual, (3) situational, and (4) dyadic. These variables are discussed (albeit briefly) because of the implications they have for intervention strategies.

Fehr (1996) notes that the first step in friendship formation is for two individuals to be in contact with one another through physical (or cyberspace) proximity. *Environmental factors*—such as proximity in residence, work, school, cyberspace, or other settings—can be instrumental in creating the condition for two people to get to know one another. However, as has been pointed out by numerous researchers in the disability area (e.g., Winstow & Schneider, 2003), physical proximity is a necessary, but not a sufficient, condition for relationships to be formed.

Another environmental factor that has been predictive in the formation of friendships is social network or communication network proximity (Fehr, 1996). Individuals often meet potential friends through friends they already have; thus current friends can often be a source for new friendships. Although this variable can be unintentional (e.g., a person may go to a friend's party and hit it off with the host's friend), it may also be intentional, such as a host of a party introducing two people because he or she thinks they may become friends.

Individual factors, such as physical attractiveness, social skills, and similarity, also predict friendship formation (Fehr, 1996). As Fehr notes, most might think that physical attractiveness plays a role only in romantic relationships, but it also plays a role in the formation of friendships. Several reasons have been postulated for the importance of physical attractiveness, including the belief that physically attractive people are more like us and have similar attitudes and personalities. Additionally, it may be more enjoyable to interact with individuals who are physically attractive, and we may believe that these individuals have better social skills.

Social skills—such as responding appropriately to what others say, following turn-taking rules during conversations, being responsive and showing interest, and using appropriate nonverbal behaviors—have been identified as being important to friendships. However, it is interesting to note that social skills are more important during the initial formation of friendships than during the later stages (Fehr, 1996). Once a friendship has been formed, the ability to self-disclose, provide support, and manage conflict (which arguably might also be defined as social skills) are viewed as being more important.

The individual factor of similarity is also significant for friendship formation; we tend to form relationships with people who are similar to us. In her review of research, Fehr (1996) stated that demographic factors (e.g., age, education, religion, health, family background), social status, and attitudes all play a role not only in the initial forma-tion of a friendship but also in the continuation of the friendship.

Situational factors are also important (Fehr, 1996). We are more likely to form a rela-tionship with someone if we know that there is a high probability of future interactions with the individual. If future interactions seem unlikely, then the amount of effort devoted to the relationship will probably be smaller.

Similarly, both individuals need to have time available for the relationship. This entails having time for interactions with one another and for engagement in mutually enjoyed activities and events. As odd as it might seem, not everyone is available for addi-tional social relationships; individuals may already have enough friends or be busy with work and family, which lessens time for getting to know others.

Another situational factor that can have a positive impact on the formation of friendships is the frequency of exposure. As Fehr (1996) notes, we are more likely to react positively to individuals if we see them on a recurrent basis. Individuals tend to believe that they are similar to the people they see most often. Interacting frequently with others makes them more familiar, and familiarity predisposes individuals to believe that similarities exist between themselves and the people they interact with repeatedly.

The final situational variable that can influence friendships is known as "outcome dependency." As Fehr (1996) explains, we are more attracted to someone who is in a position to reward or punish us. If we are dependent on someone who influences the consequences we receive, we tend to like that person more. Just the nature of being de-pendent on someone who has the ability to deliver positive or negative consequences can affect relationship formation.

Dyadic factors, which include reciprocity of liking and self-disclosure, make up the last category of variables that influence relationships (Fehr, 1996). Dyadic factors imply that the two individuals in a relationship are linked and that the behavior of one indi-vidual in the relationship can influence the other. For example, if we believe that others like us and if we are attracted to those individuals, then we are more likely to begin lik-ing them. Reciprocity of liking implies that both individuals in the dyad must like each other, and if both believe that "liking" is present, the relationship will have a better chance of being formed.

Similarly, there must be reciprocity of self-disclosure in the relationship. According to a theory posited by Altman and Taylor (1973), relationships become more intimate and positive as the self-disclosure increases in breadth (the number of different topics discussed) and depth (the number of personal or less superficial topics discussed). Ini-tially, reciprocity of self-disclosure is very important in the formation of the relation-ship, even though self-disclosure may occur at a superficial level. Once trust is formed, self-disclosure does not need to be reciprocated on an immediate basis.

In order for relationships to form, and particularly friendships, there is ample evi-dence that these four factors (i.e., environmental, individual, situational, and dyadic) must converge (Fehr, 1996). Adults must have opportunities to interact, believe they are similar, have the available time for a relationship, like each other, and self-disclose. These factors also set the stage for acquaintanceships to form, but friendships will develop only if individuals are more fully engaged in each of these four factors.

Much of the research associated with the formation of adult friendships is based on nonexperimental research designs; among adults without disabilities, few experimental studies have tested interventions that lead to friendship formation. Similarly, in the dis-ability literature, most of the studies of adult relationships are also nonexperimental. I review representative samples of the disability literature next because the variables identified in these studies, along with the factors associated with friendship formation, may provide a blueprint for intervention studies. I review literature from the two social contexts of employment and community.

NONEXPERIMENTAL STUDIES OF RELATIONSHIPS BETWEEN ADULTS WITH DEVELOPMENTAL DISABILITIES

Employment Contexts

Summary of Nonexperimental Studies

In a keynote address to the International Association for the Scientific Study of Intellectual Disabilities (IASSID), Chadsey (2004) reviewed and analyzed literature on social integration and inclusion in employment settings to determine strategies that might enhance social inclusion. Chadsey (2004) categorized the independent variables in 31 nonexperimental studies into six categories: workplace contact, workplace culture, vocational competence, social competence, coworker training, and role of the employment-training specialist, or job coach.

The category *workplace contact* refers to Allport's (1954) theory, a predominant theory used in a study by Novak (2002). This theory details conditions under which personal contact improves attitudes toward groups that are usually stereotyped. Workplace contact theory comprises several features: equality of status with coworkers, opportunities to interact, interdependent and dependent working relationships, and opportunities for stereotype disconfirmation. A number of studies have been reported in the literature that show support for workplace contact as a category. For example, several studies have indicated that coworkers are more likely to be accepting of employees with disabilities if they perceived their status to be equal (e.g., employees followed the same chain of command, had job responsibilities equal in importance, had a similar compensation package, and received the same type of training; e.g., Butterworth, Hagner, Helm, & Whelley, 2000; Novak, 2002). Mank and his colleagues referred to this phenomenon as "typicalness" (e.g., Jenaro, Mank, Bottomley, Doose, & Tuckerman, 2002; Mank, Cioffi, & Yovanoff, 1998). Although there seems to be empirical support for the idea that typicalness is associated with increased social integration, Riches and Green (2003) cautioned that even if coworkers and employees with disabilities have the same job title, it does not mean that coworkers will perceive employees with disabilities as being equal. Equality or typicalness needs to be "practiced" within the work setting rather than just labeled as such.

Working similar hours and being in physical proximity (additional features of workplace contact) were also related to having more opportunities for interaction or social participation with coworkers (e.g., Chadsey, Shelden, Horn De Bardeleben, & Cimera, 1999; Novak, 2002). Opportunities for social interactions were also central to the perceptions that employees with disabilities had of social support at work (Novak, 2002), which has been related to their job satisfaction (e.g., Test, Carver, Ewers, Haddad, & Person, 2000).

Stereotype disconfirmation, another factor associated with workplace contact, was found by Novak (2002) to be associated with social integration. Stereotype disconfirmation occurs when preexisting stereotypes about groups are not confirmed through interactions. As noted by Novak, coworkers were more accepting of an employee with a disability if the employee's work and social behavior contradicted previous negative stereotypes held by the coworkers.

Finally, Novak (2002) and others (e.g., Butterworth et al., 2000) also found that coworkers who had to rely on the work of the employee with a disability had more favorable attitudes about that employee. Consequently, coworkers had more positive attitudes about workers with disabilities if their own job tasks were dependent on or interdependent with the outcomes of employees with disabilities.

As noted, many studies investigating features of workplace contact have found it to be associated with more social integration. Chadsey (2004) stated that nonexperimental studies have also found *workplace culture* (or the behavioral norms in the work setting) to be associated with greater levels of social integration. For example, employees with disabilities who worked in settings with strong positive cultures were more likely to interact socially with coworkers (e.g., Butterworth et al., 2000; Novak, 2002). Strong positive cultures have included characteristics such as common gathering areas (Butterworth et al., 2000; Chadsey et al., 1999), supervisors who engaged in nontask work interactions (Chadsey et al., 1999), coworkers who got together outside of work (Chadsey et al., 1999), a relaxed, laid-back atmosphere (e.g., Chadsey et al., 1999; Novak, 2002), and a friendly and supportive environment (Hagner, Butterworth, & Keith, 1995).

Social integration has been associated not only with workplace contact or culture but also with the *vocational* and *social competence* of the employee with disabilities (Chadsey, 2004). Novak (2002) found positive relationships between coworker attitudes or acceptance and the vocational competence of an employee with a disability, especially when coworkers were dependent on the work of the employee. Walsh and Linehan (1997) reported that employers placed more emphasis on work productivity than on factors such as appearance and attendance and that individuals who were ranked higher on work variables were also ranked higher on social integration.

A number of nonexperimental studies have indicated that a positive relationship exists between social integration and social competence. Jenaro et al. (2002) demonstrated that a low severity of behavior problems contributed to higher number of social interactions. Walsh and Linehan (1997) found that more impaired language skills, including bizarre verbal behavior, were associated with less integration. Ohtake and Chadsey (1999) discovered that relationships between coworkers became more intimate as the depth and breadth of social disclosure increased and that self-disclosure to employees with disabilities was low. Interestingly, Novak (2002) found that job coaches rated social competence as being more important for social integration than did coworkers. Ohtake and Chadsey (2003) also found that coworkers were more accepting of some problem behaviors associated with some employees with disabilities (e.g., talking too much) than of other problem behaviors (e.g., being unable to ask for help). The results from these studies suggest that although social competence is associated with more social integration, cultural norms for acceptable social behavior may vary from workplace to workplace.

The final two categories of independent variables associated with social integration and reported by Chadsey (2004) were *coworker training* and the *role of employment-training specialists*, or *job coaches*. A number of studies found that the more coworkers were trained to work with employees with disabilities, the more social integration occurred (e.g., Jenaro et al., 2002; Mank, Cioffi, & Yovanoff, 2000). Additionally, Mank, Cioffi, & Yovanoff (1999) indicated that more integration occurred when information about workers with disabilities was provided to coworkers in their immediate work areas, when it occurred in planned, short meetings rather than big group meetings, and when it dealt with specific support needs rather than general information.

A number of researchers have reported that job coaches can interfere with social interactions between employees with and without disabilities. (e.g., Chadsey, Linneman, Rusch, & Cimera, 1997). Consequently, the role of the job coach needs to be considered when formulating strategies to increase social integration. Several studies have concluded that job coaches should shift their focus to be more business oriented by taking a problem-solving approach rather than providing direct training and involving employers and coworkers more in their decision making (Butterworth et al., 2000; Rogan, Banks, & Herbein, 2003). Ohtake and Chadsey (2003) suggested that job coaches should provide only the level of support needed in an employment setting and that the support should match the needs and skill levels of coworkers and supervisors.

Summary and Future Research

Recent nonexperimental studies have shown that several variables seem to be associated with social integration of employees with disabilities in employment settings. In her review, Chadsey (2004) sorted these variables into the categories of workplace contact, workplace culture, vocational competence, social competence, coworker training, and the role of the job coach. Unfortunately, because the studies investigating these variables were not experimental, no causality can be inferred. Research is needed to test whether these variables result in social integration and the formation of adult relationships. The field needs research that tests the individual effects of these categories of variables and examines whether treatments that combine intervention categories result in better social outcomes.

Current workplace research on social integration provides some validity for the categories of independent variables suggested by Chadsey (2004). Consider the four factors mentioned by Fehr (1996) that need to converge before friendships are formed: environmental, individual, situational, and dyadic. One could argue that many of the features associated with workplace contact and culture are similar to the environmental and situational factors suggested by Fehr. Additionally, vocational and social competence seem to be similar to Fehr's individual and dyadic factors. As with Fehr's (1996) factors, it is likely that a number of the categories need to converge in employment settings before adults with disabilities can form friendships.

Community Contexts

Similar to employment contexts, a number of nonexperimental studies conducted in community settings show that social relationships among persons with disabilities are associated with several variables, which are reviewed next. Generally, these studies seem to fall into two types: studies investigating the effects of residential size and types of support and studies of specially designed programs involving persons without disabilities.

Residential Size and Types of Support

Robertson et al. (2001) collected information on the social networks of 500 adults with mental retardation who were receiving two different types of 24-hour residential supports: those living in campus-style settings that were clustered together on one site with shared central facilities (e.g., shops) and those in community-based residential settings in more dispersed domestic-style housing. Their findings suggested that social interaction was associated with living setting and ability in several ways: (1) participants with higher skill levels and fewer challenging behaviors were more likely to have people in their social networks who were not staff members, relatives, or people with mental retardation; (2) individuals living in smaller, community-based settings had more inclusive social networks; and (3) active support practices (e.g., ongoing training and support of staff; individual and activity planning for individuals) was associated with inclusive social networks. Emerson (2004) and Barber and Hupp (1993) reported similar findings.

In a later study, Emerson and McVilly (2004) collected data from key informants on 1,542 adults with intellectual disabilities about the variables that promoted or hindered friendship activities. Overall, Emerson and McVilly (2004) found that levels of friendship activities were low and that, if they did occur, these activities most often occurred with individuals who had disabilities. They found that setting characteristics (e.g., not living in a nursing home; staff member playing role of advocate) were more related to the presence of friendship activities than were the personal characteristics of adults with disabilities; however, higher levels of adaptive behavior were associated with more participation in friendship activities.

In a study in which 96 people with intellectual disabilities were interviewed about factors that were associated with several types of satisfaction, Gregory, Robertson, Kessissoglou, Emerson, and Hatton (2001) also examined friendships and relationships. In this study, nearly half of the individuals lived in village communities (24-hour support in a campus-style setting), and most of the others lived in community-based residential facilities (24-hour support in dispersed housing for no more than eight people). Interestingly, Gregory et al. (2001) found that participants living in village communities were more satisfied with their friendships and relationships that those living in community-based housing. Additionally, higher satisfaction with friendships and relationships was associated with individuals who had more people with intellectual disabilities in their social networks. This finding was not viewed as surprising. Gregory et al. (2001) acknowledged that proximity to individuals without disabilities occurs with greater frequency for those living in community-based settings than for those living in village communities but that proximity is not a sufficient condition for friendships to form.

Specially Designed Programs

A number of nonexperimental descriptive studies have evaluated specially designed programs aimed at increasing positive social outcomes between adults with and without disabilities. For example, Green, Schleien, Mactavish, and Benepe (1995) interviewed 19 college-age students about their interactions with individuals with disabilities after they spent 6 weeks in a leisure program that paired them together on a number of variables (e.g., gender, severity of disability, living proximity, leisure interests). The students were asked to treat the individuals with disabilities as equals and to choose mutually liked, age-appropriate recreation activities. After the program ended, some students indicated that their negative preconceptions about people with disabilities were disconfirmed through positive social interactions. In addition, similarities in interests, fairly equal skill levels in activities, and appropriate social skills facilitated positive reactions. The students described their relationships as being more like big sisters or brothers than like friendships.

A similar, but later, study looked at the reactions of volunteers who had spent at least 1 year in a relationship with an individual with a disability (Jameson, 1998). In this study, volunteers were either part of the Community Access Program or Best Buddies, a nationwide university-based program. In both programs, volunteers were matched with individuals with disabilities and provided with information about disabilities and community and cultural offerings. After at least a year, 27 volunteers responded to a survey asking questions about their relationship with the persons with disabilities.

Respondents indicated that they were well matched, with the matches attributed to positive personality characteristics of the person with the disability (e.g., warmth, humor, sociability), compatible personalities, communication and cognitive skills of the person with the disability, gender, and similar recreational interests. The dyads engaged in a variety of community activities together, and most of the activities were planned by the dyads rather than by staff members. Approximately 40% of the dyads saw each other monthly, and 33% saw each other every 2–3 weeks. The volunteers thought that their relationships were reciprocal, and the majority believed that they and the individual with the disability gave each other friendship or companionship. Barriers to the relationship included logistical problems, such as work and meshing schedules.

Most recently, Hardman and Clark (2006) conducted a national survey of program participants in Best Buddies. While participating in Best Buddies, college students are supposed to make contact with their buddy (a person with a disability) on a weekly basis and go on 2–3 outings per month. Hardman and Clark (2006) surveyed 1,222 students and 1,145 individuals with disabilities who had participated in the program during a 3-year period of time. Most of the people with disabilities were 10 years older than the college students, and 80% of the students were female, resulting in mixed age and gender pairs.

Hardman and Clark (2006) reported that few college students contacted their buddies at least once a week and that less than half engaged in one-to-one outings once a month, falling short of the standards set by the Best Buddies program. The types of activities engaged in by the dyads were friendship (e.g., going to a movie or the mall, sharing a meal) or teaching (e.g., teaching the buddy social skills or personal finance; Hardman & Clark, 2006). Most of the students and individuals with disabilities reported that they would recommend the program to others, and 80% of the students reported that they enjoyed the program, that they would do it again, and that they had more positive attitudes about people with disabilities as a result (Hardman & Clark, 2006). However, even though the individuals with disabilities would recommend the program to others, Hardman and Clark (2006) stated that 37% did not feel that their lives were enhanced by the program and were concerned about the overall lack of contact with the students.

Summary and Future Research

These nonexperimental studies conducted in community contexts suggest that certain variables may be associated with positive social relationships for persons with disabilities. Although community-based living facilities, and specifically organized supports (e.g., Best Buddies), seemed to be associated with more heterogeneous social networks, it appears that friendships were associated with larger, clustered living arrangements and that these friendships typically occurred between people with disabilities. Again, considering Fehr's (1996) friendship factors, proximity in more inclusive settings is only one factor that sets the stage for friendships; other factors, such as individual, situational, and dyadic, also need to converge. Consequently, it is not surprising that friendships begin to form between adults with disabilities if they are in close proximity to each other and see each other on a regular basis, share similar interests, like each other, and begin to self-disclose.

Fehr's (1996) friendship factors seem more relevant when one considers the data from specially designed programs that promote relationships. Although programs such Best Buddies may be helpful to those without disabilities in dispelling negative stereotypes and also may be enjoyable, they do not seem to result in meaningful relationships. Again, these data are not surprising, because the programs were not long in duration and the college students and individuals with disabilities did not have much social contact. Thus, although the environmental factor of opportunity may have been somewhat adequate for friendships to form, Fehr's other factors (individual, situational, and dyadic) did not seem to be present. In the Jameson (1998) study, however, more positive results were reported; these positive results may have been due to the length of time the individuals had been together (over 1 year) and other factors, including similar interests, good social skills, and reciprocity in the relationship.

Clearly, experimental research is necessary to determine whether the presence of Fehr's (1996) factors would increase social relationships between adults with and without disabilities. Interventions need to investigate the effects of living arrangements and duration and frequency of contact, of matching individuals based on similarities and interests, and of teaching the skills needed for self-disclosure and reciprocity. The next section reviews the few experimental studies that have been conducted in employment and community contexts.

EXPERIMENTAL STUDIES ON ADULT RELATIONSHIPS
Employment Contexts

Of the nine experimental studies conducted in employment settings, Chadsey (2004) found that the majority addressed teaching social skills to employees with disabilities. Some of the skills taught included initiations, responses, conversational topics and scripts, requests for assistance, and question asking (e.g., Heller, Allgood, Ware, Arnold, & Castelle, 1996; Mautz, Storey, & Certo, 2001; Storey & Garff, 1997; Storey, Lengyel, Pruszynski, 1997). The authors of these studies used single-subject designs and generally showed replicable changes in frequencies of the social skills taught. In some studies, other measures were also employed, such as the Vocational Integration Index (Parent, Kregel, Wehman, & Metzler, 1991) and various social validation measures, such as normative comparison of interactions with coworkers (Mautz et al. 2001). Although all of these measures are important, they do not reveal much information about the formation of adult relationships.

The primary intervention strategies used to teach social skills in these single-subject-design studies were variations of systematic instructional procedures, such as role playing, modeling, practice, feedback (Storey et al., 1997), and prompting the use of specific social skills within specific social intervention contexts (Mautz et al., 2001). For example, Storey et al. (1997) incorporated systematic instructional procedures when they compared training conversational scripts with question asking. An entire conversational script about asking coworkers if they wanted a drink or a napkin was taught to workers right before break time through prompts, corrective feedback, modeling, and positive reinforcement. During the question-asking intervention, workers were given a rationale for asking questions, then were shown modeled examples of questions, asked to role-play the behavior, prompted to use questions during conversations, and reinforced for appropriate use of the behavior. Although changes in social skills were noted over baseline measures for both interventions, the data were variable and seemed dependent on the coworkers' being available for interactions and the busyness of the work schedule. Storey et al. (1997) also noted that conversational script interventions might be best for teaching new employees to initiate topics of conversation, whereas question-asking interventions might be more appropriate for employees who had been working for awhile and were already familiar with the interests of their coworkers.

Besides teaching employees with disabilities specific social skills, other types of interventions have been used, although less often (Chadsey, 2004). In one study, Chadsey et al. (1997) used a single-subject design to investigate the effects of an intervention that altered the environment by increasing the frequency of opportunities for interactions (e.g., having the employee spend time in work locations near employees without disabilities). The study also incorporated a coworker intervention in which coworkers were asked for intervention ideas and then asked to implement them. Unfortunately, neither intervention was found to be very effective, but the results may have been compromised by the presence of a job coach, which seemed to suppress interactions between the workers with and without disabilities.

Several studies have used multicomponent interventions involving social skills training, coworkers, and workplace environmental modifications (Mautz et al., 2001; Storey & Garff, 1997). Although positive results occurred in Mautz et al.'s (2001) study, they found that the job coach was essential to facilitating interactions with coworkers. This finding may seem be discrepant with other studies (e.g., Chadsey et al., 1997). Mank and his colleagues (e.g., Mank et al., 2000) reported that coworker training could go hand in hand with job-coach training of individuals with disabilities. Others have suggested that the job coach needs to act more as a consultant and social coach and should have good social skills (e.g., Rogan et al., 2003). Thus it seems that job coaches can either hinder or facilitate social relationships; it just depends on the role they assume.

Few experimental studies have incorporated group designs, and, as of this writing, no study has used a randomized control design. Lee, Storey, Anderson, Goetz, and Zivolich (1997) did use a group design (without random assignment) and found that reciprocal interactions between workers with and without disabilities increased more when using a training model involving coworkers in the intervention than when using a job-coach model (i.e., paid staff).

Community Contexts

Very few experimental studies have been conducted in community contexts. Newton and Horner (1993) and Werner, Horner, and Newton (1997) conducted two early studies on improving the social lives of adults with disabilities. Both of these studies used single-subject designs and involved individuals who had significant support needs. These two studies were unique, because, unlike most studies conducted in employment settings, the intervention strategies did not involve teaching social skills to the participants but, rather, involved making changes in environmental and situational variables.

Newton and Horner (1993) used a social-guide-modeling condition to change the social network size and composition and social integration of three individuals who lived in an apartment-based residential program. The social-guide condition was a package of strategies that consisted of: (1) changing the activity patterns of the participants so that they participated in preferred activities, (2) matching the participants with other people who had similar activity interests, and (3) helping the participants engage in reciprocal actions, such as sending thank-you notes. The intervention was found to be successful for increasing the network size, activities, and social integration of the participants.

Werner et al. (1997) used an intervention package to reduce the social barriers of three men with disabilities. Components of the package established personal schedules for the participants with scheduled weekly activities. Personal information sheets on the participants were given to people who were becoming involved in the participants' lives. A friendship form that described the people in the community who were involved with the participants was developed and was used in training new staff members. A photo address file and photo activity file of friends and activities were established so participants could choose what they wanted to do and with whom. Finally, staff met weekly to review the data on the participants' social lives. The package was explained to paid staff during a 1-hour in-service session, with support given to staff for 2 weeks after the package was implemented.

Staff members learned to implement the intervention package, and it was successful in changing the social lives of two of the participants in several ways: (1) the number of different activities engaged in with someone other than a person with a disability or paid staff member increased, (2) the number of different people who participated in activities with the participants increased, and (3) the stability of the relationships increased. Less dramatic changes in these variables were found for the third participant in the study.

Community integration (defined as talking with family or friends on the phone, visiting friends outside one's residence, and going to movies, shops, restaurants, and church) was one of the measures included in a study by Heller, Hsieh, and Rimmer (2004). This study tested the effects of a fitness and health education program on adults with Down syndrome. In this experiment, individuals were randomly assigned to either the training or the control group. Although positive results were obtained for many of the outcome measures in the study (e.g., attitudes toward exercise), there was no difference between the groups on scores of community integration.

Recently, Khemka, Hickson, and Reynolds (2005) conducted a study to test the effectiveness of an abuse prevention curriculum for 36 women with mental retardation. Although the study did not focus on facilitating social relationships per se, one might argue that healthier social relationships (particularly romantic ones) could be established when one has the ability to resist unwanted advances or abuse. In this pretest–posttest control-group design, women were randomly assigned either to a control group or to the intervention, which was a curriculum called "An Effective Strategy-Based Curriculum for Abuse Prevention and Empowerment" (ESCAPE). The curriculum taught cognitive concepts of abuse and empowerment that were intertwined with motivational and emotional considerations. The participants also learned a four-step self-instructional decision-making strategy and participated in support groups. The results showed significant differences for the intervention group on measures of knowledge, decision making, and empowerment, but not on a measure of stress management.

Summary and Future Research

Employment Contexts

It is clear from the studies conducted in employment contexts that more experimental research is needed to determine effective interventions for enhancing adult social relationships for individuals with disabilities. Few studies have been conducted, and many of them are not current. Single-subject designs have been used more frequently than other designs (e.g., group designs with random assignment).

Various systematic instructional procedures have been applied in employment studies, suggesting that social skills can be taught to employees with disabilities. Few individuals have been involved in the studies, however, and generalization and maintenance results have been limited. Future research should involve larger numbers of participants, should develop strategies that will enhance generalization and maintenance, and should extend over a longer period. Although multiple measures need to be used in any type of social intervention (e.g., social initiations, perceptions of participants and coworkers), few studies have sought to directly measure close social relationships, such as friendships or romantic relationships. Finally, most interventions were designed to change the social skills of employees with disabilities, not to change the environment or the skills of coworkers. Certainly, the nonexperimental studies reviewed from employment settings and the review of research conducted by Fehr (1996) suggests the importance of social skills in the formation of relationships. However, it was also evident that other factors seem to play a role in the development of friendships and social integration (e.g., workplace contact and culture, situational variables); thus interventions need to be designed that are comprehensive, that employ multiple variables, and that are of sufficient duration.

Community Contexts

Similar to research conducted in employment settings, there have been few experimental studies in community contexts that have sought to improve the social relationships of adults with disabilities; more research is needed. The study by Heller et al. (2004) suggests that interventions that are not specifically designed to enhance social relationships of adults with disabilities will probably be ineffective. Khemka, Hickson, and Reynolds's study (2005) demonstrated that women with disabilities could learn some aspects of complex social problem solving, which may affect their social relationships in a positive way. Although not recent, the interventions used by Newton and his colleagues (e.g., Newton & Horner, 1993) should be considered in future research because they incorporate many of the variables suggested as being important by Fehr (1996) and the nonexperimental studies reviewed in this chapter.

IMPLICATIONS FOR PRACTITIONERS

Although more experimental research is needed, there seem to be promising directions for employment and community service providers to consider when designing intervention strategies. First, a number of environmental and situational variables need to be in place for relationships to form. Across work and community settings, there must be frequent opportunities to interact with others over long periods of time (e.g., months). Work settings, in particular, should have strong positive cultures (e.g., be friendly, with supervisors who interact informally with staff) and should involve job tasks that are dependent on the skills of the employee with disabilities. In both community and employment settings, adults with disabilities should engage in roles that are valued (Lemay, 2006) and equal in status and that disconfirm previously held stereotypes. Additionally, in both settings, adults with disabilities should be taught social skills so that they can learn to initiate and respond to social interactions, to self-disclose, and to reciprocate.

Someone who is well trained may need to create and support opportunities for social interactions with others. From this review, it is clear that mere proximity to others and even specially designed social programs (e.g., Best Buddies) do not necessarily result in the formation of social relationships. Individuals with disabilities may need to be "matched" or to have opportunities to interact with others based on similarity of interests and other personal variables (e.g., religion, values, personality). There must be time available for interactions, and opportunities should be frequent and last a number of months. People who might provide these social opportunities are paid staff members, other friends, or family. Once a social relationship is established between two people, it is quite likely that external support will no longer be needed.

Can social relationships be engineered? If a multicomponent intervention package were implemented, would social relationships be established for adults with disabilities? Although people can't be "forced" to be friends (for example), the implementation of the independent variables suggested in this chapter may result in positive outcomes and are worthy of study. Practitioners must remember, however, that relationship formation is complex and that simple interventions, such as teaching two or three social skills over a short time period, will probably not be successful.

POLICY IMPLICATIONS

The formation of close social relationships is important for everyone and should be a critical outcome for adults with disabilities. The literature suggests that these adults do form relationships but that at times these relationships are with other people with disabilities, paid staff members, or family members. As noted, the field tends to devalue these types of relationships, thinking that the best relationships for adults with disabilities are with adults without disabilities who are not family members or people who are paid for support (Knox & Hickson, 2001). No one should determine other persons' social relationships; policy makers need to assert that adults with disabilities should be able to choose their own relationships and should "feel a part of a readily available, supportive and dependable social structure" (Cummins & Lau, 2003, p. 154).

Equally important, however, is for policy makers to insist that adults with disabilities have the opportunity to be a part of the typical community. Adults should live, work, and recreate in settings with people of diverse abilities. It is quite clear, though, that having the opportunity to interact with others who do not have disabilities will rarely result in social relationships forming. Because there is little evidence-based research identifying intervention strategies that result in social relationships, policy makers should push for research priorities and the needed funding in this area.

Because social relationships are essential to happiness, it is critical that intervention strategies be developed to maximize the likelihood of social relationships forming between adults with disabilities and others. Policy makers must stand firm in their commitment to promoting this complex phenomenon that contributes to everyone's overall well-being.

REFERENCES

Allport, G. W. (1954). *The nature of prejudice.* Cambridge, MA: Addison-Wesley.

Altman, I., & Taylor, D. A. (1973). *Social penetration: The development of interpersonal relationships.* New York: Holt, Rinehart & Winston.

Barber, D., & Hupp, S. (1993). A comparison of friendship patterns of individuals with developmental disabilities. *Education and Training in Mental Retardation, 28,* 13–22.

Butterworth, J., Hagner, D., Helm, D. T., & Whelley, T. A. (2000). Workplace culture, social interactions, and supports for transition-age young adults. *Mental Retardation, 38,* 342–353.

Chadsey, J. (2004, June). *Advancing social integration: Implications from research conducted in employment settings.* Keynote address presented at the World Congress of the International Association for the Scientific Study of Intellectual Disabilities, Montpellier, France.

Chadsey, J., Linneman, D., Rusch, F. R., & Cimera, R. E. (1997). The impact of social integration interventions and job coaches in work settings. *Education and Training in Mental Retardation and Developmental Disabilities, 32,* 281–292.

Chadsey, J. G., Shelden, D. L., Horn De Bardeleben, J. R., & Cimera, R. E. (1999). Description of variables impacting successful and unsuccessful cases of social integration involving co-workers. *Journal of Vocational Rehabilitation, 12,* 103–111.

Cummins, R. A., & Lau, A. L. D. (2003). Community integration or community exposure? A review and discussion in relation to people with an intellectual disability. *Journal of Applied Research in Intellectual Disabilities, 16,* 145–157.

Diener, E., Oishi, S., & Lucas, R. E. (2003). Personality, culture, and subjective well-being: Emotional and cognitive evaluations of life. *Annual Review of Psychology, 54,* 403–425.

Diener, E., & Seligman, M. E. P. (2002). Very happy people. *Psychological Science, 13,* 80–83.

Emerson, E. (2004). Cluster housing for adults with intellectual disabilities. *Journal of Intellectual and Developmental Disability, 29,* 187–197.

Emerson, E., & McVilly, K. (2004). Friendship activities of adults with intellectual disabilities in supported accommodation in northern England. *Journal of Applied Research in Intellectual Disabilities, 17,* 191–197.

Fehr, B. (1996). *Friendship processes.* Thousand Oaks, CA: Sage.

Green, F. P., Schleien, S. J., Mactavish, J., & Benepe, S. (1995). Nondisabled adults' perceptions of relationships in the early stages of arranged partnerships with peers with mental retardation. *Education and Training in Mental Retardation and Developmental Disabilities, 30,* 91–108.

Gregory, N., Robertson, J., Kessissoglou, S., Emerson, E., & Hatton, C. (2001). Factors associated with expressed satisfaction among people with intellectual disability receiving residential supports. *Journal of Intellectual Disability Research, 45,* 279–291.

Hagner, D., Butterworth, J., & Keith, G. (1995). Strategies and barriers in facilitating natural supports for employment of adults with severe disabilities. *Journal of the Association for Persons with Severe Handicaps, 20,* 110–120.

Halpern, A. (1993). Quality of life as a conceptual framework for evaluation transition outcomes. *Exceptional Children, 59,* 486–498.

Hardman, M. L., & Clark, C. (2006). Promoting friendship through best buddies: A national survey of college program participants. *Mental Retardation, 44,* 56–63.

Heller, K. W., Allgood, M. H., Ware, S., Arnold, S. E., & Castelle, M. D. (1996). Initiating requests during community-based vocational training by students with mental retardation and sensory impairments. *Research in Developmental Disabilities, 17,* 173–184.

Heller, T., Hsieh, K., & Rimmer, J. H. (2004). Attitudinal and psychosocial outcomes of a fitness and health education program on adults with Down syndrome. *American Journal on Mental Retardation, 109,* 175–185.

Jameson, C. (1998). Promoting long-term relationships between individuals with mental retardation and people in their community: An agency self-evaluation. *Mental Retardation, 36,* 116–127.

Jenaro, C., Mank, D., Bottomley, J., Doose, S., & Tuckerman, P. (2002). Supported employment in the international context: An analysis of processes and outcomes. *Journal of Vocational Rehabilitation, 17,* 5–21.

Khemka, I., Hickson, L., & Reynolds, G. (2005). Evaluation of a decision-making curriculum designed to empower women with mental retardation to resist abuse. *American Journal on Mental Retardation, 110,* 193–204.

Knox, M., & Hickson, F. (2001). The meanings of close friendship: The views of four people with intellectual disabilities. *Journal of Applied Research in Intellectual Disabilities, 14,* 276–291.

Lee, M., Storey, K., Anderson, J. L., Goetz, L., & Zivolich, S. (1997). The effect of mentoring versus job coach instruction on integration in supported employment settings. *Journal of the Association for Persons with Severe Handicaps, 22,* 151–158.

Lemay, R. (2006). Social role valorization insights into the social integration conundrum. *Mental Retardation, 44,* 1–12.

Mank, D., Cioffi, A., & Yovanoff, P. (1998). Employment outcomes for people with severe disabilities: Opportunities for improvement. *Mental Retardation, 36,* 205–216.

Mank, D., Cioffi, A., & Yovanoff, P. (1999). The impact of coworker involvement with supported employees on wage and integration outcomes. *Mental Retardation, 37,* 383–394.

Mank, D., Cioffi, A., & Yovanoff, P. (2000). Direct support in supported employment and its relation to job typicalness, coworker involvement, and employment outcomes. *Mental Retardation, 38,* 506–516.

Mank, D., Cioffi, A., & Yovanoff, P. (2003). Supported employment outcomes across a decade: Is there evidence of improvement in the quality of implementation? *Mental Retardation, 41,* 188–197.

Mautz, D., Storey, K., & Certo, N. (2001). Increasing integrated workplace social interactions: The effects of job modification, natural supports, adaptive communication instruction, and job coach training. *Journal of the Association for Persons with Severe Handicaps, 26,* 257–269.

Neumayer, R., & Bleasdale, M. (1996). Personal lifestyle preferences of people with an intellectual disability. *Journal of Intellectual and Developmental Disability, 21,* 91–115.

Newton, J. S., & Horner, R. H. (1993). Using a social guide to improve social relationships of people with severe disabilities. *Journal of the Association for Persons with Severe Handicaps, 18,* 36–45.

Novak, J. A. (2002). *Social integration of employees with disabilities: The role of workplace contact.* Unpublished doctoral dissertation, Indiana University, Bloomington.

O'Connor, G. (1983). Presidential address 1983: Social support of mentally retarded persons. *Mental Retardation, 21,* 187–196.

Ohtake, Y., & Chadscy, J. G. (1999). Social disclosure among coworkers without disabilities in supported employment settings. *Mental Retardation, 37,* 25–35.

Ohtake, Y., & Chadsey, J. G. (2003). Facilitation strategies used by job coaches in supported employment settings: A preliminary investigation. *Research and Practice for Persons with Severe Disabilities, 28,* 214–227.

Parent, W., Kregel, J., Wehman, P., & Metzler, H. (1991). Measuring the social integration of supported employment workers. *Journal of Vocational Rehabilitation, 1,* 35–49.

Pottie, C., & Sumarah, J. (2004). Friendships between persons with and without developmental disabilities. *Mental Retardation, 42,* 55–66.

Riches, V. C., & Green, V. A. (2003). Social integration in the workplace for people with disabilities: An Australian perspective. *Journal of Vocational Rehabilitation, 19,* 127–142.

Robertson, J., Emerson, E., Gregory, N., Hatton, C., Kessissoglou, S., Hallam, A., et al. (2001). Social networks of people with mental retardation in residential settings. *Mental Retardation, 39,* 201–214.

Rogan, P., Banks, B., & Herbein, M. H. (2003). Supportive employment and workplace supports: A qualitative study. *Journal of Vocational Rehabilitation, 19,* 5–18.

Seligman, M. E. P., Steen, T. A., Park, N., & Peterson, C. (2005). Positive psychology progress: Empirical validation of interventions. *American Psychologist, 60,* 410–421.

Storey, K., & Garff, J. T. (1997). The cumulative effect of natural support strategies and social skills instruction on the integration of a worker in supported employment. *Journal of Vocational Rehabilitation, 9,* 143–152.

Storey, K., Lengyel, L., & Pruszynski, B. (1997). Assessing the effectiveness and measuring the complexity of two conversational instructional procedures in supported employment contexts. *Journal of Vocational Rehabilitation, 8,* 21–33.

Test, D. W., Carver, T., Ewers, L., Haddad, J., & Person, J. (2000). Longitudinal job satisfaction of persons in supported employment. *Education and Training in Mental Retardation and Developmental Disabilities, 35,* 365–373.

Walsh, P. N., & Linehan, C. (1997). Factors influencing the integration of Irish employees with disabilities in the workplace. *Journal of Vocational Rehabilitation, 8,* 55–64.

Werner, K., Horner, R. H., & Newton, J. S. (1997). Reducing structural barriers to improve the social life of three adults with severe disabilities. *Journal of the Association for Persons with Severe Handicaps, 22,* 138–150.

Wistow, R., & Schneider, J. (2003). Users' views on supported employment and social inclusion: A qualitative study of 30 people in work. *British Journal of Learning Disabilities, 31,* 166–174.

BEHAVIOR SUPPORTS

Problem behaviors, such as aggression, self-injury, property destruction, and disruption, are a major barrier to successful inclusion of children and adults with developmental disabilities. Problem behaviors interfere with the development of successful social relationships and limit opportunities for personal independence and self-determination. Any systematic response to the challenges that developmental disabilities pose in our society must include strategies for providing support in reducing the deleterious effects of problem behaviors. The chapters in this section provide a summary of current research and encouraging directions for the future.

Dunlap and Carr describe positive behavior support as an organizing framework for the design of effective social environments. Their message is that the context in which a person behaves makes a difference. Organizing settings to enhance appropriate behavior is important. Too often our literature describes conditions in which people with developmental disabilities and limited communication, learning, or interaction skills are inadvertently placed in conditions that promote dangerous and destructive behavior. The technology of positive behavior support is in many ways the combination of behavioral, social, and cultural variables to create environments that promote and support positive behavior. The importance of individualized assessment of problem behavior is now well documented, and Dunlap and Carr define how this assessment information can be used not just to decrease problem behavior but to build the constructive behaviors that lead to a rich and independent lifestyle. Behavior support has moved beyond the initial focus on reducing undesirable behaviors and into an exciting and challenging position of building the broad supports needed for lifestyle success.

Any attention to the stability, success, and quality of individual lives, however, must address issues of mental health. Paschos and Bouras organize the current status of research on mental health variables affecting individuals with developmental disabilities. A challenging and complex feature of developmental disabilities is the comorbidity, or combination, of mental health problems and intellectual disabilities. We continue to learn about and appreciate the impact of mental health challenges such as autism, schizophrenia, depression, attention deficits, and dementia. Here again, an emphasis on efficient and solution-driven assessment becomes important. Paschos and Bouras describe an approach to support for mental health challenges that integrates and individualizes behavioral, psychopharmacological, and social therapies. For these unifying approaches to treatment to be successful, however, more targeted research is needed about basic epidemiological patterns, how best to conduct clinical assessments, and the fundamental biological issues affecting effective psychopharmacology. The theme guiding this research, however, is not development of isolated knowledge but how best to organize social systems that meet the combined needs of individuals and their families.

Both positive behavior support and mental health professionals emphasize the functional role of psychopharmacology in the design of comprehensive interventions. Although it is important to note that psychopharmacology is not required in all situations, the need for medications as part of a strategy to support individuals with developmental disabilities and problem behavior is clear. Thompson, Moore, and Symons provide a window into an innovative perspective on psychopharmacology. Their basic thesis is that medications affect how individuals experience their environment. Change how people perceive what is happening around them, and you will see changes in their behavior. Using an elegant model of behavioral, physiological, and social variables, Thompson, Moore, and Symons propose a new taxonomy for psychotherapeutic medications. They focus on how medications can change the ways antecedent events might "trigger" problem behaviors and how medications may alter the effects of "maintaining consequences" associated with other problem behaviors. They tie their taxonomy to practical approaches for comprehensive intervention and outline specific research needed to better understand the effects of medications.

Together, the chapters in this section frame an important message about moving beyond isolated interventions toward integrated systems of support. Individuals with disabilities and problem behavior can move out of destructive and disruptive cycles and toward more independent, productive, and self-determined lives with adequate support. That support will be guided both by applying current research-guided intervention strategies and by developing new strategies identified by these proposed programs of research.

Positive Behavior Support and Developmental Disabilities

A Summary and Analysis of Research

Glen Dunlap
Edward G. Carr

Individuals with developmental disabilities are at higher than ordinary risk for developing problem behaviors, such as aggression, self-injury, property destruction, intense tantrums, excessive unresponsiveness, and high levels of repetitive and stereotyped motor movements. Such behaviors can interfere with learning, socialization, and community participation, and, therefore, reduction of problem behaviors has been cited frequently as a critical priority in program development and personnel training (Horner et al., 2005). Therefore, a great deal of research has focused on problem behaviors of individuals with developmental disabilities (e.g., Conroy, Dunlap, Clarke, & Alter, 2005; Dunlap, Clarke, & Steiner, 1999) and, increasingly, much of that research has revolved around the approach known as "positive behavior support" (Carr, Horner, et al., 1999).

This chapter provides a description of positive behavior support (PBS), along with a summary and analysis of existing research on PBS with individuals who have developmental disabilities. The major components of PBS are considered, along with concise summaries of current knowledge. These components include the processes of functional assessment and planning, instructional variables and interventions, antecedent and contextual influences and manipulations, and multicomponent packages of intervention and support. Following this survey, a summary is devoted to an overall analysis of the strengths and limitations of the PBS knowledge base.

DEFINITION AND HISTORY OF PBS

PBS is an approach to intervention based on the behavioral sciences, integrated with information from biomedical and systems-change strategies, that focuses on improving individuals' quality of life and resolving problem behaviors and other challenges of behavioral adjustment (Carr et al., 2002; Dunlap, Carr, & Horner, 2006). PBS is a scientific approach that is explicitly accountable to evaluation data and a foundation of rigorous experimental and quasi-experimental procedural validation. Yet at the same time PBS is a highly pragmatic approach, open to innovation and the incorporation of strategies derived from diverse perspectives, as long as those innovations are subjected to data-based accountability (Dunlap, 2004). PBS is also a values-based approach, with overt appreciation of person-centered and family-centered perspectives on the appropriateness of intervention techniques and the specific outcomes that should be targeted and evaluated (Bambara, 2005; Kincaid & Fox, 2002).

A number of authors have elaborated on the definition of PBS by delineating descriptive features that help to identify the emphases of PBS and to differentiate the approach from other behavioral strategies (Bambara, 2005; Dunlap, 2006; Horner et al., 1990). For instance, in 2002, Carr and his associates described nine critical features the integration of which help define PBS and distinguish it from other approaches. The nine features are: (1) *comprehensive lifestyle change and improved quality of life* as the ultimate and obligatory goals of intervention; (2) a recognition that interventions and supports must be seen and implemented from a *longitudinal and lifespan perspective*; (3) a focus on *ecological validity*, meaning that strategies of intervention and support must be relevant to, and effective in, real-life settings and situations; (4) an insistence on *collaboration*, with principal stakeholders (such as parents, teachers, friends, employers, siblings) functioning as partners in the development and implementation of PBS; (5) an emphasis on the *social validity* of procedures and outcomes; (6) an acknowledgment that effective, longitudinal support requires *systems change* and *multicomponent interventions*; (7) a comprehensive *emphasis on prevention*, with an understanding that functional (proactive) intervention occurs when problem behaviors are not present; (8) a utilization of knowledge derived from *various types of methodological practices*; and, correspondingly, (9) a pragmatic appreciation for the contributions of *multiple theoretical perspectives*.

Positive behavior support began to emerge from existing approaches to problem behavior in the mid-1980s. At that time, the field associated with developmental disabilities was undergoing major transformations inspired by the rising voices of advocates and advocacy organizations. Movements had been established to promote inclusion and community participation, to prevent long-term residential hospitalization, and to ensure that people with disabilities had rights and opportunities to live, work, and participate in the full, ongoing social commerce of typical communities. Concurrent with these early movements of deinstitutionalization and school inclusion was escalating alarm regarding the treatment of individuals with disabilities accompanied by problem behaviors. It had become commonplace at that time to treat severe problem behaviors (especially aggression and self-injury but also behaviors of lesser intensity) with punitive contingencies (along with reinforcement for desirable responding). When mild punishments were ineffective, the intensity was often increased to the point that numerous individuals were exposed to highly intrusive, painful, and stigmatizing consequences in therapeutic efforts to suppress the disagreeable patterns of behavior (Guess, Helmstetter, Turnbull, & Knowlton, 1987). By the 1980s, advocates were loudly protesting this type of treatment, arguing that such aversive interventions were cruel and inhumane and, because such aversives could be used only in secluded settings, functionally inconsistent with the goals of community integration.

Fortunately, the applied behavioral sciences were beginning to elucidate alternatives to aversive behavior management. Although the necessary behavioral theory was already in place (e.g., Carr, 1977), a practical technology of "nonaversive" interventions for chronic and severe problem behaviors had not yet been developed. This began to change in the 1980s, as applied research started to reveal the functional properties of problem behaviors and the initial demonstrations of functional analysis and functional assessment were published (e.g., Carr, Newsom, & Binkoff, 1980; Iwata, Dorsey, Slifer, Bauman, & Richman, 1982/1994). This enriched, practical understanding of the motivations and the contextual governance of problem behavior led to an outpouring of new applied research that began to form the empirical basis of positive behavior support (e.g., Carr & Durand, 1985; Dunlap, Kern-Dunlap, Clarke, & Robbins, 1991; Horner & Budd, 1985). This new generation of research on problem behavior moved beyond simple contingency management and focused on assessment-based interventions composed largely of educative procedures and manipulations of environmental (antecedent and contextual) variables (Horner et al., 1990; Meyer & Evans, 1989).

Since its beginnings in the mid-1980s, PBS has been increasingly established as a popular and empirically grounded technology. The general approach, including functional assessment and positive interventions, has been endorsed in federal (e.g., the Individuals with Disabilities Education Act; IDEA) and state statutes, and hundreds of articles and books have described PBS principles and procedures. Although PBS grew from its origins in developmental disabilities, it has been applied subsequently with many different populations of individuals with and without disabilities. The remainder of this chapter is devoted to the status of research that defines the empirical basis of PBS for individuals with developmental disabilities. This research addresses a variety of problem behaviors exhibited by individuals in a wide range of settings, and it provides information on the effects of a number of PBS components. It is important to note that a good deal of the research is also aligned with affiliated disciplines, especially applied behavior analysis (ABA). The reason is that PBS recently emerged from its foundations in ABA (Carr et al., 2002; Dunlap, 2006; Risley, 1999), and a great deal of the empirical and conceptual foundation of PBS is common to both ABA and PBS.

RESEARCH ON ASSESSMENT PROCESSES IN PBS

One of the most conspicuous distinctions between PBS and earlier approaches to behavior management is that PBS is based on a functional understanding of the targeted behavior. That is, PBS requires a clear, preintervention assessment of the relationship between the behavior and the environmental events that govern the occurrence and nonoccurrence of the behavior. Such an assessment process differentiates PBS from its predecessors, which tended to rely on simple, contingency-management formulae (e.g., differential reinforcement plus extinction) or cookbook-like strategies based on behavioral topography (e.g., for aggression, use time-out and training in social skills). In contrast, the development of a PBS intervention plan is dependent on knowledge about the function of the behavior and the events in the environment that influence the behavior. It is fair to say that the advent of practical knowledge in the early 1980s about functional equivalence, the communicative motivations of many problem behaviors, and practical techniques of functional analysis and functional assessment made PBS possible. Indeed, functional assessment is widely recognized as the *sine qua non* of positive behavior support.

"Functional analysis" is the term that refers to experimental manipulations used to identify functions of problem behavior or to verify hypotheses regarding the influence of implicated variables on problem behavior. Both purposes of functional analysis have been demonstrated extensively in the behavioral literature (e.g., Repp & Horner, 1999). "Functional assessment" refers to the broader enterprise of describing functional relationships between behavior and the environment, without the requirement of experimental analysis (though functional analysis can be a part of a functional assessment). The process of functional assessment typically involves combinations of direct observations, indirect observations, and structured interviews with knowledgeable informants. At a basic level, the purpose of functional assessment is to operationally define the target behavior(s), identify the functions of the target behavior(s), and identify the specific environmental stimuli that are associated with occurrences and nonoccurrences of the behavior(s). The ultimate goal is to use the assessment information to develop an individualized behavior support plan. The technology of functional assessment has been presented in hundreds of scholarly articles and dozens of books and manuals (e.g., Dunlap & Kincaid, 2001; O'Neill et al., 1997; Umbreit, Ferro, Liaupsin, & Lane, 2007). The basic messages are that functional analysis and functional assessment are effective strategies for obtaining relevant information for intervention planning and that interventions based on functional assessments are apt to be more effective than interventions designed without the benefit of such assessment data.

Recent research has focused on efforts to make functional assessment technologies more practical for use in typical settings and by typical practitioners and to expand the breadth of data to account for additional (e.g., ecological) influences on targeted behaviors. For instance, structural analysis strategies have been developed for collecting descriptive data in ongoing classroom and residential settings in order to identify variables associated with problem behaviors (e.g., Touchette, MacDonald, & Langer, 1985). Also, as greater attention has been paid to the role of setting and ecological events in the governance of problem behaviors (McGill, 1999), there have been attempts to incorporate setting factors into the process of preintervention assessment (e.g., McAtee, Carr, & Schulte, 2004).

The explicit ambition of PBS is to develop behavior support plans that will be effective in producing quality-of-life benefits over extended periods of time. In order for this to occur, it is necessary to assess larger lifestyle variables, to develop plans for changing these variables, and to include methods for evaluating the effects of these changes (Risley, 1996). A common procedure for developing such longitudinal lifestyle plans is "person-centered planning" (Kincaid & Fox, 2002), which has become a popular component in planning and assessment for individuals with disabilities. Although some studies have shown benefits to be derived from such planning processes (e.g., Green, Middleton, & Reid, 2000), there has been an absence of large-scale research evaluating the quality-of-life effects of person-centered planning. Another element of preintervention planning and assessment relates to the notion that a behavior support plan has to "fit" with the ongoing routines, values, priorities, and overall context of the settings in which the plan is to be implemented. The concept of contextual fit is argued to be a critical determinant of the extent to which a plan will actually be implemented, and initial efforts to assess contextual fit have been advanced (Albin, Lucyshyn, Horner, & Flannery, 1996); however, there are few data as yet to inform us of the validity of such assessments or the impact that such assessments might have on plan development, implementation, and effectiveness of PBS.

A critical aspect of PBS involves carefully linking assessment information to the design of interventions, a topic to which we now turn our attention.

RESEARCH ON INSTRUCTIONAL VARIABLES IN PBS

PBS is a proactive approach that is designed to prevent problem behaviors from occurring. This is accomplished primarily through two general types of interventions: (1) environmental design—that is, manipulations of contextual and antecedent stimuli that are addressed in the next section of this chapter, and (2) instruction—that is, developing a person's competencies so that the person does not need to rely on problem behaviors to manage his or her environment. Instruction on carefully selected skills is an essential component of most PBS plans, and it is generally acknowledged that effective teaching and developmental guidance, along with reinforcement to build and maintain the use of functional skills, is the best antidote to the emergence of problem behavior. Competence in addressing life's myriad challenges and demands is inversely related to problem behaviors, and, indeed, a well-designed curriculum, with instruction occurring in all relevant activities and times of the day, has been shown to be associated with substantially reduced levels of problem behaviors (Ferro, Foster-Johnson, & Dunlap, 1996).

Two categories of skills clearly pertain to the development of adaptive performance and the reduction of problem behaviors. Both categories involve the establishment of behaviors that are intended as alternatives to undesirable responding. The first category involves teaching behaviors that serve as exact replacements for problem behaviors. Teaching replacement skills relies on the concept of functional equivalence (Carr, 1988) and the recognition that problem behaviors most often function as communicative acts. The idea is to teach the individual to use a desirable form of communication (e.g., speech, gesture) as a functionally equivalent alternative to problem behavior (e.g., aggression, tantrums). Procedures for identifying functional replacement skills, teaching those skills, and promoting the continued use of the skills have been referred to as "functional communication training" (FCT) and have been reported in a large number of journal articles, books, and manuals (e.g., Carr et al., 1994; Durand, 1990). The empirical support for FCT is compelling. Since the appearance of the initial research report on FCT (Carr & Durand, 1985), there have been hundreds of systematic replications and applications produced by dozens of authors in a variety of settings and with a range of participants (e.g., Derby et al., 1997; Dunlap, Ester, Langhans, & Fox, 2006).

The second category of instructional approaches involves teaching individuals to tolerate challenging circumstances or to engage in responses that facilitate improved coping and self-control. A number of such strategies have been discussed in the literature, including teaching individuals to endure increasing delays of gratification and teaching relaxation, social skills, and self-management (Halle, Bambara, & Reichle, 2005). Perhaps the strategy in this category that claims the most research is self-monitoring and self-management. Several authors have developed well-described procedures for teaching children with developmental disabilities to record instances of their own behavior and then applying these self-monitoring skills to reduce problem behaviors and increase adaptive performance in classrooms and other inclusive environments (e.g., Frea & Hughes, 1997; Koegel, Harrower, & Koegel, 1999). Though the literature is not voluminous, the data that exist show impressive accomplishments with self-monitoring techniques, even for children with significant intellectual disabilities.

RESEARCH ON ANTECEDENT AND CONTEXTUAL VARIABLES

Data from functional assessments have been used to determine the functions of problem behavior and to identify antecedent variables associated with occurrences and nonoccurrences of the behavior. The importance of the latter cannot be overemphasized. Manipulations of antecedent and contextual variables provide PBS practitioners with extremely powerful tools for preventing problem behaviors and promoting more desirable patterns of responding, and essentially all PBS plans include some elements of antecedent arrangements.

There is no set list of potential antecedent and contextual manipulations, because antecedent and contextual influences can be anything that affects the rate of the behavior that is present before or during the behavioral occurrence. Antecedent stimuli can include instructions, the introduction of an activity, the quality of social interactions, or any other visual, auditory, olfactory, or kinesthetic events. Contextual stimuli influence the occurrence of behavior. These stimuli may include ecological variables (including characteristics of the physical environment), the social milieu, one's physiological status (hunger, thirst, illness, arousal), and lingering effects of past events (e.g., recent disappointments). When functional assessments implicate specific events as being associated with problem behavior, then removal or amelioration of those events can serve to prevent future instances of problem behavior. Similarly, when functional assessments identify stimuli associated with desirable behavior, the intensification and amplification of those stimuli are apt to increase appropriate responding.

A great deal of research has demonstrated that individualized implementation of antecedent and contextual manipulations can produce rapid and substantial behavior change (Luiselli & Cameron, 1998). For instance, a number of studies have shown that changes in the manner in which instructions are delivered (e.g., pacing, sequencing of tasks) can affect levels of problem behavior (Dunlap & Kern, 1996). Similarly, alterations to the properties of tasks, such as modifying task difficulty and incorporating preferred stimuli in the task materials, have been demonstrated to improve behavior (Weeks & Gaylord-Ross, 1981). A related and well-developed line of antecedent research has focused on the opportunity to make choices, with the data consistently showing that giving individuals the chance to make selections among available options tends to reduce problem behavior and increase task engagement (Dunlap, Kern-Dunlap, Clarke, & Robbins, 1991). A number of reviews have documented the large amount of data that testify to the influence of instructional and curricular manipulations on problem behavior (e.g., Dunlap & Kern, 1996; Luiselli, 2006).

As mentioned previously, antecedent and contextual manipulations cover a tremendous breadth of potential interventions, as well as published research (Kern & Clarke, 2005). Studies have examined the influence of ecological factors on problem behavior and have demonstrated benefits that can accrue from adjusting various aspects of the settings. For instance, researchers have investigated the effects of enriched environments and found that settings with preferred stimuli and sufficient schedules of noncontingent reinforcement can serve to prevent problem behavior (Carr & LeBlanc,

2006). Other investigators have begun to consider the nature of interpersonal relationships as an antecedent variable that could limit the likelihood of problems. For instance, McLaughlin and Carr (2005) conducted a study in which rapport (the quality of a relationship) was the independent variable. They first showed that good rapport between a staff member and a person with developmental disabilities was associated with low levels of problem behavior, whereas poor rapport was associated with elevated problems. The authors then implemented an intervention package designed to improve the rapport that existed in some of the dyads. The intervention package succeeded in increasing the quality of the rapport, with the result that problem behaviors were reduced.

The existing research literature documents an array of antecedent and contextual manipulations that are effective in improving the behavior of individuals with developmental disabilities, and it is clear that such strategies are vitally important in the enterprise of PBS. However, antecedent interventions tend to be temporary preventives that, by themselves, are inadequate to build improved lifestyles or to be maintained over extended periods of time. For that reason, antecedent and contextual interventions are viewed almost always as components of larger and more comprehensive support plans.

RESEARCH ON MULTICOMPONENT INTERVENTIONS AND SUPPORTS

In practice, PBS interventions for individuals with developmental disabilities comprise multiple components individually selected on the basis of functional assessment and other planning data. The components most often include instruction on alternative responses, rearranged schedules of reinforcement, and antecedent and contextual manipulations. The behavior support plans may also provide for structural changes (e.g., classroom placements), social circles of support, medical assessments and treatment, heightened opportunities to access preferred community activities, and other lifestyle adjustments. In addition, PBS plans often include training for staff, scripts to assist staff in carrying out precise instructional sequences, and improved strategies for staff coordination and communication between support providers in important settings. Procedures for evaluating the effects of the intervention are also described.

Considerable research has been conducted to evaluate the effects of multicomponent PBS interventions as applied in the context of ongoing routines in typical school, home/residential, and community settings. A number of studies have used experimental or quasi-experimental case study designs, providing considerable detail regarding a small number (often only one) of participants (e.g., Carr & Carlson, 1993; Clarke, Worcester, Dunlap, Murray, & Bradley-Klug, 2002; Vaughn, Dunlap, Fox, Clarke, & Bucy, 1997). In one study, Lucyshyn, Albin, and Nixon (1997) worked with a teenage girl with multiple disabilities in a family context. In partnership with the girl's parents, the authors obtained comprehensive assessment data on the family ecology and on the functions of the problem behaviors in multiple home and community routines. Following the assessments, including an experimental analysis, a plan was developed that consisted of ecological, antecedent, instructional, reinforcement, and emergency intervention procedures, with each component tailored for application in the designated home (e.g., dinner) and community (e.g., shopping) routines. Extensive observational data were obtained, with the results indicating that the procedures were used with fidelity and that they were effective in resolving the girl's serious problem behaviors. Follow-up data collected 3 and 9 months following intervention showed that the behavior change was maintained.

In another example, Carr, Levin, and their colleagues (1999) used comprehensive PBS procedures to address the problem behaviors of three group-home residents, ages 14, 17, and 38 years old. The researchers employed a detailed process of functional assessment, verification of hypotheses, and individualized support plans that included rapport development, functional communication training, gradual shaping of increased tolerance for delay of reinforcement, choice making, and embedding (Carr et al., 1994). Intervention was conducted in multiple settings across several years, and the data showed clearly favorable outcomes with maintenance being demonstrated for years after intervention.

Although the majority of studies on comprehensive applications of PBS have included few participants, some investigations with larger samples are beginning to be conducted. One notable illustration is a study conducted by Feldman, Condillac, Tough, Hunt, and Griffiths (2002). These authors described a study of multicomponent, assessment-based PBS implemented with 20 participants (children and adults) with developmental disabilities and serious problem behaviors, including self-injury, aggression, and other destructive behaviors. The researchers found significant decreases in problem behaviors, increases in replacement behaviors, and maintenance up to 3 years following intervention.

SUMMARY OF EXISTING RESEARCH ON PBS

Creating a summary of PBS research can be a challenge because the approach is new and still evolving and because most studies have addressed the efficacy of components of PBS rather than the comprehensive interventions that truly represent PBS in practice. PBS is a multifaceted approach that begins with functional assessment and planning, the results of which lead to individualized support plans. PBS is more a dynamic process than a static program of intervention. Nevertheless, several efforts have been undertaken to synthesize existing knowledge (e.g., Carr, Horner, et al., 1999; Scotti, Ujcich, Weigle, Holland, & Kirk, 1996). In this section, we provide a very brief synopsis of what we know regarding the PBS approach, as well as a list of some key areas of knowledge that we have yet to acquire.

What We Know about PBS

Most of the knowledge that can be asserted with confidence comes from the accumulation of many years of single-subject experimental analyses of the processes of assessment and intervention. In general, the data are strong with respect to internal validity and less convincing with respect to external validity. In the general area of assessment and planning, it is fair to issue the following statements.

1. There is a wealth of compelling data indicating that experimental functional analysis, usually conducted in artificial settings, can identify the functions of problem behavior of individuals with developmental disabilities. The data are voluminous and have very strong internal validity but undetermined external validity. However, there are now also data to show that functional analyses designed to verify hypotheses from

functional assessments can be conducted in natural settings, and these latter data tend to have greater external validity and direct pertinence for intervention (e.g., Carr & Carlson, 1993; Dunlap et al., 1991).

2. There are substantial experimental data to confirm that interventions based on functional assessment information can lead to reduced problem behavior and increased levels of prosocial behavior (Carr, Horner, et al., 1999).

3. An emerging database demonstrates that assessments of broader aspects related to intervention planning, such as setting events and contextual fit, are feasible and beneficial; however, the published data remain limited (e.g., McAtee et al., 2004).

4. A very large nonexperimental literature supports the use of person-centered planning approaches (Holburn & Vietze, 2002) as part of overall planning and support; however, rigorous controlled studies have yet to be conducted.

When it comes to components of PBS interventions, the following can be said:

1. Teaching replacement behaviors is a highly effective strategy for building useful competencies and simultaneously reducing problem behavior, though it is important that the replacement behavior be functionally equivalent to the targeted problem behavior. In particular, functional communication training has been shown repeatedly to be effective with a broad range of individuals with developmental disabilities (Halle et al., 2005).

2. The development of other alternative skills (tolerance, self-control) can be a valuable strategy for addressing problem behavior. The literature on self-monitoring and self-management is especially persuasive (e.g., Koegel et al., 1999).

3. In general, building functional skills and employing a strong educational curriculum is an effective approach for behavior support and can serve to limit the frequency and intensity of problem behaviors (Ferro et al., 1996).

4. The use of differential schedules of positive reinforcement has been extensively demonstrated to increase targeted prosocial responses and to contribute to reductions in problem behavior. We do not discuss this component of PBS in this chapter, but numerous other authors have shown it to be a valuable and well-established ingredient (e.g., Cooper, Heron, & Heward, 1987).

5. Manipulations of antecedent events, identified through functional assessments, are a proven method for producing rapid behavior change. A sizable database exists with respect to antecedent variables related to curriculum and instruction; however, a large number of additional antecedent stimuli have been identified and modified in individual experimental analyses (Luiselli, 2006).

6. A few studies have examined procedures for identifying more distal and contextual stimuli (e.g., ecological, physiological events) affecting problem behavior, and there have been some successful interventions based on these identifications. Although setting events are clearly important variables and are appropriately considered in PBS plans, the database supporting a technology of setting event assessment and intervention is not as well developed as the analogous evidence for more immediate antecedent variables (e.g., McLaughlin & Carr, 2005).

7. Multicomponent PBS interventions, based on functional assessments, have been shown in numerous investigations to be associated with reductions in problem behaviors and increases in alternative, desirable responding. A number of these studies have been conducted with individuals with developmental disabilities who have long histo-

ries of severe behavior problems, and a number have shown effects that were maintained over extended periods of time (e.g., Carr et al., 1999)

Some Important Areas in Which Our Knowledge Is Limited

Naturally, there is an immense list of issues that would be important topics for future research. In the following, we identify a few areas in which we believe our lack of information is most conspicuous from the perspective of practical importance.

1. PBS has been developed to the point that efforts are under way to rapidly make the technology available for much larger numbers of individuals with disabilities. To date, however, there have been few evaluations of PBS applied on a larger scale. It is important to develop standardized protocols so that PBS can be implemented by typical intervention agents in a range of natural community settings, and it is important to systematically evaluate the process and outcomes associated with these "scaling up" efforts. This type of research will require group comparison designs, in addition to the single-case time-series analyses that have been most common in PBS studies (Dunlap, Kincaid, & Strain, 2005).

2. Comprehensive PBS is intended to be used in multiple environments over extended periods of time; however, we have little information related to the actual implementation of PBS when applied by typical support providers in their natural contexts. With some exceptions, the fidelity data currently available have been obtained in controlled and time-limited contexts. Research on implementation will be vitally important in the coming decades (e.g., Fixsen, Naoom, Blase, Friedman, & Wallace, 2005; Hieneman & Dunlap, 2000).

3. Extended fidelity of implementation is certainly related to maintenance of behavioral improvements. Although the literature contains some encouraging demonstrations of maintenance, the mechanisms underlying success as opposed to failure over time are poorly understood. Research on maintenance of PBS effects is clearly needed.

4. Thus far, PBS research in developmental disabilities has emphasized the individual as the unit of analysis, and this is altogether appropriate. However, as the focus shifts to larger scales and questions of sustainability, it will be important to look at organizational systems and the systems variables that pertain to the delivery of effective supports over extended periods of time. The recent work in schoolwide PBS (e.g., Freeman et al., 2006; Sugai et al., 2000) offers an encouraging model for this important line of research and program development.

5. An additional area in which further knowledge is needed involves the macro-variables associated with lifestyle change (Risley, 1996). Procedures for identifying needed adjustments in lifestyle, strategies for effecting those adjustments, and comprehensive evaluation of the effects of the adjustments are needed. An excellent place to begin this substantial line of research is on the processes, implementation, and outcomes of person-centered planning.

6. Finally, it is known that the problem behaviors of individuals with disabilities have serious effects on families and other caregivers (Fox, Vaughn, Wyatte, & Dunlap, 2002); yet little is known about how PBS, including family-centered PBS, might affect the well-being of those who are closest to the individual who is the focus of the support (Lucyshyn, Dunlap, & Albin, 2002). Further research on quality of life and family functioning in association with PBS interventions would be useful for further development of PBS in family contexts.

CONCLUSION

We have attempted in this chapter to provide a brief and general overview of research on positive behavior support (PBS) and developmental disabilities. This topic is so rich that we unavoidably omitted many emphases that could have warranted a chapter unto themselves. For example, there are substantial literatures under the "PBS and developmental disabilities" umbrella in the areas of early intervention, education and inclusive schooling, adults, and families, none of which we addressed directly in this chapter. Still, the vast majority of the research that we discussed has sufficient generality that the application to particular subpopulations and contexts should be apparent. And in this era of accessible information, the interested reader should find no difficulty in pursuing a refined examination of specific PBS topics.

PBS has developed in a short period of time into an approach with a substantial database to support its principal assessment and intervention components. There is also encouraging evidence to suggest that comprehensive applications of PBS can result in important lifestyle improvements for individuals with developmental disabilities. However, it is also true that PBS is still in an early stage of research that has the ultimate goal of a widely available, efficient technology of lifestyle enhancement that is demonstrably effective, appreciated by all consumers, and sustainable within preferred arrangements of active community living. As summarized in this chapter, the strong foundations for this ongoing and longitudinal research effort offer considerable reasons for optimism.

ACKNOWLEDGMENTS

Preparation of this chapter was supported by U.S. Department of Education Grant Nos. H3234P040003 to the University of South Florida and H324X010015 and H324S030002 to the University of Oregon (with contracts to the University of South Florida), though no official endorsement by the funder should be inferred.

REFERENCES

Albin, R. W., Lucyshyn, J. M., Horner, R. H., & Flannery, K. B. (1996). Contextual fit for behavior support plans: A model for "goodness of fit." In L. Koegel, R. Koegel, & G. Dunlap (Eds.), *Positive behavioral support: Including people with difficult behavior in the community* (pp. 81–98). Baltimore: Brookes.

Bambara, L. (2005). Evolution of positive behavior support. In L. Bambara & L. Kern (Eds.), *Individualized supports for students with problem behaviors: Designing positive behavior plans* (pp. 1–24). New York: Guilford Press.

Carr, E. G. (1977). The motivation of self-injurious behavior: A review of some hypotheses. *Psychological Bulletin, 84*, 800–816.

Carr, E. G. (1988). Functional equivalence as a mechanism of response generalization. In R. H. Horner, G. Dunlap, & R. L. Koegel (Eds.), *Generalization and maintenance: Lifestyle changes in applied settings* (pp. 221–241), Baltimore: Brookes.

Carr, E. G., & Carlson, J. I. (1993). Reduction of severe behavior problems in the community using a multicomponent treatment approach. *Journal of Applied Behavior Analysis, 26*, 157–172.

Carr, E. G., Dunlap, G., Horner, R. H., Koegel, R. L., Turnbull, A. P., Sailor, W., et al. (2002). Positive behavior support: Evolution of an applied science. *Journal of Positive Behavior Interventions, 4*(1), 4–16.

Carr, E. G., & Durand, V. M. (1985). Reducing behavior problems through functional communication training. *Journal of Applied Behavior Analysis, 18,* 111–126.

Carr, E. G., Horner, R. H., Turnbull, A. P., Marquis, J., Magito-McLaughlin, D., McAtee, M. L., et al. (1999). *Positive behavior support for people with developmental disabilities: A research synthesis.* Washington, DC: American Association on Mental Retardation.

Carr, E. G., Levin, L., McConnachie, G., Carlson, J. I., Kemp, D. C., & Smith, C. E. (1994). *Communication-based interventions for problem behavior: A user's guide for producing behavior change.* Baltimore: Brookes.

Carr, E. G., Levin, L., McConnachie, G., Carlson, J. I., Kemp, D. C., Smith, C. E., et al. (1999). Comprehensive multisituational intervention for problem behavior in the community: Long term maintenance and social validation. *Journal of Positive Behavior Interventions, 1,* 5–25.

Carr, E. G., Newsom, C. D., & Binkoff, J. A. (1980). Escape as a factor in the aggressive behavior of two retarded children. *Journal of Applied Behavior Analysis, 13,* 101–117.

Carr, J. E., & LeBlanc, L. A. (2006). In J. K. Luiselli (Ed.), *Antecedent assessment intervention: Supporting children and adults with developmental disabilities in community settings* (pp. 147–164). Baltimore: Brookes.

Clarke, S., Worcester, J., Dunlap, G., Murray, M., & Bradley-Klug, K. (2002). Using multiple measures to evaluate positive behavior support: A case example. *Journal of Positive Behavior Interventions, 4,* 131–145.

Conroy, M. A., Dunlap, G., Clarke, S., & Alter, P. J. (2005). A descriptive analysis of positive behavioral intervention research with young children with challenging behavior. *Topics in Early Childhood Special Education, 25,* 157–166.

Cooper, J. O., Heron, T. E., & Heward, W. L. (1987). *Applied behavior analysis.* Upper Saddle River, NJ: Merrill.

Derby, K. M., Wacker, D. P., Berg, W., DeRaad, A., Ulrich, S., Asmus, J., et al. (1997). The long-term effects of functional communication training in home settings. *Journal of Applied Behavior Analysis, 30,* 507–531.

Dunlap, G. (2004). Critical features of positive behavior support. *APBS Newsletter, 1,* 1–3.

Dunlap, G. (2006). The applied behavior analytic heritage of PBS: A dynamic model of action-oriented research. *Journal of Positive Behavior Interventions, 8,* 58–60.

Dunlap, G., Carr, E. G., & Horner, R. H. (2006). *Positive behavior support and applied behavior analysis: A familial alliance.* Manuscript in preparation.

Dunlap, G., Clarke, S., & Steiner, M. (1999). Intervention research in behavioral and developmental disabilities: 1980 to 1997. *Journal of Positive Behavior Interventions, 1,* 170–180.

Dunlap, G., Ester, T., Langhans, S., & Fox, L. (2006). Functional communication training with toddlers in home environments. *Journal of Early Intervention, 28,* 81–96.

Dunlap, G., & Kern, L. (1996). Modifying instructional activities to promote desirable behavior: A conceptual and practical framework. *School Psychology Quarterly, 11,* 297–312.

Dunlap, G., Kern-Dunlap, L., Clarke, S., & Robbins, F. R. (1991). Functional assessment, curricular revision, and severe problems. *Journal of Applied Behavior Analysis, 24,* 387–397.

Dunlap, G., & Kincaid, D. (2001). The widening world of functional assessment: Comments on four manuals and beyond. *Journal of Applied Behavior Analysis, 34,* 365–377.

Dunlap, G., Kincaid, D., & Strain, P. (2005). A randomized control group study of positive behavior support. *APBS Newsletter, 3,* 1–2.

Durand, V. M. (1990). *Severe behavior problems: A functional communication training approach.* New York: Guilford Press.

Feldman, M. A., Condillac, R. A., Tough, S., Hunt, S., & Griffiths, D. (2002). Effectiveness of community positive behavioral intervention for persons with developmental disabilities and severe behavior disorders. *Behavior Therapy, 33,* 377–398.

Ferro, J., Foster-Johnson, L., & Dunlap, G. (1996). Relation between curricular activities and problem behaviors of students with mental retardation. *American Journal on Mental Retardation, 101,* 184–194.

Fixsen, D. L., Naoom, S. F., Blase, K. A., Friedman, R. M., & Wallace, F. (2005). *Implementation research: A synthesis of the literature.* Tampa: Florida Mental Heath Institute, University of South Florida.

Fox, L., Vaughn, B., Wyatte, M. L., & Dunlap, G. (2002). "We can't expect other people to understand": The perspectives of families whose children have problem behavior. *Exceptional Children, 68,* 437–450.

Frea, W. D., & Hughes, C. (1997). Functional analysis and treatment of social-communicative behavior of adolescents with developmental disabilities. *Journal of Applied Behavior Analysis, 30,* 701–704.

Freeman, R., Eber, L., Anderson, C., Irvin, L., Bounds, M., Dunlap, G., et al. (2006). Building inclusive school cultures using school-wide PBS: Designing effective individual support systems for students with significant disabilities. *Research and Practice in Severe Disabilities, 31,* 4–17.

Green, C. W., Middleton, S. G., & Reid, D. H. (2000). Embedded evaluation of preference sample from person-centered plans for people with profound multiple disabilities. *Journal of Applied Behavior Analysis, 33,* 639–642.

Guess, D., Helmstetter, E., Turnbull, H. R., & Knowlton, S. (1987). *Use of aversive procedures with persons who are disabled: An historical review and critical analysis.* Seattle, WA: Association for Persons with Severe Handicaps.

Halle, J., Bambara, L. M., & Reichle, J. (2005). Teaching alternative skills. In L. Bambara & L. Kern (Eds.), *Individualized supports for students with problem behaviors: Designing positive behavior plans* (pp. 237–274). New York: Guilford Press.

Hieneman, M., & Dunlap, G. (2000). Factors affecting the outcomes of community-based behavioral support: Identification and description of factor categories. *Journal of Positive Behavior Interventions, 2,* 161–169.

Holburn, S., & Vietze, P. M. (Eds.). (2002). *Person-centered planning: Research, practice, and future directions.* Baltimore: Brookes.

Horner, R. H., & Budd, C. M. (1985). Acquisition of manual sign use: Collateral reduction of maladaptive behavior, and factors limiting generalization. *Education and Training of the Mentally Retarded, 20,* 39–47.

Horner, R. H., Dunlap, G., Beasley, J., Fox, L., Bambara, L., Brown, F., et al. (2005). Positive support for behavioral, mental health, communication and crisis needs. In K. C. Lakin & A. P. Turnbull (Eds.), *National goals and research for persons with intellectual and developmental disabilities* (pp. 93–107). Washington, DC: American Association on Mental Retardation.

Horner, R. H., Dunlap, G., Koegel, R. L., Carr, E. G., Sailor, W., Anderson, J., et al. (1990). Toward a technology of "non-aversive" behavioral support. *Journal of the Association for Persons with Severe Handicaps, 15,* 125–132.

Iwata, B., Dorsey, M., Slifer, K., Bauman, K., & Richman, G. (1994). Toward a functional analysis of self-injury. *Journal of Applied Behavior Analysis, 27,* 197–209. (Reprinted from *Analysis and Intervention in Developmental Disabilities,* 1982, *2,* 3–20)

Kern, L., & Clarke, S. (2005). Antecedent and setting event interventions. In L. Bambara & L. Kern (Eds.), *Individualized supports for students with problem behaviors: Designing positive behavior plans* (pp. 201–236). New York: Guilford Press.

Kincaid, D., & Fox, L. (2002). Person-centered planning and positive behavior support. In S. Holburn & P. M. Vietze (Eds.), *Person-centered planning: Research, practice, and future directions* (pp. 29–50). Baltimore: Brookes.

Koegel, L. K., Harrower, J. K., & Koegel, R. L. (1999). Support for children with developmental disabilities in full inclusion classrooms through self-management. *Journal of Positive Behavioral Interventions, 1,* 26–34.

Lucyshyn, J. M., Albin, R. W., & Nixon, C. D. (1997). Embedding comprehensive behavioral support in family ecology: An experimental, single-case analysis. *Journal of Consulting and Clinical Psychology, 65,* 241–251.

Lucyshyn, J. M., Dunlap, G., & Albin, R. W. (Eds.) (2002). *Families and positive behavior support: Addressing problem behavior in family contexts.* Baltimore: Brookes.

Luiselli, J. K. (Ed.) (2006). *Antecedent assessment intervention: Supporting children and adults with developmental disabilities in community settings.* Baltimore: Brookes.

Luiselli, J. K., & Cameron, M. J. (Eds.). (1998). *Antecedent control: Innovative approaches to behavioral support.* Baltimore: Brookes.

McAtee, M., Carr, E. G., & Schulte, C. (2004). A contextual assessment inventory for problem behavior: Initial development. *Journal of Positive Behavior Interventions, 6,* 148–165.

McGill, P. (1999). Establishing operations: Implications for the assessment, treatment, and prevention of problem behavior. *Journal of Applied Behavior Analysis, 32,* 393–418.

McLaughlin, D. M., & Carr, E. G. (2005). Quality of rapport as a setting event for problem behavior: Assessment and intervention. *Journal of Positive Behavior Interventions, 7,* 68–91.

Meyer, L. H., & Evans, I. M. (1989). *Nonaversive interventions for problem behaviors: A manual for home and community*. Baltimore: Brookes.

O'Neill, R. E., Horner, R. H., Albin, R. W., Storey, K., Sprague, J. R., & Newton, J. S. (1997). *Functional assessment of problem behavior: A practical assessment guide*. Pacific Grove, CA: Brooks/Cole.

Repp, A. C., & Horner, R. H. (Eds.). (1999). *Functional analysis of problem behavior: From effective assessment to effective support*. Belmont, CA: Wadsworth.

Risley, T. R. (1996). Get a life! In L. K. Koegel, R. L. Koegel, & G. Dunlap (Eds.), *Positive behavioral support* (pp. 425–437). Baltimore: Brookes.

Risley, T. R. (1999). Foreword: Positive behavioral support and applied behavior analysis. In E. G. Carr, R. H. Horner, A. P. Turnbull, J. Marquis, D. Magito-McLaughlin, M. L. McAtee, et al. (Eds.), *Positive behavior support for people with developmental disabilities: A research synthesis* (pp. xi–xiii). Washington, DC: American Association on Mental Retardation.

Scotti, J. R., Ujcich, K. J., Weigle, K. L., Holland, C. M., & Kirk, K. S. (1996). Interventions with challenging behavior of persons with developmental disabilities: A review of current research practices. *Journal of the Association for Persons with Severe Handicaps, 21*, 123–134.

Sugai, G., Horner, R. H., Dunlap, G., Hieneman, M., Lewis, T. J., Nelson, C. M., et al. (2000). Applying positive behavior support and functional behavioral assessment in schools. *Journal of Positive Behavior Interventions, 2*(3), 131–143.

Touchette, P. E., MacDonald, R. F., & Langer, S. N. (1985). A scatter plot for identifying stimulus control of problem behavior. *Journal of Applied Behavior Analysis, 18*, 343–351.

Umbreit, J., Ferro, J., Liaupsin, C., & Lane, K. L. (2007). *Functional behavioral assessment and function-based intervention: An effective, practical approach*. Englewood Cliffs, NJ: Merrill/Prentice-Hall.

Vaughn, B. J., Dunlap, G., Fox, L., Clarke, S., & Bucy, M. (1997). Parent–professional partnership in behavioral support: A case study of community-based intervention. *Journal of the Association for Persons with Severe Handicaps, 22*, 185–197.

Weeks, M., & Gaylord-Ross, R. (1981). Task difficulty and aberrant behavior in severely handicapped students. *Journal of Applied Behavior Analysis, 14*, 449–463.

24

Mental Health Supports in Developmental Disabilities

Dimitrios Paschos
Nick Bouras

Good mental health is an essential requirement for a good quality of life. The successful integration of people experiencing mental health problems into the community relies on the amount and quality of available mental health supports. The field of developmental disabilities has focused recently on matching appropriate supports to individual needs, so the importance of providing highly specialized mental health supports for people with developmental disabilities has become apparent. This chapter presents recent advances in the assessment and management of mental health problems in this population, discusses current trends in service provision and policy, and highlights areas for future research.

The term "developmental disabilities" is used in this chapter to mean "intellectual disabilities" or "mental retardation" (World Health Organization, 1992; American Psychiatric Association, 2000). Most of the research quoted refers to adults with developmental disabilities in the United Kingdom, Europe, and the United States, due to the limited number of large international studies and studies involving children. Where case vignettes have been used, biographical and other details have been altered to preserve confidentiality.

EPIDEMIOLOGY

Understanding that many people with developmental disabilities have mental health problems is important for planning treatment, supports, and service provision and can help increase our knowledge about the etiology of these conditions. Despite increased research activity in the past decade, results from epidemiological studies remain inconclusive and sometimes conflicting (Smiley, 2005). Kerker, Owens, Zigler, and Horwitz (2004) identified more than 200 peer-reviewed articles, government documents, national and international reports, and book chapters on the mental health of people with developmental disabilities. The analysis of the studies included in their review ($n = 52$) revealed inconsistent estimates of prevalence and discrepancies in methodologies used, populations studied, and conceptual approaches to both developmental disabilities and mental health problems. There are several reasons for the wide variation in the reported prevalence rates, the most important of which are sampling and recruitment (case ascertainment) bias. Population-based studies are rare in this field; additionally, the majority of surveys have drawn small samples from people either living in the community and receiving specialist services or living in institutional settings. It is likely, therefore, that people with mental health needs may be overrepresented in administratively defined samples and, conversely, that samples drawn from institutional settings may not be representative of the community population.

The way mental health problems are assessed can also affect the reported prevalence rates. Medical chart reviews reveal fewer cases than does the use of standardized screening instruments, and clinical interviews with experienced assessors can diagnose even more people (Horwitz, Kerker, Owens, & Zigler, 2000). There is also disagreement on whether existing psychiatric classification systems such as the ICD-10 (World Health Organization, 1992) or the DSM-IV (American Psychiatric Association, 1994) can provide a valid framework for diagnosing psychiatric disorders in people with developmental disabilities, especially in those with more severe cognitive impairments. In addition, different definitions of developmental disabilities or other related diagnostic labels have also led to inconsistencies in the reported frequencies.

Some authors have included conditions such as attention-deficit/hyperactivity disorder, autism, and behavioral disorders in their overall estimation of prevalence rates. It seems that, if these conditions are excluded, the prevalence of mental health problems in people with developmental disabilities might be comparable to that found in the general population. Deb, Thomas, and Bright (2001), using rigorous methodology and standardized assessment instruments, demonstrated an overall prevalence of mental health problems (excluding behavioral problems) of 14.4% in an administratively defined random sample of 101 adults with developmental disabilities living in the community.

Most categories of mental health problems have been reported in people with developmental disabilities. Research findings suggest an increased prevalence of anxiety and affective disorders across the whole spectrum of people with developmental disabilities and of schizophrenia spectrum disorders in those with mild developmental disabilities (Bouras et al., 2004; Cowley et al., 2004). No consensus has yet been reached on the etiology of these findings. There is, however, wider agreement on the reported syndrome-specific increased risk for certain mental disorders, such as, for example, Alzheimer's disease in people with Down syndrome, psychosis and compulsive behaviors in people with Prader–Willi syndrome, and schizophrenia in people with velocardiofacial syndrome (Murphy & Owen, 2001; Baker & Skuse, 2005). Overall, people with developmental disabilities experience common mental health problems at the same or even higher rates in comparison with the nondisabled population. Furthermore, the frequent coexistence of behavioral disturbance substantially increases the need for sufficient and effective specialist mental health supports for this population.

ASSESSMENT AND SCREENING

Diagnosing mental health problems in people with developmental disabilities is a complex and challenging process. The accuracy of such diagnosis depends on multiple factors intrinsic to both the patient and the assessor. In many ways, the assessment of mental health problems in people with developmental disabilities follows the same principles as the psychiatric assessment of people without developmental disabilities. Referral pathways, however, seem to be different, and special considerations are necessary in certain aspects of the assessment process. It is very rare for people with developmental disabilities to initiate a mental health referral themselves. Usually, they have to rely on family or residential staff to identify the problem, with most common reason for referral being behavioral disturbance. Subtle or insidiously developing changes in mood, sleep, or appetite are less likely to be detected. In many parts of the world, a further difficulty is the lack of access to specialist mental health services with expertise in the mental health of people with developmental disabilities.

Conceptualizing how the presentation might be a synthesis of vulnerability and of precipitating and maintaining factors (biological, psychological, social, and environmental) is a complex task and requires a coordinated multimodal and interdisciplinary approach to assessment (O'Hara, 2007). This biopsychosocial approach can be also applied when developing an intervention package (Hardy & Holt, 2005). In assessing mental health problems in people with developmental disabilities in a comprehensive way, the norm is to gather information from multiple sources. There is a well-documented requirement that this process be coordinated and managed by one particular team member who is able to understand and integrate the different strands of information. Confidentiality and sharing of information should always be addressed at an early stage of the assessment process.

The initial assessment interview is sometimes best conducted at the person's home. Some people may have difficulties attending an outpatient appointment; furthermore, observing the person's living environment can be very revealing. The length of the interview must also be flexible to accommodate people with memory or attention-span problems, and several short sessions may be scheduled. Special attention to the presence of sensory problems is necessary. The concepts of "psychosocial masking," "cognitive disintegration," "baseline exaggeration," and "diagnostic overshadowing" have all been reported as potential hurdles in eliciting psychiatric symptoms and signs in people with developmental disabilities (Sturmey, 1999).

Some people with developmental disabilities may be suggestible and acquiescent, and therefore leading questions are best avoided. Open questions, questions with multiple choices, and sometimes contradictory questions may be asked to ensure comprehension. Direct observation and physical examination of the person is always important. It may also be necessary to ask the person, his or her family, or residential staff members to monitor symptoms and behaviors over a period of time (Deb, Matthews, Holt, & Bouras, 2001). The degree of developmental disabilities also needs to be considered, because, for example, people with more severe developmental disabilities are more likely to show atypical signs and symptoms or behavioral problems. Developmentally appropriate phenomena, such as talking to oneself or imaginary friends, should be distinguished from psychotic phenomena, such as auditory hallucinations (Hurley & Silka, 2003).

A crucial aspect of the initial assessment is to rule out any physical cause for the mental health symptoms or behavioral problem. This is also true for the nondisabled population, but it is even more important for people with developmental disabilities, who often have significant physical health needs (U.S. Public Health Service, 2002; National Health Service Scotland, 2004). A careful physical examination, appropriate investigations (blood tests, imaging), and the review of any concurrent medical conditions are an essential part of the screening phase. Side effects from prescribed medication can sometimes mimic or cause psychiatric symptoms; therefore, a medication history, including previous dosing, duration of treatment, effectiveness, and side effects, is always necessary. A comprehensive risk assessment estimating the risk to self and/or others, as well as the risk of self-neglect, abuse, and exploitation, should also be a routine component of the assessment pathway.

Establishing a psychiatric diagnosis for a person with developmental disabilities can be particularly difficult, because of certain limitations within the current classification systems. Most psychiatric symptoms are described with the use of language-based phenomenology. Therefore, the severity of any cognitive or language deficits is bound to influence the reliability of such diagnoses. To overcome this difficulty, attempts have been made to modify criteria of existing diagnostic classifications or to describe behavioral correlates of psychiatric symptoms. In the United Kingdom, the Royal College of Psychiatrists (2001) recognized these problems and produced the *Diagnostic Criteria for Psychiatric Disorders for Use with Adults with Learning Disabilities/Mental Retardation* (DC-LD), to be used alongside ICD-10. Diagnostic accuracy can be improved with the use of structured instruments, such as the Psychiatric Assessment Schedule for Adults with a Developmental Disability (PAS-ADD) Checklist (Moss et al., 1998; Sturmey, Newton, Cowley, Bouras, & Holt, 2005); however, such instruments have psychometric limitations and should not substitute for a thorough clinical assessment.

The assessment should aim not only to arrive at a diagnosis but also to integrate information on accommodation, support networks, activities, and ability to cope with change. Revisiting the working diagnosis on a frequent basis is essential. Several times, intervention and supports will be required, even when no definite or even provisional diagnosis can be made.

MENTAL HEALTH PROBLEMS AND BEHAVIOR DISTURBANCE

Behavior supports and interventions are explored in length in Chapters 23 and 25, this volume. Before presenting common mental illness, it may be helpful to comment on the interplay of mental health problems and behavioral disturbance. Meaningful associations between problem behaviors and specific psychiatric conditions have been widely documented. For example, increased prevalence of affective symptoms (depressed or elated mood), anxiety symptoms, and higher psychopathology scores in persons with self-injurious, stereotyped, or aggressive behavior has been reported (Moss et al., 2000; Rojahn, Matson, Naglieri, & Mayville, 2004). It is also recognized that multiple other factors may predispose to, trigger, or maintain problem behaviors, such as the presence of certain genetic syndromes, physical ill health, epilepsy, communication and sensory difficulties, and autism-related social impairment (Hurley & Silka, 2004). The extent to which a psychiatric disorder contributes to behavior disturbance is sometimes impossible to ascertain, and, consequently, an integrated diagnostic and treatment approach is paramount. A behavior disorder is more likely to be due to mental illness if behavior problems occur across all settings, do not respond to well-designed behavioral interventions, and are associated with changes in biological features such as sleep, appetite, or autonomic activity.

COMMON MENTAL HEALTH PROBLEMS

People with mild developmental disabilities and good verbal skills present similar psychiatric symptoms to those presented by people without developmental disabilities. The presence of more severe cognitive impairment or autistic spectrum disorders increases the likelihood that psychiatric symptoms can present atypically and may cause or aggravate a preexisting behavior disturbance.

In relation to specific psychiatric diagnoses, a higher incidence of *schizophrenia* spectrum disorders has been consistently reported in the literature, particularly in people with mild developmental disabilities (Cowley et al., 2004). Although there are genetic conditions that increase the risk of developing psychosis (Vogels et al., 2004), the association between developmental disabilities and schizophrenia is generally not well understood. The classic symptoms of hallucinations, delusions, disorganized speech, grossly disorganized behavior, and negative symptoms may be difficult to accurately diagnose in adults with developmental disabilities. It is sometimes hard to be certain whether hallucinations are being experienced by a person with developmental disabilities (Royal College of Psychiatrists, 2001; Pickard & Paschos, 2005), especially in the presence of developmentally appropriate phenomena, such as speaking to oneself or to imaginary friends. Delusional beliefs are reported to be simpler in content. Odd behaviors, idiosyncratic speech, sensory impairments, epilepsy, and stress-related confusion can challenge assessors, and what may seem to be "negative symptoms" can in fact be the result of medication, depression, or an understimulating environment (Deb, Matthews, et al., 2001). There is, finally, evidence that people with developmental disabilities and schizophrenia spectrum disorders are more debilitated by the co-occurring disorder than are people with schizophrenia without developmental disabilities. Also, for the treatment to be beneficial, a more focused and time-consuming multimodal work is required (Bouras et al., 2004).

Depression is more common in people with developmental disabilities and, in a similar pattern to the general population, is frequently undiagnosed. Several factors are thought to increase the vulnerability of people with developmental disabilities to becoming depressed, such as higher rates of physical illness, socioeconomic adversity, and reduced life supports (Richards et al., 2001; De Collishaw & Maughan, 2004). Biological predisposition, especially in those with epilepsy, has also been suggested. In people with developmental disabilities who become depressed, the whole range of psychological and somatic symptoms of depression can be observed, but changes are often subtle and develop over time. Atypical symptoms, such as weight gain instead of weight loss, are common; moreover, self-injurious or destructive behavior may dominate the clinical picture for people with more severe developmental disabilities (Gravestock, Flynn, & Hemmings, 2005). Exclusion of medical conditions or side effects of medication and ongoing multidisciplinary assessment of the risk of self-harm or suicide is always a top priority. Structured tools, such as the Glasgow Depression Scale for People with a Learning Disability, may help increase the accuracy of such diagnosis (Cuthill, Espie, & Cooper, 2003). The treatment follows the same principles as that for people without developmental disabilities, consisting of a combination of medication and psychological treatment, alongside the provision of adequate environmental and life supports.

Bipolar affective disorder (episodes of depression and mania) can be confidently diagnosed in persons with developmental disabilities (Cain et al., 2003). Rapid-cycling bipolar disorder (more than four episodes of either mania or depression in a year) is thought to be more common among this population (Vanstraelen & Tyrer, 1999). When people with developmental disabilities experience a manic episode, it is possible that their moods are predominantly irritable rather than euphoric. Other symptoms may include overactivity, rambling speech, aggression, and disinhibition. Mixed affective states are also known to be common. Some people with developmental disabilities and/or autism appear to show cyclical changes in their behavior accompanied by altered mood. There may be other factors to account for this, such as physical factors (e.g., menstrual cycle in women) and other environmental ones (Deb, Matthews, et al., 2001).

As the life expectancy of many persons with developmental disabilities has increased in the past decades, an increasing number of people are being diagnosed with *dementia*. The higher incidence of early-onset Alzheimer's disease in people with Down syndrome is now firmly established, and several possible risk factors have been suggested (Tyrrell et al., 2001; Bush & Beail, 2004). An important part of the assessment of suspected cases of dementia is the exclusion of any treatable condition and comorbid physical (e.g., hypothyroidism) or mental (depression) illness. Equally important is establishing a "baseline"—in other words, documenting the highest level of functioning that the person had—and deciding which cognitive deficits may be longstanding. Personality change is sometimes associated with involvement of frontal lobes, and sensory deficits may complicate the clinical picture. There is still only limited research on the effectiveness of acetylcholinesterase inhibitors (the latest "antidementia" drugs) in slowing the decline of cognitive and functional ability in Alzheimer's disease in people with Down syndrome. Despite some small trials reporting beneficial results, concerns have been expressed about the tolerability of this treatment. If such agents are to be tried, a slow titration should be the norm (Stanton & Coetzee, 2004).

Anxiety disorders in psychiatric classification include a number of distinct conditions, such as phobias, generalized anxiety, panic disorder, obsessive–compulsive disorder (OCD), and posttraumatic stress disorder (PTSD). These disorders are recognized in persons with developmental disabilities and are thought to be at least as common as (and probably more common than) they are in people without developmental disabilities, but they tend to be underreported. In particular, repetitive behaviors in individuals with developmental disabilities may be difficult to categorize (Stavrakaki & Lunsky, 2007) and to distinguish from stereotyped behaviors, symptoms of OCD, or self-stimulating behaviors. Increased risk of OCD has been reported in people with Prader–Willi syndrome (Clarke et al., 2002). Anxiety that occurs in some people with autism when routines are changed should be considered part of the autism disorder and not a superimposed anxiety disorder (Deb, Matthews, et al., 2001).

People with developmental disabilities may be particularly vulnerable to PTSD because of the increased incidence of traumatic experiences, such as sexual abuse, in this population. The diagnosis of PTSD in people who do not have the communication skills to describe their experiences, feelings, and moods may be hindered, and PTSD symptoms may be attributed to other psychiatric diagnoses (McCarthy, 2001). The management and treatment of anxiety disorders parallel those used for the general population, including cognitive, psychotherapeutic, and behavioral approaches and sometimes appropriate medication (Cooray & Bakala, 2005).

Research on *substance misuse* in people with developmental disabilities shows a lower level of use of both alcohol and illicit drugs compared with the general population (McGillicuddy, 2006). Those people, however, who do misuse substances may suffer excess morbidity and mortality, mainly because of coexisting physical disorders. Gaps in service provision for people with this "triple" diagnosis have been reported.

The diagnosis of *personality disorders* in adults with developmental disabilities is particularly difficult. The reason is that it is sometimes hard to obtain an accurate baseline for behaviors and a reliable long-term account of functioning and symptoms; additionally, there is a significant symptom overlap with other psychiatric and behavior disorders (Royal College of Psychiatrists, 2001; Alexander & Cooray, 2003).

When attempting to diagnose a mental health problem in people with developmental disabilities, it is important to remember the constant and complex interplay of biological, environmental, psychological, and social factors that can shape the manifestation of such problems, as the following case illustrates.

CASE VIGNETTE 1

Mr. A is 25 years old and has a genetic syndrome and mild developmental disabilities. He lives in independent accommodation with community supports, works part time on a voluntary basis, and attends a day center for people with developmental disabilities. He also visits his family weekly and goes to a local bar to drink alcohol at least twice a week. His physical health is good. Two years ago, he was sexually assaulted and robbed while he was returning home from a bar. The perpetrator was never caught. A few months after the event, Mr. A presented with low mood, sleep disturbance, suicidal ideas, and recurrent thoughts about the attack. A provisional diagnosis of PTSD was made, and he was treated with antidepressants and counseling provided by a specialist PTSD center.

His mood initially improved, but a few months later he developed paranoid delusions about his neighbor and started hearing "voices" (auditory hallucinations). His global functioning deteriorated, and he increased his drinking. A diagnosis of schizophrenia was suggested, and an antipsychotic medication was added. In parallel, he was offered counseling for his drinking and regular support at home by a community psychiatric nurse with expertise in developmental disabilities. A couple of weeks after starting treatment, his psychotic symptoms resolved, but he developed a rash, which was thought to be a side effect of the antipsychotic medication. Careful observations by his housing support worker revealed bed bugs causing the problem, and a change of linen, rather than a change of medication, helped clear the rash. At present, Mr. A remains symptom-free, and his alcohol consumption is limited.

TREATMENT OF MENTAL HEALTH PROBLEMS IN DEVELOPMENTAL DISABILITIES

Pharmacotherapy

The treatment with psychotropic medication and relevant issues are discussed in depth in Chapter 25 in this volume; however, some basic principles on best prescribing practices are outlined here. Historically, psychotropic medications have been inappropriately and excessively used to control difficult behaviors in people with developmental disabilities. There is little controlled research on the use of medication in this population, and most of the evidence is extrapolated from studies conducted in the general population. Concomitant medical conditions, interaction with other prescribed (especially antiepileptic) medication, previous response to medication, and sensitivities and allergies, as well as consent and ethical issues, should always be considered. The prescribing physician must ensure that a thorough physical, psychological, social, and behavioral assessment has been carried out before prescribing and that a date for reviewing the need for treatment (once efficacy is established) is arranged (Einfeld, 2001). To maximize effectiveness, treatment with medication should be only part of a broader and holistic person-centered treatment plan. Routine collection of outcome data regarding target symptoms and a slow titration with frequent checks for side effects is recommended.

Polypharmacy is best avoided, because of the high risk of drug interactions and side effects and the lack of relevant evidence. Moreover, if several medications are prescribed at the same time, it is hard to clarify which medications are effective and which are causing side effects. Clear guidelines are also needed regarding the use of "as required" medication and "rapid tranquilization" regimens in residential and hospital settings. Deescalation and behavioral strategies should be used first to control difficult or violent behavior (Deb, Clark, & Unwin, 2006). Doctors prescribing psychotropic medication should remember that the relationship between mental health problems and behavior is complex and that other interventions may be effective when medication fails to control unacceptable behaviors, as shown in the following case vignette.

CASE VIGNETTE 2

Ms. M is a 35-year-old woman with a history of moderate intellectual disabilities, severe autism, and behavior disturbance, which includes verbal and physical aggression, self-injurious behavior, and inappropriate sexual behaviors. Over the years she was given an additional diagnosis of unspecified psychosis with affective symptoms. A year ago her behavior deteriorated; after that she needed constant supervision, and, on some days, more than 200 instances of problem behaviors were recorded. She was prescribed a high dose of a depot antipsychotic injection, two anticonvulsants for mood stabilization, and benzodiazepines, both regularly and on an "as required" basis. Two previous trials of antidepressants, lithium, and conventional antipsychotics had made little difference.

For many years Ms. M lived in a secure unit for people with developmental disabilities and behavioral disturbance, with little access to the community. Following a review of her care arrangements, she was transferred to a secure small residential unit for people with autism and problem behaviors. Within 4 weeks a reduction in most problematic behaviors of up to 90% was recorded. No changes in her medication had occurred. The difference in the new setting was that all care staff members had formal qualifications in positive behavior support and special training in autism and used an individually designed and consistent approach with Ms. M from day 1. Much to the disbelief of her previous care staff, Ms. M is now attending a day center in the community, and her medication is being reduced.

Psychological Interventions

Large-scale provision of psychological therapies for people with developmental disabilities has been slow to emerge because of previous assumptions about the suitability of this group for talking treatments. This attitude, previously described as "therapeutic disdain" (Bender, 1993), is now being replaced by a growing awareness that, with appropriate adaptations, people with developmental disabilities can make use of most available psychological therapies and that the therapeutic benefits can be significant for families and staff as well (Hurley, 2005). Research evidence supporting the effectiveness of these interventions is scarce, partly because of the relatively late occurrence of psychotherapies for people with developmental disabilities and partly because of methodological obstacles. Furthermore, the presence of intellectual impairment is usually an exclusion criterion in most research studies on the effectiveness of psychological treatments conducted in the general population. Case studies tend to dominate the literature, and even though very few report on outcome data, they are still useful as powerful case descriptions and as illustrations of the application and techniques of particular therapeutic modalities.

Most of the available research focuses on behavioral interventions, perhaps because, historically, this has been the mainstream approach for people with developmental disabilities. Recently, two meta-analyses of a small number of controlled and comparable studies have shown at least moderate benefit for people with developmental disabilities engaging in a wide range of psychological treatments. In particular, schema-focused cognitive work was shown to have a lasting effect on a sample of people with moderate developmental disabilities (Prout & Nowak-Drabik, 2003; Royal College of Psychiatrists, 2004b).

Despite the lack of measurable outcomes, the reported studies have helped to increase health and social care professionals' understanding of emotional and psychological issues in people with developmental disabilities. Because of the increased risk of physical and sexual abuse and the insensitive treatment and stigmatization of people with developmental disabilities, the effects of trauma on their lives have attracted particular attention (Hollins & Sinason, 2000). Several psychological treatment modalities can be employed when working with people with developmental disabilities and mental health or emotional problems.

Approaches based on *behavioral models* are the most widely researched and have been in use for several years. *Cognitive-behavioral therapy* (CBT) provides a framework for understanding the type of difficulties people with developmental disabilities can have in perceiving or identifying emotional states in themselves or others. Through adaptation of mainstream CBT interventions, models have been developed to treat depression and anxiety disorders, to teach assertiveness and other social skills, and also to inform anger management interventions. Role play, role reversal, and the inclusion of nonverbal materials, visual aids, drawings, photographs and picture storybooks are commonly used to enhance CBT techniques (Royal College of Psychiatrists, 2004b; Dangan, 2007).

Some people with developmental disabilities may find it difficult to express negative feelings, such as anger, toward people on whom they depend. *Psychodynamic theories* suggest that verbalization of such unacknowledged feelings can result in therapeutic benefit. Issues of sexuality, dependency needs, trauma, illness, and death can be too difficult to discuss for some people with developmental disabilities, and a sensitive approach is required. Psychodynamic therapists often mention the "secondary handicap," referring to the effect the primary disability has on the person (Hollins & Sinason, 2000; Parkes & Hollins, 2007). As with many other treatment modalities, there is a lack of controlled research to support the degree of effectiveness of this type of approach.

Family and systemic therapies consider the person as part of his or her family or in his or her social context. It is hoped that changing one part of the system causes a reaction in other parts, as well. Working with families may be the main focus of therapeutic supports and can enhance the effectiveness of other interventions. *Nondirective counseling* or *person-centered therapy* is also considered to be a powerful approach for people with developmental disabilities whose personal experiences are often ignored or discounted (Oliver & Smith, 2005). More recently, the application of *dialectical behavior therapy* for people with developmental disabilities has been described (Lew, Matta, Tripp-Tebo, & Watts, 2006). Finally, *art, drama*, and *music* therapy have all been used with persons with developmental disabilities at different developmental stages and with people who have autism. With the use of a variety of media and communication alternatives, these forms of therapy are thought to allow choice and to foster the growth of self-esteem. There is, however, a lack of controlled studies regarding these usually less structured interventions.

Presently, no particular type of model or approach seems to be superior. Issues other than diagnosis, such as availability of local resources, sometimes determine what type of therapy is provided. Using an array of interventions is most helpful. Moreover, modifying the approach to match individual needs makes a positive outcome more likely. Unfortunately, many generic psychotherapy services are excluding people with developmental disabilities, viewing them as a separate population. Although specialist skills may be required to work with some people with developmental disabilities, a large number should be able to benefit from generic psychotherapy services (Royal College of Psychiatrists, 2004b).

The lack of robust, empirically validated data on outcomes should not prevent providers and funding agencies from making appropriate types of therapy available to persons with developmental disabilities and emotional or psychiatric problems. However, the issues of the treatment's length and the expectations from it should be addressed early, as this is an area vulnerable to inappropriate or poor-quality therapy. It is imperative that therapists are properly supervised and have a good understanding of issues related to developmental disabilities, or, ideally, that they are dually trained.

Social Interventions and Environmental Supports

Social interventions and environmental supports have been discussed in detail in previous chapters. Environmental and social causes of psychiatric morbidity are widely reported, and there is a strong association between lower socioeconomic status, social exclusion, and mental illness. A review of the person's housing situation, daily activities, environment and life supports, and social opportunities is necessary at the beginning of assessment, and extra supports are usually necessary to effect or maintain positive change in the person's mental health.

EPILEPSY, AUTISM, AND ADHD

People with developmental disabilities have a greatly increased prevalence of up to 40% (in institutional settings) of *epilepsy* compared with the general population (0.7%). The investigation and accurate diagnosis of epilepsy and its differentiation from behavioral disorders may be particularly challenging in this population (Kerr, 2003). The impact of epilepsy on the emotional well-being of the person is related both to the disruptions and limitations in social activities caused by the seizures and to the mood disturbance associated with ictal and postictal states. The overall management of epilepsy in people with developmental disabilities, including treatment and monitoring of treatment, requires a systematic and multidisciplinary approach (International Association for the Scientific Study of Intellectual Disabilities Guidelines Group, 2001).

Relatively few studies have been done of psychiatric disorders in people with developmental disabilities and autism spectrum disorders. Anxiety, depression, and other psychiatric conditions are generally considered to be more prevalent (Bradley, Summers, Wood, & Bryson, 2004), although more recent studies cast doubt on this hypothesis (Tsakanikos et al., 2006). Antipsychotic, antidepressant, anticonvulsant, and tranquilizing medications have been used, in the absence of a psychiatric diagnosis, in an effort to reduce autism-related behaviors such as stereotypy and aggression. There is little evidence at present to support the efficacy and safety of this practice. Significant diagnostic difficulties, methodological problems, and overlap between autism-related behaviors and those relating to other disorders can limit the impact of studies that focus on narrow interventions such as pharmacotherapy alone.

Attention-deficit/hyperactivity disorder (ADHD) is considered to be common among younger people with developmental disabilities (Hastings, Beck, & Hill, 2005). Limitations in the current classification systems and the common co-occurrence of hyperactivity symptoms, especially in those with autism spectrum disorders, may hinder diagnostic attempts (Seager & O'Brien, 2003). The difficulty in diagnosing ADHD in adults without developmental disabilities is also well acknowledged. Nevertheless, open-label studies have shown promising results for the use of psychostimulants in this population (Jou, Handen, & Hardan, 2004), but larger randomized trials are needed before this treatment can be routinely recommended.

THE MENTAL HEALTH NEEDS OF CHILDREN WITH DEVELOPMENTAL DISABILITIES

The needs of children with developmental disabilities are complex and change as the child develops. They are covered extensively in Chapters 8 through 17 in this volume. With regard to mental health problems, the full array of psychiatric disorders is seen in young people with developmental disabilities. Brown, Aman, and Lecavalier (2004), using cluster analysis of behavior patterns of a sample of 601 special education students, identified clusters that bore a meaningful relationship to DSM-IV clinical variables. Younger people with developmental disabilities may need additional supports because of epilepsy, ADHD, autism spectrum disorders, and physical health problems. Serious mental illnesses such as schizophrenia and affective disorders are rarely seen before middle or late adolescence. Physical, emotional, and sexual abuse and neglect are more common in children with developmental disabilities, and their effect on the person's mental health can be detrimental.

Family therapy and other types of family work is a common component of treatment plans, and the use of psychotropic medication, although controversial in children, can sometimes be beneficial, especially in cases of comorbid ADHD (Demb & Chang, 2004; Pearson et al., 2004). "Falling between the services" provided by developmental disabilities agencies and mainstream child and adolescent psychiatric services is common experience. Potential problems have also been identified during the process of transition to adult services (Royal College of Psychiatrists, 2004a; Allington-Smith, 2006).

OFFENDERS WITH DEVELOPMENTAL DISABILITIES

People with developmental disabilities who offend pose significant philosophical, ethical, and pragmatic dilemmas for the criminal justice system and developmental disabilities services (Johnston, 2003). Despite reports of increased frequency of offending among people with developmental disabilities, it is generally believed that there is no conclusive evidence of a general causal link. One of the main methodological flaws in reported studies is that conclusions are based on samples ascertained from prison populations, with no control groups studied. However, the presence of a mental disorder (for example, personality disorder, substance misuse, or ADHD) may increase the risk of offending. Some types of offenses are reported to be more common, such as arson or sexual offenses. Sex offenders with developmental disabilities appear more likely to commit offenses across a spectrum and to be less discriminating in their victims (Lindsay, 2005). Many times the distinction between behavioral disorder and offending behavior is elusive and depends on individual, service, and societal factors.

   People with developmental disabilities are more likely to be disadvantaged by the criminal justice process because of issues of competence in following and understanding necessary legal processes. They are also known to admit to crimes they have not committed because of acquiescence and are considered unreliable witnesses when they themselves have become victims of crime. A number of people with developmental disabilities are inappropriately placed in the penal system or in conditions of higher security than they actually need (Beer et al., 2005); additionally, the capital punishment of people with developmental disabilities in some countries continues to provoke public outcry and passionate debate. Treatment and rehabilitative programs based on behavioral, educational, and cognitive models have been reported, with length of treatment appearing as a significant positive prognostic factor in reducing recidivistic reoffending (Lindsay, 2005).

SERVICE DELIVERY MODELS AND SERVICE EVALUATION

Following deinstitutionalization and the shift toward community life, there has been little consensus as to who should provide services for people with developmental disabilities and mental or behavioral disorders (Bouras & Holt, 2004). The initial, erroneous expectation that simply moving into the community would reduce the occurrence of mental health problems was followed by the realization that a significant number of people would continue to require lifelong intensive support by specialist staff, sometimes in restrictive and less integrated environments. In the past four decades, in countries in which institutional closings took place, dedicated community teams started to emerge. Different service models delivering a range of interventions for people with developmental disabilities and mental health problems have been reported in international literature. Detailed analysis of the components, function, and special characteristics of these models is beyond the scope of this chapter; however, as a general rule, the shape of services tends to reflect historical, political, and fiscal realities in the areas they serve. There has been a large geographical variation in the type and capacity of available services, sometimes even within the same state or country.

Providing a single explicit care pathway for this highly vulnerable population may not be feasible or desirable, as no particular strategy can prove successful in all cases. However, several service characteristics are considered important, such as the use of adequate clinical assessment and review methods, development and dissemination of best-practice guidelines, working across organizational boundaries, having clear funding arrangements, and strengthening interagency collaboration. At present, even though many such agreements are in place, there is a widespread sense that these agreements are less than effective (U.S. Public Health Service, 2002; DuPree, 2004; Beasley, 2004). A way to ensure that services maintain quality standards is to routinely collect outcome measures and regularly audit key service targets. In the United Kingdom, the development of the Health of the Nation Outcome Scales for People with Learning Disabilities (HoNOS-LD; Roy, Matthews, Clifford, Fowler, & Martin, 2002) and the "Green Light" audit toolkits (Foundation for People with Learning Disabilities, Valuing People Support Team, & National Institute for Mental Health in England, 2004) are positive developments in this direction.

Studies examining patterns of service utilization have produced equivocal findings, which probably reflect the great diversity and mix in expertise, staffing levels, and funding options of available services. Factors predicting both service use and need tend to vary according to service and the sociodemographic profile of local populations. People from ethnic minorities are reported to be disproportionately disadvantaged (Pruchno & McMullen, 2004).

Service-related research has also focused on people with developmental disabilities and psychiatric or behavioral disorders who require inpatient treatment. The type of unit in which the admission takes place seems to affect treatment outcomes. Admission to a specialist unit is predictive of more positive outcomes than admission to a generic mental health unit (Xenitidis et al., 2004; Charlot & Beasly, 2005). Although admissions to generic wards can be a rational response to a crisis, no comprehensive assessment, treatment, or rehabilitation can usually be provided. Moreover, people with developmental disabilities may be highly vulnerable in the environment of an acute psychiatric hospital. Assertive community treatment has been advocated as an alternative to hospital admission, but there is currently a lack of evidence with regard to cost-effectiveness (Martin et al., 2005).

Besides providing clinical care, service agencies for people with developmental disabilities and mental health problems are also required to provide liaison, consultation, support, expert advice, and training to other clinical teams, so as to enable people with developmental disabilities to access mainstream services whenever it is possible (Department of Health, England, 2001). There is some evidence that training and education interventions can yield significant gains in the ability of residential staff to recognize mental health problems in individuals with developmental disabilities (Costello, Bouras, & Davis, 2006). Psychiatrists, in particular, need special training in this field, as in many parts of the world they are likely to be asked to evaluate, prescribe, or coordinate the care of persons with developmental disabilities and mental health problems. Relevant training modules are included in training programs for psychiatry residents in the United States (Schwartz, Ruedrich, & Dunn, 2005), whereas in the United Kingdom, psychiatrists who have completed their basic psychiatric training can access a higher specialist training program (3 years) devoted exclusively to the treatment of people with developmental disabilities (Costello et al., 2007). There are similar training programs for nurses, and a number of initiatives have focused on the training needs of other health care professionals.

CONCLUSIONS AND DIRECTION OF FUTURE RESEARCH

The past four decades have brought dramatic changes in the way mental health problems in people with developmental disabilities are conceptualized, assessed, and managed. Advanced diagnostic and treatment options have improved diagnostic accuracy and helped fine-tune complex biopsychosocial interventions. A range of evidence-based supports for this population is emerging. The provision of a comprehensive range of services often depends on the careful allocation of scarce resources. Additionally, clear funding arrangements are necessary for the viability and credibility of specialized services for people with developmental disabilities and mental health problems.

Research in this area has expanded in the past decade, and more robust study designs are currently being employed to tackle previous methodological limitations. Interventions for people with developmental disabilities and mental health problems are usually highly complex. Moreover, because of the great heterogeneity of this population, "golden standard" research designs, such as randomized clinical trials may have limitations in providing the necessary evidence base. Therefore, alternative and more pragmatic designs are likely to be needed.

Future directions for research are expected to target a number of issues of importance to people with developmental disabilities. Population-based epidemiological studies are needed in order to clarify the amount of resources that is likely to be needed, whereas longitudinal studies need to examine key life transitions in order to identify risk and protective factors for mental illness. Biological research is necessary to explore the interaction between genes, brain, and behavior. Providing that the right safeguards are in place, it is important that people with developmental disabilities are included in trials of medication that could prove beneficial to them. In addition, future work should concentrate on better recruiting approaches. Finally, assessment tools need to be further refined and validated, and research networks should be developed that are not uniquely attached to a particular theoretical school but that can combine different interventions based on integrated models.

REFERENCES

Alexander, R., & Cooray, S. (2003). Diagnosis of personality disorders in learning disability. *British Journal of Psychiatry, 182,* 28–31.

Allington-Smith, P. (2006). Mental health needs of children with learning disabilities. *Advances in Psychiatric Treatment, 12,* 130–138.

American Psychiatric Association. (1994). *Diagnostic and statistical manual of mental disorders* (4th ed.). Washington, DC: Author.

Baker, K., & Skuse, D. H. (2005). Adolescents and young adults with 22q11 deletion syndrome: Psychopathology in an at-risk group. *British Journal of Psychiatry, 186,* 115–120.

Beasley, J. (2004). How well does your state serve individuals with co-occurring mental illness and intellectual disabilities? *National Association for the Dually Diagnosed Bulletin, 7*(4), 78.

Beer, D., Spiller, M. J., Pickard, M., Gravestock, S., McGovern, P., Leese, M., et al. (2005). Low secure units: Factors predicting delayed discharge. *Journal of Forensic Psychiatry and Psychology, 16,* 621–637.

Bender, M. (1993). The unoffered chair: The history of therapeutic disdain towards people with learning disability. *Clinical Psychology Forum, 54,* 7–12.

Bouras, N., & Holt, G. (2004). Mental health services for adults with learning disabilities. *British Journal of Psychiatry, 184,* 291–292.

Bouras, N., Martin, G., Leese, M., Vaustraeleh, M., Holt, G., Thomas, C., et al. (2004). Schizophrenia-spectrum psychoses in people with and without intellectual disability. *Journal of Intellectual Disability Research, 48,* 548–555.

Bradley, E. A., Summers, J. A., Wood, H. L., & Bryson, S. E. (2004). Comparing rates of psychiatric and behavioral disorders in adolescents and young adults with severe intellectual disability with and without autism. *Journal of Autism and Developmental Disorders, 34,* 151–161.

Brown, E. C., Aman, M. G., & Lecavalier, L. (2004). Empirical classification of behavioral and psychiatric problems in children and adolescents with mental retardation. *American Journal on Mental Retardation, 109,* 445–455.

Bush, A., & Beail, N. (2004). Risk factors for dementia in people with Down syndrome: Issues in assessment and diagnosis. *American Journal on Mental Retardation, 109*(2), 83–97.

Cain, N. N., Davidson, P. W., Burhan, A. M., Andolsek, M. E., Baxter, J. T., Sullivan, H., et al. (2003). Identifying bipolar disorders in individuals with intellectual disability. *Journal of Intellectual Disability Research, 47,* 31–38.

Charlot, L., & Beasly, J. B. (2005). Specialized inpatient mental health care for people with intellectual disabilities. *Mental Health Aspects of Developmental Disabilities, 8*(3), 100–103.

Clarke, D. J., Boer, H., Whittington, J., Holland, A., Butler, J., & Webb, T. (2002). Prader–Willi syndrome, compulsive and ritualistic behaviours: The first population-based survey. *British Journal of Psychiatry, 180,* 358–362.

Cooray, S. E., & Bakala, A. (2005). Anxiety disorders in people with learning disabilities. *Advances in Psychiatric Treatment, 11,* 355–361.

Costello, H., Bouras, N., & Davis, H. (2006). The role of training in improving community care staff awareness of mental health problems in people with intellectual disabilities. *Journal of Applied Research in Intellectual Disabilities* (online early article). doi:10.1111/j.1468-31482006.00320.x

Costello, H., Holt, G., Cain, N., Bradley, E., Torr, J., Davis, R., et al. (2007). Professional training for those working with people with intellectual disabilities and mental health problems. In N. Bouras & G. Holt (Eds.), *Psychiatric and behavioural disorders in intellectual and developmental disabilities* (2nd ed., pp. 400–411). New York: Cambridge University Press.

Cowley, A., Holt, G., Bouras, N., Sturmey, P., Newton, J., & Costello, H. (2004). Descriptive psychopathology in people with mental retardation. *Journal of Nervous and Mental Disease, 192*(3), 232–237.

Cuthill, F., Espie, C. A., & Cooper, S. A. (2003). Development and psychometric properties of the Glasgow Depression Scale for People with a Learning Disability: Individual and carer supplement versions. *British Journal of Psychiatry, 182,* 347–353.

Dangan, D. (2007). Psychosocial interventions for people with intellectual disabilities. In N. Bouras & G. Holt (Eds.), *Psychiatric and behavioural disorders in intellectual and developmental disabilities* (2nd ed., pp. 330–338). New York: Cambridge University Press.

De Collishaw, S., & Maughan, J. (2004). Affective problems in adults with mild learning disability: The roles of social disadvantage and ill health. *British Journal of Psychiatry, 185,* 350–351.

Deb, S., Clarke, D., & Unwin, G. (2006). The use of medication for the management of behaviour problems among adults who have learning disability: The quick reference guide (QRG). Birmingham, UK: University of Birmingham, Royal College of Psychiatrists & Mencap. Retrieved September 2006, from *www.ld-medication.bham.ac.uk/download.htm.*

Deb, S., Matthews, T., Holt, G., & Bouras, N. (2001). *Practice guidelines for the assessment and diagnosis of mental health problems in adults with intellectual disability.* Brighton, UK: Pavilion.

Deb, S., Thomas, M., & Bright, C. (2001). Mental disorder in adults with intellectual disability: 1. Prevalence of functional psychiatric illness among a community-based population aged between 16 and 64 years. *Journal of Intellectual Disability Research, 45,* 495–505.

Demb, H., & Chang, C. (2004). The use of psychostimulants in children with disruptive behavior disorders and developmental disabilities in a community setting. *Mental Health Aspects of Developmental Disabilities, 7,* 26–36.

Department of Health, England. (2001). *Valuing people: A new strategy for learning disability for the 21st century.* London: Stationery Office.

DuPree, K. (2004). Effective interagency collaboration for people with co-occurring mental illness and developmental disabilities. *National Association for the Dually Diagnosed Bulletin, 7*(1), 16.

Einfeld, S. L. (2001) Systematic management approach to pharmacotherapy for people with learning disabilities. *Advances in Psychiatric Treatment, 7,* 43–49.

Foundation for People with Learning Disabilities, Valuing People Support Team, & National Institute of Mental Health in England. (2004). *Green light: How good are your mental health services for people with learning disabilities? A service improvement toolkit.* London: Foundation for People with Learning Disabilities.

Gravestock, S., Flynn, A., & Hemmings, C. (2005). Psychiatric disorders in adults with learning disabilities. In G. Holt, N. Bouras, & S. Hardy (Eds.), *Mental health in learning disabilities: A reader* (pp. 7–17). Brighton, UK: Estia Centre and Pavilion.

Hardy, S., & Holt, G. (2005). Assessment of mental health problems. In G. Holt, N. Bouras, & S. Hardy (Eds.), *Mental health in learning disabilities: A reader* (pp. 19–26). Brighton, UK: Estia Centre and Pavilion.

Hastings, R. P., Beck, A., & Hill, C. (2005). Symptoms of ADHD and their correlates in children with intellectual disabilities. *Research in Developmental Disabilities, 26,* 456–468.

Hollins, S., & Sinason, V. (2000). Psychotherapy, learning disabilities and trauma: New perspectives. *British Journal of Psychiatry, 176,* 32–36.

Horwitz, S., Kerker, B., Owens, P. L., & Zigler, E. (2000). *The health status and needs of individuals with mental retardation.* New Haven, CT: Yale University, Department of Epidemiology and Public Health and Department of Psychology.

Hurley, A. D. (2005). Psychotherapy is an essential tool in the treatment of psychiatric disorders for people with mental retardation. *Mental Retardation, 43*(6), 445–448.

Hurley, A. D., & Silka, V. R. (2003). Identification of hallucinations and delusions in people with intellectual disability. *Mental Health Aspects of Developmental Disabilities, 6,* 153–157.

Hurley, A. D., & Silka, V. R. (2004). Aggression and maladaptive behaviors: Not necessarily symptoms of a psychiatric disorder. *Mental Health Aspects of Developmental Disabilities, 7*(1), 37–40.

International Association for the Scientific Study of Intellectual Disabilities Guidelines Group. (2001). Clinical guidelines for the management of epilepsy in adults with an intellectual disability. *Seizure, 10,* 401–409.

Johnston, S. (2003). Forensic psychiatry and learning disability. In W. Fraser & M. Kerr (Eds.), *Seminars in the psychiatry of learning disabilities* (2nd ed., pp. 287–306). London: Gaskell and Royal College of Psychiatrists.

Jou, R., Handen, B., & Hardan, A. (2004). Psychostimulant treatment of adults with mental retardation and attention-deficit/hyperactivity disorder. *Australasian Psychiatry, 12,* 376–379.

Kerker, B. D., Owens, P. L., Zigler, E., & Horwitz, S. M. (2004). Mental health disorders among individuals with mental retardation: Challenges to accurate prevalence estimates. *Public Health Reports, 119,* 409–417.

Kerr, M. (2003). Epilepsy. In W. Fraser & M. Kerr (Eds.), *Seminars in the psychiatry of learning disabilities* (2nd ed.). London: Gaskell and Royal College of Psychiatrists.

Lew, M., Matta, C., Tripp-Tebo, C., & Watts, D. (2006). Dialectical behavioral therapy for individuals with intellectual disabilities. *Mental Health Aspects of Developmental Disabilities, 9,* 1–13.

Lindsay, W. R. (2005). Model underpinning treatment for sex offenders with mild intellectual disability: Current theories of sex offending. *Mental Retardation, 43,* 428–441.

Martin, G., Costello, H., Leese, M., Slade, M., Bouras, N., Higgins, S., et al. (2005). An exploratory study of assertive community treatment for people with intellectual disability and psychiatric disorders: Conceptual, clinical, and service issues. *Journal of Intellectual Disability Research, 49,* 516–524.

McCarthy, J. (2001). Post-traumatic stress disorder in people with learning disability. *Advances in Psychiatric Treatment, 7,* 163–169.

McGillicuddy, N. B. (2006). A review of substance use research among those with mental retardation. *Mental Retardation Developmental Disability Research Review, 12*(1), 41–47.

Moss, S., Prosser, H., Costello, H., Simpson, N., Patel, P., Rowe, S., et al. (1998). Reliability and validity of the PASADD checklist for detecting psychiatric disorders in adults with intellectual disability. *Journal of Intellectual Disability Research, 42,* 173–183.

Moss, S., Emerson, E., Kiernan, C., Turner, S., Hatton, C., Alboraz, A., et al. (2000). Psychiatric symptoms in adults with learning disability and challenging behaviour. *British Journal of Psychiatry, 177,* 452–456.

Murphy, K. C., & Owen, M. J. (2001). Velo-cardio-facial syndrome: A model for understanding the genetics and pathogenesis of schizophrenia. *British Journal of Psychiatry, 179,* 397–402.

National Health Service Scotland. (2004). *People with learning disabilities in Scotland: Health needs assessment report*. Glasgow: NHS Health Scotland.

O'Hara, J. (2007). Inter-disciplinary multi-modal assessment for mental health problems in people with intellectual disabilities. In N. Bouras & G. Holt (Eds.), *Psychiatric and behavioural disorders in intellectual and developmental disabilities* (2nd ed., pp. 42–61). New York: Cambridge University Press.

Oliver, B., & Smith, P. (2005). Psychological interventions for people with learning disabilities. In G. Holt, N. Bouras, & S. Hardy (Eds.), *Mental health in learning disabilities: A reader* (pp. 41–48). Brighton, UK: Estia Centre and Pavilion.

Parkes, G., & Hollins, S. (2007). Psychodynamic approaches to people with intellectual disabilities: Individuals, groups/systems and families. In N. Bouras & G. Holt (Eds.), *Psychiatric and behavioural disorders in intellectual and developmental disabilities* (2nd ed., pp. 339–352). New York: Cambridge University Press.

Pearson, D. A., Lane, D. M., Santos, C. W., Casat, C. D., Jerger, L. W., Loveland, K. A., et al. (2004). Effects of methylphenidate treatment in children with mental retardation and ADHD: Individual variation in medication response. *Journal of the American Academy of Child and Adolescent Psychiatry*, *43*, 686–698.

Pickard, M., & Paschos, D. (2005). Pseudohallucinations in people with intellectual disabilities: Two case reports. *Mental Health Aspects of Developmental Disabilities*, *8*(3), 91–93.

Prout, H. T., & Nowak-Drabik, K. M. (2003). Psychotherapy with persons who have mental retardation: An evaluation of effectiveness. *American Journal on Mental Retardation*, *108*(2), 82–93.

Pruchno, R., & McMullen, W. F. (2004). Patterns of service utilization by adults with a developmental disability: Type of service makes a difference. *American Journal on Mental Retardation*, *109*, 362–378.

Richards, M., Maughan, B., Hardy, R., Hall, I., Strydom, A., & Wandsworth, M. (2001). Long-term affective disorder in people with mild learning disability. *British Journal of Psychiatry*, *179*, 523–527.

Rojahn, J., Matson, J., Naglieri, J., & Mayville, E. (2004). Relationships between psychiatric conditions and behavior problems among adults with mental retardation. *American Journal on Mental Retardation*, *109*(1), 21–23.

Roy, A., Matthews, H., Clifford, P., Fowler, V., & Martin, D. (2002). Health of the Nation Outcome Scales for People with Learning Disabilities (HoNOS-LD). *British Journal of Psychiatry*, *180*, 61–66.

Royal College of Psychiatrists. (2001). *DC-LD: Diagnostic criteria for psychiatric disorders for use with adults with learning disabilities/mental retardation*. London: Gaskell.

Royal College of Psychiatrists. (2004a). *Psychiatric services for children and adolescents with learning disabilities* (Council Report No. CR123). London: Royal College of Psychiatrists, College Research Unit.

Royal College of Psychiatrists. (2004b). *Psychotherapy and learning disability* (Council Report No. CR116). London: Royal College of Psychiatrists, College Research Unit.

Schwartz, S., Ruedrich, S. L., & Dunn, J. (2005). Psychiatry in mental retardation and developmental disabilities: A training program for psychiatry residents. *Mental Health Aspects of Developmental Disabilities*, *8*(1), 13.

Seager, M. C., & O'Brien, G. (2003). Attention deficit hyperactivity disorder: Review of ADHD in learning disability: The diagnostic criteria for psychiatric disorders for use with adults with LD/MR [DC-LD] criteria for diagnosis. *Journal of Intellectual Disability Research*, *47*(Suppl. 1), 26–31.

Smiley, E. (2005). Epidemiology of mental health problems in adults with learning disability: An update. *Advances in Psychiatric Treatment*, *11*, 214–222.

Stanton R., & Coetzee, R. (2004). Down's syndrome and dementia. *Advances in Psychiatric Treatment*, *10*, 50–58.

Stavrakaki, C., & Lunsky, Y. (2007). Depression, anxiety and adjustment disorders in people with intellectual disabilities. In N. Bouras & G. Holt (Eds.), *Psychiatric and behavioural disorders in intellectual and developmental disabilities* (2nd ed., pp. 113–130). New York: Cambridge University Press.

Sturmey, P. (1999). Classifications: Concepts, progress and future. In N. Bouras (Ed.), *Psychiatric and behavioural disorders in developmental disabilities and mental retardation*. Cambridge, UK: Cambridge University Press.

Sturmey, P., Newton, J. T., Cowley, A., Bouras, N., & Holt, G. (2005). The PASADD checklist: Independent replication of its psychometric properties in a community sample. *British Journal of Psychiatry*, *186*, 319–323.

Tsakanikos, E., Costello, H., Holt, G., Bouras, N., Sturmey, P., & Newton, T. (2006). Psychopathology in adults with autism and intellectual disability. *Journal of Autism and Developmental Disorders, 36*(8), 1123–1129.

Tyrrell, J., Cosgrove, M., McCarron, M., McPherson, J., Calvert, J., Kelly, A., et al. (2001). Dementia in people with Down's syndrome. *International Journal of Geriatric Psychiatry, 16*(12), 1168–1174.

U.S. Public Health Service. (2002). *Closing the gap: A national blueprint for improving the health of individuals with mental retardation.* Washington, DC: U.S. Department of Health and Human Services.

Vanstraelen, M., & Tyrer, P. (1999). Rapid cycling bipolar affective disorder in people with intellectual disability: A systematic review. *Journal of Intellectual Disability Research, 43*, 349–359.

Vogels, A., De Hert, M., Descheemaeker, M. J., Govers, V., Devriendt, K., Legius, E., et al. (2004). Psychotic disorders in Prader–Willi syndrome. *American Journal of Medical Genetics, Part A*, 127A(3), 238–243.

World Health Organization. (1992). *The ICD-10 classification of mental and behavioural disorders: Clinical descriptions and diagnostic guidelines.* Geneva, Switzerland: Author.

Xenitidis, K., Gratsa, A., Bouras, N., Hammond, R., Ditchfield, H., Holt, G., et al. (2004). Psychiatric inpatient care for adults with intellectual disabilities: Generic or specialist units? *Journal of Intellectual Disability Research, 48*, 11–18.

25

Psychotherapeutic Medications and Positive Behavior Support

Travis Thompson
Tim Moore
Frank Symons

Positive behavior supports (PBS) address all facets of the individual's physical and social environment, behavioral skills, and weaknesses, including his or her health and physical well-being. Mental health conditions are state variables that have unique stimulus properties, that change the probability of behavior, and that alter the events that will maintain behavior. In this chapter we propose a taxonomy of psychotherapeutic medications based on an analysis of the antecedent state variables, their discriminative stimulus properties, and the consequences that maintain the behavior of concern. Examples of several classes of commonly prescribed medications are explored in relation to these factors. The important relationship between physicians and other health care workers and those involved in providing PBS services is discussed. Finally, research and practice implications of recent research are examined.

BACKGROUND AND PREVALENCE

People with intellectual and related developmental disabilities receive psychotropic medications to increase learning and attention, to improve health and safety (e.g., seizure management), and for behavioral management (e.g., severe behavior problems such as aggression and self-injury). Epidemiological estimates of drug treatment prevalence vary depending on the survey instruments used and the location of the individuals surveyed. From 29 to 48% of adults residing in large long-term public residential settings receive psychoactive medication (Aman, Sarphare, & Burrow, 1995). Prevalence in community-based settings is about 10% less than that in large residential facilities (Kalachnik, 1999). Over the past decade prescribing trends have changed as a function of diagnosis and setting. Spreat, Conroy, and Jones (1997) reported in an Oklahoma sample that, overall, 22% of adults with intellectual disabilities were prescribed antipsychotics; 9.3%, anxiolytics; and 5.9%, antidepressants. However, higher percentages were reported in large public residential programs. Langworthy-Lam, Aman, and Van Bourgondien (2002) found that in North Carolina 45.7% of individuals with autism were taking psychotropic drugs;12.4%, antiepileptic drugs; and 5.7%, supplements for autism. Antidepressants were taken by 21.7%, antipsychotics by 16.8%, and stimulants by 13.9%; these were the most commonly prescribed agents. In Ohio, 45.6% of children with autism were taking some form of psychotropic agent (including St. John's wort and melatonin), whereas 11.5% were taking seizure medication and 10.3% took over-the-counter autism preparations. The most common psychotropic agents included antidepressants (21.6%), antipsychotics (14.9%), antihypertensives (12.5%), and stimulants (11.3%; Aman, Lam, & Collier-Crespin, 2003).

Growing concerns about dual diagnosis and treatment of individuals with associated behavioral challenges who also have developmental disabilities suggests that appropriate use of psychotherapeutic medications will be a concern for the foreseeable future. The role of psychotropic medications for persons with intellectual and related developmental disabilities as part of an overall support strategy remains to be explicated. In this chapter, we examine the rationale and provide a theoretical context for seeking answers to this question rather than reviewing the extensive research literature on psychotropic medications in developmental disabilities.

POSITIVE BEHAVIOR SUPPORTS AND PSYCHOTHERAPEUTIC MEDICATIONS

PBS in educational and other community settings have dramatically changed services to individuals with developmental disabilities. Emphasis has been on rearranging social and instructional environments surrounding an individual to promote more effective behavior and to make it less necessary for such individuals to engage in challenging behavior to cope with their circumstances. Many children with developmental disabilities are unable to meet instructional or social demands. A student who is a poor reader may be off-task and behave inappropriately during math seatwork because he or she is unable to adequately read and comprehend word problems. A child who needs a long processing time may seldom complete seatwork because the number of items to be completed is unrealistically large. A child with a history of escaping or avoiding assignments by behaving aggressively toward peers requires a change in the nature of his or her assignments, and consequences should be altered to reward small steps toward achievement. In none of these cases does the child have a mental health problem that requires the use of psychotropic medications. These children need carefully designed adjustments in social and academic expectations and response requirements and more thoughtful programming of consequences to promote success and discourage maladaptive coping.

However, at times general health or mental health problems play a role. Several investigators have incorporated attention to physiological events into their overall PBS strategies. Carr and Smith (1995) identified health conditions that predisposed individuals with developmental disabilities to problem behavior. In one study they used a combination of procedures to reduce discomfort and demands to decrease aggressive behavior of women with intellectual disabilities during premenstrual periods (Carr, Smith, Giacin, Whelan, & Pancari, 2003). Kennedy and Meyer (1996) and Kennedy, Meyer, Werts, and Cushing (2000) reported that sleep deprivation increases avoidance behavior, including aggressive behavior, in laboratory animals and individuals with intellectual disabilities. Internal feeling states associated with upsetting situations in a child's life or recurring mental health conditions may also have an impact on overall PBS strategy. In this chapter, we discuss the role of medications as components of PBS.

THE ROLE OF STATE VARIABLES IN CHALLENGING BEHAVIOR

Traits, States, Setting Events, and Establishing Operations

Historically within psychology, types and traits have been distinguished from transient *states*. *Types* are enduring discrete categories of characteristics, such as the somatotypes of William Sheldon (1940), that is, endomorph, ectomorph, and mesomorph. *Traits* refer to continuous dimensions of a person's characteristics, such as Hans Eysenck's introversion–extraversion dimension (1971). Traits are also enduring characteristics inferred from behavioral signs that account for consistency in individual behavior across time and circumstances and are continuous. Traits are assumed to be less influenced by situational factors. A person's *state* is usually a transient or variable condition, often induced by an identifiable antecedent, such as lack of sleep, going without food, or side effects of a drug.

Many states are induced by circumstances that have impinged on a person and that increase or decrease the efficacy of reinforcing events and change the probability of behavior maintained by those events, called *setting events* or *establishing operations*. In *The Behavior of Organisms* (1938), Skinner referred to those events as motivational or emotional operations. Bijou and Baer (1978, p. 26) wrote that "a setting event influences an interactional sequence *(of behavior and consequences)* by altering the strengths and characteristics of the particular stimulus and response functions involved in an interaction." As they used the term, an experimenter or practitioner did not necessarily control a setting event. Michael (1982, 1993) provided a formal definition of establishing operations (EOs). In 2000, he elaborated on the EO concept, stating, "The two effects of an EO are an alteration in the reinforcing effectiveness of some stimulus, object, or event (the reinforcer-establishing effect) and an alteration in the current frequency of all behavior that has been reinforced by that stimulus, object or event (the evocative effect)" (p. 403).

Feelings, Tacts, and States

Internal feelings produced by experiencing hours without eating, being subjected to hostile provocations, or losing the affection of someone important to us are familiar to everyone, leading people to say, "I'm really hungry," "That makes me mad," or "I feel terribly sad." The distinction between an EO and the internal stimuli produced by that earlier event may appear irrelevant to an average classroom teacher or parent. A teacher might say that a student hit another child *because he is angry* and that he is angry *because someone teased him on the bus on the way to school*. They tend to equate the internal feeling state of being angry with the antecedent that caused that condition, being teased on the bus. Moreover, they often assume that the feeling of being angry *caused* the behavior, rather than being correlated with the change in likelihood of problem behavior. In discussing this distinction with teachers and parents, it is useful to explain that we seldom know for sure what a child is feeling, particularly a child with a developmental delay (though we may have a good hunch), but we often know for certain what happened earlier that appears to have led to that feeling. We can often do something to change those earlier events, but seldom are we able to change a child's feelings directly.

Such verbal labels of feelings are *tacts* based on internal stimuli associated with the foregoing events that impinged on the person at some earlier time. Many people with developmental disabilities have limited ability to reliably respond discriminatively to internal feeling states, but we presume that they experience the same internal stimulus events as others. To indicate reluctance to discuss such feelings with parents or staff members ignores their importance to caregivers and creates a credibility gap between professionals and those carrying out interventions. When a parent, teacher, or counselor tells us a student arrived at school *with a chip on his shoulder*, we know that they are referring to a heightened likelihood that the youngster will behave aggressively. We believe, and we are usually right, that some event has occurred prior to the student's school arrival that changed his internal environment in ways that make hurting other people more reinforcing. It may have been lack of sleep the previous night, being constipated, or having had an altercation with his mother before leaving home. All of those events change the probability of aggressive behavior and the probability that it will be maintained by the consequences of striking out at others. In this chapter we discuss types of antecedent events that change the value of reinforcers and their mechanisms and subsequently explore psychotropic medications within the context of overall PBS strategies.

Some transient states do not have external setting events or establishing operations. Hormonal changes associated with the menstrual cycle can change the value of positive and negative reinforcers (e.g., Carr et al., 2003) but have no identifiable environmental antecedent. People with bipolar disorder undergo dramatic neurochemical changes that alter motivational functions of external environmental events, that have discriminative stimulus properties, and that typically have no clear environmental setting event or EO. At times a presumed setting event may account for a person's state, though the precise event is unknown; for example, having a bad chest cold that lowers the threshold for negative reinforcers to control behavior. We assume that the respiratory infection was caused by exposure to a bacterial or viral agent within the previous few days. More ambiguous situations involve fluctuations in a person's state that are known to be controlled by genetic factors but that may also be influenced by environmental events. For example, a person with Prader–Willi syndrome is hungry much of the time (meaning that food is a powerful reinforcer), but not within 30–60 minutes of the last large meal. In this case the interaction between a gene-regulated brain chemical event and the time since the previous meal are responsible for the state that makes access to food a powerfully reinforcing event.

In this chapter, most of the states we discuss are conditions not clearly evoked by a specific environmental event but that create a change in the internal milieu responsible for altering the value of various discriminative stimuli and controlling consequences. For that reason we use the broader term "state" to refer to those conditions of a person that seldom have a discrete setting event or EO but that nonetheless change the value of reinforcing events and often have discriminative stimulus properties for the behavior of the affected individual.

MENTAL HEALTH CONDITIONS AS STATES THAT CHANGE THE PROBABILITY OF BEHAVIOR

Psychopathological conditions, such as anxiety and depression, have discriminative properties that lead most people to use such words as "nervous," "worked up," or "unhappy" or "sad" to describe their internal states. Those internal states determine to a large extent the events that will be reinforcing. When someone is depressed, the usual social reinforcers are often ineffective. An instructional intervention that depends on teacher attention as a reinforcer may be unproductive under such conditions. When a student with autism is feeling more anxious than usual, entering a room full of strangers is an aversive event that will be avoided, by a tantrum if necessary. Practitioners occasionally attempt to override the effects of these physiological and biochemical states (such as intense feelings of anxiety) by applying behavior-analytic techniques more rigorously. By increasing the magnitude of reinforcement for appropriate responding or by making the consequence of inappropriate behavior more aversive (e.g., delaying access to a preferred commodity or activity), the teacher or therapist attempts to increase appropriate and decrease inappropriate behavior. These methods may prove effective under some circumstances; however, for children with persistent mental health problems (e.g., obsessive–compulsive disorder [OCD] associated with autism), there are often limits to their usefulness. At times some practitioners are so committed to reducing challenging behavior without using medications that they are willing to allow a child to experience considerable discomfort over days or weeks while implementing a series of minimally effective behavioral interventions. That is akin to trying to improve the mobility of a child with limited vision by differentially reinforcing improved locomotion from place to place rather than by first fitting the student with corrective eyeglasses. Just as eyeglasses are visual prostheses, psychotropic medications can be effective *behavioral prostheses.*

Most of the drugs used to treat mental health problems (as well as those that are addictive) bind to the same chemical receptors in the brain as do naturally occurring neurotransmitters (Society for Stimulus Properties of Drugs, 2005). Laboratory studies indicate that animals can reliably distinguish which brain chemical receptors are being occupied by a given drug that mimics normal brain chemical transmitter function. Not only can they distinguish one brain chemical effect from another (e.g., dopamine from GABA) but they can also distinguish between effects of dosages of the same drug and their corresponding feeling states. In his book *Verbal Behavior* (1957), Skinner called such discriminative responding based on the relative strength of tendencies to respond "autoclitics." When a stimulant drug such as amphetamine causes a person to say that he or she feels *very talkative* versus *somewhat talkative* at a lower dose, it is called an *autoclitic*, a specialized type of *tact* (see Sundberg & Partington, 1998, for further discussion of teaching of specialized tacts). When Valium binds to benzodiazepine receptors, people report feeling "relaxed" or "calm." When a child with a mental health disorder is chronically anxious, medications that act on overactive or underactive brain chemical receptors produce discernable changes in how he or she feels. Effects of naturally occurring brain chemical events, such as those associated with depressive disorder or anxiety disorder, can be reduced by medications that act on those same brain chemical receptors. Our brain chemical receptors are the eyes and ears of our internal emotional worlds. Environmental stimuli that are aversive much of the time for a child, such as teacher demands, become far less so because the brain chemical context has changed. In this way psychotropic medications can play an important role in positive behavior support.

States Change the Probability of Behavior

Psychotropic medications change how readily environmental events will be positively and negatively reinforcing. They are one of the more powerful emotional tuning devices that turn the sensitivity to reinforcers up and down. For the highly anxious, compulsive child, a selective serotonin reuptake inhibitor (SSRI) medication may allow her to feel less anxious and have less need for highly predictable routine. She may no longer need to avoid unpredictable situations, whereas, in the past, avoidance of changes in routine had served as a negative reinforcer for problem behavior. The adolescent with high-functioning autism who has few friends and seldom interacts with teachers unless spoken to may become more amenable to social reinforcement when treated with an appropriate medication.

MENTAL HEALTH CONDITIONS THAT FUNCTION AS STATE VARIABLES

One of the major difficulties in treating psychopathological conditions among individuals with developmental disabilities is that so little is known about presenting signs and symptoms in various subpopulations. In an effort to overcome this problem, the Royal College of Psychiatrists (2001) published a classification system providing operationalized diagnostic criteria for psychiatric disorders for use with adults with moderate to profound intellectual disabilities (called learning disabilities in the United Kingdom). It may also be used in conjunction with the ICD-10 (World Health Organizations, 2007) and DSM-IV-TR (American Psychiatric Association, 2000) manuals in a complementary way when working with adults with mild intellectual disabilities. Nonetheless, in the sections that follow, descriptions of major mental health disorders draw primarily on diagnostic features in typical populations, which may be useful as a starting point.

OCD in Autism Spectrum Disorders

OCD includes recurring thoughts or urges (i.e., intense tendencies to respond in particular ways) or recurring images. These are called *obsessions* and could include, for example, a recurring thought that one might not be able to breathe or repeatedly recalling an image of an advancing tornado seen on television. *Compulsions* are repetitive behaviors that reduce the fearfulness associated with the obsession, such as repeatedly lining up pencils in a row or repeatedly checking to see that the doors are locked. Compulsions are negatively reinforced responses that reduce the aversiveness of obsessions. People who do not have developmental disabilities are aware that the intruding obsessions are irrational and that there is nothing to fear. They are also aware that their rituals may appear excessive to other people. However, people with developmental disabilities may not recognize that the obsessions are not based in reality or that the rituals are dysfunctional. The subjective feelings may be so intense that they cause hyperventilation, sweating, tremulousness, or feelings of fainting. These very distinctive internal feelings are highly unpleasant to the person experiencing them, and he or she will do whatever is necessary to stop them.

In a study of 40 individuals with high-functioning autism spectrum disorders Russell, Mataix-Cols, Anson, and Murphy (2005) found that 25% of participants had clinically measurable OCD. The frequencies of obsessive and compulsive behaviors were similar among individuals with autism spectrum disorder (ASD) and psychiatric patients diagnosed with OCD but without ASD. Brain science studies have provided evidence that dysfunctional prefrontal cortex (PFC)–basal ganglia circuits are involved in the pathogenesis of OCD.

Among people with ASDs, the fear that they will be unable to engage in rituals that reduce their anxiety may be so intense that, if they are interrupted or prevented from doing so, they explode into a violent outburst. An observer who knows nothing about the individual may interpret the individual's behavior as aggression intended to hurt others, whereas in reality it is a response to feelings of panic.

At the heart of OCD is the fear of loss of control, whether it involves being touched when one does not want to be touched or being asked a question one does not understand or going into a crowded theater and fearing that one may not be able to leave. The state often involves two components that increase the likelihood of avoidance behavior: (1) the environmental circumstance that elicits fear of loss of control and (2) the physiological changes and their internal stimulus effects. Environmental accommodations can reduce the fear of loss of control, but they are often not achievable because unanticipated situations may arise before an accommodation can be made. At times, no specific environmental trigger can be identified for an OCD attack. For individuals with extreme OCD, pharmacological interventions that reduce the brain-chemical and physiological response can greatly reduce such avoidance behavior. Although OCD and associated symptoms are most extreme among individuals with ASD, they are also apparent among individuals with Prader–Willi syndrome (Feurer et al., 1998), fragile X syndrome (Bailey, Hatton, Mesibov, Ament, & Skinner, 2000), and other disabilities, as well.

Panic Attack Disorder

Panic attack disorder is closely related to OCD, and many people with OCD have panic attacks. However, some have panic attacks that are not provoked by specific environmental events. A panic attack involves a profound physiological response that the individual experiences as a feeling of impending doom and the fear that one cannot breathe and may die. Skin flushing, profuse sweating, difficulty breathing, and heart pounding are all part of panic attacks. People with panic attacks describe the fear as unbearable. Panic attacks have a storm-like quality; the attack suddenly takes over the body, runs its course, and then diminishes and stops. Some panic attacks may occur as much as a half hour after an alarming situation, for example, while the person is in a van driving home from an upsetting dentist's appointment.

As with OCD, there may be environmental triggers and physiological responses that are components of states that lead to avoidance. It is very difficult to reduce panic attacks using environmental interventions alone. In some instances, individuals can be taught to avoid specific environmental triggers (e.g., an aggressive-appearing dog), but as a practical matter that may be nearly impossible. Medications that prevent the profound physiological storm that overtakes the person during a panic attack are usually necessary.

Depression

Major depressive disorder is very difficult to diagnose among people with developmental disabilities because the DSM-IV-TR (American Psychiatric Association, 2000) diagnostic criteria require self-report of mood state. In unipolar major depression, the person has had five or more symptoms that represent definite change from usual functioning. Either depressed mood or decreased interest or pleasure must be among the five over a 2-week period. In addition to depressed mood and loss of interests, other signs or symptoms include appetite and weight changes, sleep disturbance, changed patterns of motor activity, fatigue, diminished self-worth, difficulty concentrating, and recurring thoughts about death. Some of these symptoms are nearly impossible to access in nonverbal or minimally verbal individuals.

A person with depression experiences a paucity of positive experiences in his or her daily life, and his or her threshold for positive reinforcement is greatly elevated. Even when others attempt to make positive comments, such as "I like your hair that way" or "You really did a great job," the person with depression may react to them as being negative remarks. He or she may think, "He didn't really mean it" or "I know I did a bad job." The depressed individual has a lower rate of interaction with the environment than usual and hence has fewer opportunities to experience positive consequences. In severe depression, there are unique subjective internal events that are distinctive and not easily confused with other conditions. Most people feel unremitting sadness. Some people are nauseated or feel as though they have a weight pressing down on their chests. They may feel exhausted and lose interest in things that they normally find reinforcing. Depression may not have a specific antecedent trigger.

Depression is common among people with developmental disabilities, due partially to their life circumstances and partially to genetics. Depression runs in the families of individuals with ASD. Many people with developmental disabilities experience repeated losses—for example, out-of-home placement, loss of roommates, job changes, and changing teachers or schools, all of which are antecedents to depression. Encouraging people with developmental disabilities who are experiencing mild to moderate depression to continue to actively participate in situations with high densities of potentially reinforcing experiences will often gradually change their moods and behaviors. People with more severe depression may not be able to avail themselves of the putative reinforcers in their environments. The combination of the subjective feelings of sadness, the associated physiological symptoms, and the low rate of responding in situations that could lead to positive experiences conspires to prevent them from recovering. These states make positive reinforcement unlikely, perpetuating a downward spiral of disappointment and even despair. Antidepressant medications lower the threshold for positive reinforcement and increase the operant levels of adaptive performances, making it more likely that the individual will come into contact with positively reinforcing experiences.

Bipolar Disorder

Approximately 1% of all children and adolescents experience the symptoms of bipolar disorder (BPD) or related depressive illness while they are growing up. Children with bipolar disorder are emotionally labile and often irritable and destructive. They often complain of stomachaches, headaches, or other physical ailments. They overreact to social provocations that would ordinarily produce little or no response from a peer. Children with bipolar disorder show different brain activation than controls in prefrontal cortices and in limbic and paralimbic structures in response to both negative and positive emotionally arousing stimuli. When a child with BPD is experiencing a manic episode, his or her brain chemistry changes much as it would if he or she were given a very large dose of a drug that causes excitability, irritability, and hyper-responsiveness.

If there is a trigger event for a manic episode, it often occurs several days or weeks from the epicenter of a severe manic outburst. Major family crises, child abuse, or other traumatic events may initiate the chain of events leading to a delayed manic episode. As youngsters approach the teenage years, mania increasingly resembles adult BPD. The youth will sleep progressively less, talk incessantly, and may have highly unrealistic notions of what he or she may be capable of, called *delusions of grandeur*. As a manic episode progresses, virtually nothing can be done to head it off environmentally. No amount of positive or negative consequences will change the course of the emerging crisis. Prior to the peak of a manic psychotic episode, the individual may feel euphoric and on top of the world. Once the peak passes, he or she becomes irritable and aggressive, often extremely violent. Among individuals who are nonverbal and with limited intellectual ability, the signs of mania are entirely physical, with incessant activity, destructiveness, and imperviousness to social interventions. The neurochemical states that occur during mania can usually be managed pharmacologically with one of the classic antimanic drugs (e.g., lithium, carbamazepine [Tegretol], or divalproex [Depakote]) or one of the newer medications that are increasingly used with individuals who have more frequent irregular manic episodes (called rapid cycling disorder).

Attention-Deficit/Hyperactivity Disorder

Most teachers have days when they wonder whether one of their students has attention-deficit/hyperactivity disorder (ADHD). At times they become so convinced that they talk with the child's parents about the possibility. Much of the time the answer is no. The student is going through a growth period when he or she is more curious than usual, has greater need for independence, and is more actively exploring the world around him or her. He or she may also be experiencing problems at home that are spilling over into school, but he or she does not have a true ADHD disorder. Approximately 1 in 20–30 children has a developmental disability involving either abnormalities in attention, abnormalities in activity level, or both. For a child to be diagnosed as having ADHD, he or she must exhibit at least 8 of 14 characteristics of ADHD for at least 6 months, with onset before 7 years of age (see American Psychiatric Association, 2000, and Reiff, 2004).

The brains of children with ADHD interpret and react to information differently than do those of peers the same age, especially in situations that require sustained attention (e.g., to a teacher's spoken instruction) without being distracted by other aspects of the environment (e.g., a child's voice outside the classroom, a noisy truck driving by the classroom window). Different brain areas are responsible for selective attention and sustained attention, areas that do not function properly among children with ADHD. ADHD can have many causes. Some children inherit the tendency for ADHD from their parents, usually their fathers, whereas others acquire ADHD because of damage to their brains during development inside the womb—for example, from infections or exposure to alcohol or another toxin. The end result is similar: damage to brain structures that regulate attention and activity level.

Children with *inattentive* ADHD are not adequately under the stimulus control of educational materials or adult instructions. Other distracting stimuli compete for their attention and behavior. Positive consequences that are effective in encouraging most children's behavior in a desired direction, such as teacher approval following task completion, are often not very effective. The combination of lack of stimulus control and weak reinforcement leaves the child appearing to cast about without direction. For children who also have *hyperactive* ADHD, the problem is compounded. Not only are their social and academic behaviors under poor stimulus control, but they also respond in exaggerated ways to competing stimuli. They seem unable to anticipate negative consequences at one moment and overreact to minor provocative situations at other times.

Many medications have been tried over the past 40 years in an effort to reduce the behavior problems and improve the concentration of children with ADHD. Stimulant medications are the most widely used for the management of ADHD-related symptoms. Stimulant medications change the levels of chemicals available to various adrenergic neurotransmitter systems in the brain. Attention span, impulsivity, and on-task behavior improve, especially in structured environments. Some children also have greater frustration tolerance and show greater compliance with adult requests and even improved handwriting. Relationships with parents, peers, and teachers may also improve. Often unappreciated is the fact that many children with ADHD also have learning disabilities. Children with ADHD and dyslexia have significant problems in school, are often not liked by other children, and are a source of frustration to their teachers. Affected children often realize that they are not well liked by their peers, and, not surprisingly, they are often depressed and tearful. Not only does appropriate use of stimulant medications help manage their attention and activity problems, but it also often improves their moods.

If a child with inattentive ADHD is taking a stimulant medication that wears off before the end of the school day, the teacher may notice that, as the afternoon wears on, the child switches from one activity to another, completing none of them. When asked what he or she is supposed to be working on, the child may have no idea, despite the fact that the teacher had given the child an assignment only minutes earlier. This is not willful disobedience or disregard for the teacher's authority; it reflects lack of ability to focus attention. Within a given school day, such a student may be an attentive child who accomplishes most of her or his assignments in the morning but appears confused, disorganized, and lacking direction toward the end of the school day. Under similar circumstances, a child with hyperactive ADHD becomes progressively impulsive and irritable. Parent or teacher demands that were readily followed in the morning trigger outbursts of defiance at 2 P.M. The youngster's threshold for responding to social or academic demands as aversive plummets as the day progresses and the effects of medication diminish. The neurochemical roller coaster such children ride over the course of the day is visible in their fluctuating behavior in similar circumstances.

Other Mental Health Conditions

Within the population of children with developmental disabilities, other mental health disorders exist. Older children with developmental disabilities may suffer from schizophrenia or seizure disorders that may manifest themselves as behavioral challenges (e.g., temporal and frontal lobe epilepsy). Selective mutism and specific phobias are diagnosed from time to time among children with developmental disabilities, and less common conditions such as dissociative disorders are rare but occasionally occur. Although these may be serious problems to the individual child and school personnel who must cope with them, they are beyond the scope of this chapter.

PSYCHOPHARMACOLOGICAL INTERVENTIONS THAT ALTER MENTAL HEALTH STATES

Psychopharmacology, Neuropharmacology, and Behavioral Pharmacology

Using medications to relieve sadness or anxiety isn't a new idea. In the *Odyssey*, Homer wrote of Helen, "Infusing straight a medicine to their wine/That, drowning cares and angers, did decline/All thought of ill. Who drunk her cup/could shed all that day not a tear" (Homer, 1909–1914). But the scientific study of the clinical effects of medications designed to treat mental health conditions didn't emerge until the 1950s. *Psychopharmacology* refers to the clinical science devoted to understanding and treating psychopathological conditions with medications. This discipline grows out of two basic science fields, neuropharmacology and behavioral pharmacology. *Neuropharmacology* is the science of the way drugs affect brain function at physiological, cellular, and chemical levels that contributes to their therapeutic effects. The sister discipline of *behavioral pharmacology* is the scientific investigation of the behavioral effects of drugs and understanding the behavioral processes responsible for those effects. We discuss the relationship of behavioral pharmacology to the clinical effects of medications used to treat psychopathological conditions.

Behavioral Mechanisms of Medication Effects

In *Behavioral Pharmacology* (1968), Thompson and Schuster introduced the concept of *behavioral mechanisms of drug action*. They argued that many effects of psychoactive drugs can be understood in terms of their influence on familiar processes within behavior analysis, for example, discriminative stimuli, positive and negative reinforcement, and reinforcement schedule effects. A medication may make one consequence more effective in maintaining behavior than another or may change the relative rates of reinforcement when choosing one alternative over another under a concurrent reinforcement schedule (doing math vs. bothering a neighbor). Thompson and Symons (2000) and Thompson, Hackenberg, Cerutti, Baker, and Axtell (1994) extended this reasoning, originally based on laboratory studies, to analyzing effects of psychotropic drugs on behavior of people with developmental disabilities in educational and clinical settings. A medication such as an SSRI antidepressant makes more serotonin available to bind to receptors. When that happens, stimuli that were previously powerful negative reinforcers, such as teacher task demands, may be made less aversive. Aggressive behavior that leads to avoidance of task demands is reduced. Reduced efficacy of negative reinforcers is the behavioral mechanism of drug action. In this section, we discuss examples of behavioral mechanisms of drug action specific to individuals with developmental disabilities. Before examining those mechanisms, we must first discuss how medication effects are measured in applied settings among people with developmental disabilities.

Measuring Behavioral Effects of Medications

Underlying measurement of medication effects are assumptions about what is being evaluated. For example, is the behavior of interest in and of itself (e.g., aggression), or is the purpose of measurement to assess changes in presumed underlying psychopathology?

Deciding What to Measure

Deciding what is appropriate use of psychotropic medications requires the use of valid and psychometrically sound assessment instruments to measure drug effects (Schroeder, Rojahn, & Reese, 1997; Sprague & Werry, 1971). Unknown or inadequate psychometric properties of psychopathology assessment instruments (Aman, 1991), inappropriate use of global assessment instruments (Schroeder et al., 1997), and indirect measurement strategies all plague clinical practice and research on medication effects in developmental disabilities. Schroeder et al. (1997) pointed out that most instruments used to evaluate drug effects on self-injurious behavior (SIB) are insensitive to daily rates of target behavior and that none have been evaluated for psychometric properties (i.e., reliability and validity). In fragile X syndrome the majority of psychopharmacology research has been limited to open-label trials and to surveying parents regarding their perceived efficacy, with notable exceptions for folic acid and methylphenidate (Hagerman & Cronister, 1996). Differences in assumptions about the nature of psychopathology and behavioral disorders among individuals with intellectual disabilities and corresponding differences in the selection of measures contributes to inconsistencies in outcomes regarding the clinical efficacy of medications in intellectual disabilities.

When a psychoactive medication is prescribed for a person with intellectual disabilities, it is often assumed that the person is experiencing a psychiatric disorder for which the medication is indicated. Prescribing professionals often assume that a cluster of behavior problems (e.g., aggression, self-injury, property destruction) must indicate underlying psychopathology and prescribe medications accordingly. At times mental illness is diagnosed among people with severe intellectual disabilities with little assurance that DSM diagnostic signs and symptoms are applicable. There are no well-validated diagnostic instruments suitable for dually diagnosed individuals with severe intellectual disabilities. Moreover, few doctors who provide medical care for individuals with developmental disabilities are familiar with functional assessment of problem behavior. In some cases, such an assessment could reveal that the behavior problem is environmentally caused. In some cases, individuals are diagnosed with a mental illness when, in fact, they are exhibiting maladaptive coping with their unfavorable environmental circumstances.

Michael Rutter, one of the world's leaders in child psychiatry, suggested that three measurement issues contribute to diagnostic problems. First, respondent-based interviews and questionnaires can measure only those constructs included among their items (e.g., obsessions). This limitation imposes constraints on identifying clinically relevant phenomena in cases in which the condition being evaluated is not well established within the relevant population. Recent research on behavioral phenotypes within developmental disabilities suggests that we may have a limited understanding of how psychiatric conditions are expressed (Dykkens, Hodapp, & Finucane, 2000). Moreover, there is little agreement about the nature of psychiatric conditions among nonverbal individuals with severe or profound intellectual disabilities or about their reliable and valid assessment. Second, the frequently claimed comorbidity in persons with developmental disabilities may be partially artifactual, resulting from problems in measurement and mistaken psychiatric diagnostic concepts (Mahoney et al., 1998). Third, the distinction between dimensional versus categorical measures of psychiatric disorders can be misleading (Tanguay, Robertson, & Derrick, 1998). Many measurement problems are a consequence of inappropriately using strategies designed for case identification to document treatment outcomes. Assessment instruments for behavior change need to become more refined and specifically sensitive to medication effects and to the target behaviors of interest for individuals with severe destructive behavior and developmental disabilities (Schroeder et al., 1997).

The decision to use direct rather than indirect measurement strategies can have profound consequences. This issue was encountered indirectly in evaluating the treatment of SIB with the opiate antagonist naltrexone hydrochloride. Symons et al. (2001) showed that naltrexone administration resulted in reductions of some forms of self-injury, but not others, for four adult men with severe intellectual disabilities. That fact would have been recognized only by directly measuring each form of self-injury, not by overall impressions about self-injury in general. Although the overall rate of severe forms of self-injury was reduced during naltrexone administration, a paradoxical outcome was observed. For three of the participants, self-injury became more likely (though not more frequent) while they took the medication, but only following staff prompting. It is possible that decreased self-injury leads to increased social interaction with staff, which, paradoxically, results in temporary increases in self-injury immediately following such interactions. In such cases, raters may judge self-injury to be worse during drug treatment conditions even though its overall rate declined. Treatment studies should include direct observation to corroborate staff ratings of behavior change. This may help explain outcomes of clinical psychopharmacology studies in which negative treatment outcomes have been reported from trials that rely on third-party reports for measuring self-injury at single points before and after treatment (Willemsen-Swinkels, Buitelaar, Nijhof, & van Engeland, 1995). Alternatively, weak correlations between global ratings and direct observation may not necessarily invalidate one or the other measurement strategy but could and should suggest that different aspects of the phenomena are being measured. This suggests that multiple measures sequential in time should be used in medication trials with individuals with destructive behavior and developmental disabilities.

Sequential Analysis

In 1980, Schroeder, Mulick, and Rojahn suggested that studying the sequential dependencies among social antecedents and severe destructive behavior could lead to insights into the underlying organization of behavior disorders. In addition, it could clarify the relation to the surrounding social context. In most treatment studies, the outcome measure is limited to reductions in the presenting behavior problem (i.e., self-injury, aggression, property destruction), whether it is directly observed and rated or indirectly reported on. Little is known about multiple forms of severe destructive behavior that may serve the same functions and changes in response hierarchies during pharmacological treatment. Several different responses that serve the same function (e.g., aggression and tantrums) may both decrease in frequency when a given medication is prescribed, whereas another problem behavior that serves a different function (e.g., self-injury) may remain unchanged. Component responses of sequences of behavior that escalate into a behavioral outburst may be differentially changed by a medication. This may be important practically in heading off an impending behavior problem, but it may also be theoretically important in understanding what leads to an outburst.

Social Validity

The social validation of effects of psychotropic medications on behavior of individuals with developmental disabilities has received little attention (Poling, Laraway, Ehrhardt, Jennings, & Turner, 2004; Poling, Methot, & LeSage, 1995). "Social validity" refers to the perceived importance of effects of an intervention and includes socially significant treatment goals, socially appropriate procedures to achieve the goals, and socially important effects (Wolf, 1978). A demonstration that self-injury is statistically significantly reduced by a medication when tested on a substantial sample of people may not be perceived as important to parents and other caregivers. Statistical significance may be obtained in some studies if there is a 20% reduction in self-injury on average across all people tested. If a person with a severe disability bites her hand an average of 20 times per day at baseline, that would mean that she would continue to harm herself 16 times per day after treatment. Many parents would feel that reducing self-injury by four instances per day would not enhance their daughter's overall quality of life.

Social validity is concerned with treatment acceptability and procedural viability (Schwartz & Baer, 1991). Social validity measurement does not replace directly observing and measuring target behaviors or collecting informant data through other means (i.e., checklists, rating scales) but rather augments the overall measurement strategy. In a review of social validity and quality-of-life measures used in the treatment of self-injury, Symons, Koppekin, and Wehby (1999) found that, although approximately one-third of studies included some measure related to social validity or quality of life, very little detailed information was available concerning the specific nature of the behavior change. When changes were documented, terms tended to be vague and poorly defined (e.g., "increased socialization"), and the majority of evidence was anecdotal. Objective documented changes in social relationships and support networks were minimal, which is problematic given the importance of social relationships for people with developmental disabilities (Kennedy & Shukla, 1995). Poling et al. (1995) concluded that "collecting and including social validity data would add little to the cost or difficulty of conducting a study . . . doing so, however, would allow readers to respond to the other [outcome] data in a broader, and more socially significant, context" (p. 198).

STATE INTERVENTION STRATEGIES

The first step in addressing antecedent state factors that affect the behavior of an individual with a developmental disability is to recognize that such a problem exists. If an individual's behavior is tracked over time and fluctuates widely, regardless of the educational or behavioral interventions that are in place, then an intermittent biological state variable may be operating. Part of a functional behavioral assessment (FBA) involves evaluating the role of potential biological state factors. A health checklist can be a helpful starting point that includes a record of a child's sleep patterns, toileting (constipation), eating, allergies, injuries, headaches, toothaches, and cold or flu symptoms. A corresponding parent checklist that includes a history of common mental health problems (depression, anxiety disorders) can suggest areas of attention for a child's FBA, as many mental health problems run in families. Although school personnel are not trained to diagnose psychopathology, they can collect information that may be useful for a clinical psychologist, psychiatrist, or behavioral pediatrician in arriving at such a diagnosis.

If an individual is diagnosed with one of the mental health disorders discussed here, school or related professional personnel can obtain information from the prescribing physician regarding the common signs and symptoms of that condition. Many school psychologists can also be helpful in developing a simple checklist that can be used to monitor fluctuations in mental health state. Even if a child's or adolescent's symptoms do not meet all of the criteria for a specific disorder (e.g., autistic disorder), a doctor may prescribe medication to help manage some of the symptoms (e.g., social anxiety, compulsiveness). An appreciation of the role of psychotropic medications in moderating those emotional and mental health states can assist educational personnel in interpreting a child or adolescent's behavior and plan accordingly.

FUNCTIONAL BEHAVIORAL ASSESSMENT AND DRUG EFFECTS

Over the past 20 years, observation-based assessment technology for specifying the environmental determinants of destructive behavior and designing evaluating treatments based directly on assessment outcome has expanded (Thompson, Felce, & Symons, 2000). The overall goal of this approach, referred to by several terms (functional analysis, functional assessment, functional behavioral assessment), is to identify the antecedent states, stimulus control factors, and reinforcement contingencies that maintain destructive behavior and other factors that may contribute to challenging behavior. Thus, treatment is based on behavioral processes rather than on the form of the response, such as hitting or screaming. Carr (1977) suggested that reinforcement processes, rather than psychodynamic factors, often give rise to and maintain destructive behaviors among individuals with developmental disabilities.

Iwata, Dorsey, Slifer, Bauman, and Richman (1982) provided a methodology for testing hypotheses about the effects of specific environmental consequences. The importance of identifying behavioral function to guide behavioral treatment selection has been demonstrated in numerous reports showing that interventions based on behavioral function are more likely to be effective than arbitrarily chosen treatments (Carr & Durand, 1985; Day, Horner, & O'Neill, 1994; Iwata et al., 1982; Repp, Felce, & Barton, 1988). For many individuals with intractable, apparently nonsocial, SIB, however, treatment often involves trial and error. Several pharmacological treatments reduce the SIB of some individuals but often have limited lasting efficacy.

It is relatively uncommon to find reports documenting a functional assessment prior to intervention with a pharmacological agent, despite the advantages such an approach may have in improving our ability to clarify the possible role that environmental circumstances play in determining the behavioral effect of a therapeutic drug (Schaal & Hackenberg, 1994; Thompson et al., 1994). The information gathered via such an approach could have important assessment and intervention implications. By conducting a functional assessment prior to treatment, it may be possible to show the differential effects of a given drug for different forms and functions of SIB; for example, that self-injury maintained by task avoidance is selectively affected by a given medication. Since Schaal and Hackenberg's 1994 paper called for a more integrated strategy that incorporates FBA with medication trials, only six empirical studies have been published using functional analysis as part of the medication evaluation. These studies were found using searches in the PsycInfo and PubMed databases, as well as table of contents searches in the *American Journal of Intellectual Disabilities*, the *Journal of Autism and Developmental Disorders,* and *Research in Developmental Disabilities.* In each of these studies (reviewed, in part, in the next section) functional analyses were conducted before treatment and throughout the study in multielement format. Medication and placebo were administered in a double-blind fashion. In some cases, functional analysis allowed the investigators to reveal function-specific effects of the medications.

PSYCHOTROPIC MEDICATIONS AND BEHAVIORAL MECHANISMS OF ACTION

Psychotropic Medications That Decrease Social Demand Avoidance

Hellings, Kelley, and Gabrielli (1996) evaluated effects of the selective serotonin inhibitor sertraline (Zoloft) on aggressive and self-injurious behavior of 9 adults with developmental disabilities, several of whom met diagnostic criteria for autism. Sertraline reduces depression and anxiety problems in other psychiatric populations. Using the Clinical Global Impressions Scale (Guy, 1976) in a prospective open trial, they found that the medication reduced self-injury and aggression in 8 of 9 individuals. McDougle and colleagues (1998) conducted an open trial of sertraline and found that 57% of 42 individuals showed significant improvement in repetitive and aggressive symptoms. Using other behavioral ratings, they found that 68% were responders. The behavioral mechanisms underlying these changes remain ambiguous. Reducing anxiety or depression increases tolerance for demands and reduces avoidance behavior, for example, aggression or self-injury. Because a functional assessment was not done in this study, it is difficult to know whether that was the mechanism. Lewis, Bodfish, Powell, and Golden (1995; Lewis, Bodfish, Powell, Parker, and Golden 1996) have examined effects of the cyclic antidepressant clomipramine (Anafranil) on stereotypic and self-injurious behavior of adults with intellectual disability in a state residential facility. Clomipramine is approved by the Food and Drug Administration (FDA) for treatment of obsessive–compulsive disorder in adult psychiatric patients. Whether the neurochemical and/or behavioral mechanisms are the same among people with intellectual disabilities is unclear.

Mace, Blum, Sierp, Delaney, and Mauk (2001) examined whether SIB, in participants ranging from 4 to 31 years old, was maintained by socially mediated consequences. Only participants whose behavior was found to have identifiable environmental consequences were included in the study. Through their subsequent investigation of the effects of antipsychotic medication, haloperidol (Haldol) was compared with behavioral treatment. Behavioral treatment based on identified functions of the problem behavior led to significantly greater reduction of challenging behavior than the haloperidol. These investigators did not attempt to determine whether haloperidol effects varied with the functions of challenging behavior.

Other evidence more clearly suggests that psychotropic medications can change the functions of challenging behavior. Crosland et al. (2003) found differential effects of risperidone (Risperdal) across behavioral function in an adult and a child diagnosed with autism. The adult participant's self-injury appeared more responsive to the medication than did his aggression. The participants were exposed to functional analysis conditions each day in a multielement fashion, with risperidone and placebo alternated in a double-blind fashion. In a related study, Zarcone et al. (2004) evaluated the effects of risperidone in treating 13 individuals, 10 of whom were responsive to the medication.

Seven of these individuals exhibited behavior that was not socially motivated, as identified through pretreatment functional analysis. The problem behavior of the remaining three individuals who responded to risperidone was reduced specific to the function originally identified in the pretreatment analysis.

Psychotropic Medications That Enhance Stimulus Control and Increase Value of Weak Reinforcers

Stimulants are the most widely prescribed medications for children with behavior problems. It has been estimated that approximately 70–80% of children properly diagnosed with ADHD respond favorably to one of the amphetamine medications (Dexedrine, Adderall) or methylphenidate (Ritalin, Concerta; Reiff, 2004). Because stimulant medications increase activity levels in most people (as well as laboratory subjects), it seemed paradoxical that among children with ADHD it appeared to reduce overactivity. Hill (1970) first suggested that the reason that stimulant medications improve the behavior of children with ADHD was that the drug enhanced the effectiveness of weak reinforcers (i.e., conditioned reinforcers) that were associated with academic tasks in school and compliance with parental demands at home. His initial laboratory study was suggestive but did not provide definitive proof of his hypothesis. Subsequently, Robbins (1975), Robbins and Sahakian (1979), and Cador, Robbins, and Everitt (1989) at Cambridge University published a series of laboratory studies demonstrating that stimulants have multiple effects, including enhancing stimulus control (i.e., attention mechanisms) and increasing the effectiveness of weak conditioned reinforcers. They point out that the effects of stimulant medications are not really paradoxical if one understands the underlying mechanisms of the drugs' effects.

Classroom and clinical studies are rarely designed to distinguish these two effects. A student with ADHD whose school performance improves because he or she is responding more appropriately to instructional stimuli will demonstrate even greater improvement if his or her teacher increases the frequency of positive reinforcement for compliance and task completion. It is a mistake to assume that improved attention to instructional stimuli alone will sustain improved school performance. One of the reasons stimulant medications lose their effectiveness over time for some children with ADHD is that caregivers and school personnel have not provided sufficient positive reinforcement, along with the improved attention the drug produces. The combination of stimulant medications and behavior therapy produces greater behavioral improvements than either treatment alone among many children with ADHD (Multimodal Treatment Study for Attention-Deficit/Hyperactivity Disorder Cooperative Group, 1999).

Medications That Alter Response Rate and Reinforcement Rate

As noted earlier in this chapter, individuals who suffer from depression are often less sensitive to positive reinforcers and more responsive to negative reinforcers. Lewinsohn (1992) has postulated that depression can result from a stressor that causes a low rate of response-contingent positive reinforcement. The rate of reinforcement is related to the availability of reinforcing events, personal skills to act on the environment, or the impact of certain types of events. According to this hypothesis, if an individual cannot reverse the negative balance of reinforcement, the person is likely to engage in self-criticism and behavioral withdrawal. Depressed patients have low rates of pleasant activities and obtained pleasure; their moods covary with rates of pleasant and aversive activities; their moods improve with increases in pleasant activities; and they lack social skills, at least during the depressed phase—all of which contribute to the depression. However, at times behavioral treatments alone do not seem sufficient to relieve depression in some individuals.

There is also evidence that diminished availability of the neurotransmitter serotonin in the brain is implicated in depression. Clinical studies of serotonin metabolism in major depression provide evidence for an abnormality of the serotonin brain system. Deficit in L-tryptophan appears to be the rate-limiting step in the synthesis of serotonin and is an important factor causing depression and the response of antidepressant drugs (Maes & Meltzer, 1995). Animal laboratory studies suggest that serotonin and dopamine both play a role in reinforcement. In one study, fluoxetine (Prozac), a selective serotonin reuptake inhibitor, and bupropion (Wellbutrin), a dopamine reuptake inhibitor, were given to determine their effects on behavior maintained by conditioned reinforcement. Fluoxetine, but not bupropion, enhanced performance maintained by conditioned reinforcement (Sasaki-Adams & Kelley, 2001).

Clinically, selective serotonin reuptake inhibitors (SSRIs) allow for an increased availability of serotonin, though not all individuals with depression respond to this class of drugs in treatment in the same way. Whittington et al. (2004) conducted a meta-analysis of randomized controlled trials that evaluated an SSRI versus a placebo in participants ages 5–18 years, that had been published in peer-reviewed journals or were unpublished, and that were included in a review by the Committee on Safety of Medicines (U.K.). They examined remission, response to treatment, depressive symptom scores, serious adverse events, suicide-related behaviors, and discontinuation of treatment because of adverse events. They found that two studies with fluoxetine (Prozac) yielded a positive benefit–risk profile; however, both paroxetine (Paxil) and sertaline (Zoloft) yielded equivocal results. However, subsequently, the U.K. Medicines and Healthcare Products Regulatory Authority banned SSRIs for children in the United Kingdom because of reports of suicidal ideation among children and adolescents, though no suicides had been reported. A recent review by Janowsky and Davis (2005) concluded that SSRIs are effective and safe in treating individuals with intellectual disabilities who have depression, whereas in another review, Wagner (2005) concluded that only citalopram (Celexa), Zoloft, and Prozac were more effective than placebos in treating childhood depression. Although differences of opinion exist regarding the relative efficacy of SSRI medications in treating depression among different populations, there is general agreement that as a class they are effective in enhancing positive reinforcement and reducing avoidance behavior.

Medications That Reduce Reinforcing Consequences of Self-Injury

Cataldo and Harris (1982) first suggested that a naturally occurring painkilling substance such as beta-endorphin, if released in the brain when an individual with a developmental disability injures her- or himself, might serve as a reinforcer by binding to the same opiate receptors in the brain to which addictive drugs such as heroin or morphine bind. Several investigators have demonstrated that drugs that block these receptors (naloxone and naltrexone) often reduce self-injury (e.g., Thompson et al., 1994). According to this reasoning, if the person whose opiate receptors are blocked by an antagonist injures him- or herself, the reinforcing event of opiate receptor binding cannot occur.

There have been inconsistencies in the clinical research literature regarding the outcome of naltrexone trials in self-injury, suggesting either that different measures yield different results or that there is variability within people who injure themselves that may account for the differences. Symons, Fox, and Thompson (1998) evaluated the efficacy of the opiate antagonist naltrexone combined with functional communication training (FCT) for self-injury in a 12-year-old boy with autism, intellectual disability, and communication deficits. Initial reductions in the overall rate of SIB were reported during a placebo-controlled double-blind medication trial, with further reductions noted following the addition of FCT. Similarly, Garcia and Smith (1999) evaluated the effects of naltrexone on the self-injurious behavior of two women diagnosed with profound intellectual disabilities. Both participants were exposed to pretreatment functional analyses to determine possible social reasons for their behavior at baseline. The treatment phase consisted of continued exposure to analog assessment procedures in a multi-element format, paired with daily administration of naltrexone or a placebo in a double-blind format. Naltrexone produced function-specific effects on self-injury between and within participants. For one participant, socially mediated head slapping (negatively reinforced) decreased with naltrexone administration, but non–socially mediated head banging did not. For the other participant, only her non–socially mediated self-injury was reduced with naltrexone. This study was the first to evaluate the effects of naltrexone using analog functional analysis measures.

Sandman, Touchette, Lenjavi, Marion, and Chicz-DeMet (2003) obtained a blood sample immediately after SIB. A significant number of the participants (1) reduced their SIB at least 25% at all doses of naltrexone (NTX) and (2) reduced their SIB over 50% at at least one dose of NTX. There was a correlation of .67 between elevation in beta-endorphin in blood and amount of reduction in SIB produced by naltrexone, a finding consistent with the opioid self-administration hypothesis of self-injury.

Recently, Symons, Thompson, and Rodriguez (2004) conducted a quantitative synthesis of the peer-reviewed published literature from 1983 to 2003 documenting the use of naltrexone for the treatment of SIB. Individual-level results were analyzed. Twenty-seven research articles involving 86 participants with self-injury were reviewed. Eighty percent of participants were reported to improve relative to baseline (i.e., SIB reduced) during naltrexone administration, and for 47% of participants, SIB was reduced by 50% or greater. In studies quantitatively reporting dose, males were more likely than females to respond. Collectively, the foregoing data suggest that for some people with developmental disabilities, self-injury is maintained by beta-endorphin or some similar form of opioid peptide-like activity binding to opiate receptors following SIB and that the behavioral mechanism of action of naltrexone is extinction of the self-injurious behavior.

WORKING WITH PHYSICIANS, NURSES, AND ALLIED HEALTH CARE PROFESSIONALS

Establishing and maintaining positive relationships with colleagues in medicine and allied professional fields is an important part of including medications within a PBS strategy. Though some of the following suggestions may seem self-evident, in our experience they are often not appreciated or acted on and rarely discussed. It is important to treat physicians and health care workers with respect. A psychiatrist, neurologist, or pediatrician, for example, has received an average of 14 years of postgraduate years of education and training (some 16 years). It is reasonable that they expect their expertise to be acknowledged and respected. Try putting yourself in their shoes. If a physician questioned your choice of Picture Exchange System over an AlphaSmart keyboarding communication system for one of your students, you would wonder on what basis he or she was questioning your judgment. When you are a good listener and ask informed questions, the physician's reasoning usually becomes more evident. In medicine, treatments must follow from established diagnoses and be supported by published evidence of effectiveness and safety. Treatment decisions must be made expeditiously and must not be unduly time-consuming to provide. A treatment can have demonstrated efficacy but not be effective. A treatment that reduces a behavior problem within a well-controlled clinical setting with ideal staff ratios of well-trained personnel may be impractical under most circumstances.

Information must be presented understandably. Physicians are accustomed to interpreting blood pressure and white blood counts, not behavioral or educational data. Briefly explain what is being graphed and make certain that graphs are clearly labeled. Explain why the measure you've graphed is important (e.g., words per minute, percentage correct, outbursts per hour). Physicians know what a dark spot on an MRI image represents, but not the results of a functional assessment.

To be effective you must be perceived as an affirmative, helpful colleague, not a critic or obstacle. One way to ensure this is to ask physicians or their nursing staff directly what information would be helpful to them in making treatment decisions. They may not know what you have to offer. You can facilitate this by providing examples of the kind of data you can make available to them and, more important, its relevance and how it might be used. In some cases, it may be useful to offer to train nursing staff to review graphs sent to the physician's office to save them time. Physicians are decision makers accustomed to relying on lab reports, radiologists' findings, and neurologist's electroencephalogram reports, so why not the findings of psychologists, special education specialists, or behavior analysts? Make objective behavioral and side-effect information available to physicians so they can use that information in making treatment decisions.

In the United States, physicians must cope with managed care; they do not have a choice. Treatment decisions must be justified to insurance companies or Medicaid. Third-party payers must be convinced of the correctness of the diagnosis and the most valid, realistic, and least costly course of treatment. It is not helpful for you to try to tell physicians, physician's assistants, and nurses how to do their jobs. Present objective, quantitative information, not uninformed conclusions. Accompany treatment discussions with reprints or abstracts of articles. Physicians get their information from medical journals, not behavioral or educational publications. Be professional. You are not talking with the physician as an advocate for PBS, applied behavior analysis (ABA), or any other theoretical approach to solving problems. You are exploring the best course of treatment for the individual based on evidence. Behave like an objective professional giving your informed opinion.

It is important to be realistic about expectations. Despite wanting a "yes" or "no" answer regarding treatment outcomes, often "probably" or "it's very likely" is the best a physician or physician's assistant can provide. Be wary of seeming to quiz a physician about a recently reported treatment, especially in the presence of the patient or the patient's family. Regardless of how well trained and experienced he or she may be, a physician or nurse cannot possibly know every finding in the latest subspecialty publication or appearing on the World Wide Web. If you have a question, leave them with print information and get back to them after they have had an opportunity to look into the new findings. Avoid siding with parents in efforts to convince the physician to change treatment. Though some parents may be enthusiastic about complementary or alternative treatments, most physicians are alienated by the suggestion that they employ treatments for which there is scant objective evidence of effectiveness or safety.

Common courtesy goes a long way. Write a follow-up note to the physician thanking him or her for taking time to talk with you and offering to be of assistance in the future. If you treat physicians and their staff members with the respect you hope others will accord you, much more will be accomplished on behalf of the student or client with whom you are working.

IMPLICATIONS FOR RESEARCH AND PRACTICE

Dr. J. Bronchus Croup publishes a paper indicating that Tussis-CD, a hypothetical cold medication, significantly reduces coughing in 37% of people who cough, as compared with 11% who receive a placebo cough medicine. How helpful is that information? It would be important to know whether the 37% of people who improved were coughing because they had a common cold, pneumonia, allergies, or asthma or whether they were extremely anxious. Doctors might decide to treat people with an antibiotic, an antihistamine, or an antianxiety medication, depending on the reason they coughed, and they need to know how Tussis-CD produced its effects. Patients would want to know whether Tussis-CD would help with their particular kind of cough. The results of Dr. Croup's study would not be enlightening to either group. Knowing that any given treatment reduces symptoms in a percentage of people is of very little interest unless the vast majority of people receiving the treatment dramatically improved or unless more were known about the reasons the treatment was effective for some but not others.

The time will come in the not too distant future when researchers and most well-trained clinicians will stop asking, "What psychotherapeutic medication is most effective for autism or aggression or anxiety?" Instead they will ask the question more like this: "What medication is most effective for a prepubertal child who meets the ADOS diagnostic criteria for autism and has a deletion of the XYZ gene and whose challenging behavior in the classroom is maintained by social escape–avoidance?" And they will also ask, "In what *specific ways* is the medication effective? Is it associated with improvements in joint attention, effectiveness of social reinforcers, or the semantic appropriateness of the child's verbal utterances?" The more interesting and valuable information will concern which people with what underlying neurochemical and functional behavioral profiles are improved in what ways by a medication that specifically acts on those neurochemical and functional behavioral mechanisms.

Several promising developments have occurred in research on neurodevelopmental disabilities that have implications for use of psychotherapeutic medications. Research on behavioral phenotypes and their relationships with genotypes has begun to shed light on subtypes of individuals who appear to meet the same or similar diagnostic criteria using DSM or other standardized assessment tools but who differ in reliable ways (Dykens, 1995; Flint, 1998). This research begins to provide a way to identify which people who on the surface may appear similar will respond differentially to treatments (e.g., intensive behavior therapy, atypical antipsychotic medications, or peer tutors in the classroom).

A second development is the search for *endophenotypes*. Gottesman and Shields (1967) introduced the endophenotype concept in connection with understanding subtypes of schizophrenia, but the same reasoning applies to neurodevelopmental disabilities, as well. Disabilities that are influenced by a combination of several genes and environmental factors, such as social learning histories and stressors, are usually highly heterogeneous. They vary in types and severity of symptoms. That makes identifying subtypes that are differentially responsive to treatments very difficult. Gottesman and Shields (1967) argued that simpler clues to genetic underpinnings than the complex array of symptoms seen in the clinical syndrome itself can be found, which can result in more successful genetic analysis and, ultimately, improved treatments. An endophenotype may be neurophysiological, biochemical, endocrinological, neuroanatomical, cognitive, or neuropsychological. It is also likely that functional behavioral assessments can add to predictive power of endophenotypes. Once endophenotypes are identified, it becomes far more likely that we will be able to predict which people will respond to specific treatments.

A third development is the recognition that social learning history produces permanent changes in the brain, especially during the first 5 years of life. Consider a hypothetical developmental disability that is most commonly caused by deletion of three genes located near one another on a specific human chromosome. A child is born with two of those genes missing, not three. That child has a lower dose of the genetic error that may make him or her at less risk for some of the symptoms of the developmental disorder than those missing all three genes, but *if and only if* the child is also exposed to an early social learning environment that fails to adequately promote development of social skills and language. A child of parents who are abusive or who have significant mental health or drug abuse problems that makes them unresponsive, or who are socially less competent (e.g., have borderline symptoms of autism) may increasingly develop symptoms of pervasive developmental disorder, not otherwise specified over his or her preschool years. Such factors are called "social potentiators" (Meehl, 1990) or "epigenetic factors" (Thompson, 2005). The challenge is how best to compensate for the combined disadvantage and therefore prevent the symptoms of a disability. A medication that could prolong the period during which new synapses are rapidly formed could increase the window of opportunity within which to overcome some of the effects of the gene defect and early social learning disadvantage. The enduring effects of intensive early behavior therapy on a subset of children diagnosed with autism (Lovaas, 1987), combined with what is known about the optimal period of new synapse development and their consolidation in the brain (Huttenlocher & de Courten, 1987), leads us to conclude that behavioral intervention can be a form of brain intervention. Perhaps the effectiveness of social, language, and cognitive development interventions could be enhanced by use of appropriate medications that prolong high levels of synapse formation.

FBA as a diagnostic tool (alone and together with other endophenotypic information) to predict response to treatment is another very promising research area. Earlier evidence discussed in several studies suggested that an FBA approach could improve our ability to tailor-make interventions for individual children and youth with behavioral challenges. More focused efforts using more carefully characterized cohorts of people with specific developmental disability subtypes are more likely to yield improved predictions of response to intervention.

Funding for services to individuals whose habilitative care and education are among the most costly to deliver are going to come under increasing scrutiny at all levels of government and among private insurers. Schools and human service agencies are going to be subject to increasing pressure to use the least expensive services. Prescribing and administering a pill is much less costly than employing highly trained staff to provide optimal human services for such individuals. Medications are more likely to be used appropriately and less likely to be substituted for appropriate educational or habilitative services *if service providers employ evidence-based practices.* It will be increasingly necessary to demonstrate that intervention methods used by teachers and other human service practitioners significantly contribute to child outcomes (Dixon et al., 2001; Powell, Fixsen, & Dunlap, 2003). School personnel and other human service workers will find it necessary to document effects of each intervention, alone and in combination. Interventions whose effects cannot be demonstrated persuasively are likely to be reduced or eliminated.

Governmental and private funders have grown impatient with administrative barriers to collaboration (e.g., between education and mental health). Best practices will be mandated, including monitoring effects of medications at school or in other nonmedical settings and working closely with medical personnel. That implies that physicians will need to know more about educational and social interventions, and school and social service staff will find it necessary to understand much more about medications and medical aspects of disabilities. Demonstration projects designed to develop decision-making intervention algorithms will become more common in these fields, as they are in medicine. Their purpose is to encourage more timely evidence-based intervention decisions contingent on demonstrated progress (or lack of progress).

The reasoning presented in this paper may be helpful to researchers and practitioners by providing tools with which to develop intervention strategies for the whole child based on solid evidence of effectiveness.

CONCLUSIONS

Much of the time, when people with intellectual or other developmental disabilities exhibit behavioral challenges, those problems are due to environmental antecedents (including setting events or establishing operations), skill deficits, task characteristics, or inopportune behavioral consequences. In those instances, psychotropic medications are seldom necessary. However, increasing evidence suggests that *state variables* less clearly linked to specific environmental events also contribute to problem behavior by increasing or decreasing efficacy of specific types of consequences. Some of these conditions are psychopathological states such as anxiety, depression, mania, or other health variables (e.g., certain types of seizure disorders). Psychotropic medications do not eliminate behavioral challenges—as the pest-control man vanquishes vermin in the television advertisement with the spray from his pesticide bottle. Medications that change brain chemistry produce their effects by altering the way the environment functions in its relation to behavior. *Behavioral mechanisms of drug action* involve analyzing and changing the functions of environmental events that set the occasion for behavior or maintain it. Determining whether a behaviorally active medication produces desired therapeutic effects requires multiple measures, ideally including some level of direct observational data recorded repeatedly over time. Functional assessments of events surrounding problem behavior can be useful in determining which behavioral processes are being affected and which are not. Psychotropic medications can be an important part of an overall PBS strategy if they are appropriately used based on an understanding of those behavioral mechanisms and if their effects are carefully monitored to assess outcome.

ACKNOWLEDGMENTS

Portions of the work reported here were supported, in part, by National Institutes of Health Grant No. 44763 to the University of Minnesota, Frank Symons, Principal Investigator.

REFERENCES

Aman, M. G. (1991). Review and evaluation of instruments for assessing emotional and behavioural disorders. *Australia and New Zealand Journal of Developmental Disabilities, 17*(2), 127–145.

Aman, M. G., Lam, K. S., & Collier-Crespin, C. (2003). A prevalence and patterns of use of psychoactive medicines among individuals with autism in the Autism Society of Ohio. *Journal of Autism and Developmental Disorders, 33*(5), 527–534.

Aman, M. G., Sarphare, G., & Burrow, W. (1995). Psychoactive drugs in group homes: Prevalence and relation to demographic/psychiatric variables. *American Journal on Mental Retardation, 99*, 500–509.

American Psychiatric Association. (2000). *Diagnostic and statistical manual of mental disorders* (4th ed., text rev.). Washington, DC: Author.

Bailey, D. B., Hatton, D. D., Mesibov, G., Ament, N., & Skinner, M. (2000). Early development, temperament, and functional impairment in autism and fragile X syndrome. *Journal of Autism and Developmental Disorders, 30*(1), 49–59.

Bijou, S. W., & Baer, D. M. (1978). *Behavior analysis of child development.* Engelwood Cliffs, NJ: Prentice-Hall.

Cador, M., Robbins, T. W., & Everitt, B. J. (1989). Involvement of the amygdala in stimulus-reward associations: Interaction with the ventral striatum. *Neuroscience, 30*, 77–86.

Carr, E. G. (1977). The motivation of self-injurious behavior: A review of some hypotheses. *Psychological Bulletin, 84*, 800–816.

Carr, E. G., & Durand, V. M. (1985). Reducing behavior problems through functional communication training. *Journal of Applied Behavior Analysis, 18*, 111–126.

Carr, E. G., & Smith, C. E. (1995). Biological setting events for self-injury. *Mental Retardation and Developmental Disabilities Research Reviews, 1*, 94–98.

Carr, E. G., Smith, C. E., Giacin, T. A., Whelan, B. M., & Pancari, J. (2003). Menstrual discomfort as a biological setting event for severe problem behavior: Assessment and intervention. *American Journal of Mental Retardation, 108*, 117–133.

Cataldo, M. F., & Harris, J. (1982). The biological basis of self-injury in the mentally retarded. *Analysis and Intervention in Developmental Disabilities, 7*, 21–39.

Crosland, K. A., Zarcone, J. R., Lindauer, S. E., Valdovinos, M. G., Zarcone, T. J., Hellings, J. A., et al. (2003). Use of functional analysis methodology in the evaluation of medication effects. *Journal of Autism and Developmental Disabilities, 33*(3), 271–279.

Day, H. M., Horner, R. H., & O'Neill, R. E. (1994). Multiple functions of problem behaviors: Assessment and intervention. *Journal of Applied Behavior Analysis, 27*, 279–289.

Dixon, L., McFarlane, W. R., Lefley, H., Lucksted, A., Cohen, M., Falloon, I., et al. (2001). Evidence-based practices for services to families of people with psychiatric disabilities. *Psychiatric Services, 52*(7), 903–910.

Dykens, E. M. (1995). Measuring behavioral phenotypes: Provocations from the "new genetics." *American Journal on Mental Retardation, 99*, 522–532.

Dykens, E., Hodapp, R. M., & Finucane, B. M. (2000). *Genetics and mental retardation syndromes: A new look at behavior and interventions.* Baltimore: Brookes.

Eysenck, H. (1971). Relationship between intelligence and personality. *Perceptual and Motor Skills, 32*, 637–638.

Feurer, I. D., Dimitropoulos, A., Stone, W. L., Roof, E., Butler, M. G., & Thompson, T. (1998). The latent variable structure of the compulsive behaviour checklist in people with Prader–Willi syndrome. *Journal of Intellectual Disabilities Research, 42*(6), 472–480.

Flint, J. (1998) Behavioral phenotypes: Methodological and conceptual issues. *American Journal of Medical Genetics (Neuropsychiatric Genetics), 81*, 235–240.

Garcia, D., & Smith, R. G. (1999). Using analog baselines to assess the effects of naltrexone on self-injurious behavior. *Research in Developmental Disabilities, 20*(1), 1–21.

Gottesman, I. I., & Shields, J. (1967). A polygenic theory of schizophrenia. *Proceedings of the National Academy of Sciences of the USA, 58*, 199–205.

Guy, W. (1976). Clinical Global Impressions Scale. *ECDEU assessment manual for psychopharmacology, revised* (DHEW Pub. No. ADM 76-338; pp. 218–222). Rockville, MD: U.S. Department of Health, Education, and Welfare, Public Health Service, Alcohol, Drug Abuse, and Mental Health Administration, National Institute of Mental Health. Psychopharmacology Research Branch, Division of Extramural Research Programs.

Hagerman, R. J., & Cronister, A. (Eds.). (1996). *Fragile X syndrome: Diagnosis, treatment, and research* (2nd ed.). Baltimore: Johns Hopkins University Press.

Hellings, J. A., Kelley, L. A., & Gabrielli, W. F. (1996). Sertraline response in adults with mental retardation and autistic disorder. *Journal of Clinical Psychiatry, 57*, 333–336.

Hill, R. T. (1970). Facilitation of conditioned reinforcement as a mechanism of psychomotor stimulation. In E. Costa & S. Garattini (Eds.), *Amphetamines and related compounds*. New York: Raven Press.

Homer. (1909–1914). *The odyssey of Homer* (S. H. Butcher & A. Lang, Trans.). Retrieved February 5, 2007, from *www.bartleby.com/22/4.html.*

Huttenlocher, P. R., & de Courten, C. (1987). The development of synapses in striate cortex of man. *Human Neurobiology, 6*, 1–9.

Iwata, B. A., Dorsey, M. F., Slifer, K. J., Bauman, K. E., & Richman, G. S. (1982). Toward a functional analysis of self-injury. *Analysis and Intervention in Developmental Disabilities, 2*, 3–20.

Janowsky, D. S., & Davis, J. M. (2005). Diagnosis and treatment of depression in patients with mental retardation. *Current Psychiatry Reports, 7*(6), 421–428.

Kalachnik, J. E. (1999). Measuring side effects of psychopharmacologic medication in individuals with mental retardation and developmental disabilities. *Mental Retardation and Developmental Disabilities Research Reviews, 5*(4), 348–359.

Kennedy, C. H., & Meyer, K. A. (1996). Sleep deprivation, allergy symptoms, and negatively reinforced problem behavior. *Journal of Applied Behavior Analysis, 29*, 133–135.

Kennedy, C. H., Meyer, K. A., Werts, M. G., & Cushing, L. S. (2000). Effects of sleep deprivation on free-operant avoidance. *Journal of the Experimental Analysis of Behavior, 73*(3), 333–345.

Kennedy, C. H., & Shukla, S. (1995). Social interaction research for people with autism as a set of past, current, and emerging propositions. *Behavioral Disorders, 21*, 21–36.

Langworthy-Lam, K. S., Aman, M. G., & Van Bourgondien, M. E. (2002). Prevalence and patterns of use of psychoactive medicines in individuals with autism in the Autism Society of North Carolina. *Journal of Child and Adolescent Psychopharmacology, 12*(4), 311–321.

Lewinsohn, P. (1992). *Control your depression* (rev. ed.). New York: Fireside.

Lewis, M. H., Bodfish, J. W., Powell, S. B., & Golden, R. N. (1995). Clomipramine treatment for stereotypy and related repetitive movement disorders in mental retardation: A double-blind comparison with placebo. *American Journal on Mental Retardation, 100*(3), 299–312.

Lewis, M. H., Bodfish, J. W., Powell, S. B., Parker, D. E., & Golden, R. N. (1996). Clomipramine treatment for self-injurious behavior in individuals with mental retardation: A double-blind comparison with placebo. *American Journal on Mental Retardation, 100*(4), 654–665.

Lovaas, O. I. (1987). Behavioral treatment and normal educational and intellectual functioning in young autistic children. *Journal of Consulting and Clinical Psychology, 55*, 3–9.

Mace, F. C., Blum, N. J., Sierp, B. J., Delaney, B. A., & Mauk, J. E. (2001). Differential response of operant self-injury to pharmacologic versus behavioral treatment. *Developmental and Behavioral Pediatrics, 22*(2), 85–91.

Maes, M., & Meltzer, H. Y. (1995). The serotonin hypothesis of major depression. In F. Bloom & D. Kupher (Eds.), *Psychopharmacology: The fourth generation of progress* (pp. 933–944). New York: Raven Press.

Mahoney, W. J., Szatmari, P., MacLean, J. E., Bryson, S. E., Bartolucci, G., Walter, S., et al. (1998). Reliability and accuracy of differentiating pervasive developmental disorder subtypes. *Journal of the American Academy of Child and Adolescent Psychiatry, 37*(3), 278–285.

McDougle, C. J., Holmes, J. P., Carlson, D. C., Pelton, G. H., Cohen, D. J., & Price, L. H. (1998). A double-blind, placebo-controlled study of risperidone in adults with autistic disorder and other pervasive developmental disorders. *Archives of General Psychiatry, 55*(7), 633–641.

Meehl, P. E. (1990). Toward an integrated theory of schizotaxia, schizotypy, and schizophrenia. *Journal of Personality Disorders, 4*, 1–99.

Michael, J. L. (1982). Distinguishing between discriminative and motivational functions of stimuli. *Journal of the Experimental Analysis of Behavior, 37*, 149–155.

Michael, J. L. (1993). Establishing operations. *Behavior Analyst, 16*, 191–206.

Michael, J. L. (2000). Implications and refinements of the establishing operation concept. *Journal of Applied Behavior Analysis, 33*, 401–411.

Multimodal Treatment Study for Attention-Deficit/Hyperactivity Disorder Cooperative Group. (1999). A 14-month randomized clinical trial of treatment strategies for attention-deficit/hyperactivity disorder: A multimodal treatment study of children with ADHD. *Archives of General Psychiatry, 56*(12), 1073–1086.

Poling, A., Laraway, S., Ehrhardt, K., Jennings, L., & Turner, L. (2004). Pharmaceutical interventions in developmental disabilities. In W. L. Williams (Ed.), *Developmental disabilities: Etiology, assessment, intervention, and integration.* Reno: Context Press.

Poling, A. D., Methot, L. L., & LeSage, M. G. (1995). *Fundamentals of behavior analytic research.* New York: Plenum Press.

Powell, D., Fixsen, D., & Dunlap, G. (2003). *Pathways to service utilization: A synthesis of evidence relevant to young children with challenging behavior.* Tampa, FL: Louis de la Parte Florida Mental Health Institute, Center for Evidence-based Practice: Young Children with Challenging Behaviors.

Reiff, M. I. (2004). *ADHD: A complete and authoritative guide.* Elk Grove Village, IL: American Academy of Pediatrics.

Repp, A. C., Felce, D., & Barton, L. E. (1988). Basing the treatment of stereotypic and self-injurious behaviors on the hypotheses of their causes. *Journal of Applied Behavior Analysis, 21*, 281–289.

Robbins, T. W. (1975). The potentiation of conditioned reinforcement by psychomotor stimulant drugs: A test of Hill's hypothesis. *Psychopharmacologia, 45*, 103–114.

Robbins, T. W., & Sahakian, B. J. (1979). "Paradoxical" effects of psychomotor stimulant drugs in hyperactive children from the standpoint of behavioural pharmacology. *Neuropharmacology, 18*, 931–950.

Royal College of Psychiatrists. (2001). DC-LD: Diagnostic criteria for psychiatric disorders for use with adults with learning disabilities/mental retardation. London: Gaskell.

Russell, A. J., Mataix-Cols, D., Anson, M., & Murphy, D. G. M. (2005). Obsessions and compulsions in Asperger syndrome in high-functioning autism. *British Journal of Psychiatry, 186*, 525–528.

Sandman, C. A., Touchette, P., Lenjavi, M., Marion, S., & Chicz-DeMet, A. (2003). Beta-endorphin and ACTH are dissociated after self-injury in adults with developmental disabilities. *American Journal of Mental Retardation 108*(6), 414–424.

Sasaki-Adams, B. S., & Kelley, A. E. (2001). Serotonin-dopamine interactions in the control of conditioned reinforcement and motor behavior. *Neuropsychopharmacology, 25*, 440–452.

Schaal, D. W., & Hackenberg, T. (1994). Toward a functional analysis of drug treatment for behavior problems of people with developmental disabilities. *American Journal of Mental Retardation, 99*(2), 123–124.

Schroeder, S. R., Mulick, J. A., & Rojahn, J. (1980). The definition, taxonomy, epidemiology, and ecology of self-injurious behaviors. *Journal of Autism and Developmental Disorders, 10*, 417–432.

Schroeder, S. R., Rojahn, J., & Reese, R. M. (1997). Brief report: Reliability and validity instruments for assessing psychotropic effects on self-injurious behavior in mental retardation. *Journal of Autism and Developmental Disorders, 27*(1), 89–102.

Schwartz, I. S., & Baer, D. M. (1991). Social validity assessments: Is current practice state of the art? *Journal of Applied Behavior Analysis, 24*, 189–204.

Sheldon, W. H. (with Stevens, S. S., & Tucker, W. B.). (1940). *The varieties of human physique: An introduction to constitutional psychology.* New York: Harper.

Skinner, B. F. (1938). *Behavior of organisms.* New York: Appleton.

Skinner, B. F. (1957). *Verbal behavior.* New York: Appleton Century Crofts.

Society for Stimulus Properties of Drugs, Drug Discrimination Database. (2005). Retrieved February 7, 2007, from *www.sspd.org.uk*.

Sprague, R. L., & Werry, R. S. (1971). Methodology of psychopharmacological studies with the retarded. In N. R. Ellis (Ed.), *International review of research in mental retardation* (Vol. 5, pp. 148–220). New York: Academic Press.

Spreat, S., Conroy, J. W., & Jones, J. C. (1997). Use of psychotropic medication in Oklahoma: A statewide survey. *American Journal of Mental Retardation, 102*(1), 80–85.

Sundberg, M. L., & Partington, J. W. (1998) *Teaching language to children with autism or other developmental disabilities.* Danville, CA: Behavior Analysts.

Symons, F. J., Fox, N. D., & Thompson, T. (1998). Functional communication training and naltrexone treatment of self-injurious behavior: An experimental case report. *Journal of Applied Research and Intellectual Disabilities, 11*(3), 273–292.

Symons, F. J., Koppekin, A., & Wehby, J. H. (1999). Treatment of self-injurious behavior and quality of life in persons with mental retardation. *Mental Retardation, 37,* 297–307.

Symons, F. J., Tapp, J., Wulfsberg, A., Sutton, K. A., Heeth, W. L., & Bodfish, J. W. (2001). Sequential analysis of the effects of naltrexone on the environmental mediation of self-injurious behavior. *Experimental and Clinical Psychopharmacology, 9*(3), 269–276.

Symons, F. J., Thompson, A., & Rodriguez, M. C. (2004). Self-injurious behavior and the efficacy of naltrexone treatment: A quantitative synthesis. *Mental Retardation and Developmental Disabilities Research Reviews, 10,* 193–200.

Tanguay, P., Robertson, J., & Derrick, A. (1998). A dimensional classification of autism spectrum disorder by social communication domains. *Journal of the American Academy of Child and Adolescent Psychiatry, 37*(3), 271–277.

Thompson, T. (2005). Paul E. Meehl and B. F. Skinner: Autotaxia, autotypy and autism. *Behavior and Philosophy, 33,* 101–131.

Thompson, T., Felce, D., & Symons, F. (Eds.) (2000). *Behavioral observation: Technology and applications in developmental disabilities.* Baltimore: Brookes.

Thompson, T., Hackenberg, T., Cerutti, D., Baker, D., & Axtell, S. (1994). Opioid antagonist effects on self-injury: Response form and location as determinants of medication effects. *American Journal on Mental Retardation, 99,* 85–102.

Thompson, T., & Schuster, C. R. (1968). *Behavioral pharmacology.* Englewood Cliffs, NJ: Prentice Hall.

Thompson, T., & Symons, F. (2000). Psychotropic medication treatment for destructive behavior based on neurobehavioral mechanisms of drug action. In N. Wieseler & R. Hanson (Eds.), *Challenging behavior in persons with mental health disorders and severe developmental disablities.* Washington, DC: American Association on Mental Retardation.

Wagner, K. D. (2005). Pharmacotherapy for major depression in children and adolescents. *Progress in Neuropsychopharmacology and Biological Psychiatry, 5,* 819.

Whittington, C. J. Kendall, T., Fonagy, P., Cottrell, D., Cotgrove, A., & Boddington, E. (2004). Selective serotonin reuptake inhibitors in childhood depression: Systematic review of published vs. unpublished data. *Lancet, 363,* 1341–1345.

Willemsen-Swinkels, S. H., Buitelaar, J. K., Nijhof, G. J., & van Engeland, H. (1995). Failure of naltrexone hydrochloride to reduce self-injurious and autistic behavior in mentally retarded adults: Double-blind, placebo-controlled studies. *Archives of General Psychiatry, 52*(9), 766–773.

Wolf, M. M. (1978). Social validity: The case for subjective measurement or how applied behavior analysis is finding its heart. *Journal of Applied Behavior Analysis, 11,* 203–214.

World Health Organization. (2007). *ICD-10 classification of mental and behavioral disorders: Clinical descriptions and diagnostic guidelines. International Classification of Diseases.* (10th ed.). Geneva: Author.

Zarcone, J. R., Lindauer, S. E., Morse, P. S., Crosland, K. A., Valdovinos, M. G., et al. (2004). Effects of risperidone on destructive behavior of persons with developmental disabilities: III. Functional analysis. *American Journal of Mental Retardation, 109*(4), 310–321.

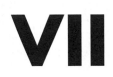

FAMILY ISSUES

Of families, the well-known columnist and essayist Anna Quindlen wrote: "I can't think of anything to write about except families. They are a metaphor for every other part of society." We might add, "So, too, for families of children with developmental disabilities."

Only a few decades ago, the concept of the "scientific study of families," especially with respect to developmental disabilities, would have been unheard of. Indeed, the topic of "families research" was not considered integral to our understanding of disability. Today, not only do family interactions prepare children (with or without disabilities) for later inclusion into the larger community, but they are also influenced by the behaviors of other individuals and groups.

Bronfenbrenner (1978) articulated this concept of multiple and reciprocal influences on families in his ecological model. Using concentric circles, as in a target, Bronfenbrenner (1978) placed the individual at the center, with other circles of influence, including family (parents, siblings), schools, and finally the broader influences of society, politics, and culture, surrounding each. Researchers who focused on families and disability found that extensions of Bronfenbrenner's (1978) ecological approach could accommodate the numerous child characteristics in the case of mental retardation and other developmental disabilities (e.g., Crnic, Friedrich, & Greenberg, 1983).

As demonstrated by the chapters included in this section of the *Handbook*, research on families and disability both affects and has been affected by the work of scientists, practitioners, and policy makers. Thus the role of families is one of the emerging strengths of the field of developmental disabilities, and, as a cognate research area, one with exciting opportunities for development and application. The three chapters included in this section cover a number of theoretical and practical themes. As diverse as these three chapters may appear at first blush, common themes emerge. Among them are: (1) the resilience of families; (2) recognition that the effect of a child or adult with developmental disabilities on a family may have both positive and negative dimensions; (3) the importance of cultural context and diversity in understanding the complexity of families; and (4) the emerging role of etiology in family adjustment. The chapters included are written by different investigators with diverse training and perspectives on the field, but together they "tell a story" about family experiences and the impact of having a child with developmental disabilities.

Chapter 26, by Blacher and Hatton, brings the reader up-to-date on family coping with and adaptation to a child with an intellectual and/or developmental disability. This chapter provides a historical perspective on family adjustment and takes both cultural context and etiological perspectives of families and disability into account. Of course, coping is a lifelong endeavor, and this fact is highlighted by Lounds and Seltzer in Chapter 27, on family impact in adulthood. Their chapter incorporates a lifespan perspective and draws heavily on family systems theory in the presentation of data pertaining to developmental disabilities and adulthood. An important focus is on maternal well-being. Finally, in Chapter 28, A. Turnbull, Zuna, H. R. Turnbull, Poston, and Summers review research and policies on families and schooling. Their chapter represents a different approach to the literature and is organized around the specific family roles associated with the current principles for educating students with developmental disabilities under the Individuals with Disabilities Education Act.

A careful reading of these chapters will underscore the tremendous momentum that the scientific study of families has brought to the field of developmental disabilities. Whether or not the reader agrees that families are a metaphor for every other part of society, he or she surely will conclude from these writings that family interactions with children with developmental disabilities must be understood within a broader societal or contextual field.

REFERENCES

Bronfenbrenner, U. (1978). *The ecology of human development: Experiments by nature and design.* Cambridge, MA: Harvard University Press.

Crnic, K. A., Friedrich, W. N., & Greenberg, M. T. (1993). Adaptation of families with mentally retarded children: A model of stress and copying. *American Journal on Mental Deficiency, 88,* 125–138.

Families in Context

Influences on Coping and Adaptation

Jan Blacher
Chris Hatton

In the short years since the turn of the century, research on families and developmental disability (DD) has not just grown, it has blossomed into a more scientific field. Three changes in the family research field are especially noteworthy: (1) Methodologies for the study of families have grown more sophisticated, both theoretically and statistically; (2) our understanding of families is becoming more comprehensive, with research foci on both positive and negative outcomes and a consideration of the broader cultural context; and (3) new genetic advances prompt a more complex approach to studying environmental influences.

Although researchers are now encouraged to "think etiologically," this still leaves room for the crucial importance of families. Despite the impact of genetic counseling on reproductive planning, generations of children will be born with disorders such as fragile X, autism, and Down syndrome. These children usually have hundreds of thousands of interactions with family members before entering intervention programs. There are genetic and environmental determinants that children and parents bring to the mix. Yet relatively little attention has been paid to the family context. Thus the focus of this chapter is on family coping and adaptation and the influences of culture, phenotype, and social support on family well-being.

HISTORICAL PERSPECTIVES ON FAMILIES, RESEARCH, AND DEVELOPMENTAL DISABILITY

Children with intellectual or developmental disability (IDD), like all children, are born into families. From the last half of the 20th century, researchers have examined the role of parents in the child's development, as well as the impact of a child with IDD on the family. However, this has not always been the case. Up until about 1940, the family was essentially "invisible" in U.S. research journals that pertained to intellectual disability, with parents or biological family members basically excluded from "treatment" of persons with IDD (Blacher & Baker, 2002). This was due to prevailing beliefs that both genetics and poor parenting practices or a maladaptive family environment were causal factors for mental retardation (MR; Vaux, 1936). Institutional care was often suggested by professionals, a practice later labeled "parentectomy," as the intent was to remove parental influences (and to preclude the child's subsequent childbearing; Turnbull & Turnbull, 1978).

Even at the height of the eugenic movement in the 1920s and 1930s, a different perspective was expressed by some professionals that emphasized the value of living at home:

> In the past it may have been assumed that because the child was mentally defective, the parents were probably mentally defective also, and therefore unfit guardians for the child, but with the latest evidence as to the heredity of mental deficiency indicating that much mental deficiency is of the non-hereditary type, it is apparent that many mentally defective children may have entirely normal and intelligent parents. (Davies, 1925, p. 213)

Ironically, we now know that some parents who have IDD may have children who do not. Whether or not we know the heritability of a particular type of retardation or IDD, we argue here that, overall, there is no place like the family home when it comes to an optimal environment. It took several decades, however, for this conclusion to be accepted by family researchers.

Although the mid-20th century brought a burst of interest in families, "scientific papers" focused on negative outcomes, characterized by Blacher and Baker (2002) as the "woe is me" years. At that time, the birth of a child with any disability, but especially retardation, was considered a tragedy, imbuing the family with hardship, anger, economic distress, and negative attitudes toward the child (e.g., Grebler, 1952). Reflecting the prevalence of psychoanalysis at the time, some authors wrote that parents themselves needed "fixing" (Schonell & Watts, 1956), with Olshansky (1962) speaking of "chronic sorrow," a lifelong sense of loss of the hoped-for child.

Other theorists characterized family reactions to having a child with IDD in terms of stages of adjustment similar to Kübler-Ross's (1970) stages of grief, such as shock or disbelief, followed by emotional disorganization (e.g., denial, blame, anger), and finally a stage of emotional organization (e.g., adjustment and acceptance). For example, Wikler, Wasow, and Hatfield (1981) combined the chronic-sorrow and stages notions and theorized that parents would recycle through these stages at later, particularly stressful, points in the life course. However, the empirical basis and usefulness of such stage models in understanding families was later questioned (Blacher, 1984; Eden-Pearcy, Blacher, & Eyman, 1986), with some viewing the stages concept as a way of stereotyping, rather than helping, parents (Allen & Affleck, 1985).

When considering family coping and adaptation in historical context, one is struck that the main source of stress for families may not have been their child's disability but the attitudes of professionals toward the child and the family. Prior to the 1970s in the United States, parents had limited access to publicly funded educational services for their children with IDD. There were few types of family support and no federal legislation ensuring rights to persons with IDD. Subsequent legislative changes in the realm of education (Individuals with Disabilities Education Act [IDEA], 2004) have mandated equal access for persons with disabilities. To a certain extent, social and legal changes taking place in broader society have been paralleled by changes in research approaches to our understanding of family coping and adjustment.

EMERGENCE OF THEORIES OF FAMILY ADJUSTMENT AND COPING

The research of Bernard Farber (1959, 1960) set the stage for the empirical study of families with children with MR. Farber, a sociologist, described what he saw as the processes by which families adapted to a child with MR, writing about forms of family accommodation and the equilibrium or disequilibrium that might ensue when there was a child with MR. His original study (Farber, 1959) involved 249 white, two-parent, married families who had one "severely mentally deficient" child age 16 or younger. Possibly the best-known conclusion drawn from this study was that placing a male child out of the home had a beneficial effect on the parents' marriage and on nondisabled sisters, who were relieved of child care duties on placement.

Many researchers since have tried to either replicate Farber's findings or expand the scope of the investigation, for example, in investigating the potential impact of IDD on the parents' marriage. A meta-analysis of marital satisfaction studies published between 1975 and 2003 (Risdal & Singer, 2004) found a small but significant effect size, indicating less marital satisfaction in parents of children with IDD than in parents of typically developing children. Thus Farber's work was seminal in that it highlighted families who had children with MR as being of legitimate scientific interest. His work focused on the main effects of having a child with retardation, but it also reinforced negative perceptions of having a child with MR, that is, of the child as the cause of any family disintegration or pathology. However, his work spawned a number of investigations and continues today to influence researchers interested in families and IDD.

Development of Conceptual Models

Empirical research with families, which expanded dramatically in the 1980s, was largely influenced by two theoretical papers. McCubbin and Patterson (1983) proposed a theoretical model of adjustment and adaptation as a mechanism for explaining family stress. Based on Hill's (1949) original ABCX family-crisis model, this new "double ABCX model" could be understood specifically with reference to children with disabilities. Unique to McCubbin and Patterson's model was the emphasis on parent appraisal of the situation, or parents' cognitive style, a component influenced largely by the work of stress and coping researchers (Lazarus, 1993). For example, the double ABCX model suggests that family stress (X) is influenced by child disability and other characteristics (A), by resources available for dealing with the stressor crisis (B), and by parental coping strategies, as well as the meaning given to the stressful event (C). The idea that it isn't just the "event" itself (e.g., a child's MR) but parents' cognitive appraisal of it that determines family stress has had a large influence on later studies of family impact of DD, as exemplified by research assessing locus of control (Hassall & Rose, 2005), parental personality variables or traits reflecting optimism, sense of coherence (Baker, Blacher, & Olsson, 2005; Olsson & Hwang, 2002), and resilience (Heiman, 2002).

The ABCX is a multivariate model appropriate for assessing normative and nonnormative events or crises. Thus this model identified potential explanatory mechanisms for the main effects found by others. Indeed, the ABCX model has been used in many studies of families and IDD. The notion that families can experience child stressors but can successfully adapt to them was fairly unique at the time. This research group also hypothesized that stress could also result in positive adaptation ("bonadaptation") to serve as a counterpoint to the maladaptation that was previously presumed to characterize families facing a major stressor. The ABCX model allowed researchers to look at mediators of the child stressor–parent stress relationship (mechanisms through which the relationship occurs), as well as moderators (buffers) that might explain the conditions under which the main stress effects occur.

In the same year, Crnic, Friedrich, and Greenberg (1983) published the most widely cited *American Journal of Mental Deficiency* family article of the 20th century, presenting a model of stress, coping, and family ecology with specific reference to children with IDD. Their model expanded on earlier approaches to the study of families in a number of ways, and it was prescient with regard to family research issues of the 21st century. For example, Crnic et al. (1983) present a literature review in their paper that focuses on fathers, siblings, and parent–child interaction systems, rather than a singular focus on mothers. Their model also accounts for a range of possible outcomes, both positive and negative, associated with having a child with MR. Finally, like the ABCX model, Crnic et al. (1983) incorporate family coping resources and what they call the ecological environment.

The consideration of "context" in the study of families and MR is expanded on in subsequent sections of this chapter. However, cultural context, in particular, has a main role in Blacher's (2001) model of family adjustment and coping during the transition to adulthood, which builds on the model of Crnic et al. (1983). Cultural context is hypothesized to moderate the relationship between the adolescent stressor (defined as behavior challenges or psychiatric disorder) and family well-being. Here, "well-being" is defined as including physical and mental health outcomes, as well as cognitive appraisals of the positive and negative impact of the son or daughter with IDD. Considerations of well-being go beyond the traditional focus on mothers and can include fathers or siblings. Cultural context has been shown to be important in the assessment of positive outcomes in IDD for Latina mothers (Blacher & Baker, 2007; Blacher & McIntyre, 2006) and in understanding Latina mothers' attributions about IDD (Chavira, Lopez, Blacher, & Shapiro, 2000).

Residential Placement and Family Coping

A unique challenge for families of children with IDD involves out-of-home placement, that is, the decision to have a child with IDD live outside of the family home. Farber (1959, 1960) set the stage for the study of placement with mainly descriptive work reporting on adjustment issues in families who had placed their sons or daughters, in comparison with families who chose to keep their sons or daughters at home. Issues of residential placement and community supports, as well as independent living, are covered elsewhere in this *Handbook* (see Chapters 20 and 21). Here we focus on the family issues that led to the placement and on the few studies that pertain specifically to postplacement family adjustment.

During much of the 20th century, placement was viewed as a solution for families who could no longer "cope" with their son or daughter with IDD. Parents rarely report "triggering events" (Bruns, 2000); more often there is a snowball of mounting stresses and concerns, the two most pressing being difficulties balancing child and family needs and maladaptive child behaviors (Llewellyn, McConnell, Thompson, & Whybrow, 2005;

Pfeiffer & Baker, 1994). As parents age, their own health, in tandem with the daily care needs of their child, become causal factors in placement (Seltzer, Greenberg, Krauss, & Hong, 1997; Seltzer, Krauss, Choi, & Hong, 1996). Yet the most pressing need for out-of-home placements continues to be challenging behavior. Alborz (2003) developed a model to account for the experiences of families whose sons or daughters with severe maladaptive behaviors move out of the family home. This model has three "transition routes": (1) "forensic," in which the individual's challenging behaviors involved police contact; (2) problems in the "family," that is, severe family stress; and (3) "service," that is, deficits in service provision that lead to placement.

Several studies have compared families who had placed a child with families who had a similar child with IDD at home at one point in time, although, to our knowledge, only Blacher's Families Project at the University of California, Riverside, has studied postplacement family adjustment longitudinally. Blacher, Baker, and Feinfield (1999) summarized some of the project's findings when they wrote about "leaving vs. launching" to differentiate families who "placed" their offspring during the child's early childhood or school years from families who tried to "launch" their son or daughter into adulthood by moving him or her into a community residential setting. This was an important distinction, because the family dynamics and stresses would likely be very different in these two circumstances.

Blacher et al. (1999) tracked the adjustment of parents postplacement using indices of parental emotional, cognitive, and behavioral involvement with their sons or daughters. Emotional involvement included assessments of parents' feelings of continued attachment to the child; cognitive involvement included assessments of how much parents worried about or thought about the child; behavioral involvement included assessments of visits to the child, visits home by the child, and phone calls by the parent to the residential placement (Baker & Blacher, 1993). Although these involvement indices were all based on parent report, Baker, Blacher, and Pfeiffer (1993) found high correspondence between parent and staff reports of these indices of parental adjustment.

Of particular importance were the findings that initial preplacement involvement predicted postplacement involvement and that parents developed a pattern of postplacement involvement early on and tended to maintain that through the 4-year period studied (Blacher et al., 1999). Indeed, there was no evidence of "detachment"—a strong lessening of attachment to the child—which was a key element of the Families Project theoretical model (Blacher & Baker, 1994). Parents reported continuing strong attachment to the offspring who was "launched," but despite this, they overwhelmingly reported more advantages than disadvantages to the family from having placed the son or daughter with IDD (Baker & Blacher, 2002). Subsequent studies have found similar advantages and disadvantages with adults moving into placements (Schwartz, 2005), including adults with autism spectrum disorder (Krauss, Seltzer, & Jacobson, 2005).

In sum, whether residential placement occurs during childhood, adolescence, or adulthood, parents seem to adjust well in the postplacement period. The few studies addressing issues of postplacement involvement indicate that placement out of the home is indeed *not* placement out of the family (Blacher, 1994), although more research on the postplacement adjustment of the individuals being placed is needed.

Families Are More Than Mothers

Theories of adjustment to a child with IDD could well be described as theories of "mother adjustment," as the overwhelming body of research excludes other family members. Many researchers now include analyses from fathers, siblings, the child with

IDD, and even the whole family in order to present a more complete picture, with some myths being debunked as a result of these studies. For example, mothers and fathers generally appear to be far less discrepant than was originally suggested. Many earlier concerns about family pathology, especially among nondisabled siblings, have also proven to be without merit. Although siblings do have particular concerns about their brothers or sisters with IDD, there is little support for the supposition of psychopathology or other serious adverse outcomes (Eisenberg, Baker, & Blacher, 1998).

POSITIVE EXPERIENCES OF FAMILIES WITH A PERSON WITH DEVELOPMENTAL DISABILITIES

Researchers are increasingly recognizing that the birth of a child with IDD can have many positive effects on families, and it is crucial to set these positive experiences against the better researched negative effects if we are to develop a fuller understanding of family life (Hastings & Taunt, 2002). Families have consistently reported positive experiences associated with a person with IDD being part of the family, although dominant research paradigms have, until recently, given families limited opportunities to express these experiences.

Research on positive family experiences is not yet well developed or integrated within prevalent models of family functioning and therefore lacks cross-study coherence within clear theoretical frameworks. Influenced by the "positive psychology" movement, family researchers have looked to related fields for theoretical perspectives, such as Taylor and colleagues' positive perceptions in understanding health outcomes (Taylor, 1983; Taylor, Lerner, Sherman, Sage, & McDowell, 2003) or Antonovsky's (1987, 1998) sense of coherence. Antonovsky argued that individuals with a strong sense of coherence (SoC) would be more likely to define a stressful event as a nonstressor, even a challenge, and thus less contentious or dangerous. A person with a weak SoC would be more likely to perceive a stressor as a threat.

Recent reviews have begun to map out the terrain concerning the dimensions of positive experiences in families with a person with IDD. In a review of five largely qualitative studies, Hastings and Taunt (2002) produced a list of 14 key positive perceptions commonly mentioned by parents (more recent studies with qualitative components also report similar dimensions of positive parental experience; e.g., Krauss et al., 2005; Poehlmann, Clements, Abbeduto, & Farsad, 2005). As Table 26.1 shows, these 14 key themes can be usefully mapped onto the six domains of psychological well-being recommended by Dykens (2005) as a framework for considering positive family experiences, taking into account whether these positive parental perceptions are within the parent, relational, or within the child (cf. Grant, Ramcharan, McGrath, Nolan, & Keady, 1998).

This initial mapping suggests some starting points for considering positive parental perceptions. First, the broadest range of themes mentioned by parents concern the changes that the child has brought about within them as parents and people, rather than positively mentioning specific characteristics of the child. Second, parents believe that the child can be the occasion for positive changes across a whole range of relationships both within and beyond the family. Third, positive parental perceptions concerning the impact of their child with IDD are relevant to every area of psychological well-being. Although the themes generated by Hastings and Taunt (2002) concerned parents, the literature concerning positive sibling experiences (see Dykens, 2005; Stoneman, 2005) may well be amenable to a similar mapping exercise. The relevance of

TABLE 26.1. Key Positive Parental Perceptions and Their Relationship to Psychological Well-Being

Dimension of psychological well-being	Within the parent	Relational	Within the child
Self-acceptance	Becomes a better person (more compassionate, less selfish, more tolerant) Makes the most of each day, living life at a slower pace		
Positive relations with others	Gets pleasure/satisfaction in providing care for child	Shares love with the child Strengthens family and/or marriage Expands social and community networks	Becomes source of joy/happiness
Autonomy	Increases personal strength or confidence		
Environmental mastery	Gains sense of accomplishment in having done one's best for one's child		
Purpose in life	Gives a new or increased sense of purpose in life Changes one's perspective on life (e.g., clarified what is important in life, more aware of the future)		
Personal growth	Leads to development of new skills, abilities, or new career opportunities Increases spirituality		Provides a challenge or opportunity to learn and develop

Note. Data from Dykens (2005), Grant et al. (1998), and Hastings and Taunt (2002).

such a framework to the positive experiences of the people with IDD in the family is less clear.

Table 26.1 suggests many research questions concerning positive experiences within families with a person with IDD yet to be answered. First, it is unclear how specific positive family perceptions, broader domains of psychological well-being, and global constructs such as satisfaction with life are related to each other. Are they in essence the same construct described at different levels of detail, or are specific positive perceptions distinct from constructs of well-being, and, if so, how are they related conceptually and empirically (Hastings, Beck, & Hill, 2005)?

Second, how common are positive family perceptions? Although much of the current research has been qualitative, some multimethod studies that include quantitative components have reported that positive perceptions can be extremely common. Grant et al. (1998), in a survey of the sources of satisfaction experienced by 120 family caregivers for people with IDD across the lifespan, reported that 8 of 28 items concerning sources of satisfaction were endorsed by 90% or more of family caregivers, and that 24 of 28 items were endorsed by 50% or more. Broadly speaking, rewards linked to perceived gains for the person with IDD were most commonly endorsed, and rewards that were more personal to the family caregiver were less commonly endorsed. Scorgie and Sobsey (2000), in a survey of positive personal transformations experienced by 79 parents of children with disabilities, reported that 4 of 16 items were endorsed by 90% or more of parents and that 15 of 16 items were endorsed by 50% or more. Parents reported positive changes in the areas of personal growth, improved relationships with others, and changes in their own spiritual values or philosophy.

Third, which factors are associated with either positive perceptions or psychological well-being in families with a person with IDD? For both parents and siblings of a family member with IDD, there may be variations in the nature and extent of positive perceptions that depend on many factors, including gender (e.g., Hastings et al., 2005; Orsmond & Seltzer, 2000), the age of the person with developmental disabilities, and the stage of the family life cycle (Poehlmann et al., 2005; Seltzer, Greenberg, et al., 2004), and whether the person with IDD is living at home or outside the home (Krauss et al., 2005). All these potential dimensions of variation in positive family experiences, along with others such as socioeconomic position, family culture, and the extent and nature of the family member's disability, require further investigation.

Fourth, are the "special benefits" of positive perceptions noted earlier unique to disability, or are they also reported by parents raising typically developing children? Although reports from studies of positive impact have some heuristic value in identifying themes that might serve as "special benefit" to parents of children with DD, any conclusions must be considered in light of the positive bias in the way questions have been asked, because without adequate control groups, we cannot know whether these are special benefits (Blacher & Baker, 2007).

Fifth, are there cultural differences in perceived positive benefits of having a child with DD? This question was addressed in two studies (Blacher & McIntyre, 2006; Blacher & Baker, 2007) in which Latina mothers reported more positive impacts of their son or daughter with DD than Anglo mothers, regardless of whether the target child was a preschooler or young adult. This finding is notable because in these studies, Latina mothers were more disadvantaged with regard to education and income than the Anglo mothers.

Finally, how do positive and negative family perceptions relate to each other? Parents in several studies have reported both positive and negative parental experiences alongside each other (Blacher &McIntyre, 2006; Grant et al., 1998; Krauss et al., 2005; Poehlmann et al., 2005; Scorgie & Sobsey, 2000). There appears to be no simple inverse relationship between positive and negative family experiences, suggesting that they are not the opposite ends of a single dimension of family experience but are distinct phenomena that both require investigation (Hastings & Taunt, 2002). Beyond this general statement, however, the relationship between positive and negative family experiences is murky and little explored, and it begins to touch on a final fundamental question about the status of positive family experiences within general models of family functioning (Hastings & Taunt, 2002).

There are many ways that positive family perceptions can be considered conceptually within more general theories of family functioning, none of which are mutually exclusive and all of which are likely to function in causally complex ways. For example, the role of positive perceptions within family stress and coping models has been given some attention, although little theoretical clarity has emerged (Hastings & Taunt, 2002). Coping strategies such as reframing and accommodative coping have been associated with dimensions of positive psychological well-being among parents of people with IDD (Hastings, Allen, McDermott, & Still, 2002; Seltzer, Abbeduto, et al., 2004). However, it is unclear whether positive perceptions and psychological well-being are best conceptualized as resources that underpin the selection and use of adaptive coping strategies, as examples of adaptive coping strategies, or as the result of adaptive coping strategies.

An alternative lens for viewing positive perceptions and psychological well-being comes from family resilience models (e.g., Heiman, 2002). Parents of children with disabilities have described how positive transformations in their family lives have been partly the result of a drive to attain positive psychological well-being through the processes of achieving a new identity after the birth of the child with disabilities, of deriving a sense of meaning from the situation, and of developing a sense of personal control (King et al., 2006; Scorgie, Wilgosh, & McDonald, 1999).

Current research on positive aspects of family experience, although at an early stage, suggests exciting avenues for further research, theory, and intervention. Over time, researchers have become progressively less negative about the situation of families with a person with developmental disabilities (Blacher & Baker, 2002). We may be at the point of another conceptual shift; rather than thinking about how families can avoid catastrophe, we might begin to think about how families can achieve positive well-being. Families will inevitably face stresses and challenges, but the successful negotiation of these challenges, along with enjoyment of the good times, may be a crucial part of the development of positive well-being.

BEHAVIORAL PHENOTYPES AND FAMILY ETIOLOGICAL RESEARCH

Historically, family researchers have paid little attention to the potential influence on family adjustment of the etiology associated with the child's IDD. However, the "new genetics" is having a major impact on family research, as more specific genetic and chromosomal etiologies associated with IDD are being discovered and their impact on the phenotype (how the genes express themselves in appearance or behavior) of the child with IDD becomes better understood (Dykens, Hodapp, & Finucane, 2000; Hodapp & Dykens, 2004). Much of this work is rooted in the concept of behavioral phenotypes. Prototypically, "a behavioral phenotype should consist of a distinct behavior that occurs in almost every case of a genetic or chromosomal disorder, and rarely (if at all) in other conditions" (Flynt & Yule, 1994, p. 666). This strict definition would limit the study of behavioral phenotypes to a small number of genetic/chromosomal conditions with clear behavioral consequences (e.g., self-mutilation in Lesch–Nyhan syndrome; hyperphagia in Prader–Willi syndrome). This original concept of behavioral phenotypes has been broadened to a more probabilistic definition, for example, "the heightened probability or likelihood that people with a given syndrome will exhibit certain behavioral and developmental sequelae relative to those without the syndrome"

(Dykens, 1995, p. 523). More broadly still, there is a recent recognition that the research designs and methods applied to behavioral phenotypes may be a particular instance of etiology-based research (Hodapp & Dykens, 2006), in which nongenetic/chromosomal etiologies associated with IDD (e.g., perinatal asphyxia) may be relevant to a child's subsequent behavior and development. There may also be an argument for including phenomenologically defined syndromes (such as autism spectrum disorder) in such a research endeavor, even though the etiology(ies) of autism is as yet unknown.

Although etiology-based research in a family context is in its early stages and although there are formidable methodological challenges involved, the etiology of the child's condition may be important in understanding families with a person with IDD in several ways.

First, the characteristics of the child associated with the etiology may have a direct impact on family well-being. For example, several studies have found that different levels of child behavior problems and psychopathology can partly account for variations in parental distress and mental health problems across child syndromes (e.g., Down syndrome vs. fragile X syndrome vs. autism; Abbeduto et al., 2004). Other characteristics of the child are likely to have indirect effects on family adjustment via the reactions of other people (including family members) to the child. For example, the facial characteristics of children with Down syndrome are rated by others as friendlier, more social, and more compliant (Fidler & Hodapp, 1999).

Second, the etiology of the child's condition interacts with broader contexts and systems in several ways that may have an impact on the family. For example, the length of time taken to reach a diagnosis, and the certainty of that diagnosis, varies across etiologies, with consequent impacts on family adjustment (e.g., Fidler, Hodapp, & Dykens, 2000; Seltzer, Krauss, Orsmond, & Vestal, 2000). The provision of effective health, education, and social services also varies according to the etiology of the child (Hodapp & Dykens, 2006), and many child etiologies are associated with different socioeconomic profiles among families.

Third, there are likely to be complex interactions between these various factors (Baker & Donelly, 2001). For example, the socioeconomic context within which families live may moderate the relationship between child behavior problems and parental well-being (Emerson, 2003), and parents' understandings of the child's condition may influence their attributions for the child's behavior and their consequent interactions with the child in ways that may be helpful or unhelpful over the family life course (Dykens et al., 2000).

As befits transactional models of family functioning, there are also numerous ways in which the family can have an impact on the child with a specific etiology, although these impacts have been little studied by family researchers (Hodapp & Dykens, 2006). General models of family impact on child development will apply (e.g., Harris, Kasari, & Sigman, 1996), although parental understandings of their child and her or his likely trajectory through life may be strongly influenced by a diagnostic label attached to a syndrome and may result in patterns of parental interactions with their children that are partly based on these understandings rather than on the individual characteristics of the child (Ly & Hodapp, 2002, 2005). In the case of genetic/chromosomal disorders, such parental understandings may be helpful (e.g., an understanding of the child's condition helps the parent to build on the child's likely strengths and ameliorate areas of likely weakness) or unhelpful (e.g., an understanding of negative sequelae of a syndrome as inevitable, resulting in a lack of parental intervention) and are likely to be influenced by all the other factors discussed in this chapter: social support, socioeconomic position, cultural context, and more.

Taken together, these findings suggest that the etiology associated with the child's IDD cannot be ignored by researchers working with families, and much work remains to be done to understand the complexities of the transactions involved. However, it is also important to remember that etiology is only one factor among many when considering child development and family adjustment. For example, Cahill and Glidden (1996) found that etiology-based differences in parental functioning disappeared when families were matched on four variables: child level of functioning, child age, parental marital status, and family income. It is also likely that the behavioral phenotypes associated with most genetic/chromosomal etiologies will themselves change over time, as education, health, and social supports improve. Finally, the importance of how families (and other people in other contexts) understand the etiology and its impact on their child is likely to be crucial, and reflexive feedback loops between research knowledge and parental understandings are likely to occur (research findings will influence parental understandings, which will in turn influence parental behavior toward the child).

CONSIDERATIONS OF CULTURAL CONTEXT IN UNDERSTANDING ADJUSTMENT

Researchers are increasingly attending to the cultural context of families (Blacher & Mink, 2004; Hatton, 2002; Mink, 1997). Culture has been defined as "a shared organization of ideas that includes the intellectual, moral, and aesthetic standards prevalent in a community and the meaning of communicative actions" (LeVine, 1984, p. 67). As many of the world's wealthier countries become more ethnically diverse (Castles & Miller, 1998), the disadvantages and discrimination experienced by many ethnic communities have been increasingly highlighted as a social problem (Modood et al., 1997; Shinagawa & Jang, 1998). Projected increases in the ethnic diversity of populations of people with developmental disabilities, particularly in the United Kingdom due to more efficient identification and documentation of disability (Emerson & Hatton, 1999), have also been accompanied by increased attention paid to the disadvantages and discrimination experienced by families from ethnic communities other than white Anglo communities (see Hatton, 2002; Mink, 1997, for reviews). Much of the research with these families has rightly focused on documenting the disadvantages and discrimination that they face, with the aim of improving policy and service practices (e.g., Blacher, Shapiro, Lopez, Diaz, & Fusco, 1997; Hatton, Akram, Shah, Robertson, & Emerson, 2004; Shapiro, Monzo, Rueda, Gomez, & Blacher, 2004). However, this strand of family research, in addition to highlighting policy and practice issues, is beginning to ask searching questions of traditional family research and theory.

Cultural Perspectives

Some family researchers have conducted in-depth studies concerning the culture of families from a specific ethnic and/or cultural group, using qualitative (e.g., Gabel, 2004; Harry, 1992; Magana, 1999), quantitative (e.g., Bailey et al., 1999; Rogers-Dulan, 1998), or mixed (e.g., Hatton et al., 2004) methods. The aim of these studies has been to build up detailed pictures of families' lives, while allowing important constructs to emerge that are not emphasized in mainstream research with families with a member with IDD. For example, family religiosity and religious connectedness have been found to be an important, and largely positive, aspect of the lives of African American families (Rogers-Dulan, 1998; Rogers-Dulan & Blacher, 1995), U.S. Latino families (Skinner, Correa, Skinner, & Bailey, 2001), U.S. family members of the Church of Jesus Christ of Latter-Day Saints (Dollahite, 2003), and U.K. South Asian families (Hatton et al., 2004). The construct of familism, "a cultural value including interdependence among nuclear and extended family members for support, loyalty and solidarity" (Magana, 1999, p. 466) has been found to be highly relevant to U.S. Latino families (Magana, 1999), as has the related construct of filial piety to Chinese American families (Blacher & Mink, 2004). Acculturation (the extent to which families adopt practices of the majority culture or maintain their heritage, culture, and identity, and the extent to which relationships are sought with people from other ethnic groups; Berry, Poortinga, Segall, & Dasen, 2002) has been explored with U.S. Latino families (Blacher & Mink, 2004) and U.K. South Asian families (Hatton et al., 2004). Finally, several studies have shown that many families consider the competence of their child's behavior in social terms, such as fulfilling family roles and duties, knowing social customs, and showing ties of affection (e.g., Rao, 2006; Rueda, Monzo, Shapiro, Gomez, & Blacher, 2005), rather than emphasizing the importance of behaviors that demonstrate independence.

In cross-cultural psychology terms, constructs such as religious connectedness and familism emphasize a collective dimension to family experience that may be underrepresented in theories of family adjustment developed for families in more individualist cultures. Individualist (as opposed to collectivist) cultures have been defined in terms of: (1) the definition of the self as personal versus collective and as independent versus interdependent; (2) personal goals having priority over group goals (or vice versa); (3) emphasis on exchange rather than on communal relationships; (4) the relative importance of personal attitudes versus social norms in a person's behavior (Triandis, 1995). It is important that family research includes a collectivist dimension and tests some of these constructs across all families; religiosity, familism, and socially embedded judgments of child behavior may well be important for families across all cultural groups, with cultural patterning in the way these constructs are played out within family systems.

Cultural Relevance of Measures

Family researchers have begun to critically appraise the cross-cultural relevance of many measures and constructs used in family research (Blacher & Mink, 2004; Hatton, 2004). Many of the terms used within family research, even such fundamental terms as "mental retardation" or "intellectual disability," may have very different meanings and connotations across cultural groups, particularly when translated across languages (e.g., Blacher & Mink, 2004; Gabel, 2004; Harry, 1992). Measures commonly used within family research have proved problematic when translated for use across cultural groups (Blacher & Mink, 2004), partly because some of the constructs that frame these measures are not equally applicable across cultures. Family researchers have adopted a number of research strategies to assess the cross-cultural equivalence of measures and constructs across cultures and languages.

One strategy has been to directly test the cross-cultural equivalence of measures using rigorous translation and back-translation procedures and extensive pilot testing of measures with families (e.g., Blacher & Mink, 2004; Hatton et al., 2004). This initial testing can be followed at the analysis stage by investigations of structural equivalence; for example, examining the factor structure of a measure separately for different cultural groups (e.g., Hatton et al., 2004) or examining whether associations between the measure of interest and other measures or constructs are similar when analyses are conducted separately within different cultural groups (e.g., Chavira et al., 2000; Magana & Smith, 2006). The structural equivalence strategy concerning measures overlaps with structural equivalence strategies concerning theories that are beginning to be adopted by family researchers; are patterns of findings replicable with different cultural groups? If they are, then there are greater grounds for considering a theory as being cross-culturally valid (e.g., Blacher, Lopez, Shapiro, & Fusco, 1997; Chavira et al., 2000; Hatton et al., 2004).

Cultural Differences

Family researchers also have begun to critically evaluate the mechanisms underpinning differences across ethnic groups, recognizing that ethnic differences are the beginning rather than the end of a search for an explanation. Many factors of great relevance to family adjustment, such as socioeconomic position, household size, and composition and language differences between families and service professionals, commonly co-occur with ethnic differences (e.g., Fujiura & Yamaki, 1997) and need to be factored into any cross-cultural study of families and IDD. Further, the specific cultural mechanisms underpinning ethnic differences in family adjustment need to be theorized and examined directly rather than relying on ethnic group as a proxy indicator of cultural difference (Hatton, 2004).

Developing a proper cross-cultural understanding of family adjustment will require the adoption of the three main research strategies that underpin a universalist approach, which assumes that basic human characteristics are universal and that culture influences the development and display of these characteristics (Berry, 1999): (1) to transport and test current knowledge and perspectives by using them in other cultures; (2) to explore and discover new aspects of the phenomenon being studied in local cultural terms; and (3) to integrate what has been learned from the first two strategies to generate theories of cross-cultural applicability that can be tested (Hatton, 2004). Researchers may also want to heed the advice of Lopez and Guarnaccia (2000), who pointed out that what is often missing in the study of culture is its existence in a "social world," that culture is dynamic and not a static variable. Family researchers are making substantial progress with the first two research strategies; more integrative theorizing is now required for the study of culture to become fully integrated into mainstream family adjustment theories.

ROLE OF FAMILY SUPPORT AS ENHANCING FAMILY COPING AND ADAPTATION

A wealth of literature attests to the importance of family support for the well-being of parents of children with IDD. This literature spans the life course and includes the delivery of such formal services as early intervention and parent training through adult services. Indeed, in the year 2000, the total spending for family support services from state developmental disability agencies in the United States exceeded $1 billion (Parish, Pomeranz-Essley, & Braddock, 2003). Other agencies (e.g., educational and health departments) also provide services to families, so the actual amount is likely much higher. Although large-scale studies of statewide databases are critical to track service delivery patterns to determine access and equity (Parish et al., 2003; Widaman &

Blacher, 2003), asking individual family members about how family support contributes to their well-being has also been useful.

Many family researchers have included the role of support in their conceptual models of family adjustment. Armstrong, Birnie-Lefcovitch, and Ungar (2005) discussed pathways between parental social support and parental well-being. They underscored the beneficial effects of social support on well-being, whether or not the person (here, parents) was under stress—a main effects model. In addition, social support may have a protective function by buffering potentially negative effects from stressors—a moderation model.

Informal support, that is, the provision of help with daily child care or counsel in the form of "listening," likely also contributes to higher family well-being. Freedman and Boyer (2000), in focus groups with parents of children with DD, reported that family support enhanced family well-being, in part by averting future crises. Families viewed knowledge about programs, resources, and supports as empowering. As in other studies, the investigators noted the need for cultural and ethnic minority groups to have similar access to support services in their own language that are sensitive to their cultural values and family backgrounds. Ethnic and minority families report unmet service and support needs more often than do European Americans (Blacher & Widaman, 2004; Pruchno & McMullen, 2004), though this finding is confounded by socioeconomic status and the actual availability of services.

Recently, Emerson, Hatton, Llewellyn, Blacher, and Graham (2006) have identified the critical role of low socioeconomic status indicators in predicting poorer well-being among mothers of children with IDD. In a nationally representative sample, British mothers with dependent children with IDD reported lower levels of happiness, self-esteem, and self-efficacy than mothers of children who did not have IDD. Statistically controlling for differences in socioeconomic factors between groups accounted for observed differences in maternal well-being. Thus Emerson et al. (2006) concluded that low socioeconomic status places mothers of children with IDD or DD at risk of poor overall well-being.

The literature on family support and its relationship to maternal well-being includes two other specific subgroups—mothers of children with autism spectrum disorder and aging mothers. With regard to autism, Bromley, Hare, Davison, and Emerson (2004) found that half (34) of 68 mothers of children with autism indicated significant psychological distress, and this was associated with high levels of challenging child behavior and low levels of family support. Poorer parental well-being was also associated with the diagnosis of autism in a study by White and Hastings (2004). These investigators cautioned that multiple measures of social support may produce a more accurate assessment of need and that parents of adolescents with disabilities may be especially vulnerable to disruptions in ongoing support.

With regard to aging parents, it is well known that most adults with IDD are still being cared for by their parents and that aging parents of adults with IDD or DD are themselves at risk for lower psychological and physical well-being (McConkey, 2005). However, researchers also have identified the beneficial and reciprocal nature of support, both emotional and instrumental, provided by adults with IDD to their parents and vice versa (Heller, Miller, & Factor, 1997).

In sum, examination of the growing body of research related to support yields an understanding of pathways among the child or adult with DD, family environment, family and social supports, and parental well-being (or adjustment). The studies mentioned here and others indicate both main and buffering effects of support that influence family well-being, suggesting that family support acts as a protective mechanism.

IMPLICATIONS FOR RESEARCH ON FAMILIES

While the search for cause and cure of disability continues, we must be mindful of the importance of studying the family context. After all, children with DD first are born into the family, and most of them spend many years there. Recent research on family coping and adjustment attests to the resilience of families and to the need for researchers to incorporate more aspects of resilience and positivity into their conceptual models. Another finding that is well substantiated in the literature is that most families cope better with the assistance of social support, although we know little about cultural variation in its influences on family well-being.

Ultimately, findings pertaining to behavioral phenotypes will likely necessitate more targeted family interventions. For example, research on the process and trajectory of family impact will need to evolve in response to new information about the genetic underpinnings of certain neurodevelopmental disorders. Fragile X syndrome (FXS) is a case in point, in which genetic counseling efforts are now influencing reproductive planning for families. Genetic testing used to detect FXS in newborns might save some families a great deal of stress but perhaps produce anxiety in others (Bailey, 2004; Hagerman, Ono, & Hagerman, 2005). We know, too, that negative impact, or stress, varies by specific syndromes, but this can be accounted for by syndrome-specific behavioral challenges (Eisenhower, Baker, & Blacher, 2005), whereas positive impact, which varies only modestly by specific syndromes, is related more to cultural characteristics (Blacher, 2006; Blacher & McIntyre, 2006).

Some newly emerging research attests to the increasing importance of behavior–environment interactions. For example, research in the area of autism suggests that family members other than the child with IDD may themselves have more subtle characteristics of the disorder, referred to as the broader autism phenotype by Piven and Palmer (1999). Such findings illustrate the complexity of studying the child with IDD in multiple contexts (such as family and school). Clearly, the newly emerging body of literature on behavioral phenotypes suggests that families will need clear, user-friendly information about their child's syndrome as early as possible. However, it is also important that the information delivered is not overly deterministic, particularly with regard to the prognosis for any given genetic syndrome. Such information should be regularly reviewed and updated.

IMPLICATIONS FOR SERVICE DELIVERY TO FAMILIES

In addition to the implications for intervention noted before, family research has equally relevant implications for service delivery, at least at this point in time. Research and service delivery contexts need to consider changing family constellations. Service providers will need to reconsider who counts as a "family" and not focus exclusively on the mother–child relationship. It is not unreasonable to expect service delivery efforts to start from the position of understanding relevant issues *from the family's perspective*, instead of from the service providers' perspective on what families need or, worse yet, on what services are available.

In addition, service providers may need to consider the socioeconomic circumstances of the families, their culture, their values, the social networks within which families exist, and the families' expectations about their child's disability across the life course.

IMPLICATIONS FOR POLICY RELATED TO FAMILIES

Finally, there is a pressing need for researchers to be more proactive in educating policy makers about the growing scientific research on families and DD. There is an empirical basis for the potential benefits of policies that support families in achieving positive, valued lives for themselves and for their family member with an intellectual or developmental disability. Too often, services are geared toward alleviating families in crisis, a practice that often amounts to too little, too late. Although it is important not to ignore the stressors and tough times that families of children with DD experience at various points during the life course (as all families do), policies should be aimed at helping families build resilience and self-determination through both the good and bad times. A strong case can surely be made for paying more attention to family well-being.

ACKNOWLEDGMENTS

The preparation of this chapter was supported in part by National Institute of Child Health and Human Development (NICHD) Grant No. 21324 (J. Blacher, Principal Investigator) and NICHD Grant No. 34879-1459 (K. Crnic, B. L. Baker, J. Blacher, & C. Edelbrock, Coprincipal Investigators).

REFERENCES

Abbeduto, L., Seltzer, M. M., Shattuck, P. T., Krauss, M. W., Orsmond, G. I., & Murphy, M. M. (2004). Psychological well-being and coping in mothers of adolescents and adults with developmental disabilities: Comparisons between autism, Down syndrome and fragile-X syndrome. *American Journal on Mental Retardation, 109,* 237–254.

Alborz, A. (2003). Transitions: Placing a son or daughter with intellectual disability and challenging behaviour in alternative residential provision. *Journal of Applied Research in Intellectual Disabilities, 16,* 75–88.

Allen, D. A., & Affleck, G. (1985). Are we stereotyping parents? A postscript to Blacher. *Mental Retardation, 23,* 200–202.

Antonovsky, A. (1987). *Unraveling the mystery of health: How people manage stress and stay well.* San Francisco: Jossey-Bass.

Antonovsky, A. (1998). The sense of coherence: An historical and future perspective. In H. I. McCubbin, E. A. Thompson, A. I. Thompson, & J. E. Fromer (Eds.), *Stress, coping, and health in families: Sense of coherence and resiliency* (pp. 3–20). Thousand Oaks, CA: Sage.

Armstrong, M. I., Birnie-Lefcovitch, S., & Ungar, M. T. (2005). Pathways between social support, family well-being, quality of parenting, and child resilience: What we know. *Journal of Child and Family Studies, 14,* 269–281.

Bailey, D. B. (2004). Newborn screening for fragile X syndrome. *Mental Retardation and Developmental Disabilities Research Reviews, 10,* 3–10.

Bailey, D. B., Jr., Skinner, D., Correa, V., Arcia, E., Reyes-Blanes, M., Rodriguez, P., et al. (1999). Needs and supports reported by Latino families of young children with developmental disabilities. *American Journal on Mental Retardation, 104,* 437–451.

Baker, B. L., & Blacher, J. (1993). Out-of-home placement for children with mental retardation: Dimensions of family involvement. *American Journal on Mental Retardation, 98,* 368–377.

Baker, B. L., & Blacher, J. (2002). For better or for worse? Impact of residential placement on families. *Mental Retardation, 40,* 1–13.

Baker, B. L., Blacher, J., & Olsson, M. B. (2005). Preschool children with and without developmental delay: Behavioural problems, parents' optimism and well-being. *Journal of Intellectual Disability Research, 49,* 575–590.

Baker, B. L., Blacher, J., & Pfeiffer, S. (1993). Family involvement in residential treatment of children with psychiatric disorder and mental retardation. *Hospital and Community Psychiatry, 44,* 561–566.

Baker, K., & Donelly, M. (2001). The social experiences of children with disability and the influence of environment: A framework for intervention. *Disability and Society, 16,* 71–85.

Berry, J. W. (1999). On the unity of the field of culture and psychology. In J. Adamopoulos & Y. Kashima (Eds.), *Social psychology and cultural context* (pp. 7–15). London: Sage.

Berry, J. W., Poortinga, Y. H., Segall, M. H., & Dasen, P. R. (2002). *Cross-cultural psychology: Research and applications* (2nd ed.). Cambridge, UK: Cambridge University Press.

Blacher, J. (1984). Sequential stages of parental adjustment to the birth of a handicapped child: Fact or artifact? *Mental Retardation, 22,* 55–68.

Blacher, J. (1994). Placement and its consequences for families with children who have mental retardation. In J. Blacher (Ed.), *When there's no place like home: Options for children living apart from their natural families* (pp. 213–243). Baltimore: Brookes.

Blacher, J. (2001). The transition to adulthood: Mental retardation, families, and culture. *American Journal of Mental Retardation, 106,* 173–188.

Blacher, J. (2006, August). *Families and phenotypes: Cultural context and environmental influences on wellbeing.* Paper presented at the European Meeting of the International Association for the Scientific Study of Intellectual Disability, Maastricht, The Netherlands.

Blacher, J., & Baker, B. L. (1994). Family involvement in residential treatment of children with retardation: Is there evidence of detachment? *Journal of Child Psychology and Psychiatry, 35,* 505–520.

Blacher, J., & Baker, B. L. (2002). *The best of AAMR: Families and mental retardation: A collection of notable AAMR journal articles across the 20th century.* Washington, DC: American Association on Mental Retardation.

Blacher, J., & Baker, B. L. (2007). Positive impact of intellectual disability on families. *American Journal on Mental Retardation, 112.*

Blacher, J., Baker, B. L., & Feinfield, K. A. (1999). Leaving or launching? Continuing family involvement with children and adolescents in placement. *American Journal on Mental Retardation, 104,* 452–465.

Blacher, J., Lopez, S., Shapiro, J., & Fusco, J. (1997). Contributions to depression in Latina mothers with and without children with retardation: Implications for caregiving. *Family Relations, 46,* 325–334.

Blacher, J., & McIntyre, L. L. (2006). Syndrome specificity and behavioural disorders in young adults with intellectual disability: Cultural differences in family impact. *Journal of Intellectual Disability Research, 50,* 184–198.

Blacher, J., & Mink, I. T. (2004). Interviewing family members and care providers: Concepts, methodologies, and cultures. In E. Emerson, C. Hatton, T. Thompson, & T. Parmenter (Eds.), *International handbook of applied research in intellectual disabilities* (pp. 133–159). Chichester, UK: Wiley.

Blacher, J., Shapiro, J., Lopez, S., Diaz, L., & Fusco, J. (1997). Depression in Latina mothers of children with mental retardation: A neglected concern. *American Journal on Mental Retardation, 101,* 483–496.

Blacher, J., & Widaman, K. F. (2004). *Final report: Determination of purchase of services variation across regional centers: Implications for clients and policy.* A report to the Legislature, State of California.

Bromley, J., Hare, D. J., Davison, K., & Emerson, E. (2004). Mothers supporting children with autistic spectrum disorders: Social support, mental health status and satisfaction with services. *Autism, 8,* 409–423.

Bruns, D. A. (2000). Leaving home at an early age: Parents' decisions about out-of-home placement for young children with complex medical needs. *Mental Retardation, 38,* 50–60.

Cahill, B. M., & Glidden, L. M. (1996). Influence of child diagnosis on family and parental functioning: Down syndrome versus other disabilities. *American Journal on Mental Retardation, 101,* 149–160.

Castles, S., & Miller, M. J. (1998). *The age of migration: International population movements in the modern world* (2nd ed.). London: Macmillan.

Chavira, V., Lopez, S. R., Blacher, J., & Shapiro, J. (2000). Latina mothers' attributions, emotions, and reactions to the problem behaviors of their children with developmental disabilities. *Journal of Child Psychology and Psychiatry, 41,* 245–252.

Crnic, K. A., Friedrich, W. N., & Greenberg, M. T. (1983). Adaptation of families with mentally retarded children: A model of stress, coping, and family ecology. *American Journal of Mental Deficiency, 88,* 125–138.

Davies, S. P. (1925). The institution in relation to the school system. *Journal of Psycho-Aesthenics, 30,* 210–226.

Dollahite, D. C. (2003). Fathering for eternity: Generative spirituality in Latter-Day Saint fathers of children with special needs. *Review of Religious Research, 44,* 237–251.

Dykens, E. M. (1995). Measuring behavioral phenotypes: Provocations from the "new genetics." *American Journal on Mental Retardation, 99,* 522–532.

Dykens, E. M. (2005). Happiness, well-being, and character strengths: Outcomes for families and siblings of persons with mental retardation. *Mental Retardation, 43,* 360–364.

Dykens, E. M., Hodapp, R. M., & Finucane, B. M. (2000). *Genetics and mental retardation syndromes: A new look at behavior and interventions.* Baltimore: Brookes.

Eden-Pearcy, G. V. S., Blacher, J. B., & Eyman, R. K. (1986). Exploring parents' reactions to their young child with severe handicaps. *Mental Retardation, 24,* 285–291.

Eisenberg, L., Baker, B. L., & Blacher, J. (1998). Siblings of children with mental retardation living at home or in residential placement. *Journal of Child Psychology and Psychiatry, 39,* 355–363.

Eisenhower, A., Baker, B. L., & Blacher, J. (2005). Preschool children with intellectual disability: Syndrome specificity, behavior problems, and maternal well-being. *Journal of Intellectual Disability Research, 49,* 657–671.

Emerson, E. (2003). Mothers of children and adolescents with intellectual disability: Social and economic situation, mental health status, and the self-assessed social and psychological impact of the child's difficulties. *Journal of Intellectual Disability Research, 47,* 385–399.

Emerson, E., & Hatton, C. (1999). Future trends in the ethnic composition of British society and among British citizens with learning disabilities. *Tizard Learning Disability Review, 4,* 28–32.

Emerson, E., Hatton, C., Llewellyn, G., Blacher, J., & Graham, H. (2006). Socio-economic position, household composition, health status and indicators of the well-being of mothers of children with and without intellectual disability. *Journal of Intellectual Disability Research, 50,* 862–873.

Farber, B. (1959). Effects of a severely mentally retarded child on family integration. *Monographs of the Society for Research in Child Development, 24,* 1–112.

Farber, B. (1960). Perceptions of crisis and related variables in the impact of a retarded child on the mother. *Journal of Health and Human Behavior, 1,* 108–118.

Fidler, D. J., & Hodapp, R. M. (1999). Craniofacial maturity and perceived personality in children with Down syndrome. *American Journal on Mental Retardation, 104,* 410–421.

Fidler, D. J., Hodapp, R. M., & Dykens, E. M. (2000). Stress in families of young children with Down syndrome, Williams syndrome, and Smith–Magennis syndrome. *Early Education and Development, 11,* 395–406.

Flynt, J., & Yule, W. (1994). Behavioural phenotypes. In M. Rutter, E. Taylor, & L. Hersov (Eds.), *Child and adolescent psychiatry: Modern approaches* (3rd ed., pp. 666–687). London: Blackwell Scientific.

Freedman, R. I., & Boyer, N. C. (2000). The power to choose: Supports for families caring for individuals with developmental disabilities. *Health and Social Work, 25,* 59–68.

Fujiura, G. T., & Yamaki, K. (1997). Analysis of ethnic variations in developmental disability prevalence and household economic status. *Mental Retardation, 35,* 286–294.

Gabel, S. (2004). South Asian Indian cultural orientations toward mental retardation. *Mental Retardation, 42,* 12–25.

Grant, G., Ramcharan, P., McGrath, M., Nolan, M., & Keady, J. (1998). Rewards and gratifications among family caregivers: Towards a refined model of caring and coping. *Journal of Intellectual Disability Research, 42,* 58–71.

Grebler, A. M. (1952). Parental attitudes toward mentally retarded children. *American Journal of Mental Deficiency, 56,* 475–483.

Hagerman, R. J., Ono, M. Y., & Hagerman, P. J. (2005). Recent advances in fragile X: A model for autism and neurodegeneration. *Current Opinion in Psychiatry, 18,* 490–496.

Harris, S., Kasari, C., & Sigman, M. (1996). Joint attention and language gains in children with Down syndrome. *American Journal on Mental Retardation, 100,* 608–619.

Harry, B. (1992). An ethnographic study of cross-cultural communication with Puerto Rican–American families in the special education system. *American Educational Research Journal, 29,* 471–494.

Hassall, R., & Rose, J. (2005). Parental cognitions and adaptation to the demands of caring for a child with an intellectual disability: A review of the literature and implications for clinical interventions. *Behavioural and Cognitive Psychotherapy, 33,* 71–88.

Hastings, R. P., Allen, R., McDermott, K., & Still, D. (2002). Factors related to positive perceptions in mothers of children with intellectual disabilities. *Journal of Applied Research in Intellectual Disabilities, 15,* 269–275.

Hastings, R. P., Beck, A., & Hill, C. (2005). Positive contributions made by children with an intellectual disability in the family. *Journal of Intellectual Disabilities, 9,* 155–165.

Hastings, R. P., & Taunt, H. M. (2002). Positive perceptions in families of children with developmental disabilities. *American Journal on Mental Retardation, 107,* 116–127.

Hatton, C. (2002). People with intellectual disabilities from ethnic minority communities in the United States and the United Kingdom. *International Review of Research in Mental Retardation, 25,* 209–239.

Hatton, C. (2004). Cultural issues. In E. Emerson, C. Hatton, T. Thompson, & T. Parmenter (Eds.), *International handbook of applied research in intellectual disabilities* (pp. 41–60). Chichester, UK: Wiley.

Hatton, C., Akram, Y., Shah, R., Robertson, J., & Emerson, E. (2004). *Supporting Asian families with a child with severe disabilities.* London: Kingsley.

Heiman, T. (2002). Parents of children with disabilities: Resilience, coping, and future expectations. *Journal of Developmental and Physical Disabilities, 14,* 159–171.

Heller, T., Miller, A. B., & Factor, A. (1997). Adults with mental retardation as supports to their parents: Effects on parental caregiving appraisal. *Mental Retardation, 35,* 338–346.

Hill, R. (1949). *Families under stress: Adjustment to the crises of war separation and return.* Oxford, UK: Harper.

Hodapp, R. M., & Dykens, E. M. (2004). Studying behavioral phenotypes: Issues, benefits, challenges. In E. Emerson, C. Hatton, T. Thompson, & T. R. Parmenter (Eds.), *International handbook of applied research in intellectual disabilities* (pp. 203–220). Chichester, UK: Wiley.

Hodapp, R. M., & Dykens, E. M. (2006). Mental retardation. In K. A. Reininger & I. E. Sigel (Eds.), *Handbook of child psychology* (6th ed., Vol. 4, pp. 453–496). New York: Wiley.

Individuals with Disabilities Education Act Amendments of 2004, 20 U.S.C. § 1400 *et seq.*

King, G. A., Zwaigenbaum, L., King, S., Baxter, D., Rosenbaum, P., & Bates, A. (2006). A qualitative investigation of changes in the belief systems of families of children with autism or Down syndrome. *Child: Care, Health and Development, 32,* 353–369.

Krauss, M. W., Seltzer, M. M., & Jacobson, H. T. (2005). Adults with autism living at home or in non-family settings: Positive and negative aspects of residential status. *Journal of Intellectual Disability Research, 49,* 111–124.

Kübler-Ross, E. (1970). *On death and dying.* New York: Collier Books/Macmillan.

Lazarus, R. S. (1993). Coping theory and research: Past, present, and future. *Psychosomatic Medicine, 55,* 234–247.

LeVine, R. A. (1984). Properties of culture: An ethnographic view. In R. A. Shweder & R. A. LeVine (Eds.), *Culture theory: Essays on mind, self, and emotion* (pp. 67–87). Cambridge, UK: Cambridge University Press.

Llewellyn, G., McConnell, D., Thompson, K., & Whybrow, S. (2005). Out-of-home placement of school-age children with disabilities and high support needs. *Journal of Applied Research in Intellectual Disabilities, 18,* 1–6.

Lopez, S. R., & Guarnaccia, P. J. (2000). Cultural psychology: Uncovering the social world of mental illness. *Annual Review of Psychology, 51,* 571–598.

Ly, T. M., & Hodapp, R. M. (2002). Maternal attribution of child noncompliance in children with mental retardation: Down syndrome versus other etiologies. *Journal of Developmental and Behavioral Pediatrics, 23,* 322–329.

Ly, T. M., & Hodapp, R. M. (2005). Children with Prader–Willi syndrome versus Williams syndrome: Indirect effects on parents during a jigsaw puzzle task. *Journal of Intellectual Disability Research, 49,* 929–939.

Magana, S. (1999). Puerto Rican families caring for an adult with mental retardation: The role of familism. *American Journal on Mental Retardation, 104,* 466–482.

Magana, S., & Smith, M. J. (2006). Health outcomes of midlife and older Latina and Black American mothers of children with developmental disabilities. *Mental Retardation, 44,* 224–234.

McConkey, R. (2005). Fair shares? Supporting families caring for adult persons with intellectual disabilities. *Journal of Intellectual Disability Research, 49*, 600–612.

McCubbin, H. I., & Patterson, J. M. (1983). The family stress process: The double ABCX model of family adjustment and adaptation. *Marriage and Family Review, 6*, 7–37.

Mink, I. T. (1997). Studying culturally diverse families of children with mental retardation. *International
Review of Research in Mental Retardation, 20*, 75–98.

Modood, T., Berthoud, R., Lakey, J., Nazroo, J., Smith, P., Virdee, S., et al. (1997). *Ethnic minorities in
Britain: Diversity and disadvantage.* London: Policy Studies Institute.

Olshansky, S. (1962). Chronic sorrow: A response to having a mentally defective child. *Social Casework,
43*, 190–193.

Olsson, M. B., & Hwang, C. P. (2002). Sense of coherence in parents of children with different developmental disabilities. *Journal of Intellectual Disability Research, 46*, 548–559.

Orsmond, G. I., & Seltzer, M. M. (2000). Brothers and sisters of adults with mental retardation:
Gendered nature of the sibling relationship. *American Journal on Mental Retardation, 105*, 486–
508.

Parish, S. L., Pomeranz-Essley, A., & Braddock, D. (2003). Family support in the United States:
Financing trends and emerging initiatives. *Mental Retardation, 41*, 174–187.

Pfeiffer, S. I., & Baker, B. L. (1994). Residential treatment for children with dual diagnoses of mental
retardation and mental disorder. In J. Blacher (Ed.), *When there's no place like home: Options for children living apart from their natural families* (pp. 273–298). Baltimore: Brookes.

Piven, J., & Palmer, P. (1999). Psychiatric disorder and the broad autism phenotype: Evidence from a
family study of multiple-incidence autism families. *American Journal of Psychiatry, 156*, 557–563.

Poehlmann, J., Clements, M., Abbeduto, L., & Farsad, V. (2005). Family experiences associated with a
child's diagnosis of fragile X or Down syndrome: Evidence for disruption and resilience. *Mental
Retardation, 43*, 255–267.

Pruchno, R. A., & McMullen, W. F. (2004). Patterns of service utilization by adults with a developmental disability: Type of service makes a difference. *American Journal on Mental Retardation, 109*,
362–378.

Rao, S. (2006). Parameters of normality and cultural constructions of "mental retardation": Perspectives of Bengali families. *Disability and Society, 21*, 159–178.

Risdal, D., & Singer, G. H. S. (2004). Marital adjustment in parents of children with disabilities: A historical review and meta-analysis. *Research and Practice for Persons with Severe Disabilities, 29*, 95–103.

Rogers-Dulan, J. (1998). Religious connectedness among urban African American families who have a
child with disabilities. *Mental Retardation, 36*, 91–103.

Rogers-Dulan, J., & Blacher, J. (1995). African American families, religion, and disability: A conceptual
framework. *Mental Retardation, 33*, 226–238.

Rueda, R., Monzo, L., Shapiro, J., Gomez, J., & Blacher, J. (2005). Cultural models of transition: Latina
mothers of young adults with developmental disabilities. *Exceptional Children, 71*, 401–414.

Schonell, F. J., & Watts, B. H. (1956). A first survey of the effects of a subnormal child on the family
unit. *American Journal of Mental Deficiency, 61*, 210–219.

Schwartz, C. (2005). Parental involvement in residential care and perceptions of their offspring's life
satisfaction in residential facilities for adults with intellectual disability. *Journal of Intellectual and
Developmental Disability, 30*, 146–155.

Scorgie, K., & Sobsey, D. (2000). Transformational outcomes associated with parenting children who
have disabilities. *Mental Retardation, 38*, 195–206.

Scorgie, K., Wilgosh, L., & McDonald, L. (1999). Transforming partnerships: Parent life management
issues when a child has mental retardation. *Education and Training in Mental Retardation and Developmental Disabilities, 34*, 395–405.

Seltzer, M. M., Abbeduto, L., Krauss, M. W., Greenberg, J., & Swe, A. (2004). Comparison groups in
autism family research: Down syndrome, fragile X syndrome, and schizophrenia. *Journal of Autism
and Developmental Disorders, 34*, 41–48.

Seltzer, M. M., Greenberg, J. S., Floyd, F. J., & Hong, J. K. (2004). Accommodative coping and well-
being of midlife parents of children with mental health problems or developmental disabilities.
American Journal of Orthopsychiatry, 74, 187–195.

Seltzer, M. M., Greenberg, J. S., Krauss, M. W., & Hong, J. (1997). Predictors and outcomes of the end of co-resident caregiving in aging families of adults with mental retardation or mental illness. *Family Relations: Interdisciplinary Journal of Applied Family Studies, 46,* 13–22.

Seltzer, M. M., Krauss, M. W., Choi, S. C., & Hong, J. (1996). Midlife and later-life parenting of adult children with mental retardation. In C. D. Ryff & M. M. Seltzer (Eds.), *The parental experience in midlife* (pp. 459–489). Chicago: University of Chicago Press.

Seltzer, M. M., Krauss, M. W., Orsmond, G. I., & Vestal, C. (2000). Families of adolescents and adults with autism: Uncharted territory. In L. M. Glidden (Ed.), *International review of research on mental retardation* (Vol. 23, pp. 267–294). San Diego, CA: Academic Press.

Shapiro, J., Monzo, L. D., Rueda, R., Gomez, J. A., & Blacher, J. (2004). Alienated advocacy: Perspectives of Latina mothers of young adults with developmental disabilities on service systems. *Mental Retardation, 42,* 37–54.

Shinagawa, L. H., & Jang, M. (1998). *Atlas of American diversity.* Walnut Creek, CA: Altamira.

Skinner, D., Correa, V., Skinner, M., & Bailey, D. B., Jr. (2001). Role of religion in the lives of Latino families of young children with developmental delays. *American Journal on Mental Retardation, 106,* 297–313.

Stoneman, Z. (2005). Siblings of children with disabilities: Research themes. *Mental Retardation, 43,* 339–350.

Taylor, S. E. (1983). Adjustment to threatening events: A theory of cognitive adaptation. *American Psychologist, 38,* 1161–1173.

Taylor, S. E., Lerner, J. S., Sherman, D. K., Sage, R. M., & McDowell, N. K. (2003). Are self-enhancing cognitions associated with healthy or unhealthy biological profiles? *Journal of Personality and Social Psychology, 85,* 605–615.

Triandis, H. C. (1995). *Individualism and collectivism.* Boulder, CO: Westview.

Turnbull, A. P., & Turnbull, H. R. (1978). *Parents speak out: Views from the other side of the two-way mirror.* Columbus, OH: Merrill.

Vaux, C. L. (1936). Family care. *Proceedings. American Association on Mental Deficiency, 41,* 82–88.

White, N., & Hastings, R. P. (2004). Social and professional support for parents of adolescents with severe intellectual disabilities. *Journal of Applied Research in Intellectual Disabilities, 17,* 181–190.

Widaman, K. F., & Blacher, J. (2003). *Modeling variation in per capita purchase of services for Coffelt and non-Coffelt consumers.* A report to the Legislature, State of California.

Wikler, L., Wasow, M., & Hatfield, E. (1981). Chronic sorrow revisited: Parent vs. professional depiction of the adjustment of parents of mentally retarded children. *American Journal of Orthopsychiatry, 51,* 63–70.

Family Impact in Adulthood

Julie J. Lounds
Marsha Mailick Seltzer

This chapter examines the family impact of caregiving for an adult child with a developmental disability. To address these issues, we summarize a program of research that examines how specific elements of the caregiving context and the family system influence family relationships and the psychological well-being of each family member. Finally, we focus on a key transition among families of adult children with mental retardation and developmental disabilities (MR/DD) that has implications for the entire family system; namely, the transition out of parental care and into an alternate-care context for the adult with MR/DD.

The research presented in this chapter is informed by two overarching theoretical frameworks. The first is a lifespan perspective on development. Four assumptions are made according to this perspective: (1) Development is lifelong, (2) development is multidimensional and multidirectional, (3) development is highly plastic, and (4) development is embedded in multiple contexts (Baltes, Lindenberger, & Straudinger, 1998; Smith & Baltes, 1999). Although researchers recognize that development is a lifelong process, the majority of work concerning the family impact of developmental disabilities has focused on the early childhood years. The importance of considering development across the lifespan is particularly salient among families who have a member with a developmental disability, as the care provided by families to their members with developmental disabilities often spans five or six decades (Krauss & Seltzer, 1993). The multidirectional nature of development is also an important consideration when conducting research with families who have a member with a developmental disability. As parents and family members become more accustomed to caregiving for developmentally disabled members, they often acquire specialized skills and competencies (Kling, Seltzer, & Ryff, 1997). Gains in caregiving competence may in some cases co-occur with declines in other developmental domains due to the aging process, such as declining physical health. Therefore, to truly measure the family impact over the lifespan, it is important to consider development in multiple domains and contexts.

Finally, according to the lifespan perspective, a number of distinct influences combine to affect the life course. These tend to fall under the categories of non-normative and normative events (Baltes, 1987). Non-normative events are unshared and do not follow a predictable timetable. The experience of parenting a child with a developmental disability is an example of this type of influence. Normative experiences, on the other hand, tend to be experienced by most individuals with fairly high predictability and are mainly governed by biological maturation or sociocultural timetables. Normative influences interact with non-normative events to influence development, such as when an individual who has a sibling with a developmental disability (non-normative event) makes decisions about marriage and childbearing (normative events). These types of influences work together to produce unique developmental trajectories among families who have a member with a developmental disability. As these developmental trajectories are influenced by events throughout the life course, it is important to take a lifespan approach when observing the family impact of having a member with a developmental disability.

Our research is also informed by family systems theory. According to this theory, bidirectional influences exist in which the behaviors of each family member influence those of all others in the family (Bronfenbrenner, 1989). Although developed in the context of the general population, this theory also applies to families who have a member with a developmental disability, as the disability has ripple effects on all family members (Pruchno, Patrick, & Burant, 1996). Mothers are often the focus in studies of family impact because they typically function as the primary caregivers. There is growing recognition, however, of the importance of fathers in the family system (Essex, Seltzer, & Krauss, 2002), as well as of the impact of nondisabled siblings on the development of other members of the family. For example, Seltzer, Begun, Seltzer, and Krauss (1991) found that mothers whose other children provided support to the adult with MR/DD had better psychological well-being than mothers who had no nondisabled children or whose nondisabled children were not involved.

This chapter integrates these two perspectives by examining the family impact of having a child with a developmental disability when that child reaches adulthood. In addition, the influences of all family members are discussed, with an emphasis on how these influences interact to affect the family system.

DESCRIPTION OF OUR PROGRAM OF RESEARCH

Our longitudinal research on families who have an adult son or daughter with MR/DD began in 1988 (Seltzer & Krauss, 1989). We have studied 461 families in which the mother was between the ages of 55 and 85 at the start of the study and had a son or daughter with MR/DD living at home with her. The average age of the son or daughter with MR/DD was 34 years. Most of the sample members had mild (38%) or moderate (41%) mental retardation, and 21% had severe or profound retardation. Most of the mothers were married (66%) and had other children in addition to the son or daughter with MR/DD (93%).

Each family was visited every 18 months, with eight waves of data collected between 1988 and 2000. At each wave, the mother (the primary respondent) was interviewed in the home and completed a self-administered set of standardized measures. Data were also collected from the father and up to two nondisabled siblings in each family (for a description of the study design, see Krauss & Seltzer, 1993; Seltzer & Krauss, 1989). Families continued to participate in the study even after the death or incapacitation of the mother. In such instances, if the father survived the mother, he became the primary respondent. If the father predeceased the mother, then another family member, generally a sibling, took on this role in the study.

In the next section, results from our research on two issues are presented. The first concerns the impact of having a child with MR/DD on individual members within the family system. We present findings on caregiving activities and relationship closeness among families and examine how these variables and others (characteristics of the child with MR/DD and coping) influence psychological well-being for each family member. Finally, we summarize our research concerning the transition of caregiving to other sources. We begin by discussing the transition out of the home and into placement settings and end with a discussion of the transition to the next generation of caregivers. These particular transition points were chosen because of their salience for all members of the family system. A family member's moving from the home and into a placement setting often necessitates a reorganization of family and caregiving roles. Furthermore, as we discuss, planning for future caregiving of the individual with MR/DD is a process that often involves each member of the family system.

FINDINGS REGARDING THE FAMILY IMPACT OF HAVING A MEMBER WITH MR/DD

Caregiving Activities

Caregiving Activities Provided by Family Members

Past research among parents of young children with MR/DD has suggested that, despite the extra caregiving needs of these children, fathers do not take on a larger share of child care or housework than fathers of children without disabilities (Barnett & Boyce, 1995; Erickson & Upshur, 1989). In fact, several studies have suggested that fathers of children with MR/DD are less involved than fathers of typically developing children (Bristol, Gallagher, & Schopler, 1988; Levy-Shiff, 1986). We were interested in whether these patterns of caregiving for mothers and fathers remained evident when the individual with MR/DD reached adulthood. Specifically, we examined the division of labor within the family when the adult child with MR/DD lived in the home with his or her parents (Essex et al., 2002). Of a possible 31 instrumental and personal activities of daily living with which the adult child may need assistance (such as personal care or household maintenance), mothers helped with an average of 11 caregiving tasks. Fathers helped with significantly fewer tasks, with an average of 4 caregiving tasks. There was only one caregiving task in which fathers were more likely to help out than mothers—simple home repairs. Three tasks were equally likely to be assisted by mothers and fathers, including helping the adult child with ambulation difficulties to walk indoors, to use stairs, and to move in and out of automobiles. For the remaining 27 caregiving tasks, fathers were less likely than mothers to provide assistance.

Other studies have reported differential patterns of caregiving between mothers and fathers of adults with MR/DD. One example is a study by Heller, Hsieh, and Rowitz

(1997), who reported that mothers spent more time than fathers providing care for their adult child with MR/DD and offered their child more types of personal and instrumental supports (such as encouragement or personal care). It seems as though the patterns of caregiving that emerge in childhood, characterized by the mother as primary caregiver, continue when the child with MR/DD reaches adulthood.

We used a different measure of caregiving activities to measure the extent of sibling involvement. The amount of instrumental support offered by nondisabled siblings to the individual with MR/DD was assessed by four types of caregiving activities—direct caregiving, transportation, financial assistance, and running errands. In addition, emotional support to the sibling with MR/DD was measured using two items that assessed the extent of provision of companionship and general emotional support. Our findings indicated that adult siblings of individuals with MR/DD were more likely to provide emotional support than instrumental support (Greenberg, Seltzer, Orsmond, & Krauss, 1999).

Although mothers of adults with MR/DD were mainly responsible for the provision of care, the importance of caregiving involvement by other members of the family system demonstrates the interdependence of family members (Essex et al., 2002; Seltzer et al., 1991). As noted earlier, mothers with children who were involved with the adult child with MR/DD evidenced more favorable well-being than both mothers who had no other children and mothers with children who were not involved with the adult with MR/DD. Mothers with involved children showed better physical health, higher morale, less burden, and less stress associated with caregiving. Furthermore, mothers reported better morale when their husbands provided at least some care for their son or daughter with MR/DD than when their husbands provided no care at all. It may not be the objective amount of care provided by fathers that is most important for maternal mental health but the amount of care provided in relation to mothers' expectations for paternal care. Research on families with young children with developmental disabilities has found that mothers reported more psychopathology when a discrepancy existed between the amount of caregiving activities and household help they expected from fathers and the amount that fathers actually provided (Bristol et al., 1988; Milgram & Atzil, 1988).

Predicting Caregiving Activities

Because of the importance of father involvement for maternal well-being, we examined characteristics of the mother and father (employment, health, and age) and characteristics of the adult with MR/DD (level of retardation, gender, and age) that might influence fathers' caregiving activities. Interestingly, characteristics of neither the mother nor the father's lives influenced father involvement. A father was no more likely to help in caregiving activities whether he was employed or retired, healthy or in declining health, or over or under 65 years of age, nor whether his wife was employed or not, healthy or in declining health, or over or under 65 years of age (Essex et al., 2002).

Factors related to the child with MR/DD, however, did influence the amount of father involvement. Fathers were more likely to help with caregiving activities when the adult had severe or profound retardation as opposed to mild or moderate retardation. Fathers were also more likely to help a son with MR/DD than a daughter. Interestingly, the gender difference in help was present for issues of personal care (e.g., dressing and bathing), in which one might expect gender similarity to be important, as well as more gender-neutral tasks, such as running errands and managing finances. The gender bias in provision of care was present only for fathers; mothers' assistance was largely unrelated to the adult child's gender (Essex et al., 2002).

Similar to the findings for mothers, the amount of caregiving provided by siblings was not affected by the gender of the individual with MR/DD. The gender of the nondisabled sibling, however, played a predictive role (Orsmond & Seltzer, 2000). Sisters of individuals with MR/DD felt more knowledgeable than brothers about the skills and needs of their sibling with MR/DD (e.g., daily living skills, financial needs, physical health needs). Sisters also reported more frequent discussions with parents about the well-being of their sibling with MR/DD. The relationship between the unaffected sibling's gender and caregiving is not surprising; general developmental theory suggests that women, more so than men, are socialized from childhood to care for others (Chodorow, 1978).

Although the gender of the nondisabled sibling was an important determinant of the amount of sibling caregiving, we hypothesized that other factors related to the nondisabled sibling (whether or not the sibling had children under age 18 at home), to the individual with MR/DD (gender, residence with parents, and number of behavior problems), and to closeness to the family of origin (residential proximity to the sibling with MR/DD, emotional closeness of siblings during adolescence, and emotional closeness of the nondisabled sibling to the mother) could affect the amount of instrumental and emotional support provided by siblings (Greenberg et al., 1999). Results indicated both similarities and differences in the patterns of prediction for the two types of support. Nondisabled siblings were more likely to provide both instrumental and emotional support when they did not have children under the age of 18 living at home, when they lived in closer proximity to their brother or sister with MR/DD, and when they were more emotionally close to their mothers. In addition, siblings were less likely to provide instrumental support when the adult with MR/DD was not living with his or her parents, but only if the siblings had minor children at home.

In terms of emotional support, sisters of individuals with MR/DD were more likely to provide support. Siblings were also more likely to provide emotional support when the individual with MR/DD had fewer behavior problems and when there had been more emotional closeness between the siblings during adolescence. These findings point to the importance of strong, emotional bonds between family members that promote the involvement of the nondisabled sibling in the life of the individual with MR/DD. We now turn to a discussion of relationship closeness among family members, as well as the factors that predict closeness.

Relationship Closeness

Relationship Closeness among Family Members

The Positive Affect Index (Bengtson & Schrader, 1982) was used to measure relationship closeness between each family member (mother, father, sibling) and the individual with MR/DD. Five items ask the family member to rate his or her feelings of trust, intimacy, understanding, fairness, and respect toward the individual with MR/DD, and five items ask the family member's perception of the extent to which the individual with MR/DD displays feelings of trust, intimacy, understanding, fairness, and respect toward him or her. Summing these 10 items created an overall relationship closeness score. When comparing mothers and fathers of coresiding adults with MR/DD, fathers were found to be less close than mothers to their adult children with MR/DD (Essex et al., 2002).

Predicting Relationship Closeness

The majority of our research on the prediction of relationship closeness to the adult with MR/DD has focused on the mother, because she is often the primary caregiver. One factor that has emerged as an important correlate of relationship closeness is coping (Kim, Greenberg, Seltzer, & Krauss, 2003). We examined two major types of coping strategies: problem-focused coping and emotion-focused coping (Lazarus & Folkman, 1984). Problem-focused coping involves strategies, both cognitive and behavioral, that are aimed at altering or managing the stressful situation. Emotion-focused coping involves efforts to reduce emotional distress without focusing on solving the problem. In general, we have found that for mothers of adults with MR/DD, increasing the use of problem-focused coping strategies was related to more relationship closeness, whereas using more emotion-focused coping strategies was associated with less relationship closeness (Kim et al., 2003).

A related study examining family functioning among families that have an adolescent child with autism, fragile X syndrome, or Down syndrome further explored the factors that promote relationship closeness among mothers of individuals with developmental disabilities (Abbeduto et al., 2004). This study extended the previously discussed findings by separately examining the two components of relationship quality, namely, the maternal rating of relationship closeness and the amount of reciprocated closeness the mother felt from the son or daughter with the developmental disability. In terms of coping, results from this study supported the findings from Kim et al. (2003). Increased use of problem-focused coping strategies was related to more emotional closeness felt by the mother and more reciprocated closeness. Interestingly, increased use of emotion-focused coping strategies was related to maternal emotional closeness but not to reciprocated closeness. An additional factor, the number of behavior problems manifested by the individual with the developmental disability, was strongly related to both measures of relationship closeness. Mothers felt less close to their children, and perceived that their children felt less close to them when those children had more behavior problems. These findings point to the importance of effective coping strategies in promoting positive relationship quality between mothers and their adolescent or adult children with developmental disabilities.

We know far less about the factors that predict relationship closeness among fathers and siblings of adults with MR/DD. As we noted earlier, one factor that seems to be important in the sibling relationship is gender (Orsmond & Seltzer, 2000). Nondisabled sisters reported higher levels of closeness to their siblings with MR/DD than did brothers. However, in terms of feelings about their involvement with their siblings and their worries about their siblings' futures, it appears that the genders of both the disabled and nondisabled siblings are important. Brothers who had sisters with MR/DD had fewer positive feelings and more negative feelings about their involvement with their siblings than did brothers who had brothers with MR/DD, but the gender of the siblings with MR/DD did not affect nondisabled sisters' feelings about involvement. These findings suggest different patterns of relationship closeness than are often observed among normative sibling pairs. Same-gender sibling relationships tend to be characterized by a more intense exchange of both positive and negative emotion than cross-gender dyads (Akiyama, Elliott, & Antonucci, 1996). When one member of the sibling dyad has MR/DD, our results indicate more intense exchange of positive emotion for same-sex brothers. Furthermore, the exchange of negative emotions was the opposite of what would be expected for brothers, with less negative emotion exchanged when a nondisabled male had a brother with MR/DD. Finally, the gender-pair composition did not seem to affect the exchange of emotion for nondisabled sisters.

Although caregiving activities and relationship closeness have important implications for the family system in their own right, their greatest impact may lie in their influence on mental health and psychological well-being.

Mental Health and Psychological Well-Being

Mental Health and Psychological Well-Being among Family Members

Mental health and psychological well-being have been measured a number of ways in our program of research, including indices of both psychopathology and positive mental health. Depressive symptoms were measured using the Center for Epidemiological Studies Depression Scale (Radloff, 1977). We have also examined subjective caregiving burden using the Burden Interview (Zarit, Reever, & Bach-Peterson, 1980), which represents the potential problems a caregiver may experience as a result of caring for the impaired person. Pessimism about the prospects of the adult with MR/DD achieving self-sufficiency was measured using the Pessimism subscale of the Questionnaire on Resources and Stress (Friedrich, Greenberg, & Crnic, 1983). Positive well-being was assessed using Ryff's (1989) Psychological Well-Being scales, which measure such domains as self-acceptance, personal growth, and purpose in life.

There are a number of reasons to suspect that mothers of adults with MR/DD would experience more psychological distress than fathers. Mothers tend to be the primary caregivers for their adult children with MR/DD, even after their husbands have retired from the workforce, which puts them at greater risk for distress and strain (Heller et al., 1997). Furthermore, in the general population, women are more at risk for depression and high caregiving burden than men (Miller & Cafasso, 1992; Nolen-Hoeksema, 1990). The only manifestation of distress that one might expect, from previous research, to affect a father more than a mother is pessimism about the future of their child with MR/DD (Brubaker, Engelhardt, Brubaker, & Lutzer, 1989). Fathers tend to have less familiarity with the formal service systems that provide long-term care and may hold themselves responsible for the financial requirements of long-term care, leading to more pessimism about the prospects of independence for their children with MR/DD.

Contrary to what would be suggested by previous research (e.g., Heller et al., 1997), we did not find differences in depressive symptoms or subjective burden between mothers and fathers of adults with MR/DD (Essex, Seltzer, & Krauss, 1999). The data suggest that the lack of differences was due to lower-than-average psychopathology in the mothers rather than to higher-than-average psychopathology among the fathers. By exploring the predictors of psychological well-being in the family system, we have uncovered some of the mechanisms that seem to be suppressing the emergence of psychopathology among mothers of adults with MR/DD in our sample. Specifically, we have examined the relationships between psychological well-being and (1) adaptive and maladaptive coping styles, (2) characteristics of the adult child with developmental disabilities, and (3) relationship closeness.

Predicting Well-Being from Coping Mechanisms

One reason for the lack of difference in psychopathology among mothers versus fathers of adults with MR/DD may be that mothers have become "expert copers." In our sample, mothers were more likely to use adaptive problem-focused coping strategies than fathers (Essex et al., 1999). Furthermore, these strategies were particularly important in relieving psychological distress when mothers were experiencing high caregiving demands. For example, problem-focused coping strategies alleviated maternal depressive symptoms most effectively when the adult children with MR/DD had a high number of functional limitations. Similarly, higher usage of problem-focused coping among mothers of adults with MR/DD was related to decreases in maternal pessimism when children had high levels of behavior problems, but not at lower levels of behavior problems. These findings suggest that mothers of adults with MR/DD, but not fathers, use problem-focused coping strategies to buffer the effects of stress on psychological well-being. It may be that mothers of adults with MR/DD, who have been the primary caregivers for their children for a number of decades, have become highly skilled in using coping techniques to alleviate the stress associated with caregiving. Fathers, who tend to have less experience with caregiving, have not developed these strategies as effectively. More effective usage of problem-focused coping among caregiving mothers may be responsible for the similar levels of psychological well-being between mothers and fathers, even though mothers have more caregiving responsibilities.

A related analysis from our study provides further evidence for mothers of adults with MR/DD becoming "expert copers." Mothers of adults with MR/DD were compared with similar-age women who were experiencing a different type of stressor, namely residential relocation (Kling et al., 1997). Although the relocation sample used higher levels of problem-focused coping than our caregiving sample did, the relationships between problem-focused coping and positive psychological well-being were much stronger for mothers of adults with MR/DD. Furthermore, an examination of the mean levels of psychological well-being revealed few differences between the relocation sample, which was experiencing a short-term stressor, and the caregiving sample, which was experiencing a long-term, chronic stressor. These findings suggest that although mothers of adults with MR/DD were using less problem-focused coping, they were using these coping mechanisms more efficiently and effectively, as evidenced by the stronger consequences of coping on psychological well being in the caregiving sample compared with the relocation sample.

Although mothers of adults with MR/DD may be more skilled at using problem-focused coping to buffer the impact of stress, it is important to note that coping also has a direct influence on psychological well-being for both mothers and fathers. For both mothers and fathers, refraining from the use of emotion-focused coping strategies was associated with less subjective burden (Essex et al., 1999; Kim et al., 2003). Furthermore, increased use of problem-focused coping strategies and decreased use of emotion-focused coping were related to fewer depressive symptoms among mothers of adults with MR/DD (Seltzer, Greenberg, & Krauss, 1995). In sum, our findings demonstrate the importance of using adaptive coping mechanisms to buffer the impact of parenting a child with MR/DD on psychological well-being and psychopathology.

Predicting Well-Being from Characteristics of the Adult Child

A number of characteristics of the adult child with MR/DD were examined in order to determine which characteristics were associated with psychological well-being of mothers, fathers, and siblings (Essex et al., 1999; Seltzer, Greenberg, Krauss, Gordon, & Judge, 1997). These characteristics included age and gender of the adult with MR/DD, whether he or she was living in the parental home, and the number of functional limitations and behavior problems he or she had. Different patterns emerged depending on the family member; for mothers of adults with MR/DD, higher depressive symptoms and more subjective burden were associated with a greater number of behavior problems manifested by the son or daughter. In fact, a more recent study by McIntyre, Blacher, and Baker (2002) found that even after controlling for other characteristics of the adult child with MR/DD, such as age, gender, and whether or not he or she was in school, the adult child's having more behavior problems was associated with higher maternal burden. Behavior problems did not, however, influence well-being for fathers and siblings. In fact, characteristics of the adult with MR/DD were unrelated to well-being for siblings. Fathers, however, experienced more depressive symptoms when their adult children were male and older. They also reported more subjective burden and pessimism when their adult children had more functional limitations.

The differential relations between children's characteristics and well-being for mothers and fathers are not surprising when considering the caregiving roles each parent is likely to take. Because mothers tend to be the primary caregivers, they are more involved than fathers in the day-to-day behavior management of their adult children. It follows, then, that more behavior problems exhibited by the son or daughter would take a particular toll on the mental health of mothers. Fathers may be more worried about providing financially for their adult children with MR/DD; therefore, when their children have severe functional limitations, fathers may foresee more long-term financial burden and subsequently may feel more pessimistic about the likelihood of their children being able to live independently.

A related study of mothers of adolescent children with autism, fragile X syndrome, and Down syndrome provides further evidence for the importance of children's behavior problems in predicting maternal well-being (Abbeduto et al., 2004). Children's behavior problems were a strong predictor of both maternal pessimism and depression for all three groups. In fact, differences between diagnostic groups in maternal pessimism and depression were accounted for by behavior problems.

These findings suggest that children's behavior problems may be the phenotypic aspect of these developmental disabilities that is most important in determining maternal distress. Studies from the child literature have come to a similar conclusion, finding that differences in parental functioning according to child diagnosis tend to be minimized when controlling for behavior problems and that behavior problems are a better predictor of parenting stress than is IQ (Cahill & Glidden, 1996; Hodapp, Dykens, & Masino, 1997).

When examining relationships from a family systems perspective, it is important to consider that effects can be bidirectional (Bronfenbrenner, 1989). Although studies have reported that elevated behavior problems among adults with MR/DD are associated with more maternal distress (Abbeduto et al., 2004; Essex et al., 1999; Heller et al., 1997), it is also plausible that higher levels of maternal distress could influence children's behavior problems. We explored this question longitudinally by examining the bidirectional relationships between well-being of mothers and their adult children's behavior problems (Orsmond, Seltzer, Krauss, & Hong, 2003). Results suggested that both directions of influence were important. That is, an increase in adult behavior problems over time was associated with more subjective burden and pessimism felt by mothers, and an increase in maternal pessimism and burden over time was associated with more behavior problems in the adult child with MR/DD. Although the influence of behavior problems on maternal well-being was not surprising, the reverse relationship demonstrates the sensitivity of the adult with MR/DD to the psychological state of the mother. It may be that mothers who are experiencing more depression and more burden are not interacting as effectively with their adult child with MR/DD, which may in turn lead to more behavior problems in the adult child (Orsmond et al., 2003).

Predicting Well-Being from Relationship Closeness

Although we have not yet examined the associations between relationship closeness and well-being for fathers of adults with MR/DD, we have explored these relationships for both mothers and siblings. In terms of maternal well-being, we examined the mediating role of dispositional optimism on depression and positive well-being among mothers of adults with autism and Down syndrome (Greenberg, Seltzer, Krauss, Chou, & Hong, 2004). Our results indicated that relationship closeness between the mother and the child with a developmental disability was especially important for mothers of adults with autism. Higher ratings of closeness were associated with more dispositional optimism, fewer depressive symptoms, and more positive psychological well-being. For these mothers, optimism seemed to be a mechanism through which relationship closeness affected well-being. That is, increased feelings of closeness to the child with autism led to mothers feeling more optimistic and subsequently reporting better psychological well-being and fewer depressive symptoms. Although research is often focused on the burden that adults with disabilities place on their families, this study suggests that a more positive relationship between the mother and her child with a developmental disability can serve as a protective mechanism against psychopathology and low levels of well-being.

Relationship closeness is also an important determinant of well-being for siblings of individuals with MR/DD. In fact, after controlling for a number of variables related to positive psychological well-being, such as income, gender, and marital status, siblings of adults with MR/DD showed higher levels of well-being when they reported more relationship closeness in the sibling pair (Seltzer, Greenberg, Krauss, Gordon, & Judge, 1997).

In sum, our research on factors that predict psychological well-being in families that have a member with MR/DD show some patterns of similarity among family members, as well as patterns of differences. The utilization of adaptive coping mechanisms was important for parents, although mothers tended to use problem-focused coping most effectively. Feeling close to the adult with MR/DD was related to better well-being for both mothers and siblings, and it is reasonable to assume that this would be the case for fathers as well. We observed different patterns, however, when examining the impact of characteristics of the adult with MR/DD on family members. These characteristics were unrelated to well-being for siblings of adults with MR/DD. The adult child's having fewer functional limitations was related to better well-being among fathers, likely reflecting fathers' perceptions of more intensive future care (and the financial burden associated with it) when functional limitations are high. The most consistent relationships between children's characteristics and well-being were observed for mothers. Fewer behavior problems evidenced by the adult with MR/DD were consistently associated with less maternal psychopathology and better positive well-being.

TRANSITIONS IN THE FAMILY LIFE COURSE

We now focus in on two specific events in the life course of families that have a member with MR/DD: the launching of the adult with MR/DD out of the family home and into alternate care settings and the transition to the next generation of caregivers. Although these may appear to be two separate times of transition among families, initiating the search for alternate care settings is often related to feelings of mortality and planning for the care of the adult with MR/DD when mothers are no longer able to provide care. Furthermore, these are transition points of particular salience to all members of the family system. That is, launching the adult child with MR/DD out of the family home often implies a reorganization of caregiving and family roles, and decisions about the next generation of caregivers often involve all family members.

One of the central tasks of families is the launching of children from the family home (Carter & McGoldrick, 1989). For most parents, this is an expected event that has positive implications, marking the adult child's successful negotiation of adult roles such as marriage and employment. This event can have different implications for parents of adults with MR/DD, however, signifying the relinquishing of their active caregiving role. The launching stage for these families is often one of the most stressful transitions, marked by turmoil and disequilibrium in the family (Seltzer, Krauss, Choi, & Hong, 1996).

In our longitudinal study, we have examined residential plans and preferences of mothers who have adult children with MR/DD coresiding with them (Freedman, Krauss, & Seltzer, 1997). Less than 50% of mothers had a specific plan for where their son or daughter would live in the future, defined as placing the adult with MR/DD on a waiting list for residential programs, planning for the adult siblings or other relatives to take the adult with MR/DD into their own homes, or planning for siblings or other relatives to move back into the family home to care for the adult with MR/DD. Over 90% of the mothers expected their adult children with MR/DD to still be living at home with them 2 years later. Aging mothers' reluctance to make concrete alternate residential plans is consistent with other studies (Heller & Factor, 1991; Kaufman, Adams, & Campbell, 1991; Pruchno & Patrick, 1999) and likely reflects anxiety about the future of their children with MR/DD, as well as their perception of few preferable options for a high quality of life away from the family home.

There are, however, a number of factors that predict mothers' decisions to put their adult children on a waiting list for residential placement. We found that mothers are more likely to place their adult children on waiting lists when those children have Down syndrome, when a larger number of the son's or daughter's service needs were unmet, when mothers had smaller social support networks, and when mothers were in better physical health (Essex, Seltzer, & Krauss, 1997). The findings relating to physical health may seem surprising, but in fact they could be representative of a more normative launching model. Mothers with better physical health may be more invested in finding alternate placements for their adult sons or daughters with MR/DD because their health allows them to pursue roles (such as worker) outside of the caregiving context. Alternatively, mothers in better health could be using waiting-list placement as a means of proactive planning for possible future declines in health (Essex et al., 1997).

Pruchno and Patrick (1999) further explored the issue of future planning by examining the factors that predicted whether mothers planned to eventually place their adult children with MR/DD into residence within the formal service system or with a family member. They found that when adult children with MR/DD had more behavior problems, mothers reported more caregiving burden and were subsequently more likely to plan for nonfamilial residential placement. Mothers who reported less burden, however, were more likely to report having a family member who would take primary responsibility for caregiving in the future.

Different patterns were observed when examining the factors that predicted actual placement in a nonfamily residential setting (Essex et al., 1997; Seltzer, Greenberg, Krauss, & Hong, 1997). The most salient predictor was whether the adult with MR/DD had been on a waiting list; in fact, in our study almost 60% of placed adults had previously been on a waiting list. Other factors associated with placement included poorer maternal health and older age of the son or daughter with MR/DD.

Our longitudinal research made it possible to study families before and after the transition out of the family home. Although this transition is often accompanied by stress and uncertainty for family members of adults with MR/DD, findings from our study suggest that the postplacement effects on family members are generally positive.

We have found that after adult children with MR/DD are relocated away from the parental home, mothers continued to keep in frequent contact (Seltzer, Krauss, Hong, & Orsmond, 2001). Approximately 9 months after relocation, over one-quarter of the mothers reported daily contact (either by telephone or in person) with their sons or daughters with MR/DD. Almost 36% reported between five and eight contacts a month, 21% reported weekly contact, and about 14% had less than weekly contact. The general patterns of frequent contact between mothers and relocated adults with MR/DD remained constant, even up to 4 years after placement, and have been confirmed by other studies (Blacher, Baker, & Feinfield, 1999). In addition, mothers reported increasing satisfaction with the amount of contact they had with their sons or daughters over the 4-year period following placement, as well as declining contact with staff members (Seltzer et al., 2001). These findings may reflect mothers' feelings of increasing comfort following the relocation of their sons or daughters, not only in terms of the residences in which their children were placed but also in terms of relinquishing the primary caregiving role. In fact, multiple research projects have found that mothers' feelings of caregiving burden and stress significantly declined in the years following their adult children's relocation into a residential setting (Baker & Blacher, 2002; Seltzer, Greenberg, Krauss, & Hong, 1997).

To separate out the effects of residential relocation of the adult with MR/DD from age-graded influences on family relationships and well-being of family members, we compared families who experienced a relocation with families in which the adults with MR/DD continued to reside in the family homes (Seltzer et al., 2001). At the assessment immediately prior to residential placement, mothers in the relocation group had higher pessimism scores than did mothers whose sons or daughters remained living at home over the study period. After placement, however, the pessimism scores of mothers in the relocation group declined, ultimately dropping below the scores of coresiding mothers.

A similar pattern was found for siblings. Initial sibling pessimism scores were similar when the adults with MR/DD had relocated or continued to coreside with their mothers; however, pessimism scores diminished significantly over time for the relocation sample. Although higher initial levels of pessimism among mothers in the relocation sample likely reflect stress and worry that often accompany the launching of adult children (Carter & McGoldrick, 1989), the decline in pessimism over time for both mothers and siblings may be indicative of relief resulting from the implementation of long-term plans for the care of their family members with MR/DD.

Although relocation affected mothers and siblings similarly in terms of pessimism, differential effects were observed for emotional involvement with the adult with MR/DD (Seltzer et al., 2001). For both mothers and siblings, emotional involvement increased over the study period, regardless of whether or not the adults with MR/DD moved out of the family homes. For siblings, however, mean levels of emotional involvement with their brothers or sisters were higher when the adults with MR/DD continued to coreside with the mothers than when the adults relocated. Although emotional involvement was lower for siblings in the relocation group, these siblings reported an increase in shared activities with their brothers or sisters with MR/DD after relocation. The number of shared activities between siblings did not change over time when the adults with MR/DD continued to coreside with the mothers (Seltzer et al., 2001).

Considering these findings from a family systems perspective, it is likely that the relationships between mothers and their adult children with MR/DD, as well as how these relationships are affected by relocation, are influenced by the sibling relationships. It may be that maternal caregiving burden and pessimism about the future of the adult with MR/DD declines after relocation at least partly because the nondisabled sibling becomes more involved in the life of his or her brother or sister (as measured by more shared activities). Furthermore, sibling closeness may not increase substantially for the relocation group because mothers are continuing to be intricately involved in the lives of the adults with MR/DD. Because siblings were not expected to assume more of the caregiving role after relocation, and because they were not living in the family home during the relocation process, it is not surprising that their affective relationships with their brothers or sisters with MR/DD would not be significantly altered, especially while the mothers are alive.

TRANSITIONING TO THE NEXT GENERATION OF CAREGIVERS

Guided by the lifespan perspective, we end this chapter with a discussion of the issues surrounding the generational transition of caregiving for the adult with MR/DD. This is a transition that occurs at the end of the family life cycle, as it tends to be precipitated by the death or incapacitation of the primary caregiver, the mother. There are often a number of people who could assume the caregiving role, including fathers, nondisabled siblings, or the formal service sector. However, in our study, we found that in all cases in which the adult with MR/DD coresided with both parents prior to the mother's death or incapacitation, the father assumed primary caregiving responsibilities (Gordon, Seltzer, & Krauss, 1997).

Fathers' assumption of the primary caregiving role for adults with MR/DD is often a short-term transition, because aging fathers are likely nearing the end of the lifespan themselves. The next logical choice, within the hierarchy of caregiving, is often the sibling (Dwyer & Coward, 1992). To this end, we have studied the expectations of siblings of adults with MR/DD about assuming future caregiving once the primary caregiver is no longer able to do so. We found that two factors influence nondisabled siblings' likelihood of expecting to take over future caregiving responsibilities: gender and closeness. Sisters who reported feeling closer to the individual with MR/DD were more likely to expect to assume future caregiving roles than brothers or than siblings who felt more distant (Greenberg et al., 1999).

Assuming the primary caregiving role, however, does not always imply a plan to bring the brother or sister with MR/DD to live in the sibling's home. In a study by Griffiths and Unger (1994), parents and siblings were asked whether they expected the adults with MR/DD to coreside with those siblings when parents were no longer able to provide care. Although the majority of family members (49% of parents and 56% of siblings) felt strongly that families should be responsible for their members with MR/DD on a long-term basis, only 22% of parents expected the adults with MR/DD to coreside with siblings.

In fact, different processes seemed to be at work when examining whether siblings of adults with MR/DD expected to coreside with their brothers or sisters when parents were no longer able to provide primary care (Krauss, Seltzer, Gordon, & Friedman, 1996). To examine this question, we divided siblings into two groups: those who expected to coreside and felt that this was the best arrangement and those who expected that their brothers or sisters would live in out-of-home settings or with other relatives and felt that that was the best arrangement. Future plans to coreside were dependent on characteristics of the mothers, the adults with MR/DD, and the family relationship. Specifically, siblings were more likely to expect to coreside with the adults with MR/DD when their mothers were in worse health, when the disabled siblings were sisters who had less severe MR/DD, and when there was a greater number of shared activities between the sibling pair. Interestingly, characteristics of the nondisabled siblings predicted whether they expected to take over future caregiving responsibilities but did not predict whether they expected to coreside with the adults with MR/DD. Alternatively, characteristics of the mothers and the adults with MR/DD did not predict whether siblings were more likely to take over future care but did influence whether they expected to coreside with their disabled siblings after parents were no longer able to provide care.

SUMMARY

Not surprisingly, the impact of having an adult child with a developmental disability seems to be greatest for mothers. This is almost certainly because mothers tend to be the primary caregivers, which profoundly affects the life choices that they make. When considering mothers at a later point in the life course—specifically when their children reach adulthood and the mothers have been providing care for many decades—it seems that the day-to-day behavior management issues take the greatest toll on the mother–child relationship and maternal well-being. The stress of caring for a child with MR/DD over the life course is abated, at least somewhat, by maternal use of effective coping mechanisms. Those mothers who experienced the least negative impacts of caregiving are those who were most effective at using active, problem-focused coping techniques, especially in the face of intensive caregiving stresses.

It is also not surprising that the mother is the family member most affected by transitions in the life of her child with MR/DD, in particular the adult child's transition out of the parental home. Although this transition may be initially met with anxiety and pessimism about the future independence of the adult with MR/DD, mothers ultimately respond favorably to relocation of their adult children. They remain affectively close and involved in the lives of their children, and are more hopeful about their futures.

The impact of having a child with a developmental disability seems to be somewhat more limited for fathers. This is probably due, at least in part, to the greater number of roles held by fathers than by mothers of adults with MR/DD, primarily a greater involvement in the workplace. Our research has shown that mothers tend to have better psychological well-being when they occupy multiple roles, such as parent and worker (Hong & Seltzer, 1995). It might be that because fathers tend to occupy more roles than mothers, they may have more ways than mothers to measure their life success, which may lessen the intensity of the impact of parenting a child with MR/DD.

Even after adult siblings of individuals with MR/DD have families of their own, having a disabled sibling continues to have a significant impact. Nondisabled siblings seem to have the best outcomes, particularly in terms of psychological well-being, when they have close ties with their families of origin and particularly with their siblings with MR/DD. There were also strong patterns of gender differences in the sibling relationship. Nondisabled sisters participated more in caregiving, reported feeling closer to their siblings with MR/DD, and were more likely to plan to assume primary caregiving than were brothers.

FUTURE RESEARCH DIRECTIONS

As stated earlier, most of the extant research on the family impact of having an adult child with MR/DD is focused on maternal development and well-being. Although more recent studies have begun to examine the impact on other members of the family system, there is still much to learn. Although we know that a close relationship with the adult with MR/DD is associated with better psychological well-being for mothers and siblings, we have yet to uncover whether there is a relationship between closeness and well-being for fathers. Having a positive and affectively close relationship with their children with MR/DD may play a less important part in paternal well-being if fathers identify primarily with the family breadwinner role instead of the family caregiver role. On the other hand, a close relationship may be adaptive for all family members, regardless of their roles in the family system. We are also missing the fathers' voices concerning residential placement of their children with MR/DD and plans for future caregiving, although they are likely intricately involved in this process.

Future research should continue to examine the factors that influence well-being among siblings, with a particular focus on coping. Our findings suggest that adaptive coping plays significant role in maternal psychological well-being; it would be interesting to explore whether the positive effects of coping are also present for siblings. The protective role that adaptive coping plays in the amelioration of stresses associated with caregiving may be particularly salient for mothers, because they tend to deal with the day-to-day provision of care to their adult children with MR/DD. On the other hand, adaptive coping may have a more general function, promoting positive well-being among all family members regardless of the amount of caregiving they currently provide.

A related research question that has yet to be explored is the impact of assuming caregiving responsibilities for a sibling with MR/DD. Although we are accruing a significant knowledge base about factors that are associated with the assumption of caregiving, we know little about the impact of primary caregiving on siblings. By examining individual well-being, coping, and family patterns before and after this transition, we can begin to determine the impact of sibling caregiving on the life course.

Our findings demonstrate the interdependence of family members across the life course. The impact of having a child with MR/DD on the family and the subsequent impact on maternal well-being are dependent on the relationships of other family members to the adult with MR/DD. Mothers have better well-being and are less negatively affected by parenting an adult with MR/DD when fathers and siblings are more involved in caregiving activities. More research on the interdependence of family members is needed to better delineate how these processes work, as well as what types of interdependence are adaptive or maladaptive when a family member has MR/DD.

Last, a critical voice that is missing in the corpus of research on the family impact of having a member with MR/DD is that of the members with the disability themselves. Future research should explore their roles in the transitions out of the parental home and to the next generation of caregivers, as well as developing ways to collect self-reports of relationship quality and psychological well-being from the adults with MR/DD. It is likely that the subjective experiences of the adults with MR/DD have a substantial effect on the family impact of caring for them.

ACKNOWLEDGMENTS

This chapter was prepared with support from the National Institute on Aging (Grant No. R01 AG08768) and the National Institute of Child Health and Human Development (Grant Nos. P30 HD03352 and T32 HD07489).

REFERENCES

Abbeduto, L., Seltzer, M. M., Shattuck, P., Krauss, M. W., Orsmond, G., & Murphy, M. M. (2004). Psychological well-being and coping in mothers of youths with autism, Down syndrome, or fragile X syndrome. *American Journal on Mental Retardation, 109*, 237–254.

Akiyama, H., Elliott, K., & Antonucci, T. C. (1996). Same-sex and cross-sex relationships. *Journal of Gerontology: Psychological Sciences, 51B*, 374–382.

Baker, B. L., & Blacher, J. (2002). For better or worse?: Impact of residential placement on families. *Mental Retardation, 40*, 1–13.

Baltes, P. B. (1987). Theoretical propositions of life-span developmental psychology: On the dynamics between growth and decline. *Developmental Psychology, 23*, 611–626.

Baltes, P. B., Lindenberger, U., & Straudinger, U. M. (1998). Lifespan theory in developmental psychology. In R. M. Lerner (Ed.), *Handbook of child psychology: Vol. 1. Theoretical models of human development* (5th ed., pp. 1029–1143). New York: Wiley.

Barnett, W. S., & Boyce, G. C. (1995). Effects of children with Down syndrome on parents' activities. *American Journal on Mental Retardation, 100*, 115–127.

Bengtson, V. L., & Schrader, S. S. (1982). Parent–child relations. In D. J. Mangen & W. A. Peterson (Eds.), *Research instruments in social gerontology: Vol. 2. Social roles and social participation* (pp. 115–155). Minneapolis: University of Minnesota Press.

Blacher, J., Baker, B. L., & Feinfield, K. A. (1999). Leaving or launching?: Continuing family involvement with children and adolescents in placement. *American Journal on Mental Retardation, 104*, 452–465.

Bristol, M. M., Gallagher, J. J., & Schopler, E. (1988). Mothers and fathers of young developmentally disabled and nondisabled boys: Adaptation and spousal support. *Developmental Psychology, 24*, 441–451.

Bronfenbenner, U. (1989). Ecological systems theory. In R. Vasta (Ed.), *Annals of child development* (Vol. 6, pp. 187–251). Greenwich, CT: JAI Press.

Brubaker, T. H., Engelhardt, J. L., Brubaker, E., & Lutzer, V. D. (1989). Gender differences of older caregivers of adults with mental retardation. *Journal of Applied Gerontology, 8*, 183–191.

Cahill, B. M., & Glidden, L. M. (1996). Influence of child diagnosis on family and parental functioning: Down syndrome versus other disabilities. *American Journal on Mental Retardation, 101*, 149–160.

Carter, E. A., & McGoldrick, M. (Eds.). (1989). *The family life cycle: A framework for family therapy*. New York: Gardner Press.

Chodorow, N. (1978). *The reproduction of mothering: Psychoanalysis and the sociology of gender*. Berkeley: University of California Press.

Dwyer, J. W., & Coward, R. T. (1992). Gender, family, and long-term care of the elderly. In J. W. Dwyer & R. T. Coward (Eds.), *Gender, families, and elder care* (pp. 1–17). Newbury Park, CA: Sage.

Erickson, M., & Upshur, C. C. (1989). Caretaking burden and social support: Comparison of mothers of infants with and without disabilities. *American Journal on Mental Retardation, 94*, 250–258.

Essex, E. L., Seltzer, M. M., & Krauss, M. W. (1997). Residential transitions of adults with mental retardation: Predictors of waiting list use and placement. *American Journal on Mental Retardation, 101*, 613–629.

Essex, E. L., Seltzer, M. M., & Krauss, M. W. (1999). Differences in coping effectiveness and well-being among aging mothers and fathers of adults with mental retardation. *American Journal on Mental Retardation, 104*, 545–563.

Essex, E. L., Seltzer, M. M., & Krauss, M. W. (2002). Fathers as caregivers for adult children with mental retardation. In B. J. Kramer & E. Thompson (Eds.), *Men as caregivers: Theory, research and service implications* (pp. 250–268). New York: Springer.

Freedman, R. I., Krauss, M. W., & Seltzer, M. M. (1997). Aging parents' residential plans for adult children with mental retardation. *Mental Retardation, 35*, 114–123.

Friedrich, W. N., Greenberg, M. T., & Crnic, K. (1983). A short form of the Questionnaire on Resources and Stress. *American Journal of Mental Deficiency, 88*, 41–48.

Gordon, R. M., Seltzer, M. M., & Krauss, M. W. (1997). The aftermath of parental death: Changes in the context and quality of life. In R. L. Schalock (Ed.), *Quality of life: Vol 2. Application to persons with disabilities* (pp. 25–42). Washington, DC: American Association on Mental Retardation.

Greenberg, J. S., Seltzer, M. M., Krauss, M. W., Chou, R. J., & Hong, J. (2004). The effect of quality of the relationship between mothers and adult children with schizophrenia, autism, or Down syndrome on maternal well-being: The mediating role of optimism. *American Journal of Orthopsychiatry, 74*, 14–25.

Greenberg, J. S., Seltzer, M. M., Orsmond, G. I., & Krauss, M. W. (1999). Siblings of adults with mental illness or mental retardation: Current involvement and expectation for future caregiving. *Psychiatric Services, 50*, 1214–1219.

Griffiths, D. L., & Unger, D. G. (1994). Views about planning for the future among parents and siblings of adults with mental retardation. *Family Relations, 43*, 221–227.

Heller, T., & Factor, A. (1991). Permanency planning for adults with mental retardation living with family caregivers. *American Journal on Mental Retardation, 96*, 163–176.

Heller, T., Hsieh, K., & Rowitz, L. (1997). Maternal and paternal caregiving of persons with mental retardation across the lifespan. *Family Relations, 46*, 407–415.

Hodapp, R. M., Dykens, E. M., & Masino, L. (1997). Families of children with Prader–Willi syndrome: Stress-support and relations to child characteristics. *Journal of Autism and Developmental Disorders, 27*, 11–24.

Hong, J., & Seltzer, M. M. (1995). The psychological consequence of multiple roles: The nonnormative case. *Journal of Health and Social Behavior, 36*, 386–398.

Kaufman, A. V., Adams, J. P., & Campbell, V. A. (1991). Permanency planning by older parents who care for adult children with mental retardation. *Mental Retardation, 29*, 293–300.

Kim, H. W., Greenberg, J. S., Seltzer, M. M., & Krauss, M. W. (2003). The role of coping in maintaining the psychological well-being of mothers of adults with intellectual disability and mental illness. *Journal of Intellectual Disability Research, 47*, 313–327.

Kling, K. C., Seltzer, M. M., & Ryff, C. D. (1997). Distinctive late-life challenges: Implications for coping and well-being. *Psychology and Aging, 12*, 288–295.

Krauss, M. W., & Seltzer, M. M. (1993). Current well-being and future plans of older caregiving mothers. *Irish Journal of Psychology, 14*, 47–64.

Krauss, M. W., Seltzer, M. M., Gordon, R., & Friedman, D. H. (1996). Binding ties: The role of adult siblings of persons with mental retardation. *Mental Retardation, 34*, 83–93.

Lazarus, R. S., & Folkman, S. (1984). *Stress, appraisal, and coping.* New York: Springer.

Levy-Shiff, R. (1986). Mother–father–child interactions in families with a mentally retarded young child. *American Journal of Mental Deficiency, 91*, 141–149.

McIntyre, L. L., Blacher, J., & Baker, B. L. (2002). Behavior/mental health problems in young adults with intellectual disability: The impact on families. *Journal of Intellectual Disability Research, 46*, 239–249.

Milgram, N. A., & Atzil, M. (1988). Parenting stress in raising autistic children. *Journal of Autism and Developmental Disorders, 18*, 415–424.

Miller, B., & Cafasso, L. (1992). Gender differences in caregiving: Fact or artifact? *Gerontologist, 32*, 498–507.

Nolen-Hoeksema, S. (1990). *Sex differences in depression.* Stanford, CA: Stanford University Press.

Orsmond, G. I., & Seltzer, M. M. (2000). Brothers and sisters of adults with mental retardation: Gendered nature of the sibling relationship. *American Journal on Mental Retardation, 105*, 486–508.

Orsmond, G. I., Seltzer, M. M., Krauss, M. W., & Hong, J. (2003). Behavior problems in adults with mental retardation and maternal well-being: Examination of the direction of effects. *American Journal on Mental Retardation, 108*, 257–271.

Pruchno, R. A., & Patrick, J. H. (1999). Effects of formal and familial residential plans for adults with mental retardation on the aging mothers. *American Journal on Mental Retardation, 104*, 38–52.

Pruchno, R. A., Patrick, J. H., & Burant, C. J. (1996). Aging women and their children with chronic disabilities. *Family Relations, 45*, 318–326.

Radloff, L. (1977). The CES-D Scale: A self-report depression scale for research in the general population. *Applied Psychological Measurement, 1*, 385–401.

Ryff, C. D. (1989). Happiness is everything, or is it? Explorations on the meaning of psychological well-being. *Journal of Personality and Social Psychology, 57*, 1069–1081.

Seltzer, G. B., Begun, A., Seltzer, M. M., & Krauss, M. W. (1991). Adults with mental retardation and their aging mothers: Impacts of siblings. *Family Relations, 40*, 310–317.

Seltzer, M. M., Greenberg, J. S., & Krauss, M. W. (1995). A comparison of coping strategies of aging mothers of adults with mental illness or mental retardation. *Psychology and Aging, 10*, 64–75.

Seltzer, M. M., Greenberg, J. S., Krauss, M. W., Gordon, R. M., & Judge, K. (1997). Siblings of adults with mental retardation or mental illness: Effects on lifestyle and psychological well-being. *Family Relations, 46*, 395–405.

Seltzer, M. M., Greenberg, J. S., Krauss, M. W., & Hong, J. (1997). Predictors of outcomes of the end of co-resident caregiving in aging families of adults with mental retardation or mental illness. *Family Relations: Interdisciplinary Journal of Applied Family Studies, 46*, 13–22.

Seltzer, M. M., & Krauss, M. W. (1989). Aging parents with mentally retarded children: Family risk factors and sources of support. *American Journal on Mental Retardation, 94*, 303–312.

Seltzer, M. M., Krauss, M. W., Choi, S. C., & Hong, J. (1996). Midlife and later-life parenting of adult children with mental retardation. In C. D. Ryff & M. M. Seltzer (Eds.), *The parental experience in midlife* (pp. 459–489). Chicago: University of Chicago Press.

Seltzer, M. M., Krauss, M. W., Hong, J., & Orsmond, G. I. (2001). Continuity or discontinuity of family involvement following residential transitions of adults who have mental retardation. *Mental Retardation, 39*, 181–194.

Smith, J., & Baltes, P. B. (1999). Life-span perspectives on development. In M. H. Bornstein & M. E. Lamb (Eds.), *Developmental psychology: An advanced textbook* (4th ed., pp. 275–311). Mahwah, NJ: Erlbaum.

Zarit, S., Reever, K., & Bach-Peterson, J. (1980). Relatives of the impaired elderly: Correlates of feelings of burden. *Gerontologist, 20*, 649–655.

Families as Partners in Educational Decision Making

Current Implementation and Future Directions

Ann P. Turnbull
Nina Zuna
H. Rutherford Turnbull, III
Denise Poston
Jean Ann Summers

This chapter describes the current implementation of family–professional partnerships in education and discusses some future directions. It contextualizes this discussion within the six principles for educating students with disabilities as set forth in the Individuals with Disabilities Education Act (IDEA; Turnbull, Huerta, & Stowe, 2006):

- Zero reject
- Nondiscriminatory evaluation
- Appropriate education
- Least restrictive environment
- Due process
- Parent participation

Despite its many reauthorizations, these six principles remain intact (Turnbull, Huerta, & Stowe, 2006). This chapter emphasizes the roles that families assume with respect to each principle, discusses the evidence about how families and educators have carried out those roles, and describes how research can strengthen family–professional partnerships.

ZERO REJECT
Definition, Background, and Family Implications

The zero-reject principle requires state and local educational agencies to educate all students ages 3–21 who have disabilities. It implements the 14th Amendment's equal protection guarantee and was the foundation of the early right-to-education advocacy.

In 1975, when Congress enacted the law that gave students with disabilities the right to attend school, 1 million children and youth with disabilities were being excluded from public education, particularly those with significant disabilities that required extensive and pervasive medical and behavioral supports. Families were often required to create programs for their children or to find services outside of the public school system at their own expense.

The zero-reject principle has meant, and continues to mean, that families are guaranteed that their children will be enrolled in school and that, with their enrollment, the parents and their children's educators can focus their efforts on achieving student outcomes. It is no longer a matter of access but rather of the outcomes achieved from having had access.

Implementation Issues: Review of Research and Future Directions

A contemporary issue related to the implementation of the zero-reject principle is low graduation rates and high suspension and expulsion rates for students with developmental disabilities (DD).

Graduation and Dropout Rates

The most current data compare graduation rates and dropout rates for students age 14 and older for the 1993–1994 school year and the 2000–2001 school year. Students with mental retardation have the lowest graduation rate, at 35%, and students with orthopedic impairments have the highest rate, with slightly over half of these students graduating (57.4%). Practically no progress in increasing the graduation rate and decreasing the dropout rate for students with mental retardation, multiple disabilities, and orthopedic impairments occurred across the 7 years of data collection starting in 1993–1994. However, there was slight improvement in rates for students with autism and deaf–blindness. Clearly a gap exists between the reality and parental expectations; a national survey of parents of students with disabilities reported that 82% of parents of children with disabilities in high school anticipate that their children will receive standard diplomas (Johnson & Duffett, 2002).

When graduation and dropout rates are compared for students from different racial/ethnic groups, students who are Asian/Pacific Islander are most likely to graduate with standard diplomas and least likely to drop out of school (U.S. Department of Education, 2005a). Their rates are slightly better than the rates for white students. In comparing white and black students, 57% of white students graduate with standard diplomas, compared with 37% of black students. Alternatively, almost slightly less than half of black students drop out compared with approximately one-third of white students. The highest dropout rate is for American Indian/Alaskan Native students, at 52%.

In reviewing the literature, we were unable to locate model programs that have increased the likelihood that students with DD will graduate with a standard diploma. Developing such model programs is an important area for future research, especially given the extent to which the standards-based reform of No Child Left Behind Act of 2001 (NCLB; Public Law 107-110) emphasizes students' success on standardized examinations in order to receive a standard diploma.

Suspension and Expulsion

The zero-reject principle assures no cessation of a student's education if the student's behavior (for which he or she is sanctioned) is a manifestation of a disability and sets out procedures and standards for disciplinary action and manifestation determinations (Turnbull, Huerta, & Stowe, 2006).

The U.S. General Accounting Office (GAO; 2003) investigated how schools were implementing IDEA's disciplinary provisions. It reported that 91,000 special education students (1.4% of all special education students) were disciplined by being removed from their educational setting. The two most frequent disciplinary actions for students were placement in in-school suspension rooms or out-of-school suspensions at home. When students were removed from their educational settings for more than 10 days, they were usually placed in an alternative school or given homebound placement.

The report identifies factors used when making decisions about suspensions, including the total number of days a student was removed from his or her educational setting, the type of discipline problem, and the cost and availability of placement options. Not unexpectedly, the GAO report made no mention of the impact of the in-home or other disciplinary action on the students' families, particularly whether parents or other family members were available to supervise the student at home, whether they were able to take time off work, or whether they experienced any other consequences as a result of the schools' actions.

Qualitative research with parents of children and youth with disabilities has revealed that parents are frustrated that educators are not well prepared to deal with their children's problem behaviors at school and that educators apply discipline in inappropriate ways (Poston, 2002; Turnbull & Ruef, 1997; Wang, Mannan, Poston, Turnbull, & Summers, 2004). No data are available regarding reduced or lost employment time for families when their children are suspended or expelled (R. Horner, personal communication, October 24, 2005). Clearly, a major issue for families is their availability to supervise their children with disabilities when they are called to pick them up from school or when they have out-of-school suspensions and expulsions.

Research documents the efficacy of schoolwide positive behavior support (PBS) through universal, group, and individual support components (Scott & Barrett, 2004; Sugai et al., 2000; Turnbull et al., 2002). As models continue to evolve, future research should include a strong family component associated with each of the other three components. Collecting data on both the impact of suspensions and expulsions on family functioning and the fidelity with which individual PBS is carried out across school *and* home settings would be helpful, as would understanding the key community settings in which the student participates.

NONDISCRIMINATORY EVALUATION

Definition, Background, and Family Implications

The nondiscriminatory evaluation principle mandates that each student receive a fair and culturally and linguistically unbiased evaluation to determine whether the student has a disability and, if so, the nature and extent of special education and related services that the student needs (Turnbull & Turnbull, 2000). Accordingly, IDEA specifies procedural safeguards related to evaluation and its breadth, procedures, timing, and team membership and to the interpretation of evaluation data.

The evaluation is the basis for the student's claim to an appropriate education. If evaluations are biased, if decisions based on them are indefensible, or both, then there is a likely domino effect: Present erroneous decisions will produce future erroneous decisions (Fiedler, 2000). Thus families have a major stake in ensuring that the evaluation process is unbiased, thorough, and beneficial in increasing the likelihood that a student is provided an appropriate education.

The reevaluation procedure, which occurs every 3 years and is used to determine continued eligibility for special education services, was changed in the IDEA Amendments of 1997 (Public Law 105-17) to allow the use of existing evaluation data to complete this process. This change remains in effect in IDEA (2004). If the team decides that no additional data are needed (i.e., uses existing data) to determine continued eligibility for special education services, the local educational agency (LEA) is required to notify the parents of this decision, of the agencies' right not to conduct an assessment, and of their right to request an assessment if desired (IDEA, 2004). This change benefits both parents and students. Parents, especially those who have children with more significant disabilities, are relieved of increased paperwork, time commitments, and extensive communication with professionals. These parents are well aware that their children have lifelong disabilities and will continue to require special education services throughout their K–12 educations; the reduced federal paperwork honors this knowledge. Students benefit by remaining in the classroom for instruction rather than being removed for extensive testing procedures to determine continued eligibility for special education services.

Implementation Issues: Review of Research and Future Directions

Two areas of research on increasing the likelihood of a fair and meaningful evaluation include interventions related to prereferral and response to intervention.

Prereferral Intervention

From the mid-1980s through the end of the 1990s, one of the major strategies for ensuring that special education evaluations did not erroneously or disproportionately identify students as having disabilities was to prevent the evaluation process, if possible, through prereferral intervention. Prereferral intervention occurs *before* a formal referral for evaluation. Its primary purpose is to analyze the student's strengths and needs and then provide additional individualized assistance without providing special education (Bahr, Fuchs, & Fuchs, 1999; Safran & Safran, 1996).

The frequency of prereferral intervention increased dramatically in the mid-1980s. By the close of that decade, state educational agencies were typically recommending or requiring some type of prereferral intervention with students (Carter & Sugai, 1989). It was anticipated that referral rates for formal evaluation would drop when general and special education teachers collaborated in modifying instruction according to individualized student needs (Fuchs, Fuchs, Bahr, & Stecker, 1990; Graden, Casey, & Bonstrom, 1985). Some research, however, has indicated no significant decrease in referrals to special education when prereferral intervention is used (Short & Talley, 1996); other studies reported an increase in referral accuracy (Bahr et al., 1999; Yocum & Staebler, 1996).

The literature on prereferral interventions consistently describes them as largely professionally directed. The standard procedures have involved collaboration among general and special educators and typically have not included active parent (or student) participation in problem solving (Sindelar, Griffin, Smith, & Watanabe, 1992).

Responsiveness to Intervention

Currently, research and innovation related to nondiscriminatory evaluation is occurring within the field of learning disabilities rather than developmental disabilities. Over the past several years, increasing criticism has focused on the standard approach of identifying students with a learning disability through an IQ–achievement discrepancy (Francis et al., 2005; Fuchs, Mock, Morgan, & Young, 2003). These researchers began exploring a response-to-intervention model of evaluation, and research leaders within the field of learning disabilities followed suit (Bradley, Danielson, & Hallahan, 2002). Although there is variation in models being investigated, the general approach is to provide students with instruction, to monitor their progress, to provide more intensive instruction for students who are not making sufficient progress, to monitor the progress again, and then to explore the provision of a special education evaluation for students who still do not respond to more intensive instruction (Fuchs et al., 2003, p. 159).

The essence of the response-to-intervention model is individually gauging the explicitness, intensity, and supportiveness of instruction for each student (Torgesen, 2002). Response to intervention replaces the administration of formal tests (e.g., IQ and achievement tests) with the administration of multiple tiers of increasingly specialized instruction. The response-to-intervention model has the potential of not only redefining learning disabilities but also leading to a noncategorical approach to special education service delivery (including for students with developmental disabilities; Francis, et al., 2005).

A current debate within the learning disability field is the extent to which response to intervention has adequate scientific validation (Fuchs et al., 2003; Naglieri & Crockett, 2005). The outcome of this debate will likely have major implications for the identification and evaluation of students with developmental disabilities. To explore the efficacy of response-to-intervention research for a wider range of students, partnerships between DD researchers and researchers in learning disabilities would be beneficial. Furthermore, future research is vitally needed to develop models that involve partnerships with families. The role of families in response to intervention has been minimal.

As the field continues to expand on strategies and practices within special education, careful attention must be directed to newly developed practices, such as response to intervention, to avoid their narrower application within the disability field to only students with milder disabilities. Including all students in the development and design of promising practices embraces the notion of universal design and, in this case, extends it to the practice of assessment to better understand how all students respond to instruction.

APPROPRIATE EDUCATION

Definition, Background, and Family Implications

The principle of appropriate education requires an individualized education to respond to the student's specific needs, to build on the student's strengths, and to ensure that the student has an opportunity to benefit from his or her education. Generally speaking, until IDEA was reauthorized in 1997, educators focused primarily on the *processes* of delivering special education, conducting a nondiscriminatory evaluation, creating an individualized education program (IEP; IFSP for infants and toddlers), and identifying the least restrictive placement for the student. With the reauthorization of IDEA in 1997, the enactment of the NCLB Act in 2001, and the most recent reauthorization of IDEA in 2004, the process approach has begun to yield to an *outcome-oriented* approach (Turnbull, Turnbull, Stowe, & Wilcox, 2000; Turnbull, Huerta, & Stowe, 2006) .

Both NCLB and IDEA 2004 redefine "appropriate education" in two basic ways. The first redefinition emphasizes accountability for results. The two statutes operationalize this definition for the administration of standards-based assessment and their requirements for highly qualified educators. In addition, NCLB operationalizes the new definition by providing for rewards and sanctions for LEAs and by grounding those rewards and sanctions in students' performance on state and local educational agency assessments.

The second definition emphasizes the use of scientifically based methods of teaching. Indeed, the phrase "scientifically based methods" (or a derivative phrase) appears in NCLB 110 times (D. Deshler, personal communication, October 27, 2005). NCLB defines scientifically based research as "research that applies rigorous, systematic, and objective procedures to obtain relevant knowledge" (2001, Title I, Sec. 1208 [6]). IDEA additionally incorporates a similar approach (Turnbull, Huerta, & Stowe, 2006).

Implementation Issues: Review of Research and Future Directions

Before we address current family-related issues associated with accountability for results and scientifically based methods, it is worthwhile to consider research findings about parent satisfaction with special education services. These findings provide insight into parents' perspectives on the extent to which special education programs are appropriate.

Parent Satisfaction with Special Education Services

Descriptive data are available about parents' perspectives on the quality of special education services. Based on a national survey of randomly selected families of students in special education from K–12, approximately 70–80% of parents of students in special education reported that teachers were caring and knew a lot about how to teach their children and that they, as parents, were treated as members of the special education team (Johnson & Duffett, 2002).

In spite of this overall favorable view among parents, a subgroup of parents in the national sample was highly dissatisfied with special education services. (Parental dissatisfaction is discussed later in the chapter, related to the principle of due process.) One of the highest levels of dissatisfaction is parents' perceptions that their children are not being prepared for life after high school. Almost one-half of parents in the national survey indicated that this was an area of special education in need of improvement.

Increasing Academic Achievement

Students with mental retardation tend to be approximately 3 years behind grade level in math and reading, whereas students with autism tend to be about 1–1½ years behind in both subjects (Blackorby et al., 2005). In reading, 11% of fourth graders with disabilities and 6% of eighth graders with disabilities scored at or above proficiency level (National Assessment of Educational Progress [NAEP], 2005). In math, 16% of fourth graders and 7% of eighth graders scored at or above proficiency level (NAEP, 2005). Clearly a current priority is to increase the academic achievement of students with DD to ensure that these students pass standards-based assessments.

Many students with DD will be exempted from taking the standards-based assessments through NCLB requirements. In fact, NCLB now grants to states the flexibility to develop modified achievement standards for those students who qualify, and they may include up to 2% of the proficient scores from these assessments when reporting adequate yearly progress (AYP). Additionally, states may include the proficient scores in AYP progress for students with the most significant disabilities as long as these students do not exceed 1% of the total tested population (U.S. Department of Education, 2005b). Given the emphasis on standards-based reform, equitable assessment for students with DD should be a major research priority for the future.

Interestingly, the whole emphasis on *process* in the first 25 years of implementing IDEA is possibly one of the reasons for the scarcity of research on how families can partner with educators in increasing the academic achievement of students with disabilities. Much more research is needed on how family–professional partnerships can be implemented to most effectively contribute to increased academic achievement.

Access to Scientifically Based Methods

Parents who have children with significant disabilities, particularly those with complex health care needs, have lamented the lack of evidence-based information and resources to support their child's medical and educational needs (Edmond & Eaton, 2004; Kirk & Glendinning, 2004). Clearly more research is needed to ensure not only that relevant, timely, and evidence-based information is provided to families across the severity spectrum of developmental disabilities but also that this information contributes to the achievement of positive child and family outcomes.

In a qualitative study, Ruef and Turnbull (2001) explored the types of formats parents would most prefer when receiving research-based information. The family members indicated that they would most like to receive information from other families who have had similar experiences. In particular, they stressed a person-to-person approach in disseminating information. Families wanted written information to be brief, readable, and in layperson's language. They indicated that it would be helpful to have hands-on assistance in implementing the ideas from research and that multimedia formats would also be attractive options. A key theme was a preference for receiving information from someone they trust.

Future research should investigate ways to ensure that parents have full access to scientifically based information. Given the strong emphasis on this requirement in both NCLB and IDEA, the research community must ensure that "parents do not get left behind" by not having access to the very information that will enable them to form equal partnerships.

LEAST RESTRICTIVE ENVIRONMENT
Definitions, Background, and Family Implications

IDEA's principle of least restrictive environment (LRE) states that children and youth with disabilities have a right to be educated in a regular education classroom with their peers without disabilities "to the maximum extent appropriate" (2004, §1412[a][5][A]). Although IDEA favors educating students with disabilities with their peers, it extends a measure of flexibility by providing "to the maximum extent appropriate." Additionally, the LRE principle states that a student's removal from a general education setting should occur only when "the nature or severity of the disability of a child is such that education in regular education classes with the use of supplementary aids and services can not be achieved satisfactorily" (2004, §1412[a][5][A]). Therefore, an IEP team's appropriate selection and use of supplementary aids and services is crucial to ensuring that students are successful in inclusive settings. This is especially important when including a student with problem behavior in general education settings (Etscheidt & Bartlett, 1999). Further, Congress reports that the education of children with disabilities can be made more effective when students are expected to achieve, when their access to the general education curriculum is ensured to the maximum extent appropriate, and when the roles of parents are strengthened (IDEA, 2004).

Funded by the U.S. Department of Education, parent training and information centers (PTIs) have been instrumental in helping families meet high expectations for their children by providing information and support on important educational topics, such as determining appropriate placements and developing positive relationships with school personnel (Turnbull, Turnbull, Erwin, & Soodak, 2006). However, many parents still report difficulties in partnering with schools (Erwin & Soodak, 1995). These difficulties may be attributed to conflicting viewpoints that professionals and families have about LRE, as Erwin, Soodak, Winton, and Turnbull (2001) found. In their comprehensive literature review of early childhood inclusion, they reported that parents, especially those who have children with moderate to severe developmental disabilities, advocate more strongly for inclusive settings than do school personnel.

Not only do parents and educators express conflicting opinions about LRE, but there also exists a struggle over where the special education field should go next (Kavale & Forness, 2000). Both future practice directions and policy perspectives on these next steps will have great implications for students and their families.

In determining the future direction of LRE, it is not prudent to narrowly posit LRE as a decision about placement alone. Rueda, Gallego, and Moll (2000) suggest that LRE is more than a place; it is an interplay between individuals and their environment—a sociocultural context that either facilitates or restricts progress. Turnbull, Ellis, Boggs, Brooks, and Biklen (1981) more generally conceptualize it as "freedom" or "liberty"

(p. 10). To expand on this notion, the authors suggest that LRE should be contextualized as an ever-changing pursuit of freedom in which the individuals involved should have choices—choices about how they wish to pursue their lives and the choice of determining with whom, how, and to what extent they participate in specific environments. Teaching youth about their freedom of choice will no doubt have the greatest impact on their enjoying what our forefathers envisioned, a least restrictive environment in all aspects of life. More research must be directed to understanding student preferences when making placement decisions. As one teacher stated, "The IEP is a useless document unless the student buys it" (Turnbull, Turnbull, et al., 2006, p. 121).

Further, the right to choose is fundamental. It belongs to all people, including those with disabilities. The severity of a disability should not limit that right; that much is clear under IDEA and the Americans with Disabilities Act (ADA; 1990). But how the right is exercised is different for different people. Some have such an amount of cognitive and communicative ability that their choices are easily manifested. Others, however, may have so much cognitive and communicative limitation that they cannot "say" what they want. Instead, they demonstrate it by their behavior. Action is a form of communication. The "reasonable accommodation" that they are entitled to have is for others to respond to their behavior and their own idiosyncratic expression of choice. For those who have been permanently unable to act in such a way as to manifest their choices, the theory of empathetic reciprocity, or the "shoes" test, prevails (Turnbull & Turnbull, 2001). Choices on their behalf can be made only by striving in a genuine way to walk in their shoes—to experience life through their perspectives, preferences, fears, and needs. To fail to acknowledge that they, too, can partially participate in the choice process is to diminish their rights, and that is violative of our nation's policy.

Implementation Issues: Review of the Research and Future Directions

Because IDEA is relatively silent on how to implement LRE, determination of and implementation issues for LRE have been addressed by the courts (*Daniel R. R. v. State Board of Education*, 1989; *DOE v. Arlington County*, 1999; *Roncker v. Walter*, 1983; *Sacramento School District v. Rachel H.*, 1994). As an example, in *DOE v. Arlington*, the courts favored the school district's position for a more restrictive placement for a student with significant cognitive impairment and distractibility because it offered greater educational benefit than an integrated setting. Although court cases are useful in clarifying ambiguous portions of the law, the interpretation and application of legal outcomes for LRE provide only a provincial understanding of the LRE principle. Handwerk (2002) suggests that the proper implementation of the LRE principle requires a more thorough examination of the characteristics and effectiveness of various programmatic settings and a keener understanding of the attitudes of parents, children, youth, and educators. A review of research on parent perceptions of LRE and descriptive placement data follows.

Parents' Perceptions of LRE

Research on family perspectives on LRE is becoming more prevalent. Table 28.1 presents these findings. To summarize, most parents, regardless of their children's disability levels, cited academic and social outcomes, along with opportunities for their children to develop friendships and prepare for the "real world," as benefits of inclusion.

TABLE 28.1. Parent Perspectives on Inclusive Settings

Authors (date)	Method/sample	Findings
Frederickson, Dunsmuir, Lang, & Monsen (2004)	• Focus groups and telephone interviews • 107 pupils, parents, and staff (33 parents)	• Positives: Better postschool outcomes, social and behavioral role models, friendships, belonging, esteem • Concerns: Academic workload, social acceptance, organization (child and staff), home/school communication
Leyser & Kirk (2004)	• Survey • 400 families	• Positives: Prepare child for real world, more varied activities, increased self-esteem • Concerns: Less assistance, fewer services, inability of staff to adapt programs and integrate • Other: 40% of parents more satisfied with child's progress in special than general education; 30% were undecided on this issue; academic skill development higher in special classrooms
Palmer, Fuller, Arora, & Nelson (2001)	• Summary of written comments • 140 parents	• Positives: Improved academic or functional skills; additional stimulation; sensitivity to diversity for peers • Concerns: Medical/adaptive/language needs too great; overburdened general education teacher; distractions
Duhaney & Salend (2000)	• Review of literature	• Positives: Enhanced social, and behavioral development; diversity; increased role models and friendships; enhanced self-esteem; real-world experiences • Concerns: Lack of qualified personnel, fewer services for child, isolation of child; frustration in requesting inclusion; inexperienced administrators/teachers
Gallagher et al. (2000)	• Semistructured interviews • 21 families	• Inclusion initiation: Most often by parents, not schools • Why requested: Role models, social and academic benefits, real-world experiences; independence • Location: Some accepted inclusion only in elective courses; 50% felt full inclusion was the only option • Concerns: Lack of teacher training; need for energy to pursue; scheduling; long bus rides for child

In all studies, parents—particularly parents of children with severe disabilities—mentioned either inadequate staff training or school organization as barriers to inclusion. Finally, some parents expressed concern about a possible reduction in services or supports for their children when included in general education settings.

Descriptive Placement Data

Despite ideological and philosophical differences (Howard, 2004; Kavale & Forness, 2000) and numerous legal decisions (*Daniel R. R. v. State Board of Education*, 1989; *Roncker v. Walter*, 1983; *Sacramento v. Rachel H.*, 1994), determining where and how a student should be educated remains a contentious issue. Even though the courts have come out in favor of both restrictive and more inclusive environments, students with disabilities are spending more time being educated with their peers without disabilities. In fact, the percentage of students with disabilities participating in general education settings for more than 80% of their time has increased from 32% in 1989 to 50% in 2003 (Office of Special Education Programs [OSEP], 2004). For students with mental retardation, this percentage has increased from 7% in 1989 to 12% in 2003, and for students with multiple disabilities, the growth rate increased from 6% in 1989 to 12% in 2003 (OSEP, 2004).

Overall, these data are encouraging and suggest a continued positive trend toward greater participation in general education settings for individuals with disabilities. However, further research is needed in the areas of mental retardation and multiple disabilities to explain why the growth trend for inclusion is substantially lower for these two groups than it is for all other disabilities. During the same time period, only a 5–6% increase occurred for these students who spend 80% of their time in the general education settings compared with an 18% growth rate for all students with disabilities. Why does such a substantial difference in placement exist for these students? It is unknown whether differential placement decisions among these groups of students truly represents parental and student choice or whether the availability and location of district resources explain these discrepancies. This question warrants further investigation. Additionally, more research is needed to guide placement decisions for students with developmental disabilities, with a particular focus on their accessing the general curriculum within inclusive settings to achieve academic outcomes. Inclusion of students with developmental disabilities in general education settings has for the most part focused on their achieving social outcomes (Browder et al., 2004).

PROCEDURAL DUE PROCESS
Definitions, Background, and Family Implications

Procedural due process is subsumed under the due-process clause in the 5th and 14th Amendments of the U.S. Constitution, which "prohibits the government from unfairly or arbitrarily depriving a person of life, liberty, or property" (Garner, 2004, p. 539). Generally, it confers the right to a notice of charges and the right to a hearing; more specifically, with respect to the education of students with disabilities, it enforces the first four principles of IDEA as outlined in this chapter. Procedurally, parents must receive prior written notice whenever the school "proposes to initiate or change or refuses to initiate or change the identification, evaluation, or educational placement of the child" (2004, §1415 b [3] [A] [B]). If either the parents or the school district cannot reach agreement regarding the education of the student with a disability, either party may request an impartial due-process hearing to resolve the matter (2004). Further, if either party is dissatisfied with the results of the due-process hearing, the aggrieved party has a variety of appeals options, including state or district courts, U.S. Court of Appeals, and finally the U.S. Supreme Court.

In past IDEA court cases, which party (i.e., parents or school district) bears the burden of proof when parents pursue litigation against a school district has not always been clear. In the *Schaffer v. Weast* (2005) hearing, this issue was put to rest. The Supreme Court ruled that parents who pursue due-process hearings against a school district bear the burden of proof in demonstrating why their child's education is not appropriate. This ruling, as delivered by Justice O'Connor, claims that "the burden lies, as it typically does, on the party seeking relief" (*Schaffer v. Weast*, 2005, p. 3). This decision has great implications for families, especially those families who have different cultural and linguistic backgrounds and are of low socioeconomic status, as Justice Ginsburg in her dissenting opinion rightly recognized. She stated that "the vast majority of parents whose children require the benefits and protections provided in the IDEA" lack "knowledg[e] about the educational resources available to their [child]" and the "sophisticat[ion]" to mount an effective case against a district-proposed IEP" (p. 20).

Families, students, and educators are all affected by due-process hearings. In a parent focus group, Johnson and Duffett (2002) found, in general, that parents spend countless hours learning about their child's disability, commit time and expense to getting additional evaluations, relocate to other school districts, or quit their jobs. Getty and Summy (2004) report that, in addition to the emotional stress of hearings, parents may harbor anger or distrust toward educators, which may negatively influence educators' perceptions of students. Finally, special educators who would normally provide support to the student (and other students as well) may be called away from their duties to prepare and serve as witnesses, thus requiring substitutes to perform their duties (Lanigan, Audette, Dreier, & Kobersy, 2001). Collectively, all of these factors result in a reduced amount of time for families to "be families" and for educators to do their jobs. To improve the education of students with disabilities, a balance must be achieved between the competing interests of schools and parents without enduring such a high emotional cost for both parties.

Implementation Issues: Review of the Research and Future Directions

The President's Commission on Excellence in Special Education made four recommendations concerning the prevention and improvement of dispute resolution (President's Commission on Excellence in Special Education, 2002). Most of these recommendations were incorporated into IDEA 2004 to some extent; however, it must be noted that the statute language does not always include the word "required," as the Commission recommended. Following are the Commission's recommendations, and these recommendations are followed by citation to the IDEA (2004) statute that most closely relates to it (2002, p. 35).

- IDEA should empower parents as key players and decision makers in their children's education.
- IDEA should require states to develop processes that avoid conflict and promote individualized education program agreements, such as IEP facilitators (§ 1400[c][8]).

- IDEA should require states to make mediation available anytime it is requested and not only when a request for hearing has been made (§1415[e] [1]).
- IDEA should permit parents and schools to enter binding arbitration and ensure that mediators, arbitrators, and hearing officers are trained in conflict resolution and negotiation (§1415[e][F] and §1415[e][2][iii]).

The only recommendation by the Commission not specifically incorporated within IDEA was use of the phrase, "empower parents." Instead, in order for parents to be active participants and decision makers in their children's educations, IDEA ensures that parents "have training and information," that their "role and responsibility is strengthened," that their "rights are protected," that they "have the tools to improve educational results," and that they are "afforded procedural safeguards" (2004, §1400 *et. seq.*). Although providing information and legal protections are important, qualitatively distinct differences exist between empowering parents and extending resources and ensuring due-process rights. Further research is needed to explore the impact of empowerment within parent–school relationships and its effect on family quality of life and student outcomes.

One of the Commission's recommendations that appears to be gaining in popularity is the use of skilled facilitators at IEP meetings. Although IEP facilitators are not specifically mentioned in IDEA 2004, the amended law now states that parents and schools should be provided with more opportunities to resolve disagreements. The Technical Assistance Alliance for Parent Centers (2004), in cooperation with the Consortium for Appropriate Dispute Resolution in Special Education, created a guide for facilitated IEP meetings. The main purpose of this approach is to keep the IEP team focused on program development while skillfully handling any disagreements that may arise. Although some states (e.g., Minnesota and California) offer the option of facilitated IEP meetings (Markowitz, Ahearn, & Schrag, 2003), currently no research is available that documents their effectiveness in reducing the number of due-process hearings.

Procedural Due-Process Data

Fifty billion dollars was spent on special education for the 1999–2000 school year; of that amount, $146.5 million was spent on mediation, due process, and litigation cases (Chambers, Harr, & Dhanani, 2003). The most recent data reported by the National Association of State Directors of Special Education indicate that about a 10.4% average increase in due-process hearings occurred from 1996 to 2000, with 7,532 requests in 1996 and 11,068 in 2000 (Ahearn, 2002). However, a somewhat opposite trend has occurred for the number of due-process hearings actually held. Beginning in 1996, a 4% average *decrease* occurred each year from 1996 to 2000, with 3,555 hearings held in 1996 and 3,020 held in 2000 (Ahearn, 2002). These trends suggest that every year an increasing number of parents are dissatisfied with the education of their children; yet somehow these difficulties are resolved by mediation or some other alternative dispute resolution. What is significant, though, are not the discrepancies in these figures but rather the steady increase in parental dissatisfaction. Clearly, further research is necessary to investigate the continued increase in parental dissatisfactions and the underlying systemic issues related to these parental concerns.

Data from a national random sample telephone survey conducted by Public Agenda, a nonprofit, bipartisan research organization, provide a greater understanding of families' perspectives regarding special education issues. With respect to due-process issues, the authors of this study reported that 43% of the families felt that they needed to "stay on top of the school and fight for services for their child" (Johnson & Duffett, 2002, p. 23). Additionally, the study indicated that families who have children with severe disabilities considered suing more often (31%) than families who have children with mild disabilities (13%). This figure is not surprising, given that autism, one of the fastest growing developmental disabilities (Autism Society of America, 2005), also ranks as the disability with the highest growth rate in due-process claims (Etscheidt, 2003).

So what propels parents, the party most often initiating due-process complaints (Getty & Summy, 2004), to pursue legal recourse? A GAO report (2003) provided three of the most common reasons why parents and school districts reach an impasse: identification of the need for special education, placement decisions, and development and implementation of IEPs. The next section provides a brief analysis of parental perspectives regarding mediation and due-process hearings.

Parent Perspectives on Mediation and Due-Process Hearings

Throughout this entire section on procedural due process, the data clearly suggest that more research is needed on parental perspectives regarding educational issues, particularly with respect to parent–school conflict. This particular section highlights the work of Welsh (2004) and Lake and Billingsley (2000), who offer some insights on why parents decide to pursue mediation and their hopes and concerns about the results of the process.

Welsh (2004) reported that families want to have an opportunity to thoroughly express their concerns and to be treated with dignity and respect. Lake and Billingsley (2000) reported eight factors that parents described as either escalating or deescalating conflict. A few of these eight factors include families' and educators' lack of knowledge about special education and problem-solving skills; schools' lack of personnel, resources, and time; and schools' failure to plan for service delivery. Of the eight factors reported by Lake and Billingsley (2000) that were related to conflict, trust or lack of trust was most related to conflicts between parents and school personnel.

Although many suggestions were provided about the next line of research that might propel the special education field forward with respect to resolving due-process conflicts, no amount of research can instill within individuals trust, kindness, and respect; these are qualities that educators and parents must continually strive to display, especially when faced with challenges. The data indicate that establishing partnerships characterized by trust, respect, and equality truly represents the best direction the field must pursue to reduce parent–school conflict—a recommendation beneficial for all parties involved (Turnbull, Turnbull, et al., 2006).

PARENT PARTICIPATION
Definitions, Background, and Family Implications

Although inconsistencies exist in the education literature on how to define parent participation (Turnbull, Turnbull, et al., 2006), IDEA unequivocally delineates how and to what extent parents may be involved in the education of their child. The regulations implementing IDEA state that parents are expected to be equal participants with school personnel in developing, reviewing, and revising the IEP. Simply put, parents have the right to make informed decisions about their child's education. Numerous procedural safeguards, among other provisions within IDEA, confer these rights. In short, parents have the right to examine all educational records, receive notification of any changes to their child's education, and request due-process hearings or pursue legal recourse through the court system (IDEA, 2004).

Statutes (e.g., NCLB, IDEA, Head Start) and case law (*Amanda J. v. Clark County School District*, 2001; *W.G. v. Bd. of Trustees of Target Range School District*, 1992) have both had strong implications for interpreting the appropriate nature of parent participation. Laws have historically included a component involving strong parent participation in their child's education, rightly recognizing that families play a critical and central role in the lives of children and naturally have the children's best interest at stake. Case law, too, has consistently favored families' participation in their children's education, often rectifying by court order an educational agency's failure to adequately include parents, or to include them at all, in educational decision making. Clearly, Congress intended for parents to take an active participatory role in their children's education, and case law has upheld these challenges.

However, this increased participatory role, as many families have discovered, does not come without great effort, and some families feel alienated from school officials despite their attempts to participate (Rueda, Monzo, Shapiro, Gomez, & Blacher, 2005; Shapiro, Monzo, Rueda, Gomez, & Blacher, 2004). In fact, the implications of parental participation are twofold. In one respect, families and their children have greatly benefited from the increased role afforded them through federal policy; they have a greater voice in determining supports and services to accurately meet their children's needs. On the other hand, parents are now thrust into the roles of researchers (i.e., needing to understand research regarding their child's disability and programs), lawyers (i.e., synthesizing what the law means for their child's education), and diplomats (i.e., cordially interacting with an interdisciplinary team). These multiple family roles equally affect how educational services are implemented.

Implementation Issues: Review of the Research and Future Directions

Parent Partnership Models

Epstein (1995) delineated six types of parent involvement: parenting, communicating, volunteering, learning, decision making, and collaborating. Although this framework is frequently referenced in the general education literature, some researchers have been critical of Epstein's components, claiming they are too "school-centered" (Boethel, 2003, p. 19). Also, although numerous frameworks define and provide descriptive accounts of parental involvement (Parette & Brotherson, 2004; Symon, 2005; Wang et al., 2004), there is no consensus in the field concerning the conceptual components of parental participation. Further, only a modicum of studies have documented rigorous methodology in their analyses (Baker & Sodden, 1997).

Barton and colleagues (Barton, Drake, Perez, St. Louis, & George, 2004) propose a different model unlike the traditional models of parent participation, which define parental involvement as parent engagement in various activities at school (e.g., chaperoning on field trips), home (e.g., assisting with homework), or community (e.g., participating in fund-raising efforts). In their ecological model (Barton et al., 2004), they advocate moving away from what parents do toward an understanding of how parents' actions affect parent–school relationships, using a mediated process involving capital (e.g., social, material, human), space (school, home, community), and expression. Their model illustrates how "parent engagement . . . is more than an outcome" (p. 6) (e.g., participation in parent conferences) but is instead "a set of relationships and actions that cut across individuals, circumstances, and events" (p. 6) in which "parents activate nontraditional resources and leverage relationships with teachers, other parents, and community members in order to author a place of their own in the schools" (p. 11).

Blue-Banning, Summers, Frankland, Nelson, and Beegle (2004) also conceptually posit parents and other family members as actors on the educational scene. They demonstrate how parental engagement is more than a discrete end result but is rather an ongoing partnership represented by commitment, equality, respect, professional competence, communication, and trust (Blue-Banning et al., 2004). In this collaborative process, parents do not have to "go it alone." Together parents and educators can explore research, different programs, and the laws to ensure that meaningful results are achieved for students and their families.

Parent Participation Data

National data provide a general overview of IDEA implementation and assist in policy decisions. The data reported next are from the second wave of the National Longitudinal Transition Study (NLTS-2; 2003) in the topical area of parent involvement. For those children with disabilities in secondary settings, a greater percentage of parents whose household income was above $50,000 attended IEP meetings (94%) than of parents whose household income was below $25,000 (82%; NLTS-2, 2003). Additionally, greater percentages of parents of children who were white attended IEP meetings (92%) than parents whose children were black (82%) or Hispanic (79%). When parents were asked about their feelings about their involvement in IEP decisions, only 27% of families who were white wanted to be more involved, whereas 51% of black and 43% of Hispanic families wanted to be more involved in the decision making. Not all families are afforded the same opportunities to participate. Gorman (2001) reports that schools listen to vociferous parents but that those parents who rarely speak up, perhaps due to work schedules or language barriers, lose out. Given that parent involvement is strongly related to student outcomes (NLTS, 2003), it is imperative to ensure equal participation for all families.

Differences were also noted for families who had children with mental retardation. Forty percent of families who had children with mental retardation desired higher levels of participation in IEP decision making compared with only 24–35% of families who had a child with any other type of disability. More specifically, nearly 53% of families who had a child with mental retardation and 46% of families who had a child with autism reported that the school mostly developed the IEP goals for their child. Surprisingly, this trend was noted across all disability levels. Clearly, at the secondary level, regardless of IDEA's intent of increased parent participation in their child's education, this goal is not being realized with respect to development of IEPs. Further research is warranted to uncover the reasons behind these data.

Outcomes of Partnerships

Many benefits accrue from positive parent–educator partnerships. In a replication of a national study examining occupational therapists' relationships with parents of preschool children with cerebral palsy, Hinojosa, Sproat, and Anderson (2002) found that parental partnerships with therapists had the greatest impact on children's progress over and above any other intervention. In another study, Brookman-Frazee (2004) reported that parent confidence increased, parent stress decreased, and child affect and engagement increased when parents worked collaboratively with providers to provide treatment for their children with autism compared with providers providing treatment alone. Clearly, these studies demonstrate that parent involvement in children's education produces beneficial child and family outcomes. Further research is needed to discover the types of parental involvement that are linked to positive academic outcomes for youth in secondary settings.

A next step could be to refine such models to more explicitly address the needs of families who have children with disabilities. For the past two decades, research on inclusion of children with disabilities has been available, yet little is known about the inclusion of their families in school-related activities. A large portion of the research on parent involvement in the education of children with disabilities has focused on parent participation in IEP-related activities. Further research is needed to gain a better understanding of these families' involvement in school-related activities and the extent to which these families feel welcomed in schools and wish to participate in such activities.

CONCLUSION

IDEA's six principles provide a framework for research related to family–professional partnerships in educational decision making. Clearly, there has been tremendous progress in the 30 years since IDEA's initial implementation in 1978, and that is a fact that warrants celebration. Notwithstanding that progress, current challenges remain that warrant scientifically based approaches in seeking successful resolution. A theme throughout the discussion of each of the six principles is that families from culturally and linguistically diverse backgrounds are at particular risk for having greater barriers and fewer facilitators related to partnerships with educators. Thus we conclude with a clarion call for greater partnerships in educational decision making for all families—especially families characterized by diversity. Even greater strides can be made through research on strengthening family–professional partnerships. All too often, families of privilege and prestige, partly due to their articulate and persuasive language, secure better quality services than do underprivileged families (Gorman, 2001; Shapiro et al., 2004). Research must additionally focus on families with culturally and linguistically diverse backgrounds to ensure their equal access as well.

REFERENCES

Ahearn, E. M. (2002). *Due process hearings: 2001 update*. Alexandria, VA: National Association of State Directors of Special Education.

Alliance for Parent Centers. (2004). Facilitated IEP meetings: An emerging process. Retrieved November 4, 2005, from *www.taalliance.org/publications/index.htm*.

Amanda J. v. Clark County School District and Nevada State Department of Education (NE) (9th Cir. 2001).

Americans with Disabilities Act (ADA) of 1990, Pub. L. 101–336, 42 U.S.A. §12101 *et seq.* (2000).

Autism Society of America. (2005). Facts and statistics. Retrieved November 10, 2005, from *www.autism-society.org/site/PageServer?pagename=FactsStats*.

Bahr, M. W., Fuchs, D., & Fuchs, L. S. (1999). Mainstream assistance teams: A consultation-based approach to prereferral intervention. In S. Graham & K. Harris (Eds.), *Teachers working together: Enhancing the performance of students with special needs* (pp. 87–116). Cambridge, MA: Brookline Books.

Baker, A. J. L., & Sodden, L. M. (1997, March). *Parent involvement in children's education: A critical assessment of the knowledge base.* Paper presented at the annual meeting of the American Education Research Association, Chicago, IL.

Barton, A. C., Drake, C., Perez, J. G., St. Louis, K., & George, M. (2004). Ecologies of parent engagement in urban settings. *Educational Researcher, 33*(4), 3–12.

Blackorby, J., Wagner, M., Cameto, R., Davies, E., Levine, P., Newman, L., et al. (2005). *Engagement, academics, social adjustment, and independence: The achievements of elementary and middle school students with disabilities.* Washington, DC: U.S. Department of Education, Office of Special Education Programs.

Blue-Banning, M., Summers, J. A., Frankland, H. C., Nelson, L. L., & Beegle, G. (2004). Dimensions of family and professional partnerships: Constructive guidelines for collaboration. *Exceptional Children, 70*(2), 167–184.

Boethel, M. (2003). *Diversity: School, family, and community connections.* Austin, TX: Southwest Educational Development Laboratory.

Bradley, R., Danielson, L., & Hallahan, D. P. (2002). *Identification of learning disabilities.* Mahwah, NJ: Erlbaum.

Brookman-Frazee, L. (2004). Using parent–clinician partnerships in parent education programs for children with autism. *Journal of Positive Behavior Interventions, 6*(4), 195–213.

Browder, D., Flowers, C., Ahlgrim–Delzell, L., Karovonen, M., Spooner, F., & Algozinne, R. (2004). The alignment of alternate assessment content with academic and functional curricula. *Journal of Special Education, 37,* 211–223.

Carter, J., & Sugai, G. (1989). Survey on prereferral practices: Responses from state departments of education. *Exceptional Children, 55*(5), 298–302.

Chambers, J. G., Harr, J. J., & Dhanani, A. (2003). *What are we spending on procedural safeguards in special education, 1999–2000?* Retrieved November 4, 2005, from *www.csef-air.org/pub_seep_national.php.*

Daniel R.R. v. State Board of Education, 874 F.2d 1036 (5th Cir. 1989).

Doe v. Arlington County, 41 F. Supp. 599 (E.D. VA. 1999).

Duhaney, L. M. G., & Salend, S. J. (2000). Parental perceptions of inclusive educational placements. *Remedial and Special Education, 21*(2), 121–128.

Emond, A., & Eaton, N. (2004). Supporting children with complex health care needs and their families: An overview of the research agenda. *Child: Care, Health and Development, 30*(3), 195–199.

Epstein, J. (1995). School/family/community partnerships: Caring for the children we share. *Phi Delta Kappan, 76,* 701–712.

Erwin, E., & Soodak, L. C. (1995). I never knew I could stand up to the system: Families' perspectives on pursuing inclusive education. *Journal of the Association for Persons with Severe Handicaps, 20*(2), 136–146.

Erwin, E., Soodak, L., Winton, P., & Turnbull, A. (2001). I wish it wouldn't all depend upon me: Research on families and early childhood inclusion. In M. J. Guralnick (Ed.), *Early childhood inclusion: Focus on change* (pp. 127–158). Baltimore: Brookes.

Etscheidt, S. (2003). An analysis of legal hearings and cases related to individual education programs for children with autism. *Research and Practice for Persons with Severe Disabilities, 28*(2), 51–69.

Etscheidt, S., & Bartlett, L. (1999). The IDEA amendments: A four-step approach for determining supplementary aids and services. *Exceptional Children, 65,* 163–174.

Fiedler, C. R. (2000). *Making a difference: Advocacy competencies for special education professionals.* Boston: Allyn & Bacon.

Francis, D. J., Fletcher, J. M., Stuebing, K. K., Lyon, G. R., Shaywitz, B. A., & Shaywitz, S. E. (2005). Psychometric approaches to the identification of LD: IQ and achievement scores are not sufficient. *Journal of Learning Disabilities, 38*(2), 98–108.

Frederickson, N., Dunsmuir, S., Lang, J., & Monsen, J. J. (2004). Mainstream–special school inclusion partnerships: Pupil, parent, and teacher perspectives. *International Journal of Inclusive Education, 8,* 37–57.

Fuchs, D., Fuchs, L. S., Bahr, M. W., & Stecker, P. M. (1990). Prereferral intervention: A prescriptive approach. *Exceptional Children, 56,* 493–513.

Fuchs, D., Mock, D., Morgan, P. L., & Young, C. L. (2003). Responsiveness-to-intervention: Definitions, evidence, and implications for the learning disabilities construct. *Learning Disabilities: Resource and Practice, 18*(3), 157–171.

Gallagher, P. A., Floyd, J. H., Stafford, A. M., Taber, T. A., Brozovic, S. A., & Alberto P. A. (2000). Inclusion of students with moderate or severe disabilities in educational and community settings: Perspectives from parents and siblings. *Education and Training in Mental Retardation and Developmental Disabilities, 35,* 135–147.

Garner, B. A. (Ed.). (2004). *Black's law dictionary* (8th ed.) St. Paul, MN: West.

General Accounting Office. (2003). *Special education: Clearer guidance would enhance implementation of federal disciplinary provisions* (Report No. GAO-03-550). Washington, DC: Author.

Getty, L. A., & Summy, S. E. (2004). The course of due process. *Teaching Exceptional Children, 36,* 40–43.

Gorman, S. (2001). Navigating the special education maze: Experiences of four families. In C. E. Finn, A. J. Rotherham, & C. R. Hokanson, Jr. (Eds.), *Rethinking special education for a new century* (pp. 233–258). Washington, DC: Thomas B. Fordham Foundation and the Progressive Policy Institute.

Graden, J. E., Casey, A., & Bonstrom, O. (1985). Implementing a prereferral intervention system: II. The data. *Exceptional Children, 51,* 487–496.

Handwerk, M. L. (2002). Least restrictive alternative: Challenging assumptions and further implications. *Children's Services: Social Policy, Research, and Practice, 5*(2), 99–103.

Hinojosa, J., Sproat, C. T., & Anderson, J. (2002). Shifts in parent–therapist partnerships: Twelve years of change. *American Journal of Occupational Therapy, 56*(5), 556–563.

Howard, P. (2004). The least restrictive environment: How to tell? *Journal of Law and Education, 33*(2), 167–180.

Individuals with Disabilities Education Act Amendments of 2004, 20 U.S.C. §1400 *et seq.*

Johnson, J., & Duffett, A. (2002). *When it's your own child: A report on special education from the families who use it.* New York: Public Agenda.

Kavale, K. A., & Forness, S. R. (2000). History, rhetoric, and reality: Analysis of the inclusion debate. *Remedial and Special Education, 21,* 279–296.

Kirk, S., & Glendinning, C. (2004). Developing services to support parents caring for a technology-dependent child at home. *Child: Care, Health and Development, 30*(3), 209–218.

Lake, J. F., & Billingsley, B. S. (2000). An analysis of factors that contribute to parent–school conflict in special education. *Remedial and Special Education, 21,* 240–251.

Lanigan, K. L., Audette, R. L., Dreier, A. E., & Kobersy, M. R. (2001). Nasty, brutish . . . and often not very short: The attorney perspective on due process. In C. E. Finn, A. J. Rotherham, & C. R. Hokanson, Jr. (Eds.), *Rethinking special education for a new century* (pp. 213–231). Washington, DC: Thomas B. Fordham Foundation and the Progressive Policy Institute.

Leyser, Y., & Kirk, R. (2004). Evaluating inclusion: An examination of parent views and factors influencing their perspectives. *International Journal of Disability, Development and Education, 51*(3), 271–285.

Markowitz, J., Ahearn, E., & Schrag, J. (2003). *Dispute resolution: A review of systems in selected states.* Alexandria, VA: National Association of State Directors of Special Education, Project Forum.

Naglieri, J. A., & Crockett, D. P. (2005). Response to intervention (RTI): Is it a scientifically proven method? *MASP Communiqué, 34*(2), pp. 38–42.

National Assessment of Educational Progress. (2005). *Average scale scores and achievement-level results in reading for students with disabilities.* Retrieved October 10, 2005, from *nces.ed.gov/nationsreportcard/.*

National Longitudinal Transition Study-2. (2003). *NLTS-2 data tables.* Retrieved November 1, 2005, from *www.NLTS2.org.*

Office of Special Education Programs. (2004). *Part B trend data.* Retrieved October 18, 2005, from *www.ideadata.org/PartBTrendDataFiles.asp.*

Palmer, D. S., Fuller, K., Arora, T., & Nelson, M. (2001). Taking sides: Parent views on inclusion for their children with severe disabilities. *Exceptional Children, 67,* 467–484.

Parette, H. P., & Brotherson, M. J. (2004). Family-centered and culturally responsive assistive technology decision making. *Infants and Young Children, 17*(4), 355–367.

Poston, D. J. (2002). *A qualitative analysis of the conceptualization and domains of family quality of life for families of children with disabilities,* Unpublished doctoral dissertation, University of Kansas, Lawrence.

President's Commission on Excellence in Special Education. (2002). *A new era: Revitalizing special education for children and their families.* Retrieved July 16, 2002, from *www.ed.gov/inits/commissionsboards/whspecialeducation/.*

Roncker v. Walter, 700 F.2d 1058 (6th Cir. 1983).

Rueda, R., Gallego, M. A., & Moll, L. C. (2000). The least restrictive environment: A place or a context? *Remedial and Special Education, 21,* 70–78.

Rueda, R., Monzo, L., Shapiro, J., Gomez, J., & Blacher, J. (2005). Cultural models of transition: A view from Latina mothers of young adults with developmental disabilities. *Exceptional Children, 71,* 401–414.

Ruef, M. B., & Turnbull, A. P. (2001). Stakeholder opinions on accessible informational products helpful in building positive, practical solutions to behavioral challenges of individuals with mental retardation and/or autism. *Education and Training in Mental Retardation and Developmental Disabilities, 36*(4), 441–456.

Sacramento City School District v. Rachel H., 14 F.3d 1398 (9th Cir. 1994), *cert. denied sub nom., Sacramento City Unified School Dist. v. Holland,* 114 S. Ct. 2679 (1994).

Safran, S. P., & Safran, J. S. (1996). Intervention assistance programs and prereferral teams: Direction for the twenty-first century. *Remedial and Special Education, 17*(6), 363–369.

Schaffer v. Weast, 546 U.S. (2005). Retrieved on November 16, 2005, from *www.supremecourtus.gov/opinions/05pdf/04-698.pdf.*

Scott, T. M., & Barrett, S. B. (2004). Using staff and student time engaged in disciplinary procedures to evaluate the impact of school-wide PBS. *Journal of Positive Behavior Interventions, 6*(1), 21–27.

Shapiro, J., Monzo, L. D., Rueda, R., Gomez, J. A., & Blacher, J. (2004). Alienated advocacy: Perspectives of Latina mothers of young adults with developmental disabilities on service systems. *Mental Retardation, 42*(10), 37–54.

Short, R. J., & Talley, R. C. (1996). Effects of teacher assistance teams on special education referrals in elementary schools. *Psychological Reports, 79*(3, Pt. 2), 1431–1438.

Sindelar, P. T., Griffin, C. C., Smith, S. W., & Watanabe, A. K. (1992). Prereferral intervention: Encouraging notes on preliminary findings. *Elementary School Journal, 92*(3), 245–259.

Sugai, G., Horner, R. H., Dunlap, G., Hieneman, M., Lewis, T. J., Nelson, C. M., et al. (2000). Applying positive behavior support and functional behavioral assessment in schools. *Journal of Positive Behavior Interventions, 2*(3), 10.

Symon, J. B. (2005). Expanding interventions for children with autism: Parents as trainers. *Journal of Positive Behavior Interventions, 7*(3), 159–173.

Torgesen, J. K. (2002). The prevention of reading difficulties. *Journal of School Psychology, 40*(1), 7–26.

Turnbull, A., Edmonson, H., Griggs, P., Wickham, D., Sailor, W., Freeman, R., et al. (2002). A blueprint for schoolwide positive behavior support: Implementation of three components. *Council for Exceptional Children, 68*(3), 377–402.

Turnbull, A. P., & Ruef, M. (1997). Family perspectives on inclusive lifestyle issues for individuals with problem behavior. *Exceptional Children, 63*(2), 211–227.

Turnbull, A. P., & Turnbull, H. R. (2001). Self-determination for individuals with significant cognitive disabilities and their families. *Journal of the Association for Persons with Severe Handicaps, 26*(1), 56–62.

Turnbull, A. P., Turnbull, R., Erwin, E., & Soodak, L. (2006). *Families, professionals, and exceptionality: Positive outcomes through partnerships and trust.* Upper Saddle River, NJ: Merrill/Prentice Hall.

Turnbull, H. R., Ellis, J. W., Boggs, E. M., Brooks, P. O., & Biklen, D. P. (1981). Introduction and statement of concepts. In H. R. Turnbull (Ed.), *The least restrictive alternative: Principles and practices* (pp. 3–19). Washington, DC: American Association on Mental Deficiency.

Turnbull, H. R., Turnbull, A. P., Stowe, M., & Wilcox, B. L. (2000). *Free appropriate education: The law and children with disabilities* (6th ed.). Denver, CO: Love.

Turnbull, R., Huerta, N., & Stowe, M. (2006). *The Individuals with Education Act as amended in 2004.* Upper Saddle River, NJ: Merrill/Prentice Hall.

U.S. Department of Education. (2005a). *Twenty-fifth annual report to Congress on the implementation of the Individuals with Disabilities Education Act.* Washington, DC: Author.

U.S. Department of Education. (2005b). *Raising the achievement of students with disabilities.* Retrieved January 28, 2006, from *www.ed.gov/admins/lead/speced/achievement/factsheet.html.*

Wang, M., Mannan, H., Poston, D., Turnbull, A. P., & Summers, J. A. (2004). Parents' perceptions of advocacy activities and their impact on family quality of life. *Journal of Research and Practice in Severe Disabilities, 29*(2), 144–155.

Welsh, N. A. (2004). Stepping back through the looking glass: Real conversations with real disputants about the place, value, and meaning of mediation. *Ohio State Journal on Dispute Resolution, 19*(2), 574–678.

W. G. v. Board of Trustees of Target Range School District, 960 F.2d 1479 (9th Cir. 1992).

Yocom, D. J., & Staebler, B. (1996). The impact of collaborative consultation on special education referral accuracy. *Journal of Educational and Psychological Consultation, 7*(2), 179–192.

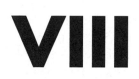

INTERNATIONAL PERSPECTIVES AND FUTURE DIRECTIONS

In this concluding section, authors draw closure to this comprehensive review of research on developmental disabilities by determining international issues and reflecting on the future directions for research and development. Although much of the research on developmental disabilities has occurred in English-speaking countries and been published in English language journals, developmental disabilities and their implications for individuals and societies are worldwide. In their circumspect and provocative chapter, Emerson, Fujiura, and Hatton examine issues that contribute to the occurrence of developmental disabilities in the range of economic and cultural contexts that exist on this planet. First documenting factors that raise the risk of developmental disabilities, such as undernutrition, birth injury, infectious diseases, and even genetics, they also describe the variations in societal response and life experiences (i.e., laws, supports, education, employment, and families) that affect individuals. Returning to the theme of social construction introduced in the first chapter, Emerson et al. describe well the variation in beliefs about developmental disabilities and their meaning in different cultures. They propose that the generators of the wealth of research and knowledge on developmental disabilities, most often the resourced nations of the Western world, should provide leadership but in a style that is respectful of local capacities, indigenous supports, and values. Viewing developmental disabilities through a "nuanced lens" of culture should be a critical feature of such leadership.

From the volume of information presented in the chapters of this *Handbook*, Warren's concluding chapter "looks forward, in a broad sense, toward the future." He

591

reflects that much of the basic and theoretical research on developmental disabilities and the applied research on practices reflect Western values, extending a theme from the previous chapter by Emerson et al. The applied research, spurred on by the interest of scientifically based practices, has consisted of relatively small, controlled studies and has been largely unidisciplinary. In looking toward the future, Warren notes the great strides currently underway in understanding the genetic contributions to human development and behavior and sees great promise in future research that examines gene–environment interactions and their relationship to different developmental disabilities. A major trend that will contribute to future development of knowledge is the elaboration of scientific methodology, such as randomized controlled trials, on the identification of biomedical, behavioral, and educational practices that have a scientific efficacy base. Such research, he proposes, will be enhanced by the future applications of technology to assessment, data collection, and analysis. The ever-increasing web-based technology will provide a powerful tool for conveying such new knowledge locally and internationally. However, as Emerson et al. also noted, Warren warns that such knowledge should not be applied unchecked, rather, critical to the utility of such knowledge is its translation into the society, culture, and community contexts in which it will be applied.

International Perspectives

Eric Emerson
Glenn T. Fujiura
Chris Hatton

As illustrated throughout this volume, the vast majority of our knowledge concerning developmental disabilities has been derived from research undertaken in the United States and other Anglophone high-income economies. Yet, of the 6.35 billion people in the world today, just 16% live in high-income economies, and only 6% live in high-income Anglophone economies (World Bank, 2005b).

The concentration of research and knowledge generation in high-income economies is neither surprising nor particular to developmental disabilities. Indeed, it is characteristic of health-related research in general (Global Forum for Health Research, 2004, 2006). It is, however, potentially problematic if the problems, issues, and solutions on which research focuses are specific to particular cultures and societies. There is, of course, a considerable risk of such social and cultural specificity in a world characterized by social and economic inequalities (United Nations, 2005a).

For example, the per capita gross national income in 2004 in the United States was $41,400. It was less than $400 in Burkina Faso, Burundi, Cambodia, Chad, Congo, Eritrea, Ethiopia, Ghana, Haiti, Laos, Malawi, Mali, Madagascar, Mozambique, Nepal, Niger, Nigeria, Rwanda, Sierra Leone, Tajikistan, Tanzania, Togo, and Uganda (World Bank, 2005b). These economic inequalities are reflected in the health and well-being of the population and the scope of educational, health, and welfare services. Life expectancy at birth for women in the United States is currently 80 years. It is less than 40 years in Malawi, Sierra Leone, Zambia, and Zimbabwe (World Bank, 2005b). Young people in the United States spend an average of 14 years in full-time education. The time span is less than 3 years for young people in Benin, Burkina Faso, Burundi, Chad, Ethiopia, Guinea, Mali, Morocco, Mozambique, Nepal, Niger, Senegal, Sierra Leone, and South Africa.

Our aim in this chapter is to place current knowledge about developmental disabilities in a wider global context. Given the paucity of research that has addressed issues relating to developmental disabilities in low- and middle-income economies, much of what follows is necessarily speculative. However, we briefly address three issues: international variation in the causes and prevalence of developmental disabilities, international variation in the life experiences of people with developmental disabilities, and international variation in the understanding and meaning of developmental disabilities.

INTERNATIONAL PERSPECTIVES ON THE INCIDENCE, CAUSES, AND PREVALENCE OF DEVELOPMENTAL DISABILITIES

No reliable data exist on the global distribution of developmental disabilities (Durkin, 2002; Institute of Medicine, 2001). There are, however, very plausible reasons to suggest that exposure to potential *environmental* causes of developmental disabilities is likely to show substantial regional and international variation, thereby leading to variations in incidence and, perhaps, prevalence. Key environmental causes of developmental disabilities include: transplacental infections (toxoplasmosis, rubella, cytomegalovirus, herpes, HIV); prenatal exposure to toxins and teratogens (e.g., alcohol, lead, mercury, maternal phenyketonuria); prenatal undernutrition (e.g., maternal iodine deficiency); birth injury, hypoxia, and rhesus incompatibility; childhood infections, especially malaria and the various types of meningitis and encephalitis; childhood exposure to environmental toxins (e.g., lead); head injury during childhood; severe dehydration and undernutrition (Durkin, 2002; Institute of Medicine, 2001; Walker et al., 2007). Reasonably reliable data exist on the global distribution of some of these risk factors; for others, it is possible to derive indirect estimates.

Risk of Undernutrition

Undernutrition, which is a major determinant of underweight and stunting, has been widely recognized as a major determinant of child survival and cognitive development (Berkman, Lescano, Gilman, Lopez, & Black, 2002; Black, 2003; Chang, Walker, Grantham-McGregor, & Powell, 2002; Grantham-McGregor et al., 2007; Pelletier & Frongillo, 2003; Walker et al., 2007). Indeed, the importance of undernutrition is reflected in the United Nations Millennium Development Goal target of reducing by 50% the prevalence of children under 5 years of age who are underweight. Figure 29.1 uses data extracted from UNICEF's *State of the World's Children 2007* to illustrate the extent of the current variation in one of the consequences of undernutrition (severe underweight) among children under the age of 5 (United Nations Children's Fund [UNICEF], 2006).

As can be seen, the reported range of children under the age 5 who are severely underweight[1] is considerable (from 0% in the United States to 18% in India). Similar variations are apparent in the distribution of severe to moderate underweight[2] (1% in

---

[1]More than 3 standard deviations below median weight for the age and reference population.
[2]More than 2 standard deviations below median weight for the age and reference population.

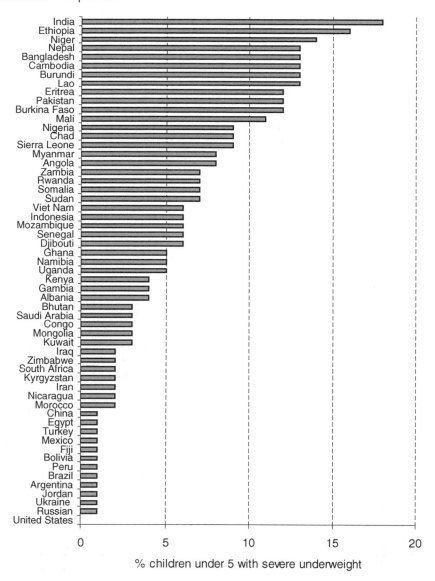

FIGURE 29.1. Percentage of children under 5 with severe underweight in selected countries. *Note.* Data from United Nations Children's Fund (2006).

the United States to 48% in Nepal, Bangladesh, and Ethiopia) and severe to moderate stunting[3] (2% in the United States to over 50% in Nepal, Ethiopia, Afghanistan, Yemen, and Burundi; UNICEF, 2004). Global and regional estimates for underweight and stunting are provided in Table 29.1. Recent estimates suggest that, whereas the global prevalence of underweight is expected to fall by 34% between 1990 and 2015, it is expected to *rise* by 12% over the same period in Africa (de Onis, Blossner, Borghi, Frongillo, & Morris, 2004).

---

[3]More than 2 standard deviations below median height for the age and reference population.

TABLE 29.1. Indicators of Risk of Developmental Disabilities Due to Undernutrition, Birth Injury, and Undetected Rh Incompatibility

	Undernutrition indicators			Birth injury and undetected Rh incompatibility indicators	
	Moderate and severe underweight	Severe underweight	Moderate and severe stunting	Antenatal care coverage (%)	Skilled attendant at delivery (%)
Regions					
Sub-Saharan Africa	29	8	38	66	41
Middle East and North Africa	14	2	21	72	72
South Asia	46	16	44	54	35
East Asia and Pacific	17	3	19	88	87
Latin America and Caribbean	7	1	16	86	82
CEE/CIS	6	1	16	80	92
Development					
Industrialized countries	—	—	—	—	99
Developing countries	27	8	31	70	59
Least developed countries	36	10	42	56	32
World	27	8	31	70	62

Note. Data from UNICEF (2004). CEE, Central and Eastern Europe; CIS, Commonwealth of Independent States.

Severe stunting in the first 2 years of life has been associated with a 10-point deficit in IQ in later childhood (Berkman et al., 2002; Grantham-McGregor, 2002) and moderate to severe stunting with a 6- to 16-point deficit in IQ (Grantham-McGregor, 2002; Grantham-McGregor et al., 2007). On the basis of a rather conservative assumption (moderate to severe stunting leads to a 7.5-point deficit in IQ), we can estimate the impact of undernutrition (as evidenced by rates of stunting) on the percentage of children expected to have an IQ of less than 70. This would range from 2.36% of children in the United States (with a reported prevalence rate for stunting of approximately 2%) to 3.64% in developing countries and 4.12% in the least developed countries. That is, on the basis of rather conservative assumptions, undernutrition alone may be responsible for a 54% increase (when compared with the United States) in the incidence of developmental disabilities during childhood in developing countries and a 75% increase in incidence in the least developed countries.

Risk of Birth Injury

The prevalence of birth injuries and the detection of rhesus incompatibility are likely to be related to access to antenatal care and the presence of skilled birth attendants during labor and at birth. Table 29.1 also presents regional and global estimates for these two indicators of risk. Again, variation is marked: Access to antenatal care ranges from 100% in Australia, Cuba, Finland, and Oman (among others) to 27% in Ethiopia and Laos, 28% in Nepal, and 32% in Somalia; and the presence of skilled birth attendants ranges from 100% in Australia, Sweden, Ukraine, Japan, and Fiji (among others) to 6% in Ethiopia and between 10 and 20% in Nepal, Afghanistan, Bangladesh, Niger, Chad, and Laos.

Risk of Infectious Disease

Table 29.2 presents a number of indicators related to the risk of infectious disease, including access to improved drinking water, sanitary conditions, HIV/AIDS prevalence in the adult population, and rates of childhood immunizations. As before, variation is marked: Access to improved drinking water ranges from 100% in high-income countries to less than 30% in Ethiopia and Somalia and less than 20% in Afghanistan; immunization against measles ranges from close to 100% in (among many others) Iran, Japan, and Brazil to less than 50% in Laos, Papua New Guinea, and Somalia and less than 30% in Nigeria and the Central African Republic; HIV/AIDS prevalence ranges from 0.1% or less in Australia, Cuba, and Laos (among many others) to over 20% in Namibia, South Africa, Zimbabwe, and Lesotho and over 30% in Botswana and Swaziland.

Genetic Factors

There is also some evidence to suggest that some genetic causes of developmental disabilities may also be unequally distributed (Institute of Medicine, 2001). For example, thalassemia (an inherited disorder in which the production of normal hemoglobin is partly or completely suppressed), which is prevalent in 2–3% of all children in West Africa, has been linked to high rates of mild intellectual disability (Steen, Xiong, Mulhern, Langston, & Wang, 1999). In low-income countries a higher proportion of

TABLE 29.2. Indicators of Risk of Contracting Infectious Disease

	% population using improved drinking water	% population with access to adequate sanitation	Prevalence of HIV/AIDS in adult population (%)	Childhood immunization rates				
				TB	DPT3	Polio	Measles	HepB3
Regions								
Sub-Saharan Africa	57	36	7.5	74	60	63	62	30
Middle East and North Africa	87	72	0.3	88	87	87	88	71
South Asia	84	35	0.7	82	71	72	67	1
East Asia and Pacific	78	50	0.2	91	86	87	82	66
Latin America and Caribbean	89	75	0.7	96	89	91	93	73
CEE/CIS	91	81	0.6	95	88	89	90	81
Development								
Industrialized countries	100	100	0.4	—	95	93	92	62
Developing countries	79	49	1.2	85	76	77	75	40
Least developed countries	58	35	3.2	79	68	68	67	20
World	83	58	1.1	85	78	79	77	42

Note. Data from UNICEF (2004). DPT3, percentage of infants who received three doses of diphtheria, pertussis (whooping cough), and tetanus vaccine; HepB3, percentage of infants who received three doses of hepatitis B vaccine.

births are to mothers age 35 and older, possibly increasing the incidence of Down syndrome (Institute of Medicine, 2001). Finally, high rates of consanguineous marriage has been associated with increased rates of child disabilities (Institute of Medicine, 2001; Teebi & El-Shanti, 2006).

Summary

A clear pattern is evident in the preceding sections: Most environmental risk factors for developmental disabilities (and some genetic risk factors) are markedly more prevalent in low-income countries. The same pattern of global inequality in risk factors is also evident for other potentially important factors, such as exposure to warfare and conflict and access to primary education (UNICEF, 2004). Indeed, it has recently been estimated that undernutrition (as evidenced by stunting) and income poverty together lead to over 200 million children failing to realize their developmental potential (Grantham-McGregor et al., 2007). Most of these children live in Africa and South Asia. The association between poverty and exposure to environmental risk factors is also evident within countries. For example, in many low-income countries, stunting is significantly more prevalent among poorer rural communities, and access to childhood immunization is associated with household wealth (World Bank, 2005b). These within-country patterns of inequality are, of course, consistent with epidemiological studies of developmental disabilities, which show a clear association between relative deprivation and the overall prevalence of developmental disabilities in both higher income countries (Emerson, Graham, & Hatton, 2006; Fujiura, 1998; Leonard et al., 2005) and lower income countries (Durkin, 2002; Durkin et al., 2000; Ganguli, 2000; Yaqoob et al., 1995).

The preceding evidence strongly suggests that the *incidence* of developmental disabilities due to environmental causes is likely to be significantly higher in low-, and, to an extent, middle-income countries. What is unclear, however, is what impact these variations in incidence will have on overall prevalence, as the same pattern of inequality is also evident in rates of child and adult mortality (Black, Morris, & Bryce, 2003; Durkin,

TABLE 29.3. Under-5 Mortality and Life Expectancy at Birth in 2003

	Under-5 mortality (death in first year per 1,000 live births)	Life expectancy at birth (years)
Regions		
Sub-Saharan Africa	175	46
Middle East and North Africa	56	67
South Asia	92	63
East Asia and Pacific	40	69
Latin America and Caribbean	32	70
CEE/CIS	41	70
Development		
Industrialized countries	6	78
Developing countries	87	62
Least developed countries	155	49
World	80	63

Note. Data from UNICEF (2004).

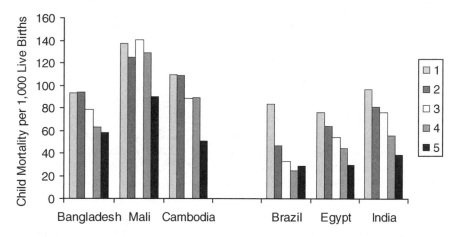

FIGURE 29.2. Under-5 mortality per 1,000 live births by asset quintile (1 = lowest, 5 = highest) for selected low- and middle-income countries. Data from World Bank (2005b).

2002; Institute of Medicine, 2001; UNICEF, 2004; World Bank, 2005b; World Health Organization, 2005). Table 29.3 presents under-5 mortality rates and life expectancy at birth for the same regions presented in Tables 29.1 and 29.2. As indicated in Figure 29.2, within-country inequalities in child survival are also evident in both middle- and low-income countries (World Bank, 2005b). Given the evidence for higher mortality rates among people with developmental disabilities (Ouellette-Kuntz, 2005), it is likely that selective mortality will serve to reduce, to a certain extent, the impact on prevalence of global inequalities in the incidence of developmental disabilities. It is also quite possible that progress in reducing child mortality in lower income countries could lead to an increased prevalence of developmental disabilities (Institute of Medicine, 2001). Nevertheless, the available information does point to markedly elevated prevalence rates for severe developmental disabilities in low- and middle-income countries such as Pakistan, India, and Jamaica (Durkin, 2002).

VARIATIONS IN THE LIFE EXPERIENCES OF PEOPLE WITH DEVELOPMENTAL DISABILITIES

We know very little about the lives and the worlds occupied by persons with developmental disabilities. Much of the knowledge base is represented in fragmented portraits of etiology, funding, population estimates, and program statistics that are largely limited to the wealthiest nations of North America, the European Union, and parts of the Pacific Rim. A modest ethnographic literature has developed, but primarily from North American and Western European studies (Bogdan & Taylor, 1994; Edgerton, 1967; Goode, 1995; MacEachen & Munby, 1996) and the far rarer cultural analysis of disability in a developing country (Devlieger, 1998; Edgerton, 1970; Ingstad, 1995).

How are life experiences encapsulated and compared internationally? Not well and not yet. In order to truly understand international variations, one must grasp the interplay of the daily dramas of individual lives played out against the institutional infrastructure of political systems, economies, and cultures. Our brief review is far less ambitious, anchored on conventional indicators of inclusion that are embodied in international disability policy: legal protections and availability and access to services and supports.

Rights under Law

Legal instruments on behalf of persons with developmental disabilities are now common and largely embedded in the ratification by nations of international conventions related to the rights of persons with disabilities generally. A small number of countries have implemented constitutional protections. International disability instruments include six major resolutions by the United Nations (U.N.) General Assembly, beginning with the *Declaration on the Rights of Mentally Retarded Persons* (United Nations, 1971) through the *Standard Rules on the Equalization of Opportunities for Persons with Disabilities* (U.N., 1993). There are numerous other international and regional agreements focused on employment and rehabilitation organized through the International Labor Organization and on education and primary prevention via the United Nations Educational, Scientific, and Cultural Organization (UNESCO). As of 2002, 46 nations had enacted legislation outlining the basic civil rights of citizens with disabilities (Degener & Quinn, 2002). International agreements on disability rights are not legally binding instruments; rather, the intent is to establish a framework of norms and expectations for government policies (Langenbach, 2003). Whether the protections arise from a country's being a signatory to an international resolution or are explicitly encoded in national law, enforcement of protections is rare throughout the world. The European Union Monitoring and Advocacy Program (EUMAP, 2005a), in its review of the educational and employment status of persons with intellectual disabilities in Europe, found a network of laws and regulatory provisions related to disabilities but little evidence of enforcement.

Supports and Infrastructure

Not unexpectedly, the character and organization of services and supports is highly idiosyncratic across nations. For the purposes of our review we organize countries according to the World Bank's classification of national economies as high income (e.g., Australia, Japan, North America, Western Europe), middle and lower-middle income (e.g., China, Mexico, Russia), and low income (e.g., Bangladesh, India, Zimbabwe). Two features of developmental-disabilities supports and infrastructure are common to all countries: Availability and access is inadequate, and reliable information on the status and prospects of citizens with developmental disabilities is extremely limited or simply not available.

Among middle- and lower-middle-income nations, the infrastructure of services appears to be a fragmented mixture of programs provided through specialized ministries supplemented in large measure by the work of nongovernmental organizations (NGOs). Access is severely limited. NGOs are typically funded through religious or other international organizations such as UNICEF, Save the Children, the World Bank, the United States Agency for International Development (USAID), and the United Nations Educational, Scientific and Cultural Organization (UNESCO), among others, and a host of private service foundations such as the Kiwanis, Lions, and Rotary. NGO supports tend to be structured around specialized services for groups of different impairments, such as physical, visual, hearing, or intellectual disabilities, and are often linked to hospitals or schools. In the world's poorest nations, there are few if any public services, and NGOs provide the vast majority of formal developmental-disabilities supports; most persons with developmental disabilities rely on traditional tribal or village-based accommodations and, of course, on family and kinship relations. The dearth of formal services and supports in rural areas has long been identified as an important issue for developmental-disabilities services in all nations and is exacerbated in the world's middle- and low-income nations (Christianson et al., 2002; Kalyanpur, 1996; United Nations, 1999). A 2002 inventory identified 205 government-sponsored programs and NGOs working with people with disabilities in Bangladesh; 159 were located in only one of the nation's 64 districts, and the majority were concentrated around the capital city of Dhaka (Danish Bilharziasis Laboratory, 2004). Even where NGO supports are established, sustainability is a challenge. In a review of disability services in Sri Lanka, Rajapaksa and Liyanage (2004) noted that NGO success often hinged on the "dedication and commitment of a few individuals" (p. 22). An important agenda is the integration and thus stabilization of disability initiatives into the broad spectrum of international developmental initiatives and funding.

In the early 1980s, a community-based rehabilitation (CBR) model was promoted as a cost-effective strategy for redressing the lack of supports in low-income nations (World Health Organization, 1981). In its most general form, CBR consists of small programs implemented through the combined efforts of those with disabilities, their families, and the community using indigenous supports (McConkey & O'Toole, 1995). The model remains the centerpiece of international development strategies (World Bank, 2005a), though numerous critiques have been directed toward the more formal, hierarchically organized programs that emphasize application of external expertise and practices (Hartley, 2002; Miles, 1996; Thomas & Thomas, 2002).

Education

Educational opportunity ranges from total exclusion to legal and (technically) enforceable mandates for access to mainstream opportunities. Not unexpectedly, the scope of educational opportunity is reflected in the degree of development in the national educational system, though full inclusion remains a distant promise in even the high-income nations of the world. The recently enacted 2001 Special Education Needs and Disability Act of Great Britain parallels the Individuals with Disabilities Education Act (IDEA) legislation in the United States. Education in mainstream schools is mandated if deemed appropriate, but, among children formally identified as eligible for educational services, a significant proportion (40%) are in segregated schools or classes (EUMAP, 2005b). Similarly, the Japanese have a highly organized special education system with national mandates (since 1979), but it remains organized around segregated classes. The EUMAP summary of educational services in Eastern Europe typifies the experiences of middle-income nations—policy commitments have been made, but significant changes have yet to occur in what are resource-poor, highly exclusionary, or segregated educational systems. In Bulgaria, children with mild intellectual disabilities were educated in segregated, primarily residential schools, whereas those children with more severe disabilities were excluded from receiving any educational services. A regulatory change in 2002 established the universal right to education in a mainstream school, but the chronic lack of money and shortages of trained staff impede implementation (EUMAP, 2005c). The Chinese profile illustrates how variable accessibility to education can be; despite regulatory safeguards and a recent expansion of special schools and classes, those with severe developmental disabilities or in rural areas are largely excluded from any educational opportunity (Chen & Simeonsson, 1993; Piao, Gargiulio, & Yun, 1995; Sonnander & Claesson, 1997; Xu, 1994).

In the poorest countries of the world, central governments set the broad contours of educational policy and may provide limited funding, but they largely devolve the administration of education to regional or local authority or, more commonly, to NGOs. NGO educational services are typically provided via residential schools or residential facilities (Rajapaksa & Liyanage, 2004). As Kalyanpur notes (1996), questions about educational services in the poorest nations tend not to be about appropriateness or quality but rather about availability.

Employment

Employment represents one of the most important proxies for assessing progress in the equalization of opportunity agenda (United Nations, 2002). Despite widespread implementation of work initiatives across high-income nations since the 1980s, the employment status of persons with developmental disabilities remains marginal at best (Yamaki & Fujiura, 2002), and integrated work options are severely limited (International Labor Organization, 2003; Jenaro, Mank, Bottomley, Doose, & Tuckerman, 2002). The EUMAP analysis reported unemployment rates in Eastern Europe at nearly 100%, and the few who were employed were isolated in government- or NGO-operated sheltered workshops that function as much as day program options as they do as employment training (EUMAP, 2005a). Fujiura, Park, and Rutkowski-Kmitta's (2005) exploratory study of four mid- to low-income nations (Albania, Bulgaria, Nicaragua, and South Africa) found dramatic disparity in rates of employment between those with intellectual disability and with other types of disabilities. The reasons for the differences most certainly varied across the countries, but the consistency of the differences suggest that underemployment is a common experience for persons with developmental disabilities internationally.

Comparing employment status across national borders is a difficult task under the best of circumstances due to variations in the base economies and cultural differences in the form of work (Desrosieres, 1996). The challenge is compounded when drawing comparisons across the established industrial economies and transitional economies that are still linked to their traditional agricultural base. Use of wage-based occupation statistics may obscure or distort the extent to which persons with developmental disabilities are included in the network of productive activity. Mpofu (2001), for example, describes the greater marginalization of persons with disabilities in the urban centers of Zimbabwe compared with the traditional village or rural community economy. Despite this caveat, the general profile of employment, at least in terms of formal wage-based occupation, is uniformly discouraging.

Role of Families

Ironically, the least is known about the largest group with developmental disabilities in the world—those living with families in their home communities. Studies conducted in high-income nations with established long-term-care residential systems find only small proportions of the population with developmental disabilities living in residential settings (Braddock, Emerson, Felce, & Stancliffe, 2001; Cabinet Office, 2001; Fujiura, 1998). Similar observations have been made in the less developed nations (Goldbart & Mukherjee, 1998; Handicap International Regional Office for Southeast Europe, 2004;

Mittler, 1990; McConkey, 2005; Stratford & Ng, 2000). For those living in low-income developing nations, the family and the network of kinship relations often represent the only basis of support; Western conceptions of independence may need to be refined or revisited when applied to the impoverished rural regions of the world (Whyte, 1998). The role of the family is one clear message in the global profile—the life experiences of the world's population of persons with developmental disabilities is defined in the ordinary daily routines of support by millions of parents, siblings, relatives, friends, and other benefactors (Miles, 2000).

Summary

Although much is unknown about the life experiences of persons with developmental disabilities throughout the world, the general contours of the international experience suggest a population that is largely marginalized, regardless of national wealth. Cautious optimism is warranted, however, as international bodies and governments appear ready, in word if not deed, to assume greater responsibility for persons with developmental disabilities. Less clear are the directions such responsibilities would take. A great deal of programmatic and policy experimentation and deliberation has occurred over the past half century, but it has occurred in the West; we must remain open to the possibility that a developmental-disabilities agenda may travel many different roads to achieve the goal of human rights and human dignity.

INTERNATIONAL UNDERSTANDINGS OF DEVELOPMENTAL DISABILITIES

As we have seen, the available evidence suggests substantial variations in the incidence, prevalence, and causes of developmental disabilities and in the lives of people with developmental disabilities around the world. This section outlines the role that cultural understandings of developmental disabilities may play in determining the experiences of people with developmental disabilities and their families. As with the rest of the chapter, only a brief sketch of the relevant issues is provided; relevant evidence concerning cultural understandings is sparse, scattered, and largely concerned with particular ethnic communities within high-income countries rather than communities within middle- and low-income countries.

Constructing Developmental Disabilities

It is now a commonplace to accept that disabilities, including developmental disabilities, are socially constructed. For example, the population identified as developmentally disabled has varied enormously within high-income societies over time (Cocks, Fox, Brogan, & Lee, 1996; Trent, 1994; Wright & Digby, 1996), partly as a function of broader social and cultural changes within these societies. Goffman (1963) suggests that these variations in constructions of developmental disabilities partly depend on changing social judgments of "obtrusiveness," behaviors that interfere with the flow of social interactions and the normal routine of everyday cultural practices. For example, largely rural, agrarian societies had different expectations of which behaviors (and therefore people) were obtrusive compared with those of the same societies after they became largely urban and industrialized (Wright & Digby, 1996). The concept of obtrusiveness is also helpful when considering developmental disabilities in an international context, as high-, middle-, and low-income societies are likely to have very different expectations of which behaviors count as obtrusive and therefore which people are likely to be identified as developmentally disabled. Anthropological work suggests that all societies may make distinctions between competent and incompetent people, with "competence" broadly defined as "the capacity or potential for adequate functioning-in-context as a socialized human" (Jenkins, 1998, p. 1), although there seems to be very little consistency across societies in what counts as competent or incompetent (Jenkins, 1998).

Over the past hundred years or more, high-income Anglophone countries have developed highly systematized methods for identifying incompetence, partly through shaping the construct of intellectual disabilities itself and partly through developing associated measurement tools. This construct of intellectual disability typically contains three elements: limitations in intellectual functioning, limitations in the display of adaptive behaviors that are necessary and appropriate to participation in the person's environment, and an age of onset before cultural norms of adulthood are reached (American Association on Mental Retardation [AAMR], 2002). As professional associations such as AAMR recognize, intellectual disability is not an inherent characteristic of individuals but is instead a product of interactions between a person and his or her community. The wide diversity of communities around the world, particularly when considering middle- and low-income countries, makes the elements of the intellectual-disability construct and the construct itself of questionable relevance internationally.

For example, within the classification systems used in high-income countries, intellectual functioning is assumed to be a unitary construct that can be assessed quantitatively (typically by using IQ tests). The cross-cultural validity of IQ tests (both across ethnic groups within countries and across countries) has been vigorously contested, with better IQ test performance robustly associated with the nature and duration of experience of formal education, familiarity with the type of stimuli used in IQ tests, and socialization into the situation of being tested (Flynn, 1987; Van de Vijver, 1997). There have also been more fundamental challenges to the construct of unitary intelligence from a cross-cultural perspective. For example, proponents of the construct of cognitive style (Sternberg & Grigorenko, 1997) do not consider intelligence to be a universally valid construct that is easily separable from the construct of adaptive behavior. Instead, different cultural groups require different cognitive styles for its members to deal effectively with problems encountered in daily living; these styles fall along a continuum from "field independence" (or autonomous functioning that relies on internal cues to shape the environment) to "field dependence" (or functioning that relies more on the external environment and is more socially oriented). Such cross-cultural conceptions of cognition suggest that the distinction between intelligence and adaptive behavior is blurred if not absent; cognitive styles develop and are used to enable a person to adapt to his or her immediate environment.

Understanding Incompetence in a Global Context

It seems clear that the construct of intellectual disability that is currently used in high-income Anglophone societies has been developed to meet the needs of a specific group of largely urban and industrialized countries at a particular point in history. For example, the construct of intelligence places a great emphasis on the abstract reasoning skills required for economic productivity within societies that value literacy and numeracy. Similarly, the construct of adaptive behavior emphasizes autonomous functioning within high-income societies.

As well as meeting particular societal needs, the construct of intellectual disability also reflects dominant values within high-income societies such as the United States and the United Kingdom (Angrosino, 1998; Devlieger, 1998; van Maastricht, 1998). In cross-cultural terms, these societies have been characterized as highly individualist (as opposed to collectivist), defined in terms of: (1) the definition of the self as personal or collective, independent or interdependent; (2) personal goals having priority over group goals (or vice versa); (3) emphasis on exchange rather than on communal relationships; (4) the relative importance of personal attitudes versus social norms in a person's behavior (Triandis, 1995).

Even within high-income countries with dominant individualist cultures, substantial variations exist in conceptualizations of competence. There is some evidence within countries such as the United States and the United Kingdom that middle-class cultures have conceptualizations of intellectual disability that are closest to professional definitions and that family members become highly involved in service systems and sometimes become professionals themselves (Gabel, 2004; Grant, 2005; Mink, 1997). Although people labeled as intellectually disabled in these countries may act in ways that reject the label, they seem less likely to reject the construct of intellectual disability itself. Instead, people so labeled seem more likely to place themselves on the competent side of the competence–incompetence divide, defined in terms of dominant individualist cultural values (Angrosino, 1998; Devlieger, 1998; Edgerton, 1967), although there is also evidence that people with this label may report more radical discontinuities between the label and their lived experience (Finlay & Lyons, 2005).

Studies of ethnic minority groups thought to be more collectivist within high-income Anglophone societies have revealed understandings of intellectual disability that reflect more collectivist values, although it is important to remember that ethnic minority cultures are diverse, constantly changing due to acculturation processes, and commonly intertwined with socioeconomic disadvantage (Hatton, 2002; McCallion, Janicki, & Grant-Griffin, 1997).

First, translated terms thought to be equivalent to "intellectual disability" have diverse connotations for different ethnic groups; for example, the Hindu term *mundh buddhi* was conceptualized by U.S. Hindu family members as including "slow brain" (having the capacity to learn as much as other people, but at a slower rate); as having a good mind but choosing not to use it; and as "bad desires" (the person wanting or pursuing something that is unhealthy, sinful, or dangerous; Gabel, 2004). Similarly, the term *ritardo* has been reported as connoting mental illness or derangement to many U.S. Latino parents of a child with intellectual disabilities (Harry, 1992). It is unclear whether these results reflect a simple translation issue or whether they capture constructions of incompetence that are broader than professional constructs of "intellectual disability."

Second, family members within some ethnic minority groups seem more likely to value and define their children's competence in terms of collectivist values based on interdependence, appropriate social behavior within the family context, and showing respect for family members and their cultural practices (Hatton, Akram, Shah, Robertson, & Emerson, 2004; Magana, 1999). The dimensions of competence valued by these family members can conflict with dominant values within high-income

Anglophone countries, for example, in the transition from education services to services for adults with disabilities, particularly in terms of out-of-home placement for the person with disabilities (Blacher, 2001; Rueda et al., 2005). However, these conflicts are also likely to be a function of the socioeconomic position of families, language issues, and racism on the part of service systems, as well as clashes of values (Hatton, 2002).

Some of the issues raised by studies of ethnic minority groups within high-income Anglophone societies are also apparent in the sparse literature concerning societies in middle- and low-income countries, in particular diverse conceptions of competence that emphasize social and relational competence rather than abstract intellectual functioning and conflicts between cultural practices and imposed professional classificatory and service practices. This literature also highlights some issues concerning living in societies without pervasive professional systems for the identification, classification, and provision of services for incompetent people.

For example, a study of two central African cultural groups showed that social perceptions of competence were largely a function of social embeddedness (recognition and observance of local social practices) and willingness to try to overcome one's difficulties (Devlieger, 1998). Bengali families living in Kolkata, India, also emphasize the importance of being able to fulfill social responsibilities as central to a definition of competence in terms of fulfilling family roles and duties, knowing how to show respect to whom, knowing social customs, looking after guests, and showing ties of affection (Rao, 2006). Similar cultural perceptions of competence have been reported in Greece (Van Maastricht, 1998), Uganda (Whyte, 1998) and Greenland (Nuttall, 1998), with sophisticated and diverse constructions of the cause, nature, and consequences of incompetence.

Several studies have reported that in middle- and low-income countries, professional classification and service support systems typically impose "Western" constructions of incompetence that often conflict with local cultural perceptions (Mpofu, 2002). Such an imposition of these Western constructions of incompetence, when allied to sufficient professional infrastructure and power, can result in the person judged to be incompetent being separated from family and local communities in the face of resistance from the person and family that can be seen as obstructive, simultaneously overprotective and in denial about the person's status, and based on superstition or other false beliefs (Lundgren, 1998; Nuttall, 1998).

Seen in this light, it is tempting to assume that professional services are the problem rather than the solution. Indeed, some studies suggest that living in societies without dominant cultural values of individualism and the professional infrastructure associated with high-income societies may have some advantages to set against the range of increased risks reported earlier in this chapter. For example, a study of rural and urban children defined as intellectually disabled in South Africa reported that rural children had much greater social maturity than would be expected from their IQ scores, possibly as a result of the increased social responsibilities such children have in their rural communities (Pillay, 2003). Edeh and Hickson (2002) reported that Nigerian students labeled as intellectually disabled performed better on tasks assessing interpersonal problem-solving performance than did African American and European American students, with Nigerian students reporting more cooperative (as opposed to individualistic) problem-solving styles. In Greece, it has been suggested that the lack of reach of formal services may allow people who would be judged to be incompetent within formal classification systems to live valued social lives embedded within local communities (Van Maastricht, 1998).

However, local cultural constructions of incompetence can also be highly stigmatizing for those individuals judged to be incompetent. In countries with limited or no services for people judged to be incompetent, this stigma may result in pervasive neglect and indifference toward the lives of people with intellectual disabilities, as has been reported in Indonesia (Komardjaja, 2005). In countries with claims to an all-encompassing professional reach but highly stigmatizing social attitudes, such as China, some countries in Eastern Europe, and Russia, the result is likely to be limited services in the form of segregated institutions (Bridge, 2004; Special Olympics, 2003). Substantial local social and family resources are required in the face of such professional indifference; changing patterns of employment, urbanization, and family structure as a result of global economic changes are likely to diminish these resources (Hartley et al., 2005).

Summary

The constructs of developmental or intellectual disability, together with instruments for the measurement of these constructs, have been developed largely within high-income, individualist, Anglophone societies. Although the evidence is extremely limited, these constructs appear to have little relevance for most of the world's population, including much of the population living within these high-income countries. Instead, most societies seem to construct competence in more socially and culturally situated terms rather than in terms of an abstract conception of intelligence, with substantial diversity in these constructions according to the specific needs and cultural mores of different cultural groups. When classification practices and service supports based on constructions of intellectual disability are imposed on societies with different conceptions of competence, tension, conflict, and resistance are likely to arise. Seen from a global context, the provision of classification systems and services based on conceptions of intellectual disability may be misguided; classification systems and services that start from local conceptions of competence and the proper social role of a competent person may be more productive.

SUMMARY AND SOME IMPLICATIONS FOR POLICY, PRACTICE, AND RESEARCH

The preceding review suggests that much of the existing knowledge about developmental disabilities is specific to high-income nations and thus may have questionable relevance for the majority of the world today. Three implications for future policy, practice, and research emerge from our review: (1) improving our understanding of risk and prevention, (2) expanding our conceptions of support and program development in resource-poor environments, and (3) incorporating cultural variations in our conceptions of developmental disability.

The higher overall *incidence* of developmental disabilities due to environmental and other causes in low-, and, to a lesser extent, middle-income economies suggests an entirely different policy and programmatic agenda beyond the borders of the high-income nations. Such an effort will entail a vastly improved understanding of the character and extent of risk and programs for their reduction. In this context, progress toward the millennium development goals is particularly important for people with developmental disabilities and their families (Inclusion International, 2005; UNICEF, 2004; United Nations, 2005b; World Bank, 2005b). It is also clear that technological solutions to many of the likely causes of developmental disabilities are already available (cf. Engle et al., 2007). The main challenges for policy, practice, and research are improvements in the quality of surveillance and the development and implementation of effective systems for delivering solutions (Black et al., 2003; Bryce et al., 2003; Jones et al., 2003; Victora et al., 2003). Some examples of possible pro-poor delivery systems and interventions include: the development of women's self-help groups to reduce child and maternal mortality (Manandhar et al., 2004); the provision of micronutrients during pregnancy (Osrin et al., 2005) and preschool (Attanasio & Vera-Hernandez, 2004); the use of tax transfers linked to maternal achievement of goals regarding nutrition, health, and education (Attanasio, Meghir, & Santiago, 2005). Finally, as Fujiura et al. (2005) previously noted, a policy priority focused on prevention of developmental disabilities will require a thoughtful dialogue about the contradictory messages of prevention and human rights.

Our review of life experiences suggests commonalities, as well as vast differences, between low-, middle-, and high-income nations. However defined, the population of persons with developmental disabilities is largely marginalized, even in the wealthiest of nations. How best to confront these enormous inequities? A critical question raised in this chapter is the global relevance of our base of research, policy, and practice; to what extent are these approaches and concepts applicable to other cultural contexts? Do the vast differences in the character of supports and infrastructure between rich and poor nations indicate greater inequity and deprivation? Certainly the resource-intensive models of high-income nations are not viable options for much of the world, at least for the near future. Understanding models of indigenous support and identifying and expanding on local innovations may be key to our agenda of improving the lives and prospects of persons with developmental disabilities while remaining responsive to, and respectful of, traditional cultures.

Finally, this chapter considered the very fundamental question "Who are the 'developmentally disabled'?" The central point of our review of international understandings is that our established conceptions have largely emerged from the measurement and cultural traditions of the Anglophone nations. It appears that these conceptions have little relevance for most of the world's population, and we have not yet systematically considered the research, policy, and practice implications of these varying constructions of developmental disabilities. What are the implications of these elastic boundaries for international priorities and development activities?

A strong case can be made on both humanitarian and economic grounds that high-income Anglophone countries have a responsibility to help address issues of developmental disabilities internationally. Indeed, the core concepts and terminology emerged from the leadership of the Western nations in the 1960s; much of the knowledge base in research, policy, and practice has developed there. Western culture's reframing of disability concerns into a human and civil rights agenda has dramatically changed the international discourse on disability. These are important achievements. But this chapter suggests the importance of viewing developmental disability through a nuanced lens when looking outward. We should lead, but lead with the understanding that effective leadership requires more than the export of ideals and models; it will require a truly international perspective.

REFERENCES

American Association on Mental Retardation. (2002). *Mental retardation: Definition, classification, and systems of supports* (10th ed.). Washington, DC: Author.

Angrosino, M. V. (1998). Mental disability in the United States: An interactionist perspective. In R. Jenkins (Ed.), *Questions of competence: Culture, classification and intellectual disability* (pp. 25–53). Cambridge, UK: Cambridge University Press.

Attanasio, O., Meghir, C., & Santiago, A. (2005). *Education choices in Mexico: Using a structural model and a randomised experiment to evaluate PROGRESA.* London: Institute for Fiscal Studies.

Attanasio, O., & Vera-Hernandez, M. (2004). *Medium and long run effects of nutrition and child care: Evaluation of a community nursery programme in rural Colombia.* London: Institute for Fiscal Studies.

Berkman, D. S., Lescano, A. G., Gilman, R. H., Lopez, S. L., & Black, M. M. (2002). Effects of stunting, diarrhoeal disease, and parasitic infection during infancy on cognition in late childhood: A follow-up study. *Lancet, 359,* 564–571.

Blacher, J. (2001). Transition to adulthood: Mental retardation, families, and culture. *American Journal on Mental Retardation, 106,* 173–188.

Black, M. M. (2003). Micronutrient deficiencies and cognitive functioning. *Journal of Nutrition, 133*(11, Suppl. 2), 3927S–3931S.

Black, R., Morris, S., & Bryce, J. (2003). Where and why are 10 million children dying every year? *Lancet, 361,* 2226–2234.

Bogdan, R., & Taylor, S. J. (1994). *The social meaning of mental retardation: Two life stories.* New York: Teachers College Press.

Braddock, D., Emerson, E., Felce, D., & Stancliffe, R. J. (2001). Living circumstances of children and adults with mental retardation or developmental disabilities in the United States, Canada, England and Wales, and Australia. *Mental Retardation and Developmental Disabilities Research Reviews, 7,* 115–121.

Bridge, G. (2004). Disabled children and their families in Ukraine: Health and mental health issues for families caring for their disabled children at home. *Social Work in Health Care, 39,* 89–105.

Bryce, J., el Arifeen, S., Pariyo, G., Lanata, C. F., Gwatkin, D., Habicht, J. P., et al. (2003). Reducing child mortality: Can public health deliver? *Lancet, 262,* 159–164.

Cabinet Office. (2001). *White paper on people with disabilities.* Tokyo: Ministry of Health, Labor, and Welfare.

Chang, S. M., Walker, S. P., Grantham-McGregor, S., & Powell, C. A. (2002). Early childhood stunting and later behaviour and school achievement. *Journal of Child Psychology and Psychiatry, 43*(6), 775–783.

Chen, J., & Simeonsson, R. J. (1993). Prevention of childhood disability in the People's Republic of China. *Child: Care, Health and Development, 19,* 71–88.

Christianson, A. L., Zwane, M. E., Manga, P., Rosen, E., Venter, A., Downs, D., et al. (2002). Children with intellectual disability in rural South Africa: Prevalence and associated disability. *Journal of Intellectual Disability Research, 46,* 179–186.

Cocks, E., Fox, C., Brogan, M., & Lee, M. (1996). (Eds.). *Under blue skies: The social construction of intellectual disability in Western Australia.* Perth, Australia: Edith Cowan University.

Danish Bilharziasis Laboratory. (2004). *Disability in Bangladesh: A situation analysis.* Copenhagen, Denmark: Author.

Degener, T., & Quinn, G. (2002). A survey of international, comparative and regional disability law reform. In M. L. Breslin & S. Yee (Eds.), *Disability rights law and policy: International and national perspectives.* Washington, DC: Disability Rights Education and Defense Fund.

de Onis, M., Blossner, M., Borghi, E., Frongillo, E. A., & Morris, R. (2004). Estimates of global prevalence of childhood underweight in 1990 and 2015. *Journal of the American Medical Association, 291*(21), 2600–2606.

Desrosieres, A. (1996). Statistical traditions: An obstacle to international comparisons? In L. Hantrais & S. Mangen (Eds.), *Cross-national research methods* (pp. 17–27). London: Pinter.

Devlieger, P. (1998). (In)competence in America in comparative perspective. In R. Jenkins (Ed.), *Questions of competence: Culture, classification and intellectual disability* (pp. 54–75). Cambridge, UK: Cambridge University Press.

Durkin, M. (2002). The epidemiology of developmental disabilities in low-income countries. *Mental Retardation and Developmental Disabilities Research Reviews, 8*(3), 206–211.

Durkin, M. S., Khan, N. Z., Davidson, L. L., Huq, S., Munir, S., Rasul, E., et al. (2000). Prenatal and postnatal risk factors for mental retardation among children in Bangladesh. *American Journal of Epidemiology, 152*(11), 1024–1033.

Edeh, O. M., & Hickson, L. (2002). Cross-cultural comparison of interpersonal problem-solving in students with mental retardation. *American Journal on Mental Retardation, 107*, 6–15.

Edgerton, R. B. (1967). *The cloak of competence: Stigma in the lives of the mentally retarded.* Berkeley: University of California Press.

Edgerton, R. B. (1970). Mental retardation in non-Western societies: Towards a cross-cultural perspective on incompetence. In H. C. Hayward (Ed.), *Socio-cultural aspects of mental retardation.* New York: Appleton-Century-Crofts.

Emerson, E., Graham, H., & Hatton, C. (2006). Household income and health status in children and adolescents: Cross-sectional study. *European Journal of Public Health, 16*, 354–360.

Engle, P. L., Black, M. M., Behrman, J. R., de Mello, M. C., Gertler, J., Kapiriri, L., et al. (2007). Strategies to avoid the loss of developmental potential in more than 200 million children in the developing world. *Lancet, 369*, 229–242.

European Union Monitoring and Advocacy Program of the Open Society Institute. (2005a). *Main monitoring findings.* Budapest, Hungary: Author. Retrieved October 10, 2005, from *www.eumap.org/topics/inteldis/reports/main_findings/*.

European Union Monitoring and Advocacy Program of the Open Society Institute. (2005b). *Rights of people with intellectual disabilities: Access to education and employment in the United Kingdom.* Budapest, Hungary: Author.

European Union Monitoring and Advocacy Program of the Open Society Institute. (2005c). *Rights of people with intellectual disabilities: Access to education and employment in Bulgaria.* Budapest, Hungary: Author.

Finlay, W. M. L., & Lyons, E. (2005). Rejecting the label: A social constructionist analysis. *Mental Retardation, 43*, 120–134.

Flynn, J. R. (1987). Massive IQ gains in 14 nations: What IQ tests really measure. *Psychological Bulletin, 101*, 171–191.

Fujiura, G. T. (1998). Demography of family households. *American Journal on Mental Retardation, 103*, 225–235.

Fujiura, G. T., Park, H. J., & Rutkowski-Kmitta, V. (2005). Disability statistics in the developing world: A reflection on the meanings in our numbers. *Journal of Applied Research in Intellectual Disabilities, 18*, 295–304.

Gabel, S. (2004). South Asian Indian cultural orientations toward mental retardation. *Mental Retardation, 42*, 12–25.

Ganguli, H. C. (2000). Epidemiological findings on prevalence of mental disorders in India. *Indian Journal of Psychiatry, 42*, 14–20.

Global Forum for Health Research. (2004). *The 10/90 Report on Health Research.* Geneva, Switzerland: Author.

Global Forum for Health Research. (2006). *Poverty, equity, and health research.* Geneva, Switzerland: Author.

Goffman, E. (1963). *Stigma: Notes on the management of spoiled identity.* Englewood Cliffs, NJ: Prentice-Hall.

Goldbart, J., & Mukherjee, S. (1998). The appropriateness of Western models of parent involvement in Calcutta, India: 2. Implications of family roles and responsibilities. *Child: Care, Health and Development, 25*, 348–358.

Goode, D. (1995). *Quality of life for persons with disabilities.* Cambridge, MA: Brookline Books.

Grant, G. W. B. (2005). Experiences of family care. In G. Grant, P. Goward, M. Richardson, & P. Ramcharan (Eds.), *Learning disability: A life cycle approach to valuing people* (pp. 222–242). Maidenhead, UK: Open University Press.

Grantham-McGregor, S. (2002). Linear growth retardation and cognition. *Lancet, 359*, 542.

Grantham-McGregor, S., Cheung, Y. B., Cueto, S., Glewe, P., Richter, L., Strupp, B., et al. (2007). Developmental potential in the first 5 years for children in developing countries. *Lancet, 369*, 60–70.

Handicap International Regional Office for Southeast Europe. (2004). *Beyond deinstitutionalization: The unsteady transition towards an enabling system in South East Europe.* Belgrade, Serbia: The Disability Monitoring Initiative.

Harry, B. (1992). An ethnographic study of cross-cultural communication with Puerto Rican–American families in the special education system. *American Educational Research Journal, 29,* 471–494.

Hartley, S. (2002). Introduction. In S. Hartley (Ed.), *CBR: A participatory strategy in Africa* (pp. 1–11). London: University College.

Hartley, S., Ojwang, P., Baguwemu, A., Ddamulira, M., & Chavuta, A. (2005). How do carers of disabled children cope? The Ugandan perspective. *Child: Care, Health and Development, 31,* 167–180.

Hatton, C. (2002). People with intellectual disabilities from ethnic minority communities in the United States and the United Kingdom. *International Review of Research in Mental Retardation, 25,* 209–239.

Hatton, C., Akram, Y., Shah, R., Robertson, J., & Emerson, E. (2004). *Supporting South Asian families with a child with severe disabilities.* London: Kingsley.

Inclusion International. (2005). *Achieving the millennium development goals for all.* Retrieved October 18, 2005, from *www.inclusion-international.org/site_uploads/1119014250141672457.pdf.*

Ingstad, B. (1995). *Mpho ya modimo*—A gift from God: Perspectives on "attitudes" toward disabled persons. In B. I. Ingstad & S. R. Whyte (Eds.), *Disability and culture* (pp. 246–263). Berkeley: University of California Press.

Institute of Medicine. (2001). *Neurological, psychiatric, and developmental disorders: Meeting the challenge in the developing world.* Washington, DC: National Academy Press.

International Labor Office. (2003). *Employment of people with disabilities: The impact of legislation (Asia and the Pacific).* Geneva, Switzerland: Author.

Jenaro, C., Mank, D., Bottomley, J., Doose, S., & Tuckerman, P. (2002). Supported employment in the international context: An analysis of processes and outcomes. *Journal of Vocational Rehabilitation, 17,* 5–21.

Jenkins, R. (1998). (Ed.). *Questions of competence: Culture, classification and intellectual disability.* Cambridge, UK: Cambridge University Press.

Jones, G., Steketee, R. W., Black, R. E., Bhutta, Z. A., Morris, S. S., & the Bellagio Child Survival Study Group. (2003). How many child deaths can we prevent this year? *Lancet, 362,* 65–71.

Kalyanpur, M. (1996). The influence of Western special education on community-based services in India. *Disability and Society, 11,* 249–270.

Komardjaja, I. (2005). The place of people with intellectual disabilities in Bandung, Indonesia. *Health and Place, 11,* 117–120.

Langenbach, A. (2003). *Human rights of persons with disabilities.* Cambridge, MA: Human Rights Education Associates.

Leonard, H., Petterson, B., De Klerk, N., Zubrick, S. R., Glasson, E., Sanders, R., et al. (2005). Association of sociodemographic characteristics of children with intellectual disability in Western Australia. *Social Science and Medicine, 60,* 1499–1513.

Lundgren, N. (1998). Learning to become (in)competent: Children in Belize speak out. In R. Jenkins (Ed.), *Questions of competence: Culture, classification and intellectual disability* (pp. 194–221). Cambridge, UK: Cambridge University Press.

Manandhar, D. S., Osrin, D., Shrestha, B. P., Mesko, N., Morrison, J., Tumbahangphe, K. M., et al. (2004). Effect of a participatory intervention with women's groups on birth outcomes in Nepal: Cluster-randomised controlled trial. *Lancet, 364,* 790–797.

MacEachen, E., & Munby, H. (1996). Developmentally disabled adults in community living: The significance of personal control. *Qualitative Health Research, 6,* 71–89.

Magana, S. (1999). Puerto Rican families caring for an adult with mental retardation: The role of familism. *American Journal on Mental Retardation, 104,* 466–482.

McCallion, P., Janicki, M., & Grant-Griffin, L. (1997). Exploring the impact of culture and acculturation on older families caregiving for persons with developmental disabilities. *Family Relations, 46,* 347–357.

McConkey, R. (2005). Family, international. In G. L. Albrecht (Ed.), *Encyclopedia of disability* (Vol. 2, pp. 713–718). Thousand Oaks, CA: Sage.

McConkey, R., & O'Toole, B. (1995). Towards the new millenium. In B. O'Toole & R. McConkey (Eds.), *Innovations in developing countries for people with disabilities* (pp. 3–14). Lancashire, UK: Lisieux Hall.

Miles, M. (2000). High level baloney for third world disabled people. *Disability World*. Retrieved April 13, 2004, from *www.disabilityworld.org/10-12_00/news/baloney.htm*.

Miles, S. (1996). Engaging with the disability rights movement: The experience of community-based rehabilitation in southern Africa. *Disability and Society, 11,* 501–517.

Mink, I. T. (1997). Studying culturally diverse families of children with mental retardation. In N. W. Bray (Ed.), *International review of research in mental retardation* (Vol. 20, pp. 75–98). San Diego, CA: Academic Press.

Mittler, P. (1990). Prospects for disabled children and their families: An international perspective. *Disability, Handicap, and Society, 5,* 53–64.

Mpofu, E. (2001). Rehabilitation from an international perspective: A Zimbabwean experience. *Disability and Rehabilitation, 23,* 481–489.

Mpofu, E. (2002). Psychology in sub-Saharan Africa: Challenges, prospects and promises. *International Journal of Psychology, 37,* 179–186.

Nuttall, M. (1998). States and categories: Indigenous models of personhood in northwest Greenland. In R. Jenkins (Ed.), *Questions of competence: Culture, classification and intellectual disability* (pp. 176–193). Cambridge, UK: Cambridge University Press.

Osrin, D., Vaidya, A., Shrestha, Y., Baniya, R. B., Manandhar, D. S., Adhikari, R. K., et al. (2005). Effects of antenatal multiple micronutrient supplementation on birthweight and gestational duration in Nepal: Double-blind, randomised controlled trial. *Lancet, 365,* 955–962.

Ouellette-Kuntz, H. (2005). Understanding health disparities and inequities faced by individuals with intellectual disabilities. *Journal of Applied Research in Intellectual Disabilities, 18,* 113–121.

Pelletier, D. L., & Frongillo, E. A. (2003). Changes in child survival are strongly associated with changes in malnutrition in developing countries. *Journal of Nutrition, 133*(1), 107–119.

Piao, Y., Gargiulo, R. M., & Yun, X. (1995). Special education in the People's Republic of China: Characteristics and practices. *International Journal of Special Education, 10,* 52–65.

Pillay, A. L. (2003). Social competence in rural and urban children with mental retardation: Preliminary findings. *South African Journal of Psychology, 33,* 176–181.

Rajapaksa, L., & Liyanage, S. (2004). *Children with disabilities: Reaching EFA in conflict affected areas in Sri Lanka*. Columbo, Sri Lanka: World Bank Office.

Rao, S. (2006). Parameters of normality and cultural constructions of "mental retardation": Perspectives of Bengali families. *Disability and Society, 21,* 159–178.

Rueda, R., Monzo, L., Shapiro, J., Gomez, J., & Blacher, J. (2005). Cultural models of transition: Latina mothers of young adults with developmental disabilities. *Exceptional Children, 71,* 401–414.

Sonnander, K., & Claesson, M. (1997). Classification, prevalence, prevention and rehabilitation of intellectual disability: An overview of research in the People's Republic of China. *Journal of Intellectual Disability Research, 41,* 180–192.

Special Olympics. (2003). *Multinational study of attitudes towards individuals with intellectual disabilities: General findings and calls to action*. Washington, DC: Author.

Steen, R. G., Xiong, X., Mulhern, R. K., Langston, J. W., & Wang, W. C. (1999). Subtle brain abnormalities in children with sickle cell disease: Relationship to blood hematocrit. *Annals of Neurology, 45*(3), 279–286.

Sternberg, R. J., & Grigorenko, E. (1997). Are cognitive styles still in style? *American Psychologist, 52,* 700–712.

Stratford, B., & Ng, H. (2000). People with disabilities in China: Changing outlook—new solutions—growing problems. *International Journal of Disability, Development and Education, 47,* 7–14.

Teebi, A. S., & El-Shanti, H. (2006). Consanguinity: Implications for practice, research, and policy. *Lancet, 367,* 970–971.

Thomas, M., & Thomas, M. J. (2002) Some controversies in community-based rehabilitation. *Asia Pacific Disability Rehabilitation Journal, 13,* 1–6.

Trent, J. W., Jr. (1994). *Inventing the feeble mind: A history of mental retardation in the United States*. Berkeley: University of California Press.

Triandis, H. C. (1995). *Individualism and collectivism*. Boulder, CO: Westview.

United Nations. (1971). *Declaration on the rights of mentally retarded persons* (General Assembly Resolution 2856 [XXVI] of 20 December 1971). New York: Author.

United Nations. (1993). *The standard rules on the equalization of opportunities for persons with disabilities* (General Assembly Resolution 48/96 of 20 December 1993). New York: Author.

United Nations. (1999). *Empowering the rural disabled in Asia and the Pacific.* Retrieved October 5, 2005, from *www.fao.org/waicent/faoinfo/sustdev/PPdirect/PPre0035.htm/*.

United Nations. (2002). *Implementation of the United Nations millennium declaration: Report of the General Secretary* (Report No. A/57/270). New York: Author.

United Nations. (2005a). *The inequality predicament: Report on the world social situation 2005.* New York: Author.

United Nations. (2005b). *Millenium development goals.* Retrieved October 18, 2005, from *www.un.org/millenniumgoals/*.

United Nations Children's Fund. (2004). *The state of the world's children 2005: Childhood under threat.* New York: Author.

United Nations Children's Fund. (2006). *The state of the world's children 2007.* New York: Author.

Van de Vijver, F. J. R. (1997). Meta-analysis of cross-cultural comparisons of cognitive test performance. *Journal of Cross-Cultural Psychology, 28,* 678–709.

Van Maastricht, S. (1998). Work, opportunity and culture: (In)competence in Greece and Wales. In R. Jenkins (Ed.), *Questions of competence: Culture, classification and intellectual disability* (pp. 125–152). Cambridge, UK: Cambridge University Press.

Victora, C. G., Wagstaff, A., Schellenberg, J. A., Gwatkin, D., Claeson, M., & Habicht, J. P. (2003). Applying an equity lens to child health and mortality: More of the same is not enough. *Lancet, 362,* 233–241.

Walker, S. P., Wachs, T. D., Gardner, J. M., Lozoff, B., Wasserman, G. A., Pollitt, E., et al. (2007). Child development: Risk factors for adverse outcomes in developing countries. *Lancet, 369,* 145–157.

Whyte, S. R. (1998). Slow cookers and madmen: Competence of heart and head in rural Uganda. In R. Jenkins (Ed.), *Questions of competence: Culture, classification and intellectual disability* (pp. 153–175). Cambridge, UK: Cambridge University Press.

World Bank. (2005a). *Examining inclusion: Disability and community driven development* (Social Development Notes, Issue 100). Washington, DC: Author.

World Bank. (2005b). *World development report 2006: Equity and development.* Oxford, UK: Oxford University Press.

World Health Organization. (1981). *Disability prevention and rehabilitation* (Technical Report Series 668). Geneva, Switzerland: Author.

World Health Organization. (2005). *The world health report 2005: Make every mother and child count.* Geneva, Switzerland: Author.

Wright, D., & Digby, A. (1996). (Eds.). *From idiocy to mental deficiency: Historical perspectives on people with learning disabilities.* London: Routledge.

Xu, Y. (1994). China. In H. Winzer & G. Mazurek (Eds.), *Comparative study of special education* (pp. 163–178). Washington, DC: Genalland University.

Yamaki, K., & Fujiura, G. T. (2002). Employment and income status of adults with developmental disabilities living in the community. *Mental Retardation, 40,* 132–141.

Yaqoob, M., Bashir, A., Tareen, K., Gustavson, K.-H., Nazir, R., Jalil, F., et al. (1995). Severe mental retardation in 2- to 24-month-old children in Lahore, Pakistan: A prospective cohort study. *Acta Paediatrica, 84,* 267–272.

30

Reflections on the Future of Research in Developmental Disabilities

Steven F. Warren

The stated purpose of this *Handbook* noted in the Preface is to "summarize the most current information on developmental disabilities." This goal has been splendidly achieved by the editors and authors in a concise and thoughtful manner. The analyses, arguments, and speculations offered in each chapter are well reasoned and stand on their own merits. My task is not to confirm or challenge any of these but instead to look forward in a broad sense toward the future. What opportunities lay ahead that hold great promise for the field? The modest purpose of this chapter is to identify some of these opportunities and to discuss their implications in terms of directions for research and practice.

To achieve this purpose, I first briefly summarize the state of the field at present as reflected in the chapters in this book. The remainder of this chapter is focused on two general themes that I believe will play a central role in shaping the future. I conclude the chapter with a discussion of a few fundamental challenges that must be met if the field of developmental disabilities research and practice is to achieve its potential over the next half century.

Speculating about the future is, of course, a perilous undertaking. Some might view it as a foolish undertaking and wisely avoid it on principle. Nevertheless, I submit that there is plenty of evidence as to what needs to be accomplished in the future if, indeed, the field of developmental disabilities is to advance in ways that truly affect the quality of life experienced by individuals and families now and for generations to come. Much of this evidence is contained in the pages of this book in the form of the thoughtful observations and recommendations of the authors.

THE STATE OF THE ART

Taken together, the chapters in this book have captured a substantial portion of the state of the art of research on developmental disabilities. As the reader works through these chapters, certain themes emerge. First, a handful of bedrock values surface again and again. These may be captured by four concepts—*individualize, include, provide choices,* and *support. Individualize* to meet the specific needs of each person with a developmental disability. To the extent possible, seek to meaningfully *include* the individual with a developmental disability as naturally and as unobtrusively as possible in all aspects of life. Allow and support individuals with developmental disabilities to make *choices* at many levels and throughout their lives much as we do with typically developing individuals. Provide *supports* for individuals to allow them to maximize their education, participate in the life of their community, work, make choices, optimize their quality of life, and minimize their dependence on others. In addition, support and empower the family of the individual in recognition of what is often their central and lifelong multifaceted role. These bedrock principles remain subject to refinement, as noted throughout this book. Nevertheless, taken together they form the essence of what has steadily emerged over at least the past 50 years as a core set of values around which goals and practices are largely constructed for individuals with developmental disabilities, at least in the ideal.

These bedrock constructs have emerged largely in the Western industrialized world as part of larger social movements to spread the rights and privileges of liberal social democracies to various historically disenfranchised groups. They are, indeed, quintessentially "American" in many ways and are reflected in principle in the U.S. Declaration of Independence and the U.S. Constitution, as well as in the constitutions of virtually all liberal democracies throughout the world. These values will continue to be both challenged and refined in application, but in principle they will hopefully hold up against outside attack and continue to stand the test of time. They serve as an essential philosophical foundation on which to create and implement research and practice.

A second theme is the uneven and, in many cases, underdeveloped nature of research on developmental disabilities. This theme is manifested in more implicit than explicit ways in this book. Furthermore, we must acknowledge the enormous progress that has been made in a mere 50 years of research on developmental disabilities and the substantial benefits that this progress has spawned. That said, in many, perhaps most, areas it would be prudent to admit that we still have a long way to go. Indeed, much of our collective effort to this point has focused on creating foundational knowledge and inventing a wide array of interventions, procedures, techniques, approaches, and curricula, many of which have been tested only with relatively small numbers of individuals under limited conditions, if at all. In the parlance of clinical trials (Piantadosi, 1997), most of our efforts have been focused on phase 1 trials—small, controlled studies. We are just now embracing the next step—determining the efficacy and effectiveness of these phase 1 inventions through increasingly large, rigorously controlled clinical trials intended to ultimately advance practice from whatever is locally favored toward culturally informed but nevertheless scientifically validated methods. In the meantime, as many authors note in this book, the empirical validation of most practices is a work in progress.

A third common theme is implicit and occasionally explicit throughout this volume—the seemingly unbridgeable gap between research and practice. Perhaps we should not be too concerned about this, given that much of applied intervention research is just moving beyond phase I. Furthermore, we do have some nice models of how research can drive practice, as demonstrated, for example, by the positive behavior supports (PBS) approach (see Dunlap & Carr, Chapter 23). But overall the empirical foundation that should anchor "best practices" in many areas appears to be commonly ignored in practice, as acknowledged in several of the chapters of this book. There are many reasons for this and no need to point fingers at anyone. It is simply the state of the field at present. But that does not make it acceptable. Ineffective practices waste extremely precious learning time and can lead to a destructive and insidious cynicism about the potential for truly enhancing the lives of individuals with developmental disabilities. Fortunately, there is no need to simply tolerate this situation—we can change it and need to do so soon. I return to this issue later.

Finally, an implicit element of much of the work presented is that, despite the complex, biobehavioral nature of most developmental disabilities, to date most of our research has been, at best, only modestly multidisciplinary. We have plodded ahead largely within our disciplinary walls, be they behavior-analytic, developmental, or other. There appear to be few theoretical reasons for this (Rutter, 2006). Instead, this stasis probably just reflects the age-old tendency of all species to "stick with what you know." In a few areas, such as the treatment of severe aberrant behavior, we have become more biobehavioral by occasionally combining pharmacological and behavioral treatments (see Thompson, Moore, & Symons, Chapter 25). But mostly we have included only our close disciplinary cousins (e.g., psychologists, educators, speech therapists) and sometimes struggled just to do that well. How much has this hindered our progress and limited our view of what might be possible? How much progress can we make in the future if we cling to the walls of our disciplines? Certainly we can improve on our phase I research, fill in some of the gaps, and take it to scale, as the PBS researchers are doing. But in the long run, what will be required if we are to make truly major, nonlinear advances?

OUR BIOBEHAVIORAL FUTURE

It is common knowledge among life scientists that the vast majority of easy research problems have all been solved. The day of the "lone wolf" scientist isolating him- or herself in the lab and chipping away at some basic question from the perspective of his or her relatively narrow discipline is all but over. Although built solidly on the backs of thousands of lone-wolf types who toiled away for decades on "basic research," further progress in solving the major problems of human development and behavior will require an unprecedented degree of cross-disciplinary collaboration. This is especially true with regard to the kind of research it will take to achieve greater success in preventing and remediating developmental disabilities (Warren, Batshaw, Bennett, Hagerman, & Seltzer, 2005). This fact is made even more daunting by the realization that, however noble such collaborations may appear to outsiders, to those trying to "collaborate," it often feels like an unnatural act between two or more nonconsenting adults who speak different languages and look at the world through very different lenses. Will future progress be held hostage by an inability to span the distance between gene–brain–behavior–environment–culture because of ancient human emotions and reactions, such as jealousy, vanity, and protection of "turf"? Neither the conceptual nor the merely emotional challenges should be underestimated. In the end, one may hope that the powerful desire to truly make a difference and the range of awards available to those who do will help us cross these hurdles.

Driving the challenge presented by truly multidisciplinary collaboration is a profound reality that now confronts life scientists. In the world that is steadily emerging from the success of the Human Genome Project, all human genes and their common DNA variations will eventually be known. However, it is evident that biological organisms are inherently tuned to their environment. Genetic factors alone typically account for only a fraction of variance in human behavior—sometimes a relatively large fraction, sometimes a remarkably small one—but always a fraction (Warren, 2002). To account for the remaining variance, that is, to fully understand development and behavior, we must increasingly move toward analyses of functional interactions between biology, environment, and behavior (Reiss & Neiderhiser, 2000; Rutter, 2002). This is where the heavy lifting really begins because of the acknowledged complexity of human behavior. Ultimately our goal must be to understand the varied roles of multiple genes and multiple environmental influences and how they operate together cumulatively over years in ways that result in such difficult problems as, for example, self-injurious behavior and in such remarkable feats as the resilience of many children to early abusive environments. Is this a bridge too far? We must hope not. Perhaps the path forward is opening in front of us right now in the form of emerging fields that seek to create new disciplines by cobbling together the leading edges of earlier endeavors of distinct disciplines. Two obvious examples of this are the emerging fields of behavioral genetics and cognitive neuroscience, both of which are combining behavior and biology in dynamic and generative ways.

Behavioral Genetics

This is a young and rapidly growing field (e.g., Plomin, Defries, Craig, & McGuffin, 2003). It is rapidly generating knowledge on how our genetic endowments affect the probability that we will develop a wide range of abilities and disabilities. It is also helping us determine the role of environment at a molar level by revealing the interaction between specific genetic variations and general environmental features. An extraordinary example of this is the role played by the *MAOA* gene in bestowing risk from or resilience to early child neglect and abuse.

Child neglect and abuse is associated with an increased risk of mild mental retardation, as well as a long list of serious problems, from school failure to violent criminal behavior. In 2002, Caspi and colleagues reported, in a groundbreaking article in the journal *Science* (Caspi et al., 2002), that boys with a specific genetic polymorphism (i.e., common variation) of the X-linked *MAOA* gene who had experienced abuse or neglect as young children were at a high risk of exhibiting aggressive, violent antisocial behavior as adults, whereas boys with another common variation of this gene appeared to suffer relatively little long-term effects despite an early history of abuse and neglect. That is, the *MAOA* gene appears to bestow heightened risk in one common form or a remarkable degree of resilience in another common form. However, these common genetic variations have no apparent effect on development or behavior in the absence of the environmental trigger of early abuse or neglect. Studies of the *MAOA* gene under various rearing conditions in mice show similar results, perhaps because of the important role this gene plays in the regulation of dopamine.

As compelling as the *MAOA*-plus-early-abuse example is, it is but one of a steadily increasing number of important gene–environment interactions that have been discovered in recent years that have direct relevance for the prevention and treatment of conditions associated with developmental disabilities (Rutter, 2006). To conduct these studies requires a deep knowledge both of genetics and of behavior and the environment. Consequently, gene–environment studies are paving the way forward in terms of truly multidisciplinary collaborations.

The field of developmental disabilities is a natural arena for the study of gene–environment interactions. Single-gene disorders such as fragile X syndrome are particularly attractive for such research, but so are complex disorders such as autism, in which gene–environment interactions have long been suspected but not yet positively identified.

Cognitive and Behavioral Neuroscience

Cognitive and behavioral neuroscience is an inherently multidisciplinary endeavor that has been fueled over the past two decades by the rapid development of technologies that allow us to directly observe the brain in action. Neuroscience itself is the most multidisciplinary of all fields concerned with human behavior. The overarching scientific challenge is to understand in specific ways the relationships between brain and behavior and ultimately the relationships of gene, brain, and behavior. In this respect, cognitive and behavioral neuroscience and behavioral genetics are ultimately linked in our efforts to understand behavior and its causes.

One example of a cognitive neuroscience perspective brings us again to the *MAOA* gene. The *MAOA* gene encodes the brain enzyme monoamine oxidase (thus the gene is named *MAOA*). The *MAOA* gene is located on the X chromosome. The enzyme it produces breaks down several important neurotransmitters such as serotonin, norepinephrine, and dopamine, leaving them inactive. These neurotransmitters control mood, aggression, and pleasure. Individuals with low *MAOA* activity seem to react much more strongly to stress than those with high activity. In the Caspi et al. study (2002), participants who suffered early abuse *and* who carried the low-activity variation of the *MAOA* gene were nine times as likely to engage in serious antisocial behavior as young adults. Thus, although we might use behavioral genetics techniques to link specific genes with behavior, we need neuroscience to understand why and how these linkages occur. Consequently, neuroscience (cognitive, behavioral, and molecular) and genetics are rapidly partnering to identify just such gene–environment–brain relationships. But such collaborations are limited if experts in human behavior are not centrally involved in making the behavior-to-brain linkages.

Creating a Developmental Science of Developmental Disabilities

The field of developmental disabilities has historically been heavily influenced by cognitive psychology and applied behavior analysis (i.e., MacLean, 1997). These two disciplines have never been particularly compatible. Both have made important contributions and have clear strengths but also inherent limitations that make them poor vehicles in their present manifestations for steering us into a future filled with generative collaborations with neuroscience and genetics. Behavioral genetics and cognitive and behavioral neuroscience have emerged as new fields because of the enabling effects of new technologies *and* new thinking. For the behavioral side of the equation to now make its mark, contributions will be required from both a new emerging technology for monitoring and measuring the environment and an emerging "developmental–transactional" conceptual approach.

Measuring behavior has historically been a labor-intensive, tedious, and expensive task (e.g., Sackett, 1978) that has at best been assisted by various technological aids (e.g., Thompson, Felce, & Symons, 2000). It many ways our standard measurement techniques are analogous to the equally labor-intensive, tedious, and expensive lab techniques involved in "gene hunting" *prior* to the technological breakthroughs (e.g., the gene chip) that led to the Human Genome Project and related revolutions in developmental biology. Measurement instruments shape, enable, and constrain the advances of all sciences. Breakthroughs in measurement lead to breakthroughs in knowledge (Abelson, 1986). Whereas the science of human development and developmental disorders has made rapid progress due to technological breakthroughs in molecular genetics and neuroscience, the behavioral sciences have lagged behind because researchers are stuck with measurement tools that have improved only marginally in 50 years. Fortunately, this may soon change.

Consider, for example, a technology now being fine-tuned by a small, well-financed start-up company named Infoture, located in Boulder, Colorado. Infoture has embarked on a quest to perfect the world's first automatic speech monitoring and analysis system. Their first version of this measurement breakthrough is named LENA. It is a 2-ounce digital recorder that slips into a pocket on a young child's clothing. It records up to 12 hours of both a child's vocalizations and words spoken to him or her. It is then docked to a USB port on a home computer, where it recharges and uploads the digital speech files via the Internet to a supercomputer in Boulder. A software program separates child speech from adult speech while categorizing and counting it and prepares a series of reports on the amount of adult speech input the child received that day, the amount of speech the child produced, and a variety of other analyses. If LENA achieves its potential, it will represent a transformative technological breakthrough in environmental measurement without parallel. It will be our technological and conceptual gene chip.

The conceptual inspiration for LENA was Hart and Risley's (1995) seminal research on the early language environment of typical children and its effects. It took Betty Hart and many research assistants thousands of hours over many years to code and analyze just a fraction of the data (just 1 hour per month of data per family) that LENA can process in just a few hours. This same transformative technology could be used to monitor the richness of language input in the home, in a child care setting, or even in an adult day care setting or institutional setting. Do you wonder what kind of "enriched" environment your child experiences when you are not around? LENA can tell you. Are you wondering whether staff members are actually interacting with residents? LENA can tell you. Do you want to see whether the intervention under way has been implemented as intensively as called for, whether it is generating changes in the target child's language, and what those changes are? LENA can tell you. Do you want to know how the richness of environments interacts with various genetic propensities over many years? Perhaps LENA will hold the key to this as well.

Hopefully, LENA will be just the first in a line of high-technology environmental measurement systems that will fundamentally change the nature of behavioral research. The implications of this new technology for research and practice and beyond are potentially profound. Chief among these implications is how we may eventually come to understand environment–behavior interaction and ultimately environment–behavior–brain–gene interactions.

What will LENA and related breakthroughs mean for developmental science? What will they mean for more behavioral approaches (i.e., applied behavior analysis)? If examples from other branches of science are any indicator, this technological breakthrough may rapidly transform conceptual models and research, perhaps leading to a much more refined approach to human behavior that gradually separates from its predecessors. What might distinguish this new approach?

First, it will be truly developmental. That is, it will focus on development over relatively long time periods, years instead of just weeks or months. And it will no longer depend on making indirect links among early and later measures across long time periods but will directly link them through frequent measurement. And in doing this it will allow a much more precise study of cumulative effects on development, both positive and negative. This was one of the real contributions of the Hart and Risley longitudinal study: It was in essence a developmental, cumulative, transactional analysis. But it was also a singular example of this approach that was unlikely ever to be replicated until now because of the tedious, slow, expensive nature of the research.

Radically improved measurement of behavior will allow a much more precise calculation of the behavioral side of the biology–behavior equation. No longer will it be necessary to just assign the error variance in behavioral genetic studies to some ill-defined notion of "the environment." Now the tools will exist to understand gene–brain–environment–behavior interactions dynamically, developmentally, and cumulatively. The behavior sciences will become full partners in this enterprise. This possibility has profound implications for truly understanding human development and disorders and for crafting maximally effective, individualized interventions and precisely monitoring their effects. That is the ultimate promise of a biobehavioral approach to the field of developmental disabilities. It should allow us to develop much more optimal interventions that will ultimately result in large and more robust effects well beyond what we can do at present.

FROM PROMISE TO PRACTICE

The chapters in this book implicitly lay out the present scientific bases for evidence-based practices. Nevertheless, it is widely acknowledged that too much of present practice is based on little more than educated guesses. Whatever their limitations, the scientific bases of the field in most areas go well beyond "best guesses." Furthermore, it is imperative that we change the ethos that governs "practice" from one that continues to implicitly support the best-guesses approach to one that demands and requires a true "best scientific evidence" approach. Until this divide is breached, research and practice will remain far apart, and, indeed, the breach will likely grow even wider. But how do we get from the promise of this science to practice? I suggest four tools that can help cross this divide.

Requiring Evidence-Based Practice

For all the downsides associated with the No Child Left Behind initiative in the United States, one huge upside has been the focus on creating an empirical basis for education, including special education. Should not our overarching goal be to create an empirical foundation for all education and therapeutic practices that are prescribed for children? Why would we settle for anything less? We should strongly support this mandate at the local, state, national, and international levels. Nevertheless, even if we manage to do this well, we must still recognize that it may take up to two decades or more to create the empirical bases for many important clinical and education practices and that it will be expensive.

Harnessing the Power of Randomized Clinical Trials

The past 50 years have seen the development of a wide array of interventions, curricula, and treatments. Much of the empirical foundation for this development has been created using small-N designs (e.g., multiple baseline designs, reversal designs, case studies). These phase 1 and 2 small-N clinical trial designs have been a powerful tool during this initial stage of development (Warren & Yoder, 1997), and they will continue to serve this role. However, broadly speaking, the field has been gradually moving into a new stage for the past decade—the stage (or age) of the randomized clinical trial (RCT). These designs have always held the high ground in terms of rigor. But they are also typically both expensive and challenging to conduct. Nevertheless, when a treatment has shown consistent promise via single-subject designs, it is time to put it to the truly rigorous evaluation inherent in one or likely a series of carefully controlled RCT studies. These designs are the coin of the realm in the world of medicine and should be in the world of developmental disabilities, too. Because of the length of time it takes to conduct these studies (often 4 or 5 years for a single study), we must recognize that it will take many years before the power of RCTs has truly resulted in rigorously tested approaches. Finally, it will never be feasible to test every intervention individually with most types of developmental disorders. If you subtract autism and Down syndrome, virtually all remaining developmental disorders meet the definition of "rare" disorders. Even fragile X, the most common inherited cause of mental retardation, meets the definition of a rare disorder, as it apparently affects only 1 in 4,000 males. Consequently, reasonably powered RCTs for most types of interventions (excluding pharmacological interventions) will simply not be feasible, and alternative approaches will be required (Warren, Brady, & Fey, 2004).

Harnessing the Power of the Web and Related Technologies

It is certainly trendy over at least the past decade to refer to the transformative power of the World Wide Web. It is easy to see examples every day of how the Web and a wide array of related technologies have transformed business and commerce, communication, government, entertainment, and on and on. These transformations have also affected the world of developmental disabilities, at least on the margins. But how much difference has or can it make in our ability to enhance the lives of people with development disabilities and to provide more effective interventions and education? The answer is becoming clear, and it certainly looks as though the Web is going to be much more important than many of us ever imagined.

In many respects, the challenge of providing effective intervention to individuals with unique and challenging needs in fully inclusive settings is a tailor-made problem for Web-based applications. In the past decade, the Web has already been harnessed to allow practitioners to rapidly and frequently assess child development and response to intervention (e.g., individual growth and development indicators; Greenwood, Carta, Walker, Hughes, & Weathers, 2006), to directly deliver intensive, individualized interventions to enhance speech-processing skills (e.g., Fast ForWord; Agocs, Burns, De Ley,

Miller, & Calhoun, 2006), and other applications. LENA, the breakthrough technology for monitoring language input and output, is possible only because of the reach and power of the Internet. Indeed, what distinguishes these applications is the dynamic, individualized uses of the Web to collect, analyze, monitor, and direct development and intervention. Another characteristic in a growing number of cases is the entrepreneurial use of business models (such as the Infoture example) capable of quickly and efficiently developing and disseminating new applications. Given the pressure on public finances and resources at present, a considerable amount of progress in the future will depend on partnerships between researchers and businesses, particularly when it comes to scaling up and disseminating assessments and intervention.

Global Translation of Empirical Practice

Much has been and is being made about increasing globalization on a wide array of dimensions. This broad trend, enabled like so much else by the Web as well as by affordable, accessible travel, presents its own opportunities and challenges. On the one hand, we can rapidly ship information on virtually any intervention or approach anywhere in the world. But on the other hand, much of what we might send out will likely run smack into "local" differences (cultural or otherwise) that may render it unusable and ineffective. Not the least of the challenges is the well-known rule of thumb that meaningful, permanent change usually occurs when a new or transformative approach is "owned" by those who are responsible for its ultimate success. For this ownership process to occur, a certain degree of local leadership is virtually always required. The Ann Sullivan Center (CASP) in Lima, Peru, is an excellent example of this kind of translational process.

CASP is a dynamic, multifaceted creation of Liliana Mayo and her longtime mentor Judith M. LeBlanc. It is the leading program in Latin America in terms of the development and translation of effective programs and practices for children and adults with developmental disabilities. Although its programmatic efforts are concentrated in Peru, it now has affiliated centers in many other Latin American countries and in other third-world and even some so-called developed countries (i.e., Spain, Japan).

CASP developed most of its own procedures under the leadership of Mayo and LeBlanc in the 1980s. Since then it has continually sought to further improve and expand its efforts through a variety of strategies. One of these is to take evidence-based practices developed in the United States and Europe and, if they appear likely to enhance the program further, to "translate" them into culturally appropriate adaptations suitable for use in Peru and other third-world countries. As one example, poverty is widespread in Peru and truly the norm for most people. However, it is very different in some ways from poverty in the United States. In the United States, poverty tends to isolate people in ways that can complicate and undermine many intervention approaches. In Peru it is not necessarily the case that poverty is isolating. The extended nature of families in Peru and the virtual total lack of government assistance have resulted in dynamic, if materially poor, neighborhoods in which a substantial degree of mutual reciprocity and support often occurs. As a result, it can be easier to enlist community supports for impoverished people with developmental disabilities because the communities they live in, despite their low standard of living, may still function well on some critical levels. The local Peruvian experts at CASP know this, of course, and they know how to work effectively in this context by taking practices they have developed over the years on their own or as necessary selected practices from the so-called developed world and translating these practices themselves into locally suitable versions. These are then passed on to other affiliated centers throughout Latin America. The fact that they have the CASP "seal of approval" makes it more likely that they will be incorporated into these centers. Thus CASP operates as a necessary bridge between cultures by evaluating some of our so-called best practices and translating and transforming them into versions suitable for differing cultural contexts. Although the Web can certainly aid this process, the local translation-and-transformation stage remains a necessary step.

SOME FINAL THOUGHTS

What if tomorrow it were announced that a cure had been discovered for fragile X syndrome, the most common inherited cause of mental retardation and one of only two known causes of autism? Believe it or not, this could happen in our lifetimes. Clinical trials on a treatment that may promise a cure for this disorder, or at least mitigate many of its effects, could begin within a few years (Miller, 2006). Let's assume, in fact, that this will eventually happen, if not with fragile X, than with some other developmental disorder. Obviously, this will be wonderful news for many affected individuals and their families. But where will that leave everybody else? I believe that this will be an extraordinarily positive event for all of us because it should accelerate research and development that can benefit everyone, even if for many disabilities a cure may be at best decades or even centuries away. Of course the notions of "cure" or "prevention" inevitably raise a range of perplexing ethical and moral issues about how developmental disabilities are presently viewed and especially how they may be viewed in the future (Reinders, 2000). These issues require serious consideration by all of us.

Imagine that, like the fairy-tale character Rip Van Winkle, you were to sit down, lean against a tree, and fall asleep for 20 years. When you finally wake up, you soon learn that effective treatments and approaches for a wide range of developmental disorders have been enhanced tenfold over your two decades of peaceful slumber, with resulting increases in education, literacy, health, quality of life, and more. Even if such a scenario takes 40 years to achieve instead of 20, wouldn't we all be overjoyed by the recognition of this monumental advancement in science and practice and its priceless impact on the human condition? This does not need to be a fairy tale. The chapters in this volume are both a baseline from which to measure our future advances and evidence that such "priceless" outcomes are well within the realm of possibility.

ACKNOWLEDGMENTS

I wish to acknowledge the contributions to my thinking and scholarship provided throughout my career by the richly interdisciplinary environments of the Mental Retardation Research Centers at Vanderbilt University (National Institute of Child Health and Human Development [NICHD] Grant No. HD15052) and the University of Kansas (NICHD Grant No. HD002528).

REFERENCES

Abelson, P. H. (1986). Instrumentation and computers. *American Scientist, 74,* 182–192.
Agocs, M. M., Burns, M. S., De Ley, L. E., Miller, S. L., & Calhoun, B. M. (2006). Fast ForWord lan-

guage. In R. McCauley & M. Fey (Eds.), *Treatment of language disorders in children* (pp. 471–508). Baltimore: Brookes

Caspi, A., McClay, J., Moffitt, T. E., Mill, J., Martin, J., Craig, I. W., et al. (2002). Role of genotype in the cycle of violence in maltreated children. *Science, 297,* 851–854.

Greenwood, C. R., Carta, J. J., Walker, D., Hughes, K., & Weathers, M. (2006). Preliminary investigations of the application of the early communication indicator (ECI) for infants and toddlers. *Journal of Early Intervention, 28*(3), 178–196.

Hart, B., & Risley, T. R. (1995). *Meaningful differences in the everyday experience of young American children.* Baltimore: Brookes.

MacLean, W. E., Jr. (Ed.). (1997). *Ellis' handbook of mental deficiency, psychological theory and research.* Mahwah, NJ: Erlbaum.

Miller, G. (2006). A fix for fragile X syndrome? *Science, 312,* 521.

Piantadosi, S. (1997). *Clinical trials: A methodological perspective.* New York: Wiley.

Plomin, R., Defries, J. C., Craig, I. W., & McGuffin, P. (Eds.). (2003). *Behavioral genetics in the postgenomic era.* Washington, DC: American Psychological Association.

Reinders, H. S. (2000). *The future of the disabled in liberal society: An ethical analysis.* Notre Dame, IN: University of Notre Dame Press.

Reiss, D., & Neiderhiser, J. E. (2000). The interplay of genetic influences and social processes in developmental theory: Specific mechanisms are coming into view. *Development and Psychopathology, 12,* 357–374.

Rutter, J. (2002). Nature, nurture, and development: From evangelism through science toward policy and practice. *Child Development, 73,* 1–21.

Rutter, M. (2006). *Genes and behavior: Nature–nurture interplay explained.* Oxford, UK: Blackwell.

Sackett, G. P. (1978). *Observing behavior: Theory and applications in mental retardation* (Vol. 1). Baltimore: University Park Press.

Thompson, T., Felce, D., & Symons, F. J. (2000). *Behavioral observation: Technology and applications in developmental disabilities.* Baltimore: Brookes.

Warren, S. F. (2002). Genes, brains, and behavior: The road ahead. *Mental Retardation, 40*(6), 471–476.

Warren, S. F., Batshaw, M., Bennett, F., Hagerman, R., & Seltzer, M. M. (2005). Biomedical research for primary and secondary prevention. In. C. Larkin & A. Turnbull (Eds.), *National goals and research for people with intellectual and developmental disabilities* (pp. 125–148). Washington, DC: American Association on Mental Retardation.

Warren, S. F., Brady, N. C., & Fey, M. E. (2004). Communication and language: Research design and measurement issues. In E. Emerson, C. Hatton, T. Thompson, & T. R. Parmeter (Eds.), *The international handbook of applied research in intellectual disabilities* (pp. 385–406). West Sussex, UK: Wiley.

Warren, S. F., & Yoder, P. J. (1997). A developmental model of early communication and language intervention. *Mental Retardation Development and Disabilities Research Review, 3,* 358–362.

Author Index

Subject Index

"f" following a page number indicates a figure; "t" following a page number indicates a table.